LaFleur Brooks'

Health Unit
COORDINATING

evolve

∴ *To access your Student Resources, visit:*

http://evolve.elsevier.com/Gillingham/HUC/

Evolve Student Resources for *Gillingham: LaFleur Brooks' Health Unit Coordinating,* **6th Edition,** offers the following features:

Student Resources

- **Certification Review Materials**
  These review materials include comprehensive questions that are based on the material in the text. Answers to the questions are accompanied by complete rationales and references to page numbers in the main text.

- **Mock Certification Exam**
  This invaluable study tool consists of 120 questions and is written in the same format used for the national certification exam. Gain practice in taking the exam, then check your knowledge and score by reviewing the answers that are provided.

- **A Comprehensive List of Laboratory Studies and Blood Components**

- **Commonly Ordered Medications**
  A list of the most commonly ordered medications, generic and brand names with their drug classification.

- **Photographs and Forms**
  These images show additional equipment and hospital forms that students will encounter during externships and on the job.

- **Weblinks**
  Links to places of interest on the web specifically for health unit coordinating.

- **Content Updates**
  Find out the latest information on relevant issues in the field of health unit coordinating.

LaFleur Brooks'
Health Unit COORDINATING

Sixth Edition

Elaine A. Gillingham, AAS, BA, CHUC

Program Director 1993 – 2005 (retired)
Health Unit Coordinator Program
GateWay Community College
Phoenix, Arizona

Monica Wadsworth Seibel, BS, MEd, CHUC

Program Director
Health Unit Coordinator Program
GateWay Community College
Phoenix, Arizona

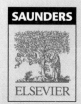

SAUNDERS

ELSEVIER

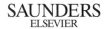

SAUNDERS
ELSEVIER

11830 Westline Industrial Drive
St. Louis, Missouri 63146

Notice

Medicine is an ever-changing field. Standard safety precautions must be followed, but as new
research and clinical experience broaden our knowledge, changes in treatment and drug therapy may
become necessary or appropriate. Readers are advised to check the most current product information
provided by the manufacturer of each drug to be administered to verify the recommended dose, the
method and duration of administration, and contraindications. It is the responsibility of the treating
physician, relying on experience and knowledge of the patient, to determine dosages and the best
treatment for each individual patient. Neither the Publisher nor the editor assume any liability for
any injury and/or damage to persons or property arising from this publication.

The Publisher

ISBN: 978-1-4160-4172-6

Publishing Director: Andrew Allen
Executive Editor: Loren Wilson
Senior Developmental Editor: Ellen Wurm-Cutter
Publishing Services Manager: Julie Eddy
Project Manager: Andrea Campbell
Designer: Julia Dummitt

Printed in Canada

Last digit is the print number: 9   8   7   6   5   4   3   2

Reviewers

Carolyn Jones, CUC
Lead Unit Coordinator, 2nd Medical
Carteret General Hospital
Morehead City, North Carolina

Lori J. H. Katz, CHUC, MEd
Hennepin Technical College
Brooklyn Park, Minnesota

Lyndee Leavitt, AS, CHUC
Dixie Regional Medical Center
St. George, Utah

Denise Carol Rezny, MSN, RN
RN Staff Nurse
Cookville Regional Medical Center
Instructor, General Education
MedVance Institute
Cookville, Tennessee

Nadine Stratford, CHUC
Dixie Regional Medical Center
St. George, Utah

Caryn Waligorski, CHUC
Health Unit Coordinator
Macomb Community College
Clinton Township, Michigan

Thank you to Myrna LaFleur Brooks for being my inspiration and mentor
Thank you to Winnie Starr for touching my life and leaving wonderful memories
and
Thank you to Bill for his love and support

Elaine A. Gillingham

Thank you, Myrna and Elaine, for being my mentors and leading me to so many wonderful opportunities
Thank you Jennifer, Erin, Colin, Aiden and Brendan Phoebe for lighting my life
and
Thank you, Scott, for love and a lifetime of companionship

Monica Wadsworth Seibel

Preface

A CAREER IN HEALTH UNIT COORDINATING

Welcome to the exciting and challenging career of Health Unit Coordinating. Individuals practicing as Health Unit Coordinators soon realize that they have far-reaching effects on the delivery of care to patients. Health Unit Coordinators manage all non-clinical tasks on hospital nursing units, making them essential members of the health care team. Responsibilities include transcribing physicians' orders for patient treatment, preparing patient charts, (when paper charts are utilized) maintaining statistical reports, dealing with visitors, and much more. The implementation of the electronic medical record with computer physician order entry has expanded the HUC responsibilities. Health Unit Coordinators will have a more efficient role of traffic control, coordination of care, and management of the electronic record. When CPOE is implemented, the Health Unit Coordinators will no longer have to interpret and transcribe physicians' orders.

As a recognized health care profession, Health Unit Coordinating has its own national organization, the National Association of Health Unit Coordinators (NAHUC), which offers certification to individuals who meet certain standards of excellence.

NEW TO THIS EDITION

Instructors and students using the 6th edition of *LaFleur Brooks' Health Unit Coordinating* will benefit from all of the quality pedagogical elements in the previous edition, plus *updated photographs* which help students envision their expected role and responsibilities on the job. Every chapter has been reviewed and updated as needed while maintaining the approach and features that make *LaFleur Brooks' Health Unit Coordinating* a success.

TOTAL EDUCATIONAL PACKAGE

The 6th edition of *LaFleur Brooks' Health Unit Coordinating* is part of a total educational package for health unit coordinating offered by Elsevier. Supplemental materials include the following:

LaFleur Brooks' Skills Practice Manual for Health Unit Coordinating, 6th edition

This printed manual contains practice activities to reinforce skills taught in the text, such as transcribing doctors' orders, communicating with co-workers, assembling a patient's chart, documenting lab values, and recording telephoned doctors' orders. Generic hospital forms and actual physicians' orders provide hands-on examples of tasks students will need to perform on the job. Also included is a clinical skills evaluation record, designed to help students objectively record and evaluate their performance during hospital rotations.

Practice Activity Software for Transcription of Physicians' Orders

This state-of-the art Windows-based CD—bound free into the *Skills Practice Manual*—simulates a hospital's computer ordering system to be used in the classroom for practice in transcribing doctors' orders, and contains printable hospital forms. The software includes mock nursing units with lists of patients, doctors' rosters, diagnostic test results, and more, offering realistic practice of transcription of doctors' orders to enhance students' skills and confidence.

LaFleur Brooks' Health Unit Coordinating Pocket Guide, 6th edition

The updated and user friendly *LaFleur Brooks' Health Unit Coordinating Pocket Guide* provides, in a portable, easy-to-read format, the material from the text that is most commonly used and referred to. Special features include a glossary, a list of abbreviations, a comprehensive list of laboratory studies and blood components, and a list of the most commonly ordered medications. Personal management pages allow users to record information that is unique to their practice situations. Students as well as practicing Health Unit Coordinators can use this tool as a quick and easy reference in clinical rotations or on the job.

TEACH for LaFleur Brooks' Health Unit Coordinating, 6th edition

This **new** instructor resource is available via Evolve. The **TEACH Lesson Plan Manual** provides instructors with customizable lesson plans and lecture outlines based on learning objectives. With these valuable resources, instructors will save valuable preparation time and create a learning environment that fully engages students in classroom preparation. The lesson plans are keyed chapter-by-chapter and are divided into 50-minute units in a 3-column format. In addition to the lesson plans, instructors will have unique lecture outlines in PowerPoint with lecture notes, thought-provoking questions, and unique ideas for lectures.

Instructor's Electronic Resource for LaFleur Brooks' Health Unit Coordinating, 6th edition

This invaluable CD-ROM contains resources to assist instructors in various education activities. It includes a 769-question test bank, an electronic image collection with all the images from the main book, and physician orders for student practice.

EVOLVE Website for LaFleur Brooks' Health Unit Coordinating, 6th edition

This feature provides free materials for both students and instructors, including an electronic image collection, physician orders for student practice, and a 769-question test bank, all with instructor-only access. For students, there is a mock certification exam, certification review materials, weblinks, information related to commonly ordered medications and comprehensive laboratory studies, forms that are commonly seen, and content updates.

MARKET-LEADING TEXTBOOK

LaFleur Brooks' Health Unit Coordinating, 6th edition, by Elaine A. Gillingham and Monica Wadsworth Seibel is the best-selling textbook of its kind on the market. It provides comprehensive coverage of the theory and practice underpinning the Health Unit Coordinator's responsibilities, introduces students to hospitals and health care, and explains non-clinical management of the nursing unit. It also offers a complete module on anatomy, physiology, and medical terminology, enabling students to learn the language of medicine so they can interact confidently with doctors, nurses, and other health care workers. Exercises in each chapter reinforce newly learned material and test students' retention and critical thinking abilities. Abundant photographs, diagrams, and illustrations further enhance understanding of the material. Students studying in programs using this text will be able to master everything they need to know to begin their career performing at a competent level.

TO THE STUDENT

How to Use This Text

This text is organized to provide theory in conjunction with hands-on activities in the *LaFleur Brooks' Skills Practice Manual for Health Unit Coordinating* to prepare you to work as a Health Unit Coordinator. The text is divided into five sections:

Section 1, *Orientation to Hospitals, Medical Centers, and Health Care,* provides a fundamental understanding of health care, including the Health Unit Coordinator position. Recent changes in health care including the electronic record with computer physician order entry and the impact on Health Unit Coordinating are discussed.

Section 2, *Personal and Professional Skills,* presents guidelines to use for effective interpersonal and intercultural communication, and management skills. Workplace behavior and appearance, confidentiality as mandated by the Privacy Rule and Security Rule contained the Health Insurance Portability and Accountability Act (HIPAA), and other ethical and legal issues are discussed.

Section 3, *The Patient's Chart and Transcription of Doctors' Orders,* provides information needed to understand written doctors' orders and enhances understanding of the various departments that carry out the orders. Activities are included that provide hands-on experience transcribing doctors' orders by using the *LaFleur Brooks' Skills Practice Manual for Health Unit Coordinating* and the *Practice Activity Software for Transcription of Physicians' Orders.* Information regarding the Health Unit Coordinators' role when the electronic medical record with computer physician order entry is implemented is outlined.

Section 4, *Health Unit Coordinator Procedures,* provides information regarding emergencies, infection control, recording vital signs, and admission, preoperative, postoperative, discharge, postmortem, and transfer procedures.

Section 5, *Introduction to Anatomic Structures, Medical Terms, and Illnesses,* presents a basic overview of human anatomy and medical terminology.

Working Your Way Through a Chapter
Read the Objectives

The objectives outline what you are expected to know when you have completed all of the exercises for the chapter. When you have read the chapter and completed the exercises, return to the objectives and quiz yourself to ensure that you have mastered the material.

Read the Vocabulary Lists

Each chapter introduces a list of words related to the material covered in that chapter. When reading the chapter, note the words in the vocabulary list to enhance your understanding of their meanings. Return to the vocabulary list after you have read the chapter and complete the exercises to quiz yourself on the definitions of the words.

Complete the Exercises that Follow the Abbreviation Lists

Most chapters include a list of abbreviations that relate to the material covered in that chapter. Exercises are included to assist you in learning those abbreviations. The abbreviations are also used throughout the chapter. It may be helpful to create flash cards for the abbreviations.

Complete the Review Questions

The review questions are written from the objectives and will assist you in learning and understanding the skills necessary to be successful as a Health Unit Coordinator.

Take Note Boxes

Pay special attention to the information provided in the Take Note boxes, as this information is especially important in performing your job accurately and efficiently. This information is emphasized to reduce the risk of errors while working as a Health Unit Coordinator.

Think About

Discussion questions related to chapter material are included at the end of chapters 1 through 22 to increase understanding of health care issues and to promote critical thinking and problem-solving skills. Discuss the questions with your classmates, friends, and family to gain others' perspectives on the topics.

Hands-On Activities

Most chapters in *LaFleur Brooks' Health Unit Coordinating* include references to activities found in *LaFleur Brooks' Skills Practice Manual for Health Unit Coordinating.* Chapters 4 and 7 have activities related to communication and management skills. Chapter 8 has activities that will familiarize you with patient chart forms and chart assembly. Chapters 10 through 19 include doctors' orders that relate to material discussed in each chapter. *Practice Activity Software for Transcription of Physicians'* Orders enables you to practice the transcription of the doctors' orders on a simulated hospital computer program. Activities are provided in Chapter 21 for other routine Health Unit Coordinator tasks, such as charting vital signs.

Use of Appendixes

Appendix A, *Abbreviations,* helps refresh your memory when you cannot recall the meaning of an abbreviation used in a doctors' order.

Appendix B, *Word Elements,* assists you in finding the definition of a word part while defining or building a medical term. You may need to find a prefix or suffix that you recognize from Chapter 23 but for which you have forgotten the definition.

Answers

Check your answers after completing exercises and review questions to ensure that you have answered them correctly.

FROM THE AUTHORS

Congratulations—you have opened the door to the health care world. By using *LaFleur Brooks' Health Unit Coordinating* as a learning tool, you may obtain a career in health care. Our hope is that you will continue to become a valuable member of the health care field and feel the pride and satisfaction that comes with helping others. Continuous advancement in technology makes working in the health care field an exciting and educational experience.

Acknowledgments

Preparing the sixth edition of *LaFleur Brooks' Health Unit Coordinating* required the expertise of many, since changes in the health care delivery system and advancement in medical technology demand new knowledge for the Health Unit Coordinator and change in the Health Unit Coordinating practice.

We thank the reviewers who helped to ensure that this was the most up-to-date revision it could be. We would also like to express our appreciation for the cooperation we received from Banner Estrella Medical Center, who allowed pictures to be taken of their facility and their employees to participate. We would like to give a special thanks to the Banner Estrella Medical Center employees who shared their knowledge and allowed their pictures to be taken. Thank you to Boswell Memorial Hospital, Del Webb Hospital and Gateway Community College in Phoenix, Arizona, who allowed access to their various departments to obtain information to prepare the manuscript. In addition, we wish to thank the following individuals for their assistance:

Edith Baie
Assistant Director
Boswell Memorial Hospital Clinical Laboratory
Sun City, Arizona

Edward Hoskins, AA, BA, RT
Faculty, Respiratory Therapy Program
GateWay Community College
Phoenix, Arizona

John Lampignano, AA, BS, MEd, RT
Faculty, Diagnostic Imaging Program
GateWay Community College
Phoenix, Arizona

Peter Zawicki, BS, MS, PT
Division Chair, Health Sciences Division
Faculty, Physical Therapy Assistant Program
GateWay Community College
Phoenix, Arizona

A special thanks to the following staff of Elsevier: Ellen Wurm-Cutter, Senior Developmental Editor, Loren Wilson, Executive Editor, and all the experts from Elsevier for their support and encouragement during the revision of this edition.

About the Authors

Elaine Gillingham started her health care career in Sandusky, Ohio, working after school at a local hospital, and was on-the-job-trained as a Health Unit Coordinator. In 1977, she moved to Phoenix, Arizona, met Myrna LaFleur Brooks and Winnie Starr who encouraged her to obtain a certificate of completion in Health Unit Coordinating and an Associate Degree in Health Services Management from GateWay Community College. She later obtained a Bachelor's degree in education from Ottawa University. Ms. Gillingham served as president of the Phoenix chapter of the National Association of Health Unit Coordinators and sat on the National Board for 2 years. In 1983, she wrote questions for and sat for the first National Certification exam sponsored by the National Association of Health Unit Coordinators. Ms. Gillingham worked at a Phoenix pediatric hospital as a Health Unit Coordinator and as an instructor for health unit coordinating for six years. After teaching on a part-time basis for five years, Ms. Gillingham was hired as a full-time instructor in the Health Unit Coordinator program in 1990. Prior to retiring in 2005, she served as the Program Director for 12 years. After retiring, she has been teaching on part-time basis and traveling. Ms. Gillingham began reviewing, consulting, and writing for the Health Unit Coordinating books in 1993.

Monica Wadsworth Seibel received her Bachelor of Science degree in Zoology from Arizona State University in 1983 and her Master of Educational Leadership degree from Northern Arizona University in 2002. After working as a health unit coordinator in the emergency and cardiovascular intensive care units at Humana Hospital in Phoenix, she acted as the data coordinator for the Heart/Lung Transplant Program administered by Humana Hospital and the Arizona Heart Institute. She met Myrna LaFleur Brooks while on the job and was given the opportunity to teach as an adjunct instructor with Elaine Gillingham in the Health Unit Coordinating Program at GateWay Community College. After teaching on a part time basis for five years, she was hired as full time residential faculty in 1992. She has served as the Program Director since the retirement of Ms. Gillingham in 2005, and is currently President-Elect for the GateWay Faculty Senate. Ms. Wadsworth Seibel was a contributing author for the fourth edition of the Health Unit Coordinating textbook. She is a member of the National Association of Health Unit Coordinators (NAHUC) as well as the American Rock Art Research Association (ARARA).

Contents

CHAPTER **1**

Health Unit Coordinating
An Allied Health Career

CHAPTER OBJECTIVES

Upon completion of this chapter, you will be able to:

1. Define the terms in the vocabulary list.
2. Write the meaning of the abbreviations in the abbreviations list.
3. Differentiate between given clinical and nonclinical tasks.
4. Describe how orders will be communicated through computer physician order entry.
5. Describe the four stages of evolution of health unit coordinating.
6. List three tasks that the health unit coordinator (HUC) may perform that relate to each of the following: the nursing staff, physicians, other hospital departments, visitors, and patients.
7. List three tasks that the HUC would perform involving implementation of the electronic record but would not do with paper charts.
8. List at least four ways to prepare for upcoming changes to the HUC position with the implementation of the electronic medical record and the computer physician order entry.
9. List three reasons why one should become a member of the National Association of Health Unit Coordinators.
10. List three reasons why the HUC should become certified.

11. List three positions in which the HUC may be cross-trained.
12. List two possible career paths for the HUC.

VOCABULARY

Career Ladder A pathway of upward mobility

Certification The process of testifying to or endorsing that a person has met certain standards

Certified Health Unit Coordinator A health unit coordinator who has passed the national certification examination sponsored by the National Association of Health Unit Coordinators (NAHUC)

Clinical Decision Support System Computerized program that provides suggestions or default values for drug doses, routes, and frequencies to the physician at the point of order entry. The program may also perform drug allergy checks, drug–laboratory value checks, drug–drug interaction checks, etc

Clinical Tasks Tasks performed at the bedside or in direct contact with the patient

Computer Physician Order Entry A computerized program into which physicians directly enter patient orders; replaces handwritten orders on an order sheet or prescription pad

Doctor A person licensed to practice medicine (used interchangeably with the term *physician* throughout this textbook)

Doctors' Orders The health care that a doctor prescribes in writing for a hospitalized patient

Electronic Medical Record An electronic record of patient health information generated by one or more encounters in any care delivery setting

Health Unit Coordinator The health care team member who performs nonclinical patient care tasks for the nursing unit (also may be called unit clerk or unit secretary)

Hospital Departments Divisions within the hospital that specialize in services, such as the nutritional care department, which plans and prepares meals for patients, employees, and visitors

Nonclinical Tasks Tasks performed away from the bedside

Nurses' Station The desk area of a nursing unit

Nursing Team A group of nursing staff members who care for patients on a nursing unit

Nursing Unit An area within the hospital that includes equipment and nursing personnel available for the care of a given number of patients (also may be referred to as a wing, floor, pod, strategic business unit, ward, or station)

Patient A person who receives health care, including preventive, promotional, acute, chronic, and all other services in the continuum of care

Policy and Procedure Manual A handbook that provides such information as guidelines for practice and hospital regulations

Recertification A process by which certified health unit coordinators exhibit continued personal and professional growth and current competency to practice in the field

Transcription A process used to communicate the doctors' orders to the nursing staff and other hospital departments; computers or handwritten requisitions are used

ABBREVIATIONS

Abbreviation	Meaning
CHUC	certified health unit coordinator
CPOE	computer physician order entry
CDSS	clinical decision support system
EMR/EHR	electronic medical (health) record
HUC	health unit coordinator
SHUC	student health unit coordinator
pt	patient

EXERCISE 1

Write the abbreviation for each term listed below.

1. certified health unit coordinator _____

2. electronic medical/health record _____

3. student health unit coordinator _____

4. patient _____

5. health unit coordinator _____

6. clinical decision support system _____

7. computer physician order entry _____

EXERCISE 2

Write the meaning of each abbreviation listed below.

1. CHUC

_____

2. EMR/EHR

_____

3. SHUC

_____

4. CDSS

_____

5. HUC

_____

6. pt

_____

7. CPOE

_____

INTRODUCTION TO HEALTH UNIT COORDINATING

The **health unit coordinator (HUC)** is usually the first person encountered when one is walking onto a hospital **nursing unit**. The HUC has always been considered essential to the effectiveness of the unit. The HUC coordinates activities on the unit, transcribes handwritten or preprinted **doctors' orders** or manages the electronic medical records, and usually functions under the direction of the nurse manager or unit manager. The overall job is usually nonclinical in nature, and the work area is the **nurses' station** (Fig. 1-1). Many health care facilities require that HUCs wear scrubs, sometimes in a particular color. Other facilities opt for professional, nonclinical wear. Everyone who works on or visits the nursing unit depends on the HUC for information and assistance.

Comments often heard in the hospital include the following:

"It's one of the most important positions on the nursing unit."
"We are so disorganized if the HUC is not here."
"The HUC creates the attitude for the entire unit."
"The HUC sets the pace for the day's work."
"Ask the HUC—she knows everything."

Whether an efficient HUC is working on a nursing unit is usually obvious to anyone who walks onto that unit. If the HUC is having a "bad day" or is in a "bad mood," the whole unit is affected because everyone has to interact with the HUC. It is important

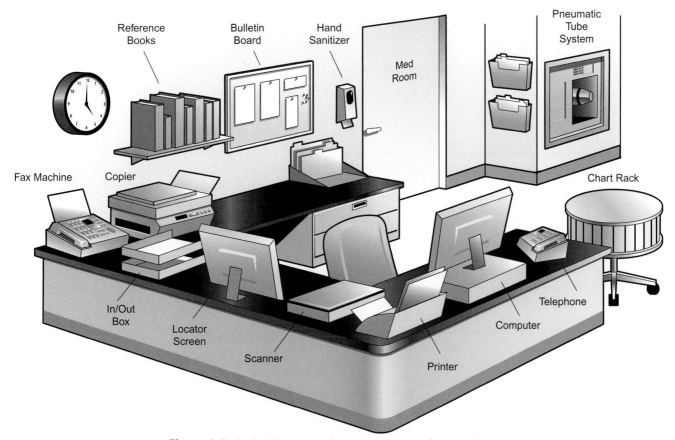

Figure 1-1 The health unit coordinator's work area is the nurses' station.

for staff members to maintain a positive, friendly attitude when working on the nursing unit. The HUC can enhance or inhibit the delivery of health care to **patients** on the nursing unit.

Although health unit coordinating was begun as a clerical position that was focused on providing assistance to the nurse, today it is a position that involves many responsibilities associated with assisting the nursing staff, **doctors**, **hospital departments**, patients, and visitors to the nursing unit (Fig. 1-2). HUCs also may be employed in doctors' offices, clinics, and long-term care facilities to assist the nurse with clerical duties related to patients' health records.

The role of the HUC has changed and expanded over the years, and the role is again changing and expanding with the introduction of electronic records and the computer physician order entry.

RECENT CHANGES IN THE HEALTH CARE SYSTEM

As electronic technology advances, hospitals move toward a paperless system. Many hospitals have replaced paper charts for patients with an **electronic medical record (EMR)**. This system allows physicians to enter orders directly into the computer rather than writing them by hand and is known as **computer physician order entry (CPOE)**. Physician orders are entered directly into the computer by the physician and are automatically sent to the appropriate departments. A **clinical decision support system (CDSS)** offers the physician assistance at the point

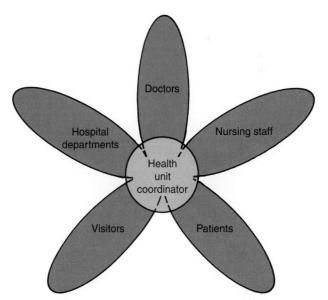

Figure 1-2 The health unit coordinator coordinates the activities of doctors, nursing staff, hospital departments, patients, and visitors on the nursing unit.

of entering patient orders. A patient's medication history is entered (by the patient's admitting nurse or by the pharmacist) into the system at the time of admission. When the physician is entering the patient's orders, the CDSS may provide prompts that warn against the possibility of drug interaction, allergy, or overdose. The system also may provide reminders to the physician, such as a reminder to order aspirin for a patient who is going home after undergoing heart surgery.

CHANGES IN HEALTH UNIT COORDINATING

The responsibilities of the HUC change with implementation of the EMR and the CPOE, allowing a greater focus on customer service. Most of the HUC's time has been spent on interpretation and **transcription** of orders and chart management. HUCs will be acquiring a more efficient role that will consist of traffic control, coordination of care, and management of the electronic record. When CPOE is implemented, HUCs will no longer have to interpret and transcribe physicians' orders but may enter an order when asked to do so by the doctor or nurse in an emergency situation. They will be involved with scheduling; coordinating ordered procedures; calling consultations; preparing consent forms; and scanning handwritten progress notes, outside reports, signed consent forms, and other documents that will become part of the patient's permanent record, as well as handling other administrative tasks to be explained in future chapters.

Comments that have been made by experienced HUCs working in hospitals that have implemented the EMR with CPOE include the following:

"It is awesome! No more trying to decipher a doctor's terrible handwriting!"

"No more hunting down charts or having them taken away from me before I am finished with them. More than one person can be viewing and working on a patient's chart at the same time."

"Patient information is always current and at your fingertips."

"I can spend more time helping visitors and staff with their needs."

"I have time to help the nurse manager with administrative work."

"I am busy from the time I get here, until I leave, but it is a less stressful busy!"

Many hospitals have implemented CPOE, but because of the expense, predictions are that it will take at least 3 to 5 years for the system to be implemented nationally. Information will be provided throughout this book for working as an HUC with and without implementation of the electronic record.

HISTORY OF HEALTH UNIT COORDINATING

Traditionally, health professions have evolved through four stages: on-the-job training, formal education, formation of a national association, and certification or licensure. Health unit coordinating is no exception to this tradition.

On-the-Job-Training

During World War II, hospitals experienced a drastic shortage of registered nurses. To compensate for this shortage, auxiliary personnel were trained on the job to assist the registered nurse. The HUC was trained to assist the nurse with nonclinical tasks, whereas the nursing assistant was trained to assist the nurse at the bedside.

EXAMPLE OF COMPETENCIES FOR AN EDUCATIONAL PROGRAM

Statement of Competency for the Health Unit Coordinator

Upon completion of this program, the student demonstrated the ability to

- perform HUC tasks and provide accountability to nursing personnel, medical staff, other hospital departments, and patients and visitors
- operate the nursing unit communication systems, including computer terminal, telephone, scanner, fax machine, intercom, locator system, pager, shredder, label printer, and conveyor system
- record diagnostic test values, vital signs, and census data
- order daily diets and daily laboratory tests
- file reports on patients' paper charts, or scan reports into the electronic record
- transcribe doctors' orders using basic knowledge of anatomy and physiology, disease processes, medical terminology, and accepted abbreviations (competent to perform this task without checking by and co-signature of the registered nurse)
- perform nonclinical tasks required for patient admission, transfer, discharge, and preoperative and postoperative procedures

- plan and execute a daily routine for the performance of nonclinical tasks for the nursing unit
- manage the nonclinical functions of the nursing unit
- listen to patient and visitor complaints and concerns, and use problem-solving skills
- maintain nursing unit supplies
- prepare patient consent forms
- maintain patients' paper charts, or manage patients' electronic records
- coordinate scheduling of patients' tests and diagnostic procedures
- transcribe medication orders, incorporating concepts of drug categories, automatic stop dates, automatic cancellations, time scheduling, and routes of administration
- practice within the professional ethical framework of health unit coordinating
- schedule radiologic procedures that require patient preparation
- communicate effectively with patients, visitors, and members of the health care team

---

After World War II ended, the nursing shortage was not as critical; however, the duties of nurses were expanding. Advancements in technology were increasing the workload of the doctor, which resulted in the shifting of many tasks, such as taking blood pressure and starting intravenous therapy, to the nursing staff. Federally sponsored health programs required more detailed record keeping, hospitals were becoming larger and more complex, and increasing numbers of specialists were required to carry out newly available tests and treatments. The nonclinical demands of every hospitalized patient increased proportionately; therefore, the need to employ HUCs continued. Today, a 500-bed hospital has approximately 50 to 60 health unit coordinating positions. The role continues to change and expand.

HUCs were trained on the job for longer than 20 years (Fig. 1-3, *A*, *B*). The first record of health unit coordinating is found in an article published in *Modern Hospital* in 1940, which discussed the implementation of health unit coordinating at Montefiore Hospital in Pittsburgh, Pennsylvania. The author, Abraham Oseroff, a hospital administrator, stated, "A new helper was introduced to the nursing unit to take care of the many details of a secretarial nature that formerly made demands on the limited time of the nurse." The title of the new helper was "floor secretary." The author wrote, "The idea of floor secretary was first met with skepticism, but it proved to be worthwhile from the beginning."

Formal Education

In 1966, one of the first educational programs for health unit coordinating was offered at a vocational school in Minneapolis, Minnesota. An article published in *Nursing Outlook* in 1966 described a research project that led to the implementation of this program (Fig. 1-3, *C*). The most popular title for "floor secretary" had become "ward" or "unit clerk." The article's author, Ruth Stryker, recommended that the title be changed to "station coordinator" because the data showed that the unit clerk "did a great deal of managing in the form of coordinating activities." Ruth Stryker wrote one of the first textbooks for health unit coordinating, *The Hospital Ward Clerk*, which was published by the C.V. Mosby Company in 1970. Today, prior to employment, most HUCs are educated in one of the many community colleges or vocational technical schools nationwide that offer HUC educational programs. The individual who completes an HUC program emerges with better preparation for the job and a greater knowledge base on which to build. Educational programs outline the competencies or job skills that students are expected to acquire by the time they have completed the program (see the Box *Example of Competencies for an Educational Program*).

Professional Association

The HUC position existed and grew for 40 years without the guidance of a professional association. The purpose of a professional association is to set standards of education and practice for peers to be enforced by peers for the protection of the public. Altruistic in nature, it is designed to enlighten its members and guide the profession to better serve the public. The constitution states the basic laws and principles of the association, and elected officers carry out the purpose listed in the constitution. By 1980, several educational programs were well established across the nation, and educators in these programs began to discuss the possibility of forming a national association.

The first organizational meeting was held in Phoenix, Arizona, on August 23, 1980. This date has since been proclaimed National Health Unit Coordinator Day by the national association. The 10 founding members represented both education and practice. In attendance were Kathy Jordan, Winnie Starr, Connie Johnston, Estelle Johnson, and Myrna LaFleur from Arizona; Kay Cox from California; Helga Hegge from Minnesota; Jane Pedersen from Wisconsin; Carolyn Hinken from New Mexico; and Velma Kerschner from Texas. During this first meeting, the founding members declared the formation of a national association for health coordinators to be called the *National Association of Health Unit Coordinators (NAHUC)* (Fig. 1-3, *D*). The founding members recognized the need to create a new title for the position that would be updated

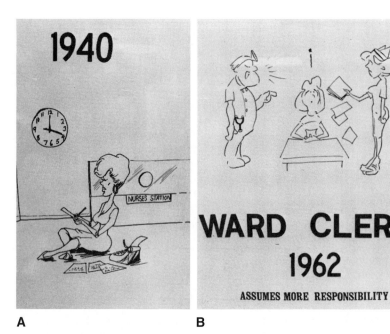

A

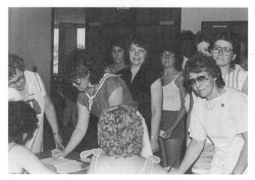

B

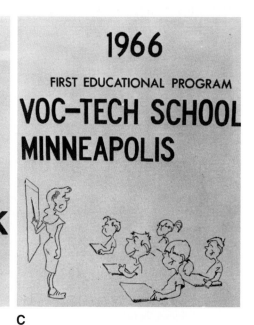

C

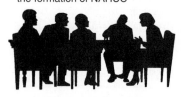

1980

August 23rd: First meeting for
the formation of NAHUC

This date has been set aside as
National Health Unit Coordinator Day

D

1983

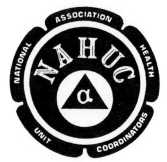

E   First certification exam

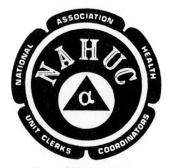

Logo prior to 1990 showing "unit clerk"

Logo as of 1990 — "unit clerks"
dropped

F

Figure 1-3 History of health unit coordinating. *A,* In 1940, health unit coordinating was first introduced as a health care occupation. The first job title was "floor secretary." *B,* In 1962, the more common title was "ward clerk." More responsibilities were added to the job. *C,* In 1966, the first vocational educational program for health unit coordinating was established. *D,* On August 23, 1980, the first meeting held to discuss the formation of the National Association of Health Unit Coordinators (Clerks) was held in Phoenix, Arizona. *E,* In 1983, the first certification examination was offered by the National Association of Health Unit Coordinators (Clerks). *F,* Logo for the National Association of Health Unit Coordinators. The five outer segments represent doctors, nursing staff, patients, visitors, and hospital departments. The circle that connects the segments is symbolic of the HUC's role in coordinating the activities of these five groups. In 1990, "unit clerk" was dropped from the name of the association, which is now known as the National Association of Health Unit Coordinators.

FIVE REASONS TO BECOME CERTIFIED

1. Enhanced credibility
2. Broader perspective on health unit coordinating (not just one specialty)—opportunity to be prepared and proactive regarding changes that are taking place in the HUC profession
3. Increased mobility, geographically and vertically
4. Peer and public recognition and respect
5. Improved self-image

FIVE REASONS TO BECOME A MEMBER OF THE NATIONAL ASSOCIATION OF HEALTH UNIT COORDINATORS

1. Professional representation
2. Forum for sharing ideas and challenges—assistance in being prepared and proactive regarding changes that are taking place in the HUC profession
3. National networking
4. National directory
5. Opportunity to develop leadership skills

---

and would be used consistently nationwide; the title "Health Unit Coordinator" was chosen. The NAHUC has worked tirelessly since that time to have this title adopted in hospitals nationwide. Because "unit clerk" was the most popular title nationwide in 1980, it was included in the title of the national association with the intent that it would be dropped when the term "coordinator" became recognized. In 1990, the national association became the "National Association of Health Unit Coordinators," after "clerk" was dropped from its name (Fig. 1-3, *F*).

At the second organizational meeting, held in San Juan Capistrano, California, the constitution was ratified and the officers elected. Today, the association has approximately 3000 members. Standards of Practice (see Chapter 6, p. 98), including educational requirements and a code of ethics (see Chapter 6, p. 96), have been adopted. The association includes three boards that govern various branches of the association. The Certification Board is responsible for offering the certification examination and maintaining records. The Education Board is responsible for conducting activities related to educational aspects of the profession. The Accreditation Board is responsible for determining and evaluating standards of educational programs nationwide (see the Box *NAHUC Membership Information*).

Certification

Certification and/or licensure is the final step in the evolution of a health profession. Certification is the process of testifying to or endorsing that a person has met certain standards. The first certification examination was offered by NAHUC in May 1983. American Guidance Service, a professional testing company, was employed to administer the test. Nearly 5000 people took the first examination (Fig. 1-3, *E*). Today, this examination is administered nationwide through an electronic system by another testing agency by the name of Applied Measurement Professionals Inc. (AMP) at testing sites. Anyone wishing to register online for the national certification exam may go to *http://www.goamp.com*. Questions are answered on a touch-sensitive computer screen, and test results are given immediately on completion of the examination. The test is available to anyone with a General Educational Development (GED) certificate or a high school diploma.

It is not necessary to be a member of NAHUC or to have completed an educational program to sit for the examination (some HUCs have been trained on the job and have years of experience). The goal of every student of health unit coordinating should be to become certified. Passing the national

certification examination indicates that one has met a standard of excellence and is competent to practice health unit coordinating (see the Box *Five Reasons to Become Certified*).

Recertification

Recertification is a process by which **certified health unit coordinators** exhibit continued personal and professional growth and current competency to practice in the field. The NAHUC requires certified HUCs to be recertified, to ensure that they stay current in their field of practice. Recertification may be achieved by taking the test every 3 years or by earning continuing education unit (CEU) hours. NAHUC offers various opportunities for acquiring CEU hours. Also, employers often offer seminars and workshops that provide CEUs to the HUCs in their health care facility or in the community.

For a group to become a profession, the following credentials must be associated:

- A national association
- A formal education
- Certification or licensure
- A code of ethics
- An identified body of systematic knowledge and technical skill
- Members who function with a degree of autonomy and authority under the assumption that they alone have the expertise to make decisions in their area of competence

Formation of the national association and the dedication of HUCs nationwide in developing and implementing these practices have advanced health unit coordinating to the level of professionalism it deserves.

Students are encouraged to join the NAHUC (see the Box *Five Reasons to Become a Member of NAHUC*). For general information or information on membership or certification testing sites, write to NAHUC at 1947 Madron Road, Rockford, IL 61107; call toll free 888-22-NAHUC (62482) or locally, 815-633-4351; or send a fax to 815-633-4438 or an e-mail to office@nahuc.org. Visit the Web site at www.nahuc.org for additional information.

Responsibilities of the Health Unit Coordinator
Responsibility to the Nursing Staff

Responsibilities of HUCs vary among health care facilities, especially between those that have implemented the electronic record and those that have not. The HUC is a member of

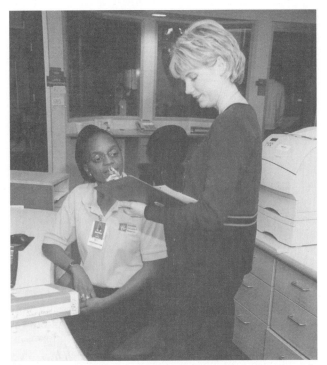

Figure 1-4 The HUC is a member of the nursing team and usually functions under the direction of the nurse manager or unit manager.

the health care team (Fig. 1-4) and usually functions under the direction of the nurse manager or unit manager. Responsibilities include (1) communicating all new doctors' orders (if paper charts with handwritten or preprinted doctors' orders are in use) or messages to the patient's nurse; (2) maintaining the patient's paper chart or managing the electronic record; (3) performing the **nonclinical tasks** required for admission, discharge, and transfer of a patient; (4) preparing the patient's chart for surgery (if a paper chart is in use); (5) handling all telephone communication for the nursing unit; (6) possibly taking responsibility for time schedules for nursing unit staff; and (7) possibly taking responsibility for monitoring and maintaining documentation required by the Joint Commission (TJC) on licenses and certifications and in-services for nursing unit staff.

Interaction with the Doctor

The HUC greets doctors on their arrival to the nurses' station and assists them, as necessary, in obtaining patients' charts (if paper charts are used) or in ordering procedures (if electronic records are used) and in procuring equipment for patient examinations. Other responsibilities include (1) transcribing the doctors' orders (if paper charts are used) (Fig. 1-5, *A*) or scanning reports or documents into the patient's electronic record (Fig. 1-5, *B*); (2) placing calls to and receiving calls from doctors' offices; and (3) obtaining information for the physician as to whether previously ordered procedures have been completed (Fig. 1-6).

Relationships With Hospital Departments

The HUC is the communicator between the doctor and nursing personnel and other hospital departments. Responsibilities include (1) ordering, scheduling, and coordinating diagnostic procedures and treatments; (2) requesting services

from maintenance and other service departments; (3) working closely with the admitting department to admit, transfer, and discharge patients; and (4) ordering supplies for the nursing unit ranging from food to paper products and patient care supplies.

Interaction with the Patient

The HUC greets new patients when they arrive on the nursing unit and may accompany them to their rooms (Fig. 1-7, *A*). The HUC may be given the responsibility of instructing new patients on how to use the call light (Fig. 1-7, *B*), turn on the television, and operate bed controls. Through the use of the intercom in each patient's room, the HUC relays patient requests to nursing personnel. The HUC usually has little bedside contact with patients.

Interaction with Hospital Visitors

The HUC (1) uses the computer to find the patient and informs visitors of patient location (Fig. 1-8); (2) provides information about the location of bathrooms, visitors' lounge, cafeteria, etc.; (3) informs visitors about the rules of visitation and explains any special precautions that may be required during their visit to a patient's room; (4) receives telephone calls from relatives or friends who are inquiring about the patient's condition; and (5) is often the first person to handle visitor concerns.

JOB DESCRIPTION

The tasks that may be performed by the HUC are many and vary greatly between hospitals and even between units within a hospital. Implementation of the EMR has resulted in the addition of many new tasks to the HUC job description.

Hospitals outline responsibilities for each category of employee in a formal written statement called a *job description*. Because health unit coordinating practices vary, it is important to look at the hospital's HUC job description to find out what responsibilities the hospital assigns to the HUC during employment. Examples of job descriptions for an HUC with and without implementation of the EMR and the CPOE are provided below.

Examples of Job Descriptions

A job description for an HUC *without EMR and CPOE* may include the following:

- Communicate all new doctors' orders to the patient's nurse.
- Maintain the patient's paper chart.
- Perform nonclinical tasks required for patient admission, discharge, and transfer.
- Prepare the patient's chart for surgery.
- Handle all telephone communication for the nursing unit.
- Greet doctors on their arrival to the nurses' station, and assist them, if necessary, in obtaining patients' charts.
- Obtain information regarding scheduling of tests.
- Locate and print out test results.
- Transcribe the doctors' orders.
- Place phone calls to and receive calls from doctors' offices.
- Schedule diagnostic procedures and treatments.
- Request services from maintenance and other service departments.

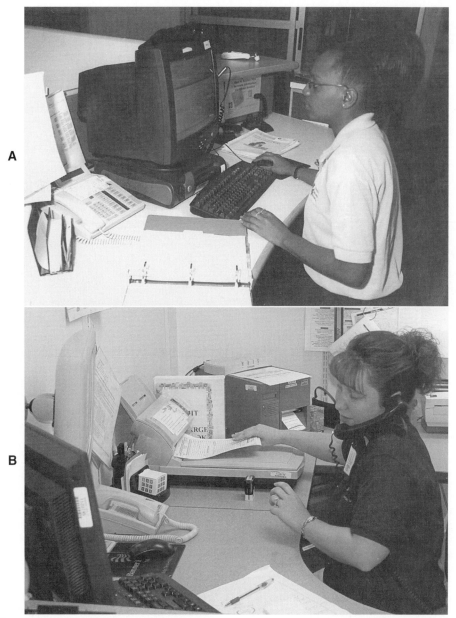

Figure 1-5 *A,* A major responsibility of the HUC when paper charts are used is to transcribe doctors' orders. *B,* A major responsibility of the HUC when the electronic record is used is to scan reports and documents into the patient's electronic record.

- Work closely with the admitting department to admit, transfer, and discharge patients.
- Order all supplies for the nursing unit ranging from food to paper products and patient care supplies.
- Recapture lost supply purchasing departmet charges.
- Greet new patients when they arrive on the nursing unit and accompany them to their rooms.
- Answer patient call lights on intercom and relay patient requests to the nurse.
- Use the intercom or locators to locate health care personnel and/or to relay patient requests to nursing staff. (The HUC usually has little bedside contact with patients.)
- Find the patient using the computer and advise visitors of patient location.
- Provide information on the location of bathrooms, visitors lounge, cafeteria, etc.

- Inform visitors of the rules of visitation and explain any special precautions required during their visit to a patient's room.
- Receive telephone calls from relatives or friends inquiring about the patient's condition.
- Handle visitor complaints.
- Advanced duties may include cardiac monitoring, some coding, or admitting responsibilities.

A job description for an HUC *with implementation of EMR and CPOE* **may include the following:**

- Coordinate administrative functions on the nursing unit.
- Make decisions and take follow-up action to ensure effective communication and information flow throughout the nursing department.

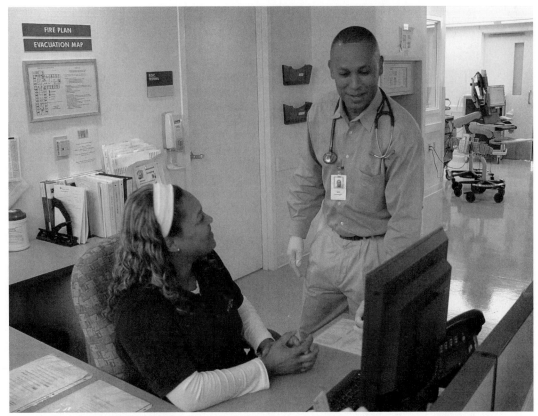

Figure 1-6 The HUC assists the doctor in obtaining information as to whether previously ordered procedures have been completed.

- Perform receptionist/clerical duties on the nursing unit.
- Handle customer problems or collect necessary data and follow through to appropriate person for problem resolution.
- Monitor and maintain the electronic record.
- Place requests to the nutritional care department and to the appropriate department for other unit supplies.
- Coordinate patient activities and patient information.
- Assist the nursing staff as needed with processing of medical records related to patient admission, discharge, and transfer.
- Maintain confidentiality of patient information.
- Integrate/scan paper documents created by caregivers into the EMR.
- Send electronic requisitions for clerical, office, nutritional care, and medical supplies, and maintain adequate supply levels on the nursing unit.
- Input data for reports, and assist in the coordination of mandatory education and skill assessment.
- Maintain the nursing bulletin board.
- Assist with staffing/scheduling.
- Compile statistical data and prepare reports.
- Provide assistance in process improvement.

Preparing for the Change to the Electronic Medical Record and the Computer Physician Order Entry

Change is most often an opportunity for growth. Be proactive! Education is essential for success in working with changing technology. Effective communication and strong organizational skills are required for interfacing with health care personnel, visitors, and patients. Suggestions for ways to prepare for ongoing changes in the HUC position are listed below:

- Complete an HUC program.
- Complete management classes related to health care.
- Attend in-services that are offered through the hospital or classes that are available at local community colleges targeted toward the development of communication or related administrative skills.
- Complete computer classes to become efficient in or gain a working knowledge of advanced word processing, databases, spreadsheets, and e-mail. (Typing skills are essential.)
- Become a member of the NAHUC. Receive and read the newsletter, and attend educational conferences.
- Become certified by taking the National Health Unit Coordinator certification test.

CROSS-TRAINING OPPORTUNITIES

Some hospitals cross-train hospital employees, so they are qualified to handle more than one position as needed. Examples of positions for which the HUC may be cross-trained include telemetry technician, case management technician, and patient care assistant. In a few hospitals, HUCs are trained to perform electrocardiography and/or phlebotomy.

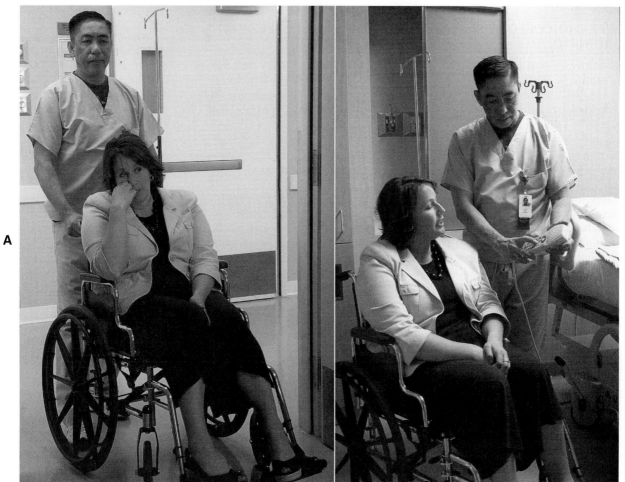

Figure 1-7 *A,* The HUC may greet the new patient on arrival to the nursing unit and may accompany the patient to the assigned room. *B,* The HUC may instruct new patients on use of the call light, television, computer Internet connection, etc.

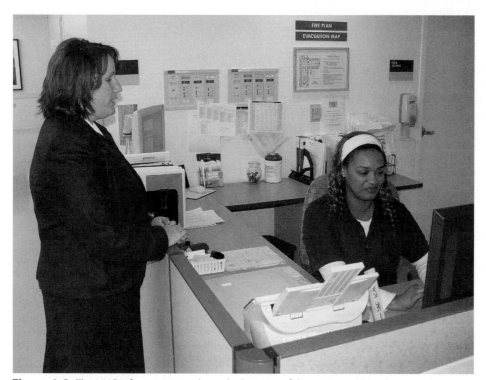

Figure 1-8 The HUC informs visitors about the location of the patient, visiting hours, and any special precautions that may be required.

CAREER CHOICES FOR THE HEALTH UNIT COORDINATOR

Health unit coordinating can be a fulfilling and rewarding career, and many HUCs have made this their career choice. Ancillary health care students or student nurses often work as HUCs, to gain health care experience, earn a salary, obtain health care benefits, and earn tuition reimbursement, while continuing to participate in educational programs in their chosen profession. Many nurses, ancillary health care workers, and doctors have worked as HUCs while working toward their degrees.

A **career ladder** is a pathway of upward mobility and is a popular concept in health care facilities. Most facilities offer employees opportunities for assisted advancement, such as prepaid on-campus education programs, college tuition reimbursement, and flexible work schedules. Many hospitals provide additional training for the HUC in areas such as cardiac monitoring, coding, and information processing.

CAREER PATHS

Health unit coordinating is recognized as the entry level job for those on a nonclinical career path. After having acquired experience and required education, the HUC can advance to a management position. Possible management positions include Health Unit/Service Manager and Health Information Manager. Employment information for both of these management positions is provided in the Box titled *Possible Career Ladder Opportunities for the Health Unit Coordinator After Implementation of the Electronic Medical Record.*

KEY CONCEPTS

Health unit coordinating is a recognized health care profession. Individuals who practice as HUCs soon realize that they can have far-reaching effects on the delivery of care to patients. The job is changing, and although change can be stressful, it can also be exciting and can provide opportunities for growth. The EMR is expanding the administrative and management roles of the HUC.

POSSIBLE CAREER LADDER OPPORTUNITIES FOR THE HEALTH UNIT COORDINATOR AFTER IMPLEMENTATION OF THE ELECTRONIC MEDICAL RECORD

(For more information about these positions and about community colleges that offer degree programs and classes for these positions, the titles may be searched on the Internet).

Position

Health Unit/Service Manager (also called Health Care Administrator)

Responsibilities

Plan, direct, coordinate, and supervise the delivery of health care services—provide leadership in a variety of health service and business office settings. Responsibilities include directing others, coordinating work activities, monitoring financial resources, and assisting in the development of an effective organization. Medical and health service managers include specialists (in charge of specific clinical departments or services) and generalists (manage or help manage an entire facility or system).

Work Environment

Most medical or health service managers work in facilities such as hospitals, nursing care facilities, or group practices. Some managers have their own offices; others share an office with other managers or staff. Some managers oversee more than one health care facility. Hours are long.

Job Outlook

Employment for health service managers is expected to grow faster than average as technology advances and health care services expand.

Educational Requirement

A Master's degree is the standard credential, although a Bachelor's degree is adequate for some entry level positions in smaller facilities and in positions involving health information management.

Position

Health Information Manager

Responsibilities

Responsible for the maintenance and security of all patient electronic records. The health information manager must keep up with current computer and software technology and with legislative requirements and developments regarding the maintenance and security of patient electronic records.

Work Environment

Health information managers work in health care settings such as hospitals, nursing homes, home health care agencies, and health maintenance organizations.

Job Outlook

Rapid employment growth is projected with implementation of the electronic medical record.

Educational Requirement

A Bachelor's degree from an accredited program and a Registered Health Information Administrator certificate from the American Health Information Management Association are required.

REVIEW QUESTIONS

1. Define the following terms:

a. clinical tasks _____

b. nonclinical tasks _____

c. career ladder _____

d. certification _____

e. transcription _____

2. Identify the following tasks as clinical or nonclinical:

a. assisting a patient to the bathroom _____

b. transcribing doctors' orders _____

c. filing reports in patients' charts _____

d. feeding a patient _____

e. answering the unit telephone _____

f. changing a patient's dressing _____

g. answering a patient's request on the intercom _____

3. The four stages of evolution of a health profession are listed below. Write the year that each stage began for health unit coordinating, and describe events that surrounded the date.

a. on-the-job training

_____

b. formal education

_____

c. professional association

_____

d. certification or licensure

_____

4. List three health unit coordinating tasks that relate to each of the following:

a. nursing personnel

i. _____

ii. _____

iii. _____

b. doctor

    i. _____

    ii. _____

    iii. _____

c. hospital departments

    i. _____

    ii. _____

    iii. _____

d. patients' visitors

    i. _____

    ii. _____

    iii. _____

e. patients

    i. _____

    ii. _____

    iii. _____

5. Explain what an *electronic medical record* is.

_____

6. Describe a *computer physician order entry*.

_____

7. Give an example of how the *clinical decision support system* could assist the physician during the ordering process.

_____

8. List three tasks that the HUC may perform when the EMR with CPOE is implemented that would not be necessary when paper patient charts are used.

a. _____

b. _____

c. _____

9. List three reasons why an HUC should become a member of the NAHUC.

a. _____

b. _____

c. _____

10. List three reasons why an HUC should pursue certification.

a. _____

b. _____

c. _____

11. List three positions for which the HUC may be cross-trained.

a. _____

b. _____

c. _____

12. List two career paths for HUCs.

a. _____

b. _____

13. List four ways to prepare for changes in the HUC position that happen with implementation of the EMR and the CPOE.

a. _____

b. _____

c. _____

d. _____

14. The date proclaimed by the NAHUC to be National Health Unit Coordinator Day is

_____

THINK ABOUT...

1. Visit the NAHUC website at www.nahuc.org. (If necessary, use a school computer or go to a library.)
   a. Locate the online *Health Unit Coordinator Certification Handbook*. Discuss the sample questions listed.
   b. Locate and print the NAHUC Standards of Practice, and discuss the significance of each standard listed.
   c. Locate the list of NAHUC representatives, and copy the name, telephone number, and e-mail address of your local representative. Discuss the advantages of knowing the name of your local NAHUC representative.
2. Discuss the importance of the HUC role in terms of promoting efficiency on the nursing unit.
3. Discuss the reasons why recertification is required by the NAHUC.
4. Discuss changes that are occurring in the HUC position, and explain how the HUC can best be prepared for these changes.

CHAPTER 2

Overview of Health Care Today

CHAPTER OBJECTIVES

Upon completion of this chapter, you will be able to

1. Define the terms in the vocabulary list.
2. Write the meaning of the abbreviations in the abbreviations list.
3. List five challenges facing today's health care system and discuss reactions to them.
4. List eight advantages of implementing an electronic medical record (EMR) system.
5. List four disadvantages of implementing an EMR system.
6. Define managed care and explain why it was created.
7. Explain the differences between Medicare A, Medicare B, and Medicare D.
8. List five functions a hospital may perform.
9. List three ways in which hospitals may be classified.
10. List five preemployment/annual in-services required by the Joint Commission.
11. Describe the general structure of a typical hospital.
12. Identify the respective roles of an attending physician and a hospital resident.
13. Identify the titles of physicians who serve in provided specialties.
14. Explain the function of the departments in finance, health information management, diagnostic and therapeutic services, additional services, and operational services.
15. List three resources that may be used for finding health care job opportunities.

VOCABULARY

Accepting Assignment Providers of medical services agreeing that the receipt of payment from Medicare for a professional service will constitute full payment for that service

Accreditation Recognition that a health care organization has met an official standard

Acute Care Level of health care, generally provided in hospitals or emergency departments, for sudden, serious illnesses or trauma

Attending Physician Term applied to a physician who admits and is responsible for a hospital patient

Capitation Payment method whereby the provider of care receives a set dollar amount per patient, regardless of services rendered

Case Manager Health care professional and expert in managed care who assists patients in assessing health and social service systems to ensure that all required services are obtained; coordinates care with doctor and insurance companies

Catastrophic Coverage Coverage a Medicare beneficiary has after reaching a certain amount of "out of pocket" monies paid for their medications during the temporary coverage gap. The beneficiary will pay a coinsurance amount (like 5% of the drug cost) or a copayment ($2.15 or $5.35 for each prescription) for the rest of the calendar year.

Chief Executive Officer Individual in direct charge of a hospital who is responsible to the governing board

Chiropractic Medicine Complementary and alternative health care profession with the purpose of diagnosing and treating mechanical disorders of the spine and musculoskeletal system with the intention of affecting the nervous system and improving health

Chronic Care Care for illnesses of long duration, such as diabetes or emphysema

Community Health Concerned with the members of a community with emphasis on prevention and early detection of disease

Coverage Gap Sometimes called a "donut hole"; a temporary coverage gap in Medicare that occurs after the beneficiary has accumulated a certain amount of money (no more than $3,850) in total prescription drug expenses. The beneficiary pays 100% of drug costs while in the gap (maximum amount, $3,051.25); then the beneficiary receives catastrophic coverage.

Custodial Care Unskilled care given for the primary purpose of meeting personal needs, such as bathing and dressing

Diagnosis-Related Group Classification system used to determine payments from Medicare by assigning a standard flat rate to major diagnostic categories. This flat rate is paid to hospitals regardless of the full cost of the services provided

Governing Board Group of community citizens at the head of the hospital organizational structure

Health Maintenance Organization Organization that has management responsibility for providing comprehensive health care services on a prepayment basis to voluntarily enrolled persons within a designated population

Home Health Equipment and services provided to patient in-home to ensure comfort and care

Homeopathic Medicine Alternative medical system. A belief that "like cures like," meaning that small, highly diluted quantities of medicinal substances are given to cure symptoms, when the same substances given at higher or more concentrated doses would actually cause those symptoms

Hospice Supportive care for terminally ill patients and their families

Hospitalist Full-time, acute care specialist who focuses exclusively on hospitalized patients

Inpatient Patient who has been admitted to a health care facility for at least 24 hours for treatment and care

Integrated Delivery Networks Health care organizations merged into systems that can provide all needed health care services under one corporate umbrella

International Statistical Classification of Diseases and Related Health Problems Detailed description of known diseases and injuries. Each disease (or group of related diseases) is described with its diagnosis and is given a unique code, up to six characters long. Published by the World Health Organization

Magnet Status Award given by the American Nurses' Credentialing Center to hospitals that satisfy a set of criteria designed to measure their strength and quality of nursing

Managed Care The use of a planned and systematic approach to providing health care, with the goal of offering quality care at the lowest possible cost

Medicaid Federal and state program that provides medical assistance to the indigent

Medical Savings Accounts (MSAs) Tax exempt bank accounts that are *owned by an individual* and managed by a financial institution. The individual must have a qualified health plan. An individual cannot use the tax benefit of an MSA until the qualified health plan is in place. The qualified health insurance policy can be applied completely independently of the MSA

Medicare Government insurance; enacted in 1965 for individuals older than age 65 and any person with a disability who has received Social Security benefits for 2 years (some disabilities are covered immediately)

Medicare Supplement Private insurance plan available to Medicare-eligible persons to cover the costs of medical care not covered by Medicare

Merger The combining of individual physician practices and small, stand-alone hospitals into larger networks

Naturopathic Medicine Alternative medical system that proposes that there is a healing power in the body that establishes, maintains, and restores health. Treatments include nutrition and lifestyle counseling, nutritional supplements, medicinal plants, exercise, homeopathy, and treatments from traditional Chinese medicine.

Outpatient Patient who receives care at a health care facility but is not admitted to the facility for 24 hours

Primary Care Physician Sometimes referred to as "gatekeepers," these general practitioners are the first physicians to see a patient for an illness

Proprietary For profit

Resident A graduate of a medical school who is gaining experience in a hospital

Robotic surgery The use of robots in performing surgery

Surfing the Web Using different websites on the Internet to locate information

Triage Nursing interventions. Classification defined as establishing priorities of patient care, usually according to a three-level model: emergent, urgent, and nonurgent

Voluntary Not for profit

Web Address (URL, or uniform resource locator) Keywords that when entered after "http://www…" on the Internet will take the user to a specified location, referred to as a *website*

ABBREVIATIONS

Abbreviation	Meaning
ANA	American Nurses Association
ANCC	American Nurses Credentialing Center
CCM	certified case manager
CEO	chief executive officer
CFO	chief financial officer
COO	chief operating officer
DO	doctor of osteopathy
DRG	diagnosis-related group
DSU	day surgery unit
ECF	extended care facility
ED	emergency department
ER	emergency room
HIMS	health information management system
HMO	health maintenance organization
HO	house officer

Abbreviation	Meaning
ICD	International Statistical Classification of Diseases and Related Health Problems
LTC	long-term care
MD	medical doctor
Neuro	neurology
OB	obstetrics
OR	operating room
Ortho	orthopedics
PACU	postanesthesia care unit
PCP	primary care physician
Peds	pediatrics
PPO	preferred provider organization
Psych	psychiatry
RR	recovery room
SAD	save a day (patient admitted the day of surgery)
SDS	same-day surgery (patient admitted on the day of surgery)
SNF	skilled nursing facility
Surg	surgical
TJC	The Joint Commission (formerly the Joint Commission on Accreditation of Health-care Organizations [JCAHO])
UCR	usual, customary, and reasonable
WHO	World Health Organization
www	World Wide Web

EXERCISE 1

Write the abbreviation for each term listed below.

1. American Nurses Association _____

2. American Nurses Credentialing Center _____

3. certified case manager _____

4. chief executive officer _____

5. chief financial officer _____

6. chief operating officer _____

7. day surgery unit _____

8. doctor of osteopathy _____

9. diagnosis-related group _____

10. extended care facility _____

11. emergency department _____

12. emergency room _____

13. health information management system _____

14. health maintenance organization _____

15. house officer _____

16. International Statistical Classification of Diseases and Related Health Problems _____

17. The Joint Commission _____

18. long-term care _____

19. medical doctor _____

20. neurology _____

21. obstetrics _____

22. operating room _____

23. orthopedics _____

24. postanesthesia care unit _____

25. primary care physician _____

26. pediatrics _____

27. preferred provider organization _____

28. psychiatry _____

29. recovery room _____

30. save a day _____

31. same-day surgery _____

32. skilled nursing facility _____

33. surgical _____

34. usual, customary, and reasonable _____

35. World Health Organization _____

36. World Wide Web _____

EXERCISE 2

Write the meaning of each abbreviation listed below.

1. ANA

_____

2. ANCC

_____

3. CCM

_____

4. CEO

_____

5. CFO

_____

6. COO

_____

7. DSU

_____

8. DO

_____

9. DRG

_____

10. ECF

_____

11. ED

_____

12. ER

_____

13. HIMS

_____

14. HMO

_____

15. HO

_____

16. ICD

_____

17. TJC

_____

18. LTC

_____

19. MD

_____

20. Neuro

_____

21. OB

_____

22. OR

_____

23. Ortho

_____

24. PACU

_____

25. PCP

_____

26. Peds

_____

27. PPO

_____

28. Psych

_____

29. RR

_____

30. SAD

_____

31. SDS

_____

32. SNF

_____

33. Surg

_____

34. UCR

_____

35. WHO

_____

_____

36. www

_____

_____

CHALLENGES FACING THE HEALTH CARE SYSTEM TODAY AND SOME REACTIONS

Challenges facing the U.S. health care system include the following:

1. **Improving quality of care**. A greater emphasis is now being placed on patient safety by regulatory agencies, especially the Joint Commission (TJC, formerly the Joint Commission on Accreditation of Healthcare Organizations). Financial incentives are available from the Federal Government to encourage hospitals to join in a national quality reporting effort. Federal leadership is encouraging the adoption of health information technology, and federal and private sector hospital pay-for-performance programs are in place.

2. **The staggering cost of advanced technology.** Hospitals strive to generate profit (surplus revenue) to purchase new technology by negotiating higher payment rates from health plans and by increasing efficiency. There is an increase in hospital group purchasing organizations and an effort to get health plans to include new technology in a benefit package and to pay the full cost. Advanced electronic technology has resulted in greater accountability in use of supplies and medications, thereby reducing misuse and waste.

3. **Increasing insurance costs**. Customers of health insurance are now assuming a greater share of premiums and are paying higher deductibles, higher copayments, and a higher percentage of coinsurance. A thinning out of health plan benefits is taking place, along with a decline in employer health plans that cover family members. **Managed care** is returning, and the concept of "consumer-driven" health care includes a **medical savings account** with defined contributions and catastrophic insurance.

4. **A growing number of people without health insurance with U.S. hospitals providing about $21 billion in uncompensated care.** The multiple, fragmented governmental and private programs currently in existence provide minimal insurance coverage for targeted populations (e.g., children).

5. **An increasing demand for care, with most emergency departments reporting that they are "at" or "over" capacity, and hospitals facing severe workforce shortages that are having an impact on patient care.** State governments are intervening to prevent the closure of emergency departments. Recruitment packages, higher wages, and incentives for nurses and other personnel in short supply are among the efforts in place to improve the workplace climate. Physician recruitment programs and advanced information technology are being implemented to minimize the impact of shortages.

ROBOTIC SURGERY

Three major advances aided by surgical robots are remote surgery, minimally invasive surgery, and unmanned surgery. Major advantages of robotic surgery include precision, miniaturization, articulation beyond normal manipulation, and three-dimensional magnification. Some surgical robots are autonomous and not always under the control of a surgeon. They are sometimes only used as tools to extend the surgical skills of a trained surgeon.

In 1985, a robot, the **PUMA 560**, was used to place a needle for a brain biopsy using CT guidance. In 1988, the **PROBOT** was used to perform prostatic surgery in England. In 1998, Dr. Friedrich-Wilhelm Mohr, using the **Da Vinci surgical robot**, performed the first robotically-assisted heart bypass at the Leipzig Heart Centre in Germany. The Da Vinci robot is currently being used nationally to perform coronary artery bypass grafts. The first unmanned robotic surgery took place in 2006 in Italy.

Current equipment is expensive to obtain, maintain, and operate. Surgeons and staff need special training. Data collection of procedures and their outcomes remains limited.

IMPLEMENTING A NATIONAL INTERCONNECTED ELECTRONIC MEDICAL RECORD SYSTEM

Ideally, a national interconnected electronic medical record (EMR) system provides an accurate, confidential, cost-effective, and accessible means of delivering appropriate, high-quality care. The EMR will allow the federal government to track the course and impact of a pandemic in real time. A spokesperson from the Center for Health Transformation reported that a national EMR system would allow for safer and more efficient care under normal circumstances, and would provide local, state, and federal governments with the necessary data to direct therapies, medical personnel, and supplies during an emergency. The EMR would also enhance patient confidentiality because a paper record is not available for just anyone to look at. Physicians and nurses have unlimited access to the patient's electronic chart, and other health care providers may have limited access to it, in accordance with their area of expertise. A patient's chart may be opened and viewed or used by more than one person at a time. If someone who is viewing the record steps away from the computer, it will turn off automatically, and when the person returns and signs onto the computer again with their code, the screen will be at the same place.

Computer physician order entry (CPOE) with a clinical decision support system (CDSS) can be remarkably effective in reducing the rate of serious medication errors. Studies conducted by the Leapfrog Group have shown that CPOE with CDSS, if implemented in all urban hospitals in the United States, could prevent as many as 907,600 serious medication errors each year

Studies have also shown that the EMR and CPOE reduce length of stay and reduce retesting and turnaround times for laboratory, pharmacy, and radiology requests while delivering cost savings. This system, once in place nationally, will provide local, state, and federal governments with the necessary data to direct therapies, medical personnel, and supplies during an emergency. Images may be downloaded and medical instruments may be interconnected, allowing diagnostic data to be entered directly into the patient's EMR.

The upfront cost of implementing CPOE is a major obstacle for hospitals. Also, cultural obstacles to CPOE implementation may exist because many physicians resist the idea of entering their orders via computer.

Some additional advantages of the EMR include access to patient information anytime and anywhere, easily tracked data, reductions in variability of care, improved communication, enhanced legibility with reduced opportunity for misinterpretation of information, simplified health information for patients, reduced medical errors, and improved coordination of care between facilities, providers, and laboratories.

The few disadvantages of the EMR include upfront costs of implementing, increased need for advanced privacy and security protection, inconsistency among systems, lack of standardization, increased potential to link health care information to the wrong patient, widespread interruption if the system goes down, and increased health care costs.

MANAGED CARE

People are living longer because of advancements in health care technology, early diagnosis, improved sanitation, improved food choices, greater emphasis on healthy lifestyle choices, better pharmacologic agents, more advanced surgical procedures, and decreased infectious disease. This increase in the older population and the cost of increased technology have caused a crisis in health care, resulting in the emergence of managed health care. **Managed care** is the use of a planned and systematic approach to providing quality health care at the lowest possible cost.

Managed care systems most often are associated with **health maintenance organizations (HMOs)**, organizations that have management responsibility for providing comprehensive health care services on a prepayment basis (**capitation**) to voluntarily enrolled persons within a designated population. Several models of HMOs are in place, and each is unique in the way it contracts for the services of physicians.

The *staff model HMO* is a multispecialty group of physicians who practice at a facility that is an HMO and whose physicians are salaried employees.

The *group model HMO* is similar to the staff model, but there is no specific facility called an HMO; physicians contract with the HMO to provide nearly all services to members.

The *individual practice association (IPA) model* is used when the HMO contracts with an association of individual physicians to provide services for members in their private offices; physicians are able to contract with large patient populations and still maintain independence (except for emergencies, members must be referred by physicians in the HMO before receiving services outside the facility; failure to do so may result in nonpayment by the HMO for care provided).

The *preferred provider organization (PPO)* is an independent group of physicians or hospitals that provide health care for fees that are 15% to 20% lower than customary rates. It is more like a traditional insurance plan (no capitation) because there is a "participating physician list," and patients usually do not need referrals.

In 1983, Congress authorized the creation of Medicare's prospective payment system (PPS) for hospitals. This changed the way physicians and hospitals receive payment in that they no longer establish their own prices. The policy required Medicare to fix prices in advance on a cost-per-case basis, with the use of 500 **diagnosis-related groups** as a measure.

HEALTH CARE PAYMENT SOURCES

Many sources provide health care payment; the most common of these are listed below.

Third-party payers are insurance companies or government programs that pay for health care services on behalf of the patient.

Medicare is government insurance that was enacted in 1965 for individuals older than age 65 or persons with a disability who have received Social Security benefits for 2 years (some disabilities, such as end-stage renal disease, are covered immediately). Three types of coverage consist of type A, hospital insurance; type B, medical insurance (premium and deductible); and type D, which started in January of 2006 and is a drug plan created for senior citizens who did not have drug coverage.

Medicaid is a federal and state program that provides medical assistance for the indigent. It has no entitlement features; recipients must prove their eligibility. Funds come from federal grants and are administered by the state; benefits are closely associated with the economic status of the beneficiary. The benefits cover **inpatient** care, **outpatient** and diagnostic services, skilled nursing facilities, physician services, and **home health** care.

Indemnity insurance is a fee-for-service plan. The patient may use any licensed physician, other health care providers, or an accredited hospital, and the plan will pay for a certain portion (usually 80%) of the cost. The annual deductible ranges from $100 to $500. Charges in excess of eligible charges (usual, customary, and reasonable [UCR]) are not covered by the plan.

Workers' compensation pays the medical bills and a significant portion of the lost wages when an on-the-job accident or illness results in injury or disability. The employer pays a premium to an insurance carrier to meet the Workers' Compensation policy. The injured worker must fill out a claim form and send it to the insurance carrier. The injured worker receives no bill, pays no deductible, and is covered 100% for medical expenses related to that injury or illness.

HEALTH CARE DELIVERY SYSTEMS AND SERVICES

History of Hospitals

The histories of early Egyptian and Indian civilizations indicate that crude hospitals were in existence 6 centuries before Christ. The early Greeks and Romans used their temples to the gods as refuges for the sick.

During the Crusades, *hospitea* were established, at which pilgrims could rest from their travels. The word *hospital* comes to us originally from the Latin noun *hospes*, which means "guest" or "host." The term **hospice**, which relates to family-centered care for the terminally ill, also is derived from *hospes*.

As Christianity progressed, the care of the sick, although it remained an important part of the work of the church, was moved out of the temples into separate buildings. During the 12th and 13th centuries, great hospital growth occurred in England and France. Members of religious orders cared for the needs of the ill. An organizational structure similar to that of the modern hospital began to emerge.

The earliest hospital in what is now the United States served sick soldiers on Manhattan Island in 1663. However, the first established hospitals were founded in Philadelphia in the early 18th century. The development of hospitals continued worldwide as more inventions and discoveries were brought to light. The middle 19th and early 20th centuries were important for hospital growth because during this period, the foundations of modern biology were laid and books on the subject were written. The early 20th century also saw substantial advances in the education of nurses and doctors and an increase in the number of people who were being trained for these professions.

Through the centuries, people's interest in the welfare of their fellow human beings continued to grow. The hospital of today continues to serve those in need during illness or injury with modern technologies, improved medical knowledge, and compassion.

Hospital Functions

The primary function of the hospital is *the care and treatment of the sick*. This is true of all hospitals, regardless of size. Other functions include the *education of physicians and other health care personnel*, *research*, and *prevention of disease*. Especially in smaller communities, the hospital also *serves as a local health center*.

Only large hospitals may find it possible to perform all five functions. The functions the hospital performs depend on many factors, including the hospital's location, the population it serves, and the size of the facility. The care and treatment of the sick or injured necessitates proper accommodations for the patient, along with adequate medical and nursing care. Services performed take into account the patient's comfort and safety. The care and treatment of each patient calls for a team effort. Each department that is involved with the patient plays an important role in assisting the patient to return to a better state of health.

Some hospitals maintain schools in various health services, such as radiology, clinical laboratory, and respiratory care. Other hospitals provide practical experience for students enrolled in university or community college educational programs at all levels of nursing, diet therapy, hospital administration, health unit coordinating, and other hospital-related fields. A hospital may have a residency program for doctors, and it may provide additional experiences for medical students.

The type of research conducted in hospitals may depend on specific services rendered by the hospital. A hospital that specializes in the care of patients with cancer would do research in cancer, whereas a hospital that specializes in the care of patients with skeletal deformities would be actively involved in research on that topic.

The trend today is toward the prevention of disease. The hospital may serve as a **community health** center, providing low-cost or free clinics for the early detection of symptoms of disease conditions and for administration of immunization programs. Doctors and other health care personnel also provide counseling and instruction in health care.

Hospital Classifications

Hospitals can be classified in many ways. The three most common classifications are (1) the type of patient service offered, (2) the ownership of the hospital, and (3) the type of accreditation the hospital has been given.

Type of service offered refers to the distinction between general hospitals and specialized hospitals. General hospitals—the most common type—render various services for patients with many disease conditions and injuries. Not all general hospitals in a community offer identical services because this would prove too costly. Specialized hospitals provide services to a particular body part (e.g., an eye hospital), to a particular segment of the population (e.g., a children's hospital), or for a particular type of care (e.g., a psychiatric or rehabilitation hospital).

Ownership of the hospital is the second type of classification. The federal government maintains hospitals for veterans and for personnel in the U.S. Navy and Air Force. The government also provides health services in hospitals for Native Americans. States, counties, and cities are also owners of hospitals. Churches and fraternal organizations may own and control general or specialized hospitals, which are usually nonprofit agencies. **Proprietary** hospitals (operated for profit and owned by a group of individuals or corporations) are also in operation.

The hospital of today is often part of a health care system. This health care system usually has a "parent" corporation that oversees the other companies within the system. The hospital is one of the subsidiary companies. Subsidiaries are designated as profit or nonprofit. Each has its own board of directors. Aside from the hospital, the system may include a company that provides durable medical equipment, another that provides home care to the community, another that operates parking facilities or linen services, and so forth. Most health care systems have a component called a *foundation*, whose purpose is to focus on donations and fundraising activities that benefit the entire system.

Accreditation refers to recognition that a hospital has met an official standard. For example, a *TJC-accredited hospital* means that the hospital has been surveyed, graded, and approved by the Joint Commission. Participation in TJC accreditation is voluntary. Several other accrediting agencies also conduct surveys, according to the services provided by the hospital. All facilities that are receiving Medicare reimbursement must receive TJC accreditation.

The hospital's license to operate usually is granted by the Department of Health Services of the individual state.

Magnet Recognition Program

The *Magnet Recognition Program* was developed by the *American Nurses Credentialing Center (ANCC)*, an affiliate of the *American Nurses Association (ANA)*. **Magnet status** is an award given by the ANCC to hospitals that satisfy a set of criteria designed to measure the strength and quality of their nursing. Magnet evaluation criteria are based on quality indicators and standards of nursing practice as defined in the *Scope and Standards for Nurse Administrators of the ANA* (1996). These criteria are similar to TJC standards. Currently, no registered nurse (RN)-to-patient ratios are required to achieve Magnet status. To obtain Magnet status, health care organizations must apply to the ANCC, must submit extensive documentation that demonstrates their adherence to ANA standards, and must undergo an on-site evaluation to verify the information provided in submitted documentation and to assess for the presence of the "forces of magnetism" within the organization. The ANCC collects a fee from hospitals for its Magnet recognition process. Magnet status is awarded for a 4-year period, after which time the organization must reapply.

This program is marketed by ANCC as a vehicle that can provide to hospitals the following benefits: enhanced nursing care, increased staff morale, appeal to high-quality physicians; reinforced positive collaborative relationships, creation of a "Magnet culture," improved patient quality outcomes, enhanced nursing recruitment and retention, and a competitive advantage. The premise is that staff nurses are more valued and more involved in data collection and decision making in patient care delivery. Nurses are rewarded for advancing in nursing practice, and open communication between nurses and other members of the health care team is encouraged. Hospitals may use their Magnet status as a promotional tool.

Operational Guidelines

The *American Hospital Association (AHA)* and the TJC determine hospital operational guidelines. AHA guidelines address confidentiality, privacy, informed consent, patient rights, and the like. TJC guidelines promote quality of care and dimensions of performance. *TJC-required annual in-services* for all health care employees include Cardiopulmonary Resuscitation (CPR), Infectious Disease Control, Fire and Safety Training, Universal (standard) Precautions, and HIPAA (Health Insurance Portability and Accountability Act) Training. TJC also requires a preemployment and an annual tuberculosis skin test. Hospitals may have additional preemployment requirements, as is discussed in Chapter 6.

Hospital Organization
Administrative Personnel

The **governing board,** which is at the top of the organizational structure of a hospital, also may be referred to as the board of trustees or the board of directors. Three of the main responsibilities of the board include establishing policy, providing adequate financing, and overseeing personnel standards. The board is composed of persons from the business and professional communities, as well as concerned citizens from all socioeconomic groups. The number of hospital board members varies with the size of the hospital. In hospitals that are part of a health care system, the hospital's governing board is responsible to the board of the parent corporation of the system.

In direct charge of the hospital and responsible to the governing board is the **chief executive officer (CEO)**. The CEO plans for the implementation of policies set forth by the governing board. The *chief operating officer (COO)* is responsible for the day-to-day operations of the hospital and reports directly to the CEO. The *chief financial officer (CFO)* is responsible for the fiscal aspects of the hospital administration and reports directly to the CEO. A vice president or a director supervises each service within the hospital. Vice presidents report to the hospital COO. Figure 2-1 is an example of a typical hospital structure.

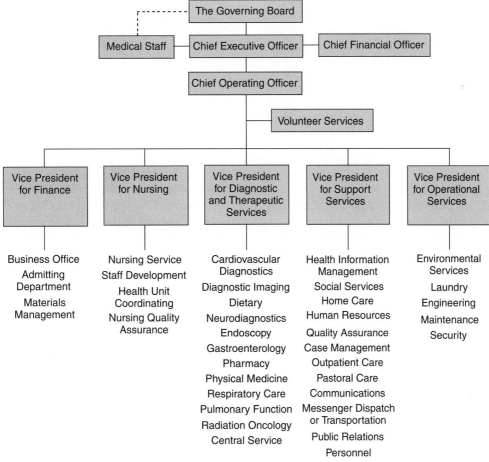

Figure 2-1 An example of a typical hospital organizational structure.

The board delegates the supervision of patient care quality and of the conduct of physicians who practice in the hospital to a committee that is representative of the medical staff.

The Medical Staff

Because the health unit coordinator (HUC) transcribes doctors' orders and acts as the receptionist for the nursing unit, there is a great deal of interaction each day with the medical staff. Therefore, it is helpful for the HUC to understand the different roles of doctors who work at the hospital.

The hospital governing board has a duty to the community to exercise care in the selection of doctors appointed to the medical staff. A doctor who has submitted credentials to the state medical board and who has a license to practice in the state may submit an application for appointment to the staff of a hospital or hospitals.

A physician who has been appointed to the medical staff and who sends patients to the hospital for admission is known as the patient's **attending physician**. The attending physician prescribes care and treatment (doctors' orders) during the patient's hospital stay. A doctor who is caring for hospital patients may be a *doctor of medicine* (MD) or a *doctor of osteopathy* (DO). Both pursue identical approved programs of study, but colleges of osteopathic medicine place special emphasis on the relationship of organs to the musculoskeletal system. Structural problems are corrected by manipulation. Attending physicians are not hospital employees and receive no salary from the hospital. A **hospitalist** is a full-time **acute care** specialist who focuses exclusively on hospitalized patients. This position was created in 1991 to enable family physicians to effectively manage their inpatient practices and treat more people in their outpatient practices. Hospitalists are employed by and receive a salary from the hospital. There may be other doctors on the staff (such as the director of medical education, the hospital pathologist, or the director of radiation oncology) who are salaried hospital employees.

Large hospitals may offer an educational program in which medical school graduates can apply their knowledge to the practice of medicine. The term *intern* rarely is used in reference to the medical school graduate. The term **resident** is applied to all medical school graduates who are gaining hospital experience. These graduates frequently are referred to as postgraduate year 1 (PGY-1) or first-year resident. Residents may be referred to as house staff or house officers (HOs).

Physicians who specialize in a particular aspect of medicine, such as pediatrics, internal medicine, or general surgery spend 3 to 5 years in a specific residency program. After completing the residency and passing a specific examination, the physician is acknowledged as certified. Often after residency, a 1- to 2-year fellowship period provides the opportunity for the clinician to become more familiar with a specific area, such as cardiology. These practitioners are referred to as fellows. Some attending physicians serve as teachers of hospital residents.

Many physicians have chosen to practice in special fields and are known by their specialties. It is common to refer to a doctor by their specialty, as in the terms *cardiologist, gynecologist,* and *pediatrician.*

In the course of work at the hospital, medical specialty terms may be required when one is referring to doctors (see the Box *Common Medical Specialties*).

Hospital Departments and Services

The HUC interacts daily with many hospital departments during the transcription or scheduling of doctors' orders or when requesting services provided by the department. Therefore, it is important to have an overall view of the departments and their functions as they relate to the role of the HUC. See the Box *Hospital Departments* for a brief description of their services. These services are divided into business services, diagnostic and therapeutic services, support services, and operational services. It is important to remember that not all hospitals have each of the departments listed, nor may the department in each hospital use the same name as is used in this text.

Business Services

The business services department deals with the financial aspects of the hospital. The HUC works closely with the admitting department during the patient's admission to, transfer within, and discharge from the hospital. The HUC orders all the unit supplies from the purchasing department.

The *business office* is in charge of patient accounts, budget planning, employee payroll, and payment of bills incurred by the hospital. This office determines the ability of the patient to pay through hospitalization insurance and Medicare or Medicaid. The business office also provides a place for safekeeping of patient valuables. In the area of budget planning, each department and nursing unit is issued a cost control center number. For example, the nutritional care department may be given number 4622. All purchases, maintenance fees, and other expenses must include the cost control center number on the request for record keeping purposes.

The *admitting department*, sometimes called patient services, admits new patients to the hospital, transfers patients within the hospital, and discharges patients from the hospital. On admission, the admitting department obtains pertinent information from patients or their relatives. When the EMR has been implemented, the admitting department will enter demographic information into the EMR. Admitting department personnel witness the signing of the admission agreement by the patient or their representative and prepare the identification bracelet and labels.

The *materials management department*, or *purchasing department*, is responsible for obtaining all supplies and equipment to be used by hospital departments. Sometimes, small hospitals band together to have greater purchasing power and to save money.

Diagnostic and Therapeutic Services

The following departments relate to the direct care of the hospitalized patient. During transcription procedures, the HUC orders tests, treatments, or supplies from these departments, according to doctors' orders.

The *cardiovascular diagnostics department* performs tests related to cardiac (heart) and blood vessel function. The diagnostic procedures ordered most often are electrocardiograms (EKG or ECG) and echocardiograms (ultrasound of the heart), which are performed at the patient's bedside. Cardiac catheterization is also performed by this department.

The *diagnostic imaging department* includes the radiology, nuclear medicine, and ultrasound departments. Diagnostic

COMMON MEDICAL SPECIALTIES

Physician's Specialty	Specialty Description
Allergist	Treats patients who have hypersensitivity to pollens, foods, medications, and other substances
Anesthesiologist	Administers drugs or gases to produce loss of consciousness or sensation in the patient; care during surgery and recovery from an anesthetic is included.
Cardiologist	Diagnoses and treats diseases of the heart and blood vessels
Dermatologist	Diagnoses and treats disorders of the skin
Emergency room physician	Diagnoses and treats patients in trauma and emergency situations
Endocrinologist	Diagnoses and treats diseases of the internal glands that secrete hormones
Family practitioner	Specializes in primary health care for all family members
Gastroenterologist	Diagnoses and treats diseases of the digestive tract
Geriatrist	Diagnoses and treats diseases and problems of aging
Gynecologist	Diagnoses and treats disorders and diseases of the female reproductive tract
Health information specialist	Obtains, posts, and analyzes medical, workload, finance, and insurance data. Ensures that this information is properly recorded into medical records, so practitioners can plan and evaluate health care provided to patients
Hospitalist	Provides acute care exclusively to hospitalized patients
Internist	Diagnoses and medically treats diseases and disorders of the internal organs of adults
Medical and health services	Plans, directs, coordinates, and supervises the delivery of health managers (also called care health care executives or health care administrators)
Neonatologist	Diagnoses and treats disorders of the newborn
Neurologist	Diagnoses and treats diseases of the nervous system
Obstetrician	Cares for women during pregnancy, labor, delivery, and after delivery
Oncologist	Diagnoses and treats cancerous conditions
Ophthalmologist	Diagnoses and treats diseases and defects of the eye
Orthopedist	Diagnoses and treats diseases or fractures of the musculoskeletal system
Otolaryngologist	Diagnoses and treats diseases of the ear, nose, and throat
Pathologist	Studies cell changes and other alterations of the body caused by disease
Pediatrician	Provides preventive care and diagnoses and treats diseases of children
Physiatrist	Diagnoses and treats diseases of the neuro-musculoskeletal system with physical elements to restore the individual to participation in society
Proctologist	Diagnoses and treats diseases of the rectum and anus
Psychiatrist	Diagnoses and treats mental illness
Radiation oncologist	Treats cancer through the use of radiation
Radiologist	Diagnoses and treats diseases with the use of various methods of imaging such as x-ray, ultrasound, radioactive materials, and magnetic resonance
Surgeon	Treats diseases and injuries through operative methods; may specialize in a particular areas, such as heart, eye, or pediatric surgery
Urologist	Diagnoses and treats diseases of the male and female urinary tracts and of the male reproductive system

studies are performed with the use of x-ray, ultrasound, computed tomography, magnetic resonance imaging, and radioactive element scanners. A radiologist, a medical doctor qualified in the use of x-ray and other imaging devices, is in charge of this department. The radiographer, a graduate of a 2- or 4-year educational program, performs many of the technical procedures.

The nutritional care department plans and prepares meals for patients, employees, and visitors and works under the direction of a registered dietitian (a graduate of a 4-year college program). Personnel within the department deliver meals and nourishment to nursing care units. Other dietitians in the department instruct patients in proper nutrition and in the use of special diets when they are ordered by the doctor. Some hospitals participate in an internship program for college students enrolled in a hospital dietitian curriculum.

The *neurology department* performs diagnostic studies of the brain. Electroencephalography (EEG) records the electric impulses of brain waves. An EEG technician performs the test, and a physician, usually a neurologist, interprets the brain wave tracings.

The *endoscopy department* performs diagnostic procedures with the use of endoscopes. These instruments permit the visual examination of a body cavity or hollow organ, such as the stomach. A specialist employed by the hospital or in private practice may perform endoscopies. Registered nurses or licensed practical nurses usually assist the doctors with these procedures.

The *gastroenterology department,* or *GI lab,* performs studies to diagnose disease conditions of the digestive system. Tests, which are usually performed on an outpatient basis, are related to problems of the esophagus, stomach, pancreas, gallbladder, and small intestine. A gastroenterologist, a doctor with additional education related to diseases of the gastrointestinal system, is in charge of the department. A laboratory technologist or an RN may assist with these procedures.

HOSPITAL DEPARTMENTS

Department	Service
Business	
Business office	Patient accounts
Admitting	Admission of new patients
Materials management, or purchasing	Obtains supplies and equipment
Diagnostic and Therapeutic	
Cardiovascular diagnostics	Tests related to heart and blood vessels
Diagnostic imaging	X-rays, nuclear medicine, and ultrasound studies
Nutritional care	Meals
Neurology	Studies of the brain
Endoscopy	Diagnostic procedures performed with the use of endoscopes
Gastroenterology or GI lab	Studies related to the digestive system
Pathology/Clinical laboratory	Diagnostic procedures on specimens from the body
Pharmacy	Medications
Physical medicine	Rehabilitation
Cardiopulmonary or respiratory care department	Treatment related to respiratory function
Radiation oncology, or radiation treatment department	Treatment of cancer growths
Support Services	
Case management	Coordinates patient care with insurance companies
Central supply department, or supply purchasing department	Storage and distribution of supplies and equipment used for patient care
Health information management, or medical records	Patient charts or electronic medical records
Quality assurance	Quality care
Social services	Assistance to patients and families
Home care, or discharge planning	Transition from hospital to home
Outpatient	Services to patients outside the hospital
Pastoral care	Spiritual support
Patient advocate	Available to patients who have concerns about their care or environment
Communications	Switchboard
Transportation department	Delivery
Public relations	Provides information to the public
Volunteer services	A variety of services provided by volunteers
Operational Services	
Housekeeping or environmental services	Housekeeping duties
Hospital information systems department	Repairs electronic equipment, including telephones, computers, printers, etc.
Mechanical	Keeps equipment in working condition
Health information systems	Repair of electronic equipment, including computers, department printers, fax machines, scanners, telephones, etc.
Laundry, or linens department	Maintains linens
Human resources	Recruitment, records, and benefits
Security	Protection

The *pathology department/clinical laboratory* is concerned with diagnostic procedures performed on specimens from the body, such as blood, tissues, urine, stools, sputum, and bone marrow. This department may be separated into several divisions that are named for the tests or substances to be examined, such as hematology, urinalysis, microbiology, chemistry, and blood bank. The pathologist also examines specimens removed during surgery. Autopsies are performed under the direction of this department. The laboratory functions under the direction of a pathologist and employs medical technologists and medical laboratory technicians who have graduated from a recognized school for laboratory personnel.

The *pharmacy* provides the medications used within the hospital or in the clinics and may be involved in instructing patients regarding the proper use of medications. The pharmacist fills the prescription ordered by the doctor. The pharmacy also may provide lotions and mouthwashes for patient use.

Intravenous solutions to which medications have been added are prepared in the pharmacy under sterile conditions. A registered pharmacist is in charge of the pharmacy.

The *physical medicine department* is composed of several smaller departments related to the rehabilitation of the patient. The physical medicine department works under the direction of a physiatrist. Physical therapy and occupational therapy are the two most common therapeutic areas within the physical medicine department. Small hospitals may have only a physical therapy department. The physical therapy department provides treatment through the use of exercise, massage, heat, light, water, and other methods. Registered physical therapists (graduates of a 4-year college program) and physical therapy technicians (graduates of a 2-year community college program) carry out prescribed evaluations and treatments.

The *occupational therapy department* provides patients with purposeful activities that are designed to evaluate and treat those who are impaired physically, mentally, and developmentally. These activities help prevent deformities, restore function to affected body parts, and preserve morale. Registered occupational therapists, graduates of a 4-year college program, are employed in the occupational therapy department.

The *cardiopulmonary*, or *respiratory care department*, performs diagnostic tests to determine lung function, provides treatment related to respiratory function, and assists in maintaining patients on ventilators (breathing machines). The department also administers respiratory physical therapy. The respiratory care therapist and the respiratory care technician, graduates of 1- to 4-year educational programs, are employed here.

The *radiation oncology department*, or *radiation therapy department*, may be a division within the diagnostic imaging department or a separate department. Its primary purpose is to treat cancerous growths. Cobalt beam units and linear accelerators are examples of equipment used in these departments. The radiation oncologist, a physician with additional education in the use of radiation for the treatment of disease, is the head of the radiation oncology department.

Support Services

The following departments are also very important in the concept of caring for all patients' needs. The HUC interacts with most of the following departments by requesting services, supplies, and/or equipment for patients on the nursing unit.

The *central service department (CSD)*, or *supply purchasing department (SPD)*, is the distribution area for supplies and equipment used by nursing personnel to perform treatments on patients. Enema kits, dressing trays, bandages, and other supplies used most frequently by nursing unit personnel may be kept on the nursing unit. When a nurse takes an item from floor stock for patient use, the item is charged (by use of computer) to the appropriate patient by scanning the bar code on the item into the patient's account. Central service department technicians replenish the unit supply daily. Figure 2-2, *A*, shows an example of a CSD or SPD supply room (also called C-locker); Figure 2-2, *B*, shows examples of floor stock. Packs of supplies used by the operating and delivery rooms may be processed and sterilized by CSD personnel.

The *health information management system (HIMS)*, or *medical records department*, manages the patient's EMR and cares for the patient's paper record after the patient has been discharged from the hospital. Records are stored here and may be retrieved for the doctor if the patient is readmitted. These records (electronic and paper) also may be used for research. This department is also responsible for coding medical and surgical conditions of patients on discharge.

This coding is related to the system of Medicare reimbursement and involves diagnosis-related groups (DRGs), whereby payment is based on the type of illness. Accurate coding of the patient's diagnosis that is based on the International Classification of Disease (ICD) system is a critical function within the department. If coding is not exact, the direct result can be financial loss for the hospital. ICDs are used world wide for morbidity and mortality statistics, reimbursement systems, and automated decision support in medicine. The World Health Organization (WHO) publishes three major and other minor updates annually.

Medical transcription (not related to transcription as used in the transcription of a doctor's orders) is another service of the health records department that is available to doctors for the dictation of patient histories, physical examination findings, and so forth. The transcriptionist prepares typewritten reports from dictated tapes. These reports are placed in the hospitalized patient's chart.

✏ TAKE NOTE

Facilities with successful electronic medical records are more likely to be those where health information management (HIM) professionals played a role, according to newly released research.

One of the health information technician's responsibilities is to certify documents scanned by HUCs before making them a permanent part of the patient's electronic record.

The *quality assurance department* provides information to various departments within the hospital for the purpose of assisting those departments to provide quality care. Through analysis of actual occurrences and practices against standards set by various departments, quality assurance continuously uses ongoing activities to suggest improvements. Individual departments, such as nursing, may have their own quality assurance component, which coordinates with the hospital-wide quality assurance department. Risk management, a system of ensuring appropriate nursing care, can be part of the quality assurance manager's responsibilities. Risk management includes identifying possible risks, analyzing them, acting to reduce risks, and evaluating the steps taken.

The *social services department* provides services to patients and to their families when emotional and environmental difficulties impede the patient's recovery. The social worker's knowledge of the community and of the agencies that provide a variety of services aids in lifting emotional and financial burdens caused by the illness. This department also can arrange nursing home and extended care facility placement. The department head holds an advanced degree in social work. This department may also be responsible, when necessary, for assisting patients in preparing for the transition from hospital to home.

The *case management department* consists of individuals who work in health care facilities to coordinate patient care with insurance companies. The **case manager,** who is an expert

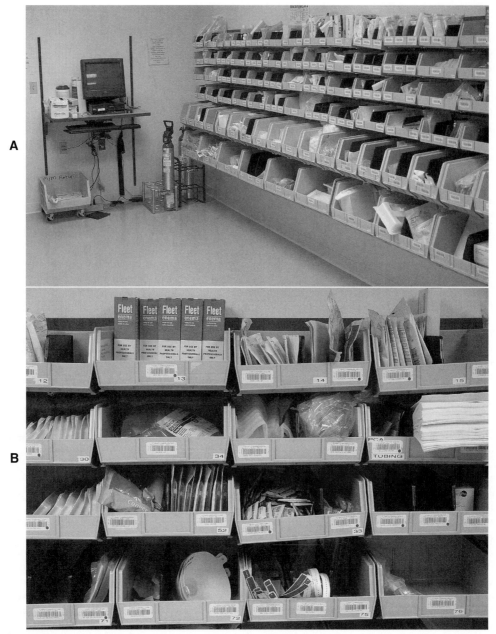

Figure 2-2 A, An example of a central service department (CSD), supply purchasing department (SPD) supply room or C-locker located on the nursing unit. **B,** An example of floor stock found in the CSD, SPD supply room or C-locker.

in managed care, acts as an advocate for the patient to most appropriately enforce the benefits and coverage of their health policy. A case managers may be certified as a CCM (certified case manager), as a nursing case manager through the American Nurses Credentialing Center (ANCC), or in a specialty area, such as rehabilitation or disability. The case manager may have assistants or a secretary to assist with the workload. The case manager, when necessary, also may be responsible for assisting patients in preparing for the transition from hospital to home.

The *home care department* assists patients in preparing for the transition from hospital to home. A registered nurse with a public health background usually heads the department. The needs of the patient who is returning to the home environment are identified. Plans for care are prepared by the visiting

nurse service, and rental of needed equipment may be arranged before the patient is discharged. Follow-up studies also are provided for the doctor.

The *outpatient department*, or clinic, provides services to patients outside the hospital. Clinics for various disease conditions, such as diabetes, allergies, and gynecologic problems, may be open weekly. Prenatal care and dental care also may be offered. Visits are usually scheduled by appointment. The outpatient area provides clinical experience for resident doctors.

The *pastoral care department* provides spiritual support to the patient and family in time of need. Some hospitals maintain a chaplaincy program for members of the clergy who are interested in becoming hospital chaplains.

The *communications department* may be called the telephone switchboard in many hospitals. Telephone operators process incoming and outgoing telephone calls and operate the doctor paging system. In emergencies, such as fire, disaster, or cardiac arrest, communications personnel alert hospital personnel in code, such as Code 1000, to announce a fire in the hospital. In some hospitals, the telephone operator also may serve as an information station for visitors to the hospital.

The *transportation department* performs multiple tasks throughout the hospital. Delivery of interdepartmental mail, carrying of specimens to the laboratory, assisting with the discharge or admission of patients, and transporting of patients from one area of the hospital to another are all carried out by personnel of this department.

The *public relations department* serves to provide the public with information concerning the hospital's activities. This may be accomplished by means of the community newspaper. Many hospitals publish a weekly, bimonthly, or monthly newspaper for patients and/or employees.

The *volunteer services department* is made up of people from the community. Members of the women's auxiliary or its counterpart, the men's auxiliary, give generously of their time and talents to staff the patient library or gift shop. Many perform tasks for the various hospital departments or on the nursing unit. High school students also may have an auxiliary organization.

Operational Services

The following services are not related to the direct care of the hospitalized patient but are concerned with the patient's hospital environment. It is the task of the HUC to request services from these departments as needed by the nursing unit.

The main responsibility of *environmental service,* or the *housekeeping department,* is to maintain a clean hospital through proper cleaning methods aimed at preventing the spread of infection. Daily cleaning of the hospital is provided by environmental services. Environmental services is responsible for cleaning the individual patient unit after a patient has been discharged and preparing it for a new admission. Another duty that this department may perform is the changing of draperies and cubicle curtains around the patient's bed. In some hospitals, environmental services also has the responsibility of delivering isolation equipment to the unit.

The *mechanical services department* of the hospital is responsible for keeping all equipment in working condition. In a large hospital, this department may be divided into various branches, such as engineering, maintenance, and electronic equipment repair. The engineering division is concerned with heating, lighting, air conditioning, power systems, water, and sewage. The maintenance division is responsible for keeping the hospital and its surroundings, equipment, and furnishings in good condition. Services rendered include painting, maintenance of televisions, carpentry, and pneumatic tube systems repair. Gardeners and groundskeepers are also members of this department.

The *hospital information systems department* is responsible for repair and maintenance of electronic equipment, including telephones, computers, printers, etc.

The *laundry department,* or *linens department,* maintains the hospital's linen supply; tasks may include the washing, drying, and repairing of linens. Many hospitals send the laundry out to a commercial laundry under the coordination of the hospital laundry department. Some hospitals may join together in ownership of a laundry service if this more economically serves the needs of all. Laundry personnel may deliver the linen to nursing care units.

The *human resources department* organizes recruitment programs, interviews new employees, conducts employee termination interviews, and maintains records for all employees. Employee benefits and retirement records are also the responsibility of the human resource department.

An employee fitness center is available in many hospitals to assist employees with their own health maintenance. Some hospitals may provide counseling services to employees to assist them in coping with personal and employment problems.

The *security department* is responsible for protecting the hospital, patients, visitors, and employees. Thefts and disturbances on the premises should be reported to this department. Whenever a threat of violence is perceived by the HUC, it must be immediately reported to security and to the nurse in charge.

Other Health Care Delivery Systems

Health care services often are provided in nonhospital settings. This is particularly true for long-term care. *Extended care facilities (ECFs)* provide care for patients who are not acutely ill and cannot be cared for at home. These facilities provide skilled or intermediate levels of care. The following facilities are providers of long-term care that offer employment opportunities for HUCs. Nursing homes are licensed by the state and may be classified by ownership and accreditation. Nursing homes provide care for those who are so sick or functionally disabled that they require ongoing nursing and support services provided in a formal health care institution. These services generally are classified as **custodial care**; however, another level of nursing home is the *skilled nursing facility (SNF),* which provides care for those too sick to go home or to a nursing home but who are not so acutely ill that they require the technologic and professional intensity of a hospital. Many hospitals also operate an SNF.

Physical medicine and rehabilitation facilities may be classified as ECFs, although such care may be given to outpatients as well. Individuals who receive care in such facilities primarily require special support services, in addition to varying levels of nursing care.

Long-term care also may be provided in the home through a home health agency. These agencies provide such services as skilled nursing, rehabilitation (for such problems as speech or language pathology or for physical or occupational therapy), pharmacy, and medical social work. *Hospice* is another form of care sometimes classified as long term. It provides palliative and supportive care for terminally ill patients and their families. Emphasis is placed on control of symptoms and preparation for and support before and after death. The hospice can be freestanding, hospital based, or home based. Hospice is a not an actual type of facility but is a concept of providing health care services wherever necessary.

EMPLOYMENT IN THE HEALTH CARE FIELD

U.S. government statistics indicate that health care is the fastest growing industry, employing more than 98 million workers. Health care is delivered in hospitals, clinics, physicians' offices, HMOs, surgi-centers, rehabilitation facilities, ECFs, mental health facilities, home care agencies, and hospice settings. More than 200 health careers have been identified, and it is a $2 billion-a-day business (see the Box *Current Health Care Professionals*). The implementation of the electronic patient record has expanded the role of the HUC and has created a greater need for non-clinical health care personnel.

Job and job training opportunities can be researched in several ways. One way is by **surfing the web**. Many national sites are available, and each state has local career websites that can be searched for information pertaining to local areas (see the Box *Health Care Employment Resources*).

KEY CONCEPTS

Administrative organizations, job titles, and job descriptions may differ in many aspects among health care facilities. Health care is constantly changing with the advancement of technology. The HUC must have knowledge about the hospital, its personnel, and the services that it renders in order to carry out assigned tasks. Being aware of trends in health care is a proactive step in preparing for change. The EMR is being implemented nationally, and the HUC, although this role is changing, remains an important part of the health care team.

CURRENT HEALTH CARE PROFESSIONALS

1. Ambulance attendant
2. Animal health technologist
3. Art therapist
4. Athletic trainer
5. Audiologist/speech–language pathologist
6. Cardiovascular technologist
7. Chiropractor
8. Clinical laboratory scientist
9. Clinical laboratory technician
10. Counselor
11. Cytotechnologist
12. Dental assistant
13. Dental hygienist
14. Dentist
15. Diagnostic medical sonographer
16. Dialysis technician
17. Dietetic technician
18. Dietitian/nutritionist
19. Electrocardiograph technician
20. Electroneurodiagnostic technician
21. Emergency medical technician/paramedic
22. Health information (medical records) administrator
23. Health information specialist
24. Health information technician
25. Health unit coordinator
26. Histotechnologist
27. Home health aide
28. Homeopath
29. Hospital admitting clerk
30. Hospital central service worker
31. Licensed practical nurse
32. Medical assistant
33. Medical biller
34. Medical coder
35. Medical and health services manager
36. Medical illustrator
37. Medical radiation technologist
38. Medical transcriptionist
39. Midwife
40. Music therapist
41. Naturopath
42. Nuclear medicine technologist
43. Nurse anesthetist
44. Nurse practitioner
45. Nursing assistant
46. Occupational therapist
47. Occupational therapist assistant
48. Ophthalmic dispensing optician
49. Ophthalmic laboratory technician
50. Ophthalmic medical technician
51. Optician
52. Optometrist
53. Orthotist
54. Patient care technician
55. Perfusionist
56. Perioperative nurse
57. Pharmacist
58. Pharmacist assistant
59. Phlebotomist
60. Physical therapist
61. Physical therapy assistant
62. Physician
63. Physician's assistant
64. Physician specialist
65. Physiotherapist
66. Podiatrist
67. Prosthetist
68. Psychologist
69. Psychology technician
70. Radiology technician
71. Radiology technologist
72. Registered nurse
73. Rehabilitation counselor
74. Respiratory therapist
75. Respiratory therapy technician
76. Surgical technician first assistant
77. Surgical technologist
78. Therapeutic recreation specialist
79. Ultrasonographer
80. Veterinarian
81. Others as identified

HEALTH CARE EMPLOYMENT RESOURCES

Internet general national websites include the following:

www.careerbuilder.com
www.monster.com
www.jobsonline.net
www.simplyhired.com
Jobs may be researched on the Internet by specific profession through various search sites by typing in keywords such as "health unit coordinator."

Other employment resources include the following:

Newspaper classified advertisements	Networking with professionals in the field
Job placement/career counselors	Instructors
Employment agencies	Health care hotlines
Library resources	Health care facility websites and bulletin boards

---

REVIEW QUESTIONS

1. List five challenges that face the health care system today.

a. _____

b. _____

c. _____

d. _____

e. _____

2. List eight advantages of the EMR system.

a. _____

b. _____

c. _____

d. _____

e. _____

f. _____

g. _____

h. _____

3. List four disadvantages of the EMR system.

a. _____

b. _____

c. _____

d. _____

4. The primary function of the hospital is

_____

5. Four other functions of a hospital are

a. _____

b. _____

c. _____

d. _____

6. The doctor who may admit and care for patients in the hospital is known as the patient's

_____

7. A doctor who is a medical school graduate who is gaining experience in the hospital is called a

_____

8. Hospitals may be classified according to

a. _____

b. _____

c. _____

9. Match the specialists listed in the left-hand column with their area of expertise by filling in the appropriate letter from the right-hand column.

_____ 1. internist	a. disorders of the newborn
_____ 2. cardiologist	b. treatment of mental disorders
_____ 3. gynecologist	c. diseases of ear, nose, and throat
_____ 4. dermatologist	d. study of cell changes and other alterations in the body caused by disease
_____ 5. allergist	e. administration of drugs or gases that cause loss of feeling or sensation
_____ 6. neonatologist	f. glandular diseases
_____ 7. pediatrician	g. hypersensitivity to foods, pollens, or medicines
_____ 8. psychiatrist	h. focuses exclusively on hospitalized patients
_____ 9. anesthesiologist	i. problems and diseases of the aged
_____ 10. otolaryngologist	j. diseases and disorders of internal organs of adults
_____ 11. geriatrist	k. diseases of children
_____ 12. endocrinologist	l. diseases of the female reproductive tract
_____ 13. pathologist	m. diseases of heart and blood vessels
_____ 14. hospitalist	n. diseases of the skin

10. Match the specialists listed in the left-hand column with their area of expertise by filling in the appropriate letter from the right-hand column.

_____ 1. surgeon	a. use of x-rays, ultrasound, and radioactive element scanners
_____ 2. urologist	b. diseases of the nervous system
_____ 3. orthopedist	c. diagnosis and treatment of cancerous conditions
_____ 4. neurologist	d. treats trauma patients
_____ 5. physiatrist	e. eye diseases
_____ 6. radiologist	f. treatment of cancer by radiation
_____ 7. oncologist	g. diseases of the male and female urinary tracts and of the male reproductive tract
_____ 8. obstetrician	h. diseases of the rectum

_____ 9. radiation oncologist i. use of operative methods

_____ 10. proctologist j. diseases of the skeletal system

_____ 11. ophthalmologist k. care of pregnant women

_____ 12. emergency room l. treatment of diseases of the neuromusculoskeletal
                 system with the use of physical elements

11. Name the hospital department in charge of each of the following tasks.

a. patient accounts _____

b. transfer, discharge, and admissions _____

c. performing blood, urine, and tissue studies _____

d. diagnostic tests that use computed tomography, ultrasound, radioactive element scanners, and radiant energy _____

e. treatment for cancerous growths _____

f. providing medications for patients _____

g. treatment with use of exercise, heat, and light _____

h. evaluation, treatment, and preservation of morale through purposeful activities _____

i. treatment related to respiratory function _____

j. food preparation and treatment with the use of foods _____

k. diagnosis through the use of instruments to view body cavities or hollow organs such as esophagus and bronchi _____

l. diagnostic procedures for diseases of the GI tract _____

m. diagnostic studies of the heart _____

n. brain studies _____

o. maintaining the patient's paper or electronic record _____

p. supplies and equipment for treatment of patients _____

q. services to patients outside the hospital _____

r. providing services for financial and social problems _____

s. planning the transition from hospital to home _____

t. maintaining a clean hospital _____

u. supplies and equipment for all hospital departments _____

v. spiritual services _____

w. keeping hospital equipment repaired _____

x. maintaining the linen supply _____

y. repairing telephone and computers _____

z. protecting patients, visitors, employees, and hospital _____

12. List five annual in-services required by TJC.

a. _____

b. _____

c. _____

d. _____

e. _____

13. Name the citizen group that is at the head of the hospital's organizational structure.

_____

14. The individual in direct charge of a hospital who is responsible to the governing board is the

_____

15. List three resources used to access employment opportunities.

a. _____

b. _____

c. _____

16. The case manager is an expert in and acts as the patient's

_____

17. Define the following terms/abbreviations:

a. inpatient _____

b. outpatient _____

c. Magnet status _____

d. accreditation _____

e. acute care _____

f. chronic care _____

g. hospitalist _____

h. merger _____

i. ICD _____

j. HMO _____

k. capitation _____

18. Provides supportive care for terminally ill patients and their families.

_____

19. Provides equipment and services to patients in their home

_____

20. Explain the purpose of managed care.

_____

_____

21. Medicare type A is

_____

22. Medicare type B is

_____

23. Medicare type D is

_____

24. Pays the medical bills and a significant portion of lost wages when on-the-job accident or illness results in injury or disability

_____

THINK ABOUT...

1. How will a national interconnected EMR system change health care?
2. Discuss the challenges that face health care today and some results or solutions.
3. What factors should be considered in choosing a health care plan?
4. Should a person interview a new physician or health care provider before choosing care for himself or his family?
5. Discuss problems that may be encountered with a health care provider, and discuss some ways to improve interaction between the consumer and health care providers.
6. Using the Internet or other employment resources, find two job openings. Discuss which one would be a good choice, and explain why.

CHAPTER 3

The Nursing Department

CHAPTER OBJECTIVES

Upon completion of this chapter, you will be able to

1. Define the terms in the vocabulary list.
2. Write the meaning of the abbreviations in the abbreviations list.
3. List three personnel commonly employed in nursing units and special care units, and briefly describe the role of each.
4. Identify the services provided by each of the nursing and special units listed in this chapter.
5. Describe the responsibilities of the nursing service department.
6. Discuss two nursing care delivery models presented in this chapter.
7. Explain what is involved in holistic nursing care.
8. List six benefits of interdisciplinary teamwork.
9. List three services that come under the general heading of perioperative services, and provide a description of each.

VOCABULARY

Acuity Level of care patients would require on the basis of their medical condition; used to evaluate staffing needs

Assignment Sheet A form completed at the beginning of each work shift that indicates the nursing staff member(s) assigned to each patient on that nursing unit

Assistant Nurse Manager A registered nurse who assists the nurse manager in coordinating activities on the nursing unit

Certified Nursing Assistant A certified health care giver who performs basic nursing tasks

Clinical Pathway A method of outlining a patient's path of treatment for a specific diagnosis, procedure, or symptom

Computerized Nurses' Notes Documentation entered directly into the patient's electronic medical record, usually at the patient's bedside on a portable computer

Director of Nursing A registered nurse in charge of nursing services (may be called director of patient services, nursing administrator, vice president of nursing services, or chief nursing officer [CNO])

Holistic Nursing Care A modern nursing practice that expresses the philosophy of total patient care that considers the physical, emotional, social, economic, and spiritual needs of the patient. Also called *comprehensive care*

Interdisciplinary Teamwork Well-coordinated collaboration across health care professionals toward a common goal (improved, efficient patient care)

Licensed Practical Nurse A graduate of a 1-year school of nursing who is licensed in the state in which he or she is practicing; provides direct care and functions under the direction of the registered nurse

Nurse Manager A registered nurse who assists the director of nursing in carrying out administrative responsibilities and is in charge of one or more nursing units (may also be called *unit manager*, *clinical manager*, or *patient care manager*)

Nursing Intervention Any act by a nurse that implements the nursing care plan or clinical pathway or any specific objective of that plan or pathway

Nursing Service Department Hospital department responsible for all nursing care administered to patients

Nursing Unit Administration Division within the hospital responsible for non-clinical patient care

Patient Care Conference Meeting of a patient's doctor or resident, primary nurse, case manager or social worker, and other health care professionals for the purpose of planning the patient's care

Patient Support Associate Nursing unit staff member whose duties may include some patient-admitting responsibilities, coding, or stocking of nursing units; job description and title may vary among hospitals

Perioperative Services Department of the hospital that provides care before (preoperative), during (intraoperative), and after (postoperative) surgery. It encompasses total care of the patient during the surgical experience

Primary Care Nursing One nurse provides total care to assigned patients

Registered Nurse Graduate of a 2- or 4-year college-based school of nursing or a 3-year hospital-based program who is licensed in the state in which they are practicing; may provide direct patient care or may supervise patient care given by others

Shift Manager Registered nurse who is responsible for one or more units during their assigned shift (also may be called *nursing coordinator* or *nursing supervisor*)

Staff Development Department responsible for orientation of new employees and continuing education of employed nursing service personnel (also may be called *educational services*)

SWAT HUC, Nurse, or SWAT Team A health unit coordinator, a nurse, or a group of health care workers that are on call for all units in the hospital to provide assistance as needed (may also be called *resource HUC, nurse,* or *resource team*)

Team Leader Registered nurse who is in charge of a nursing team (also may be called *pod leader* or *charge nurse*)

Team Nursing Consists of a charge nurse and two to three team leaders, along with four to five team members who are working under the supervision of each team leader

ABBREVIATIONS

Abbreviation	Meaning
CCU	coronary care unit
CNA	certified nursing assistant
CVICU	cardiovascular intensive care unit
Gyn	gynecology
ICU	intensive care unit
L&D	labor and delivery
LPN	licensed practical nurse
Med	medical
MICU	medical intensive care unit
Neuro	neurology
NICU	neonatal intensive care unit
Ortho	orthopedics
PICU	pediatric intensive care unit
PSA	patient support associate
Psych	psychiatry
RN	registered nurse
SICU	surgical intensive care unit

Abbreviation	Meaning
SSU	short-stay unit
TICU	trauma intensive care unit

EXERCISE 1

Write the abbreviation for each term listed below.

1. coronary care unit   _____

2. certified nursing assistant   _____

3. cardiovascular intensive care unit   _____

4. gynecology   _____

5. intensive care unit   _____

6. labor and delivery   _____

7. licensed practical nurse   _____

8. medical   _____

9. medical intensive care unit   _____

10. neurology   _____

11. neonatal intensive care unit   _____

12. orthopedics   _____

13. pediatric intensive care unit   _____

14. patient support associate   _____

15. psychiatry   _____

16. registered nurse   _____

17. surgical intensive care unit   _____

18. short-stay unit   _____

19. trauma intensive care unit   _____

EXERCISE 2

Write the meaning of each abbreviation listed below.

1. CCU

_____

2. CNA

_____

3. CVICU

_____

4. Gyn

_____

5. ICU

_____

6. L&D

_____

7. LPN

_____

8. Med

_____

9. MICU

_____

10. Neuro

_____

11. NICU

_____

12. Ortho

_____

13. PICU

_____

14. PSA

_____

15. Psych

_____

16. RN

_____

17. SICU

_____

18. SSU

_____

19. TICU

NURSING SERVICE ORGANIZATION

The Nursing Service Department

The **nursing service department** is responsible for ensuring the physical and emotional care of the hospitalized patient, providing nursing treatment, and evaluating and coordinating treatment and diagnostic studies performed by other hospital departments. Other responsibilities include patient assessment and recording, planning and implementing patient care plans, and patient teaching. Implementation of the electronic medical record (EMR) has made it possible for the nurse to enter documentation directly into the patient's record at the bedside via computer. The nursing service department is almost always the single largest component of the hospital. Often 50% or more of all hospital personnel are employed in the nursing service department.

NURSING SERVICE ADMINISTRATIVE PERSONNEL

The **director of nurses**, also called the _vice president of nursing,_ is responsible for the overall administration of nursing service. Setting nursing practice standards and staffing are two examples of the responsibilities of the director of nursing. The director of nursing is responsible to the chief executive officer of the health care facility.

The **nurse manager** (also called _clinical manager, patient care manager,_ or _unit manager_) is a **registered nurse** (RN) who usually is responsible for the patients and nursing personnel on the unit for 24 hours a day. The nurse manager reports to the director of nursing. Managerial responsibilities include the planning and coordinating of quality nursing care for patients hospitalized on the unit. Selecting, supervising, scheduling, and evaluating personnel employed on the unit are other managerial responsibilities of the nurse manager. The nurse manager works closely with physicians to coordinate nursing care with the care prescribed by the physician. Usually, an RN, titled charge nurse, **shift manager**, nursing care manager, or **assistant nurse manager** oversees the nursing unit in the absence of the nurse manager.

The director of **staff development** is responsible for the orientation and evaluation of new nursing service employees and for the continuing education (including Joint Commission on Accreditation of Healthcare Organizations, or JCAHO, requirements) of all employed nursing service personnel. The person in this position usually reports to the director of nursing.

HOSPITAL NURSING UNITS

The health unit coordinator (HUC) works at the nurses' station on the nursing unit. The hospital is divided into nursing units according to the types of services provided to patients. The HUC usually has a computer that is used for transcribing orders and for entering and retrieving information. Additional computers, including portable computers and notebooks that may be taken into the patients' rooms, are available on the unit for the use of doctors, nurses, and other health care personnel. The area where the HUC sits may be a much smaller and partially enclosed area with a computer, a scanner, and a fax machine.

Many methods are used to name the nursing units within the hospital. Sometimes, units are named according to the service offered, such as pediatrics, or the name may be derived from the floor level and direction of the hospital wing (e.g., 4 East).

Regular Nursing Units

Most nursing units are designed to accommodate 18 to 50 hospitalized patients. A regular nursing unit may provide one of the following services:

Behavioral health: Includes psychiatry (psych), which is the care of patients hospitalized for treatment of disorders of the mind or having difficulty coping with life situations; also may include programs for treatment of alcohol and drug abuse and programs related to changing destructive behaviors such as eating disorders

Cardiovascular: Care of patients who are hospitalized for the treatment of diseases of the circulatory system

Gynecology surgery (Gyn): Care of women who are hospitalized for surgery of the female reproductive tract

Medical (Med): Care of patients who are hospitalized for medical treatment

Neurology (Neuro): Care of patients who are hospitalized for treatment of diseases of the nervous system

Obstetrics (OB), labor and delivery (L&D), and nursery: Care of mothers before, during, and after labor and care of newborn infants

Oncology: Care of patients who are hospitalized for treatment of cancer

Orthopedics (Ortho): Care of patients who are hospitalized for treatment of diseases or fractures of the musculoskeletal system

Pediatrics (Peds): Care of children (12 and younger) who are hospitalized for medical or surgical treatment

Rehabilitation (Rehab): Care of patients who are hospitalized for physical handicaps; usually, these patients need long-term treatment and care

Stepdown or Progressive Care unit: Care of patients who require more specialized care than that given at regular nursing units but who do not require intensive care (also called *intermediate* or *transitional care unit*)

Surgical (Surg): Care of patients who are hospitalized for general surgical treatment

Telemetry: Care of patients with cardiac arrhythmias and other heart problems, whose electrocardiogram readings are monitored at the nurses' station. An example of telemetry screens on a telemetry unit is shown in Figure 3-1.

Urology: Care of patients who are hospitalized for treatment of diseases of the male reproductive or urinary system or of the female urinary system

Intensive Care Units

Another type of nursing unit found in the modern hospital is the *intensive care unit (ICU)* (also called *special* or *critical care units*). Its purpose is to provide constant specialized nursing care to critically ill patients. As the condition of the critically ill patient improves, the patient is transferred to the *stepdown unit* for less intense nursing care. Personnel employed in the ICUs are specially qualified for the type of nursing care offered by the unit.

ICUs are usually identified by the type of care they provide to a particular population of patients. For example, the *surgical intensive care unit (SICU)* cares for surgical patients, the *medical intensive care unit (MICU)* cares for medical patients, the *coronary care unit (CCU)* cares for patients with heart disease, the *trauma intensive care unit (TICU)* cares for patients involved in trauma, the *neonatal intensive care unit (NICU)* cares for premature and ill newborns, and the *pediatric intensive care unit (PICU)* cares for pediatric patients.

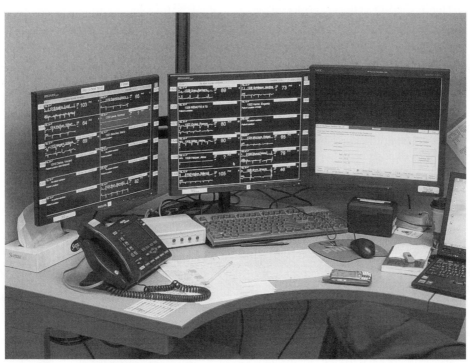

Figure 3-1 An example of telemetry screens on a telemetry unit.

Specialty Units

Specialty areas within the hospital that are usually a part of nursing services and that employ various categories of nursing personnel include the following:

Day surgery or outpatient surgery unit or ambulatory surgery: Care of patients who are having surgery or examinations but who do not require overnight hospitalization

Emergency department: Care of patients who need emergency treatment; after emergency treatment is administered, the patient is admitted to the hospital or is discharged to home, according to their medical needs

Perioperative services include the following:

Preoperative area: Area in the hospital where patients are prepared for surgery

Intraoperative area: Operating room/area in the hospital where surgery is performed

Postoperative area: Postanesthesia care unit (PACU) or recovery room/area in the hospital where patients are cared for immediately after surgery until they have recovered from the effects of the anesthesia

NURSING UNIT PERSONNEL

To maintain 24-hour coverage, nursing service personnel usually are scheduled in two shifts. An example would be one shift from 7:00 A.M. to 7:30 P.M. (day shift) and one from 7:00 P.M. to 7:30 A.M. (night shift). Three shifts also may be used; these shifts then are usually scheduled from 7:00 A.M. to 3:30 P.M., from 3:00 P.M. to 11:30 P.M., and from 11:00 P.M. to 7:30 A.M. Shifts overlap by one-half of an hour to allow communication between personnel.

Nursing personnel other than the HUC, who may be employed on the nursing unit and functioning under the supervision of the nurse manager, are discussed in the following paragraphs.

The *registered nurse* is a graduate of a 2-to 4-year college-based program or a 3-year hospital-based program and currently is licensed to practice in the state of employment. The RN performs all types of treatments, and it is usually hospital policy that only the RN can perform complex procedures, such as administering intravenous (IV) medication. The RN is responsible for applying the nursing process. This encompasses assessment, nursing diagnosis, planning, implementation, and evaluation of patient care, as well as participating in educating patients/family and teaching staff members. When the EMR is in use, the RN is responsible for reading and carrying out doctors' orders from the patient's electronic record and entering their notes directly into the computer to become part of the patient's permanent record.

The **licensed practical nurse (LPN)** is a graduate of a 1-year school of nursing and is licensed to practice in the state of employment. The LPN functions under the direction of the RN and provides direct patient care; performs technical skills, such as discontinuing an IV; and administers medication to patients, as prescribed by physicians.

 The **certified nursing assistant (CNA)** is trained on the job or has completed a short training course 6 to 12 weeks in length at a vocational school. A state examination is required for the nursing assistant to be certified. Nursing assistants perform bedside tasks, such as bathing and feeding patients. They also provide basic treatments, such as taking vital signs and giving enemas. The CNA functions under the supervision of the RN or LPN.

NURSING CARE DELIVERY MODELS

The two most common nursing care delivery models used in hospitals today are the team and total or primary patient care models, as described below.

Team Nursing Care Model

The *team nursing care model* is made up of the charge nurse who oversees the nursing unit, two to three **team leaders** (RNs), and three to four team members who work under the supervision of each team leader. Members of the team may be RNs, LPNs, and/or CNAs. The team leader assigns patients to each team member on the basis of patient **acuity** for care during a shift. Team members perform the particular tasks for their patients that they are qualified to perform. The team leader is responsible for the patients and for the members of their team. A team usually cares for 15 or fewer patients; thus, a nursing unit may have one to three teams. Many hospitals use modified forms of the **team nursing** method. An example of a team nursing model is shown in Figure 3-2.

Total Patient Care Model

The *total patient care model* sometimes is referred to as case nursing. In total patient care, the RN assigned to a patient is responsible for planning, organizing, and performing all care, including providing personal hygiene, medications, and treatments, emotional support, and education required for a group of patients during an assigned shift. An example of a total patient care model is shown in Figure 3-3.

Holistic Nursing Care

Holistic nursing care is the modern nursing practice that expresses the philosophy of comprehensive patient care (total patient care) and considers the physical, emotional, social, economic, and spiritual needs of the patient, their response to illness, and the effect of the illness on ability to meet

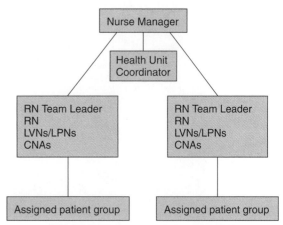

Figure 3-2 Team nursing care model.

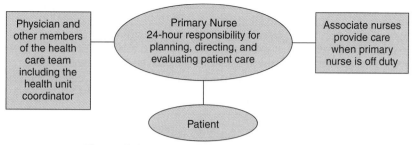

Figure 3-3 Total patient care (case nursing) model.

self-care needs. Holistic health is the concept that concern for health requires the perspective of the individual as an integrated system; rather than treating specific symptoms, all factors are considered.

INTERDISCIPLINARY TEAMWORK

Interdisciplinary teamwork is the well-coordinated collaboration across health care professionals toward a common goal (improved, efficient patient care). Planning of nursing care involves consultation with other members of the health care team. Consultations are most advantageous during planning and implementation and are based on problem solving. Often, **patient care conferences** are held with members of the health care team that may include the patient's doctor or resident, primary nurse, and case worker or social worker, as well as any other health care professional who is caring for the patient and can provide input. Benefits of interdisciplinary teamwork include the following:

- Facilitates continuous quality improvement
- Improves patient care
- Decreases errors
- Provides "total patient care"
- Maximizes resources
- Increases professional satisfaction for health care givers

There is no team without personal accountability. The HUC is a member of the health care team who plays an important role in maximizing efficiency in patient care and treatment.

CLINICAL PATHWAYS

Clinical pathways, also called *critical paths,* are used as a method of outlining a patient's path of treatment for a specific diagnosis, procedure, or symptom. Doctors' orders are usually preprinted with options from which the doctor may choose to meet a specific patient's needs. If the EMR is in use, the doctor's previously written orders will be on file, and the doctor can modify these as appropriate for each patient. Examples of preprinted or stored doctors' orders include surgical and medical orders. See Figure 3-4 for an example of a clinical pathway for a patient with a diagnosis of pneumonia. Each physician develops a protocol into the orders. If a paper chart is used, the HUC will label the appropriate preprinted doctors' orders and will place them into patients' charts. After the doctor chooses the desired options and signs the orders, the HUC transcribes the orders. If the EMR is used, the doctor will enter any modifications onto the computerized order sheet, and each order will automatically be sent to the appropriate department.

Goals for developing and using clinical pathways include the following: (1) identify patient and family needs, (2) determine realistic patient outcomes and time frames required to achieve those outcomes, (3) reduce length of stay and inappropriate use of resources, and (4) clarify the appropriate care setting, providers, and timelines of intervention. The "pathway" can be viewed as a road map for the patient and as a guide for the health care team to follow to enhance the patient's care management and recovery. As the patient progresses along the path, specified goals should be accomplished. If a patient's progress deviates or leaves the planned path, a variance has occurred. A positive variance occurs when the patient's progress is ahead of schedule, and a negative variance is noted when a predicted goal is not accomplished.

ASSIGNMENT SHEET

An **assignment sheet** is a form completed at the beginning of each work shift that indicates the nursing staff assigned to each patient on that nursing unit. The form also may include lunch times and break times for nursing personnel. The HUC keeps the assignment sheet close at hand to refer to when necessary to locate the nurse who is caring for a particular patient. If a locator system (discussed in Chapter 4) is used, the HUC can look at a computer screen to locate nursing unit personnel. Information on the assignment sheet may vary, depending on the nursing delivery system used. Refer to Figure 3-5 for an example of an assignment sheet used for the total care and team nursing models.

NURSING UNIT ADMINISTRATION

Some hospitals have a division of **nursing unit administration** that is responsible for non-clinical patient care functions. In this model, the nursing unit administration is made up of two categories of workers: the HUC and the health unit manager; the HUC is supervised by the health unit manager rather than by the nurse manager. The HUC continues to work very closely with the nursing unit team.

The *health unit manager* performs supervisory and administrative non-clinical functions, such as budgeting, research, and training of new employees, possibly for several nursing units. Health unit managers also may be RNs or may hold degrees in other disciplines. Unit management usually functions under administration rather than under the nursing services department. See Figure 3-6 for an organizational chart that includes nursing unit administration.

Diagnosis: _____

Comorbidities: ☐Angina ☐Atrial Fibrillation ☐Cardiomyopathy ☐COPD ☐CHF ☐Dehydration ☐Malnutrition
☐ Diabetes w/ Manifestations ☐ Diabetes, Insulin Dependent ☐ Diabetes, Uncontrolled
☐ Other: _____ _____

Condition:

Consults:

Treatments:
O2 via nasal prongs, titrate to maintain sats ≥ 90%, decrease as tolerated.
Vital signs q 4hrs. x 24hrs., then routine.
I&O
Incentive spirometer q 2hrs. while awake, cough and deep breathe.

Activity:
Ambulate QID, if possible.

Diet:
☐4gm Na, Low in Saturated Fat.
☐If patient is diabetic, 1800-2400 ADA.
☐Regular

Laboratory Requests: (Do not repeat if done in ER)
Stat blood culture x 2
Sputum culture
CBC, CMP, UA
☐Other:

Diagnostics: (Do not repeat if done in ER)
☐ Chest x-ray
☐ Other:

IV Fluids:
IV lock

Medications:
Antibiotics for community-acquired pneumonia (give first dose within 2hrs. of orders being noted, even if blood or sputum cultures not done). Antibiotic recommendations per updated Infectious Disease Society of America guidelines, 2000. *Please use choices from either one column or the other, not both.*

For those with low risk for complications or resistant organisms:	For those with frequent hospitalizations where resistant organisms are suspected:
☐ Ceftriaxone (Rocephin) 1gm IV q 24hrs.	☐ Levofloxacin (Levaquin) 500mg IV q 24hrs.
☐ Doxycycline (Vibramycin) 100mg IV q 12hrs.	*(monotherapy)*
(Combination therapy optimal for streptococcal and atypical organism coverage).	
☐ MD aware of Penicillin allergy, OK to give Rocephin.	If patient taking **scheduled oral medications**, will **receive oral Levaquin starting on Day 2** (per P&T decision, May 2001)

☐ Albuterol inhaler with spacer _____ puffs q _____hours.
☐ Atrovent inhaler with spacer _____ puffs q _____hours.
☐ Medication/inhaler/spacer teaching per Respiratory if on metered-dose inhaler (MDI)
  SVN's with Albuterol 2.5mg/3ml unit dose q 4hrs.
☐ Include Atrovent in SVN 500mcg/2.5ml unit dose q 4hrs.
☐ Self administer SVN's
☐ Other:

Discharge Planning:

Physician signature to activate per path: **Date:**

Opportunity Medical Center

**PNEUMONIA
ORDER SET**

Figure 3-4 Clinical pathway for a diagnosis of pneumonia.

ASSIGNMENT SHEET

Nursing Unit _3 West_   **Date** _00/00/00_   **Shift** _7 A – 7 P_

Nurse	Pager #	Lunch	Breaks
Sara	17–8234	12:30	9A & 4P

Patient Name	Rm #
Tony Garcia	321–1
Frank Gerod	321–2
Pat Smith	322
Jody Hackenheimer	327–1

Nurse	Pager #	Lunch	Breaks
Cheryl	17–8222	1:00	10A & 4:30P

Patient Name	Rm #
Carl Patell	318–1
Frances Conners	319–1
Penny Packer	319–2

	Name	Office ext	Pager #
Nurse Manager	Pat Lawson	3249	17–6000
Residents on call	Julie		17–2244
	David		17–2238
Case Managers	Jan	3245	17–5525
	Stan	3245	17–5528

A

Figure 3-5 **A,** An example of an assignment sheet for the total care nursing delivery model.

ASSIGNMENT SHEET

Nursing Unit _3 West_   **Date** _00/00/00_   **Shift** _7 A D-7 P_

Team 1		Pager #	Lunch	Breaks	Assignment	Rm #
TL	Sara	17D-8234	12:30	9A & 4P		321D-327
LPN	Elaine	17D-3749	1:30	10A & 3:30P	medications	318D-327
CNA	John		2:00	9A & 4P	T. Garcia	321D-1
					F. Gerod	321D-2
					P. Smith	322
					J. Hackenheimer	327D-1
CNA	Julie		2:30	11A & 4:30P	C. Patell	318D-1
					F. Conners	319D-1
					P. Packer	319D-2

Team 2		Pager #	Lunch	Breaks	Assignment	Rm #
Peter		17D-8222	2:30	10A & 5P	TL	316D-320
CNA	Jane		1:00	9A & 4P	T. Johns	316D-1
					T. Pratt	317D-2
					P. Smith	318D-1
					C. Luctzu	318D-2
CNA	Cynthia		2:30	11A & 4:30P	M. Peterson	318D-1
					I. Hayes	319D-1
					M. Baker	319D-2

	Name	Office ext	Pager #
Nurse Manager	Pat Lawson	3249	17D-6000
Resident on call	Julie		17D-2244
Case Manager	Jan	3245	17D-5525

B

Figure 3-5 cont'd—**B,** An example of an assignment sheet for the team nursing delivery model.

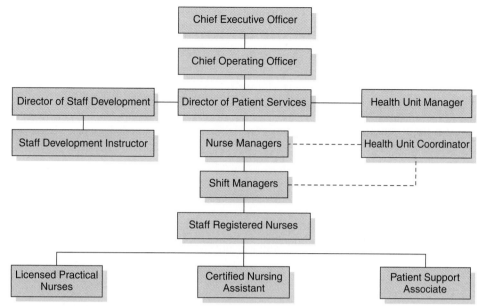

Figure 3-6 Organizational structure for the nursing services department and for nursing unit administration.

KEY CONCEPTS

Health care delivery is continually undergoing change intended to provide the most efficient and cost-effective patient care. In fact, by the time this text is published, some of this information may be obsolete. At this time, about 2% to 5% of U.S. hospitals have implemented the EMR, and it is predicted that in just 5 years, the EMR with computer physician order entry will be implemented and nationally interconnected in most or all hospitals. It is the responsibility of each HUC to keep up with and to adapt to changes as they occur at their place of employment. Although HUCs do not provide direct patient care, their performance greatly influences the quality of care delivered by other nursing team members.

REVIEW QUESTIONS

1. Match the appropriate nursing unit from the right-hand column to patients with the conditions listed in the left-hand column (choose the nursing unit where patients would likely be admitted).

_____ 1. cardiac arrhythmia	a. GYN
_____ 2. drug abuse	b. urology
_____ 3. surgical treatment	c. behavioral health
_____ 4. was critically ill, still requires specialized care, but no longer needs intensive care	d. surgical
_____ 5. disease of the circulatory system	e. telemetry
_____ 6. disease of the urinary system	f. neurology
_____ 7. 10 years old	g. cardiovascular
_____ 8. long-term treatment and care	h. pediatrics
_____ 9. cancer	i. orthopedics
_____ 10. fractured hip	j. oncology
_____ 11. surgery on the female reproductive tract	k. obstetrics
_____ 12. medical treatment	l. medical
_____ 13. disease of the nervous system	m. rehabilitation
_____ 14. pregnant and about to deliver	n. stepdown unit

2. Briefly describe the responsibilities of the nursing service department.

_____

_____

3. List three nursing personnel commonly employed on a nursing unit, and briefly describe the role of each.

a. _____

b. _____

c. _____

4. List three services that come under the general heading of perioperative services, and give a brief description of each.

a. _____

b. _____

c. _____

5. Explain why a patient would be admitted to an ICU, and why they would be transferred to a stepdown unit.

_____

_____

_____

6. Compare the total nursing care delivery model with the team nursing care delivery model.

_____

_____

_____

7. The level of care required by a patient's medical condition is referred to as the _____ and is used by nurses when assigning nursing team members.

8. _____ is the hospital department that is responsible for orientation of new employees and continuing education, including TJC requirements.

9. List three nursing personnel who could work on a nursing team.

a. _____

b. _____

c. _____

10. Explain the use of clinical pathways

_____

_____

_____

_____

11. Explain what is involved in holistic nursing care.

_____

_____

_____

_____

12. List six benefits of interdisciplinary teamwork.

a. _____

b. _____

c. _____

d. _____

e. _____

f. _____

THINK ABOUT...

1. Discuss some advantages associated with nurses taking computers into the patient's room and entering their notes directly into the patient's permanent electronic record.
2. Discuss how visiting a patient in an ICU is different from visiting a patient on a regular nursing unit.
3. Interview a doctor and/or a nurse to ask how health care has changed in the past 5 years.
4. Interview someone who has recently been a patient at a local hospital, and ask how they would rate the care received.

Communication Devices and Their Uses

CHAPTER OBJECTIVES

Upon completion of this chapter, you will be able to

1. Define the terms in the vocabulary list.
2. Write the meaning of the abbreviations in the abbreviation list.
3. State three circumstances that would require use of the hold button.
4. List and apply eight rules of telephone etiquette.
5. Describe briefly how to plan a telephone call to a doctor's office regarding a patient.
6. List six items to be recorded when taking a telephone message, and explain why it is important to accurately record messages.
7. Explain the locator system, and describe how it may be used.
8. List three methods of paging within the health care facility.
9. Discuss how the health unit coordinator (HUC) would be notified when an HUC task needs to be done on a patient's record, when the electronic record has been implemented.
10. List three types of documents or items that the HUC would scan to be entered into the patient's electronic record.
11. Discuss why a re-dial option should not be used on a fax machine in the nursing station.
12. Discuss the HUC's responsibility in maintaining the unit bulletin board.
13. Discuss the uses of computer terminals located on the nursing unit.
14. List four guidelines that should be followed when leaving a voice mail message.
15. Identify two guidelines for the use of e-mail in the workplace, and list two examples of misuse of e-mail.

VOCABULARY

Cell Phone Wireless phone that may be carried by some hospital personnel and doctors

Computer An electronic machine that is capable of accepting, processing, and retrieving information

Computer on Wheels A computer on a cart with wheels that can be taken into the patient's room

Computer Terminal Combination of three components: a keyboard, a viewing screen, and a printer

Copy Machine A machine that is used to make duplicates of typed or written materials

Cursor Flashing indicator on the computer screen that identifies the place within the viewing area that will receive the information

Doctors' Roster Alphabetic listing of names, telephone numbers, and directory telephone numbers of physicians on staff (most hospitals have made this available on computer as well)

Document Management System Computer system (or set of computer programs) used to track and store electronic documents and/or images of paper documents

Document Scanner Device used to transmit images of paper documents/pictures to be entered into the patient's electronic record

Downtime Requisition A requisition (paper order form) that is used to process information when the computer is not available for use

Dumbwaiter A mechanical device for transporting food or supplies from one hospital floor to another

E-mail (electronic mail) Method of sending and receiving messages via the computer to anyone with an e-mail address

Fax Machine Telecommunication device that transmits copies of written material over a telephone wire from one site to another

Keyboard Computer component used to type information into the computer

Label Printer Machine that prints patient labels from information entered into the computer; located near the health unit coordinator's area

Locator A small tracking device worn by nursing personnel, including health unit coordinators, so their location may be detected on the interactive console display when necessary

Menu List of options that is projected on the viewing screen of the computer

Modem Device that enables a computer to send and receive data over regular phone lines

Patient Call System Intercom Device used to communicate between the nurses' station and patient rooms on the nursing unit

Pen Tab or Tablet PC Computer that may be removed from its base, or a portable computer that can be taken into patient rooms, with a stylus used to enter information directly into a patient's electronic record, as in a notebook

Pneumatic Tube System System in which air pressure transports tubes carrying supplies, requisitions, or some lab specimens from one hospital unit or department to another

Pocket Pager Small electronic device that when activated by entering a series of numbers into a telephone delivers a message to the carrier of the pager

Shredder Machine located in most nursing stations that shreds confidential material (chart forms that have a patient's label affixed with patient name, room number, patient account number, medical record number, and the like)

Tower The system unit of the computer; houses internal components

Viewing Screen Computer component that displays information; it resembles a television, and it also may be called a monitor, a cathode ray tube, or a video display terminal

Voice Paging System System by which the hospital telephone operator pages a message for a doctor or makes other announcements; the system reaches all hospital areas (used only when absolutely necessary to keep noise level down)

ABBREVIATIONS

Abbreviation	Meaning
D or E Drive	drive/s to read CDs or DVDs
C drive	hard drive stored inside the computer
COW	computer on wheels
CPU	central processing unit; the microprocessor that is often called the computer's brain
DMS	document management system
PC	personal computer
VDT	video display terminal

EXERCISE 1

Write the abbreviation for the following terms.

1. Drive/s to read CD or DVD _____

2. Hard drive stored inside the computer _____

3. Central processing unit _____

4. Personal computer _____

5. Video display terminal _____

6. Computer on wheels _____

7. Document management system _____

EXERCISE 2

Write the meaning of each abbreviation listed below.

1. D or E drive

   _____

2. C drive

   _____

3. CPU

   _____

4. PC

   _____

5. VDT

   _____

6. COW

   _____

7. DMS

   _____

The health unit coordinator (HUC) is responsible for entering doctors' orders into the **computer**, answering the nursing unit telephone, and operating all of the other communication devices discussed in this chapter. Communication and operating the communication devices are among the most important responsibilities of the HUC.

Implementation of the electronic medical record (EMR) has made it necessary for doctors, nurses, ancillary personnel, and HUCs to be better educated in computer technology. Communication devices used in hospitals and their uses will be discussed in this chapter.

THE TELEPHONE

The telephone is probably the most used communications device at the nurses' station (Fig. 4-1). Because we are so familiar with using the telephone, often we fail to use it in a professional manner in the workplace. Speaking on the telephone requires a different interaction than occurs with face-to-face speaking (Fig. 4-2). A good attitude about telephone transactions will result in positive customer relationships, so proper telephone etiquette is essential in the health care setting to promote effective communication.

Telephone Etiquette

- Answer the telephone promptly and kindly, preferably prior to the third ring. If engaged in a conversation at the nurses' station, excuse yourself to answer the telephone.
- Identify yourself properly by stating location, name, and status. For example: "4 East, Stacey, Health Unit Coordinator." The manner in which you identify yourself and address the caller is the caller's first clue about your professional identity, self-esteem, mood, expectations, and willingness to continue the communication. At this time, you are conveying to the caller an image of the hospital. By correctly identifying yourself, the caller is saved time, and confusion is eliminated.
- Speak into the telephone—be sure the mouthpiece is not under your chin, making it difficult for the caller to hear.

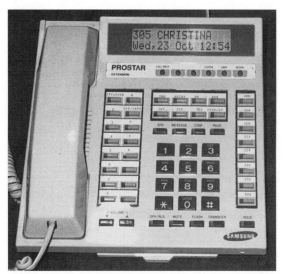

Figure 4-1 A telephone with several lines and a hold button.

- Give the caller your undivided attention—It is difficult to focus on the telephone conversation while attempting to do something else.
- Speak clearly and distinctly—do not eat food or chew gum while talking on the telephone.
- Always be courteous—say "Please" and "Thank you."
- When you do not know the answer, state that you will locate someone who can help the caller.
- If necessary to step away or answer another call, place the caller on hold after asking permission to do so and waiting for an answer. For example: "May I put you on hold, Mr. Phillips, so I can find Jane to speak to you?"

When the telephone is used for communication, an image of the nursing unit is created for the caller. Realize this, and handle each telephone conversation with care.

Use of the Hold Button

Telephones on hospital nursing units may have several incoming telephone lines plus a hold button. The hold button allows a caller to stay on the line while other calls are answered. Use the hold button for the following purposes:

- **To locate information or a person for the caller.** Always return to the person on hold every 30 to 60 seconds to ask if they wish to remain on hold, or prefer to leave a number for a return call.
- **To answer other phone lines.** Return to the first caller after asking the second caller if they would hold or instead wish to be called back.
- **To protect patient confidentiality.** Conversations held in the nursing station often involve confidential patient information and should not be overheard.

When communicating a message regarding a call on hold, include the name of the caller, the nature of the call if possible, and which line the call is on. The message may be as follows: "Susan, Dr. Harrison is on line 1 regarding Mr. Mark's medication order."

 SKILLS CHALLENGE

To practice answering the telephone and placing a caller on hold, complete Activities 4-1 and 4-2 in the *Skills Practice Manual.*

Taking Messages

When taking messages over the telephone or in person, be sure to get all the information needed for the person for whom the call is intended. Record the following:

- Who the message is for
- The caller's name
- The date and time of the call
- The purpose of the call
- The number to call if a return call is expected
- Your name

Always write the information down. As a student or a newly employed HUC, gaining the trust and confidence of nursing

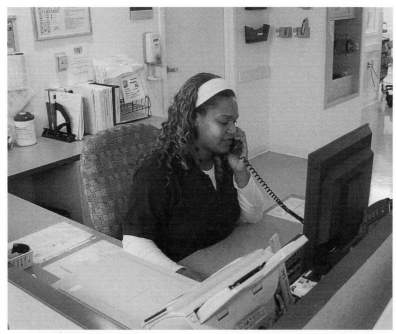

Figure 4-2 The HUC handles telephone communication for the nursing unit.

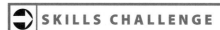

Figure 4-3 A pad for telephone messages.

team members is important. Putting messages in writing may be the first important step toward gaining the confidence of unit personnel while guaranteeing accuracy during the communication process. Always have a pad and pencil or a pen near each telephone. Deliver messages promptly. Many health care facilities have special telephone message pads (Fig. 4-3).

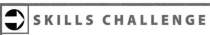
SKILLS CHALLENGE

To practice recording messages, complete Activity 4-3 in the *Skills Practice Manual.*

Placing Telephone Calls

When asked to place a call to a doctor, to another department, or outside of the health care facility, *plan the call.* If it concerns a patient, have the patient's chart handy, so that facts will be available when questions are asked. Also write down the main facts that need to be discussed and the telephone number to be called, should the line be busy and the call needed to be made later.

Anyone who requests a call to be placed regarding a patient should provide the patient's name and the reason for the call. Write down the name of the person who requested the call to be made. Before placing a call for a nurse to a doctor, alert the nurse that the call is being placed, and ask the person who requests it to stay on the unit, if possible, or to designate someone else to take the call in their place.

SKILLS CHALLENGE

To practice placing a telephone call, complete Activity 4-4 in the *Skills Practice Manual.*

Voice Mail

Voice mail is used in health care facilities, physicians' offices, and homes to receive incoming calls. To use voice mail effectively, follow these guidelines.

After listening to the recorded greeting and indicated tone, do the following:

- Speak slowly and distinctly so the person listening to the message can hear and understand what is being communicated.
- If leaving a message, include the name of the patient and/or the doctor—give the first and last names, and spell the last name.

- If the message includes a telephone number or laboratory values, speak slowly and repeat the numbers twice, allowing time for the listener to record the information.
- Always leave your name and telephone number, and repeat both twice (at the beginning of the message and at the end of the message) so the listener can call for clarification if necessary.

> **◐ SKILLS CHALLENGE**
>
> To practice leaving a voice mail message, complete Activity 4-5 in the *Skills Practice Manual*.

Telephone Directories

Many health care facilities publish a directory of extension numbers for telephones in the hospital. These are alphabetized and easy to use. Both department numbers and key personnel are listed. Hospitals using the individual pocket pager also may publish a directory of pocket pager numbers. This information may also be downloaded into the computer in some hospitals.

The **doctors' roster** is another directory frequently used by the HUC. Most health care facilities have computer access to this information, but a hard copy may also be available on the nursing units. The listing includes the names of the doctors (in alphabetical order) who have admitting or visiting privileges. It lists their medical specialty, their office telephone number, and the answering service telephone number. When placing a telephone call, select the doctor's number with care because often several doctors are listed with the same name. If two doctors have the same first and last names, refer to their specialty to select the correct telephone number. To practice placing a telephone call, complete the activities provided at the end of this chapter.

LOCATOR SYSTEM

Locators are small devices that are worn by nursing unit personnel, including HUCs (clipped on uniforms). Figure 4-4 shows an example of a locator clipped on a nurse's uniform. A display screen displays a list of the nursing unit personnel who wear the locators, along with their locations. Figure 4-5 shows an HUC who is locating and communicating with a nurse using the locator system. If the locator is flipped over or obstructed, it may not show the nurse's location. The locator system is used for communication between nursing unit personnel and the nursing station. If the person who is wearing the locator needs help, a button on the locator may be pushed to call the nursing station. The HUC may also call into a patient's room to speak to the nurse. This system is also very helpful when personnel are covering more than one unit or are working as a "SWAT," meaning, on call for all units in the hospital. Some hospitals use pagers or **cell phones** for this purpose.

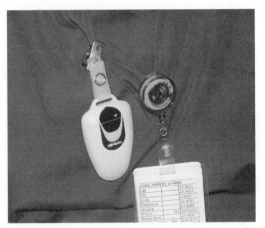

Figure 4-4 A locator device clipped to a nurse's uniform.

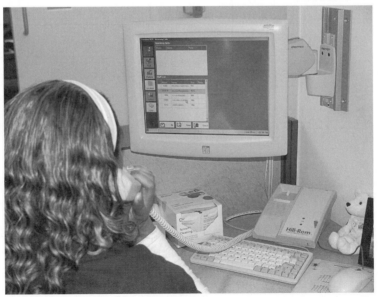

Figure 4-5 An HUC locating and communicating with a nurse using the locator system. This system may be used to answer patients' call lights and to communicate with patients in their rooms.

Locator display systems are often interactive with a device on the patient's bed. A small box with a display screen may also be located on the wall at each end of the nurses' station that displays the location of nursing personnel when pushed.

UNIT INTERCOM

An intercom or locator system is another method that is used to communicate between the nurses' station and patient rooms on a nursing unit (see Fig. 4-5). This intercom provides a method of taking patients' requests without going into their rooms. On admission, the patient should be given directions regarding use of the call light and intercom by the HUC or another member of the nursing staff.

A buzzer and/or a light on the intercom alerts the HUC or nurse at the nurses' station that someone has activated the call system. The room number button lights up on the intercom console to designate the caller's room. By pressing the appropriate button, one may converse with the patient. Always identify yourself and your location. For example, "This is Kimberly at the nurses' station. May I help you?" When two or more patients are assigned to the room, ask the patient's name.

The HUC may also use the intercom to locate nursing personnel. To page personnel on the intercom, depress the button that allows the message to be heard in each of the rooms. A simple message, such as "Susan, please call the nurses' station," is all that is needed.

The HUC should be selective about information communicated over the intercom because some types of messages may prove embarrassing to the patient. For example, do not use the intercom to ask a patient whether he has had a bowel movement. Try to keep the message as brief as possible, and do not communicate any confidential patient information to a nurse over the intercom because other patients may hear the message.

POCKET PAGER

The **pocket pager** (Fig. 4-6) is a small, electronic device that is activated by dialing a series of numbers on a telephone to deliver a message to the carrier of the pager. The pocket pager may be digital or voice. When using a voice pager, dial the pager number and state the message. Always say the message, including name and extension number, twice. A digital pager is similar in appearance to a voice pager. To contact a person by digital pager, dial the pager number from a touch-tone phone. Listen for a ring followed by a series of beeps. Dial

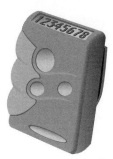

Figure 4-6 A pocket pager. (Courtesy of Motorola Communications and Electronics, Inc., Schaumburg, IL.)

the nursing unit telephone number followed by the pound sign (#). A series of fast beeps indicates a completed page. The number appears on the pager display. The receiver then calls back to the provided number for the message. Allow at least 5 minutes before paging a second time, unless it is a stat (emergency) situation.

Some nursing units use a number code entered at the end of the call-back number—number 1 indicates "stat," number 2 indicates "as soon as possible," and number 3 indicates "at one's convenience." Residents, ancillary personnel, and your instructor usually carry pocket pagers.

SKILLS CHALLENGE

To practice contacting a person using a digital pager, complete Activity 4-6 in the *Skills Practice Manual*.

VOICE PAGING SYSTEM

The **voice paging system** is a communication system by which the hospital switchboard operator, upon request, pages someone on a speaker that is heard in every area of the hospital. To locate a doctor with this system, dial the hospital switchboard operator, indicate the name of the doctor who is needed, and give the telephone extension number of the nursing unit. The operator announces the name of the doctor who is needed and the extension number to call.

The operator also uses the voice paging system to locate a doctor for calls received from outside the hospital. The HUC frequently is asked by doctors to listen for their page, especially when they are in a patient's room. When a page for a doctor is announced, the HUC may contact the operator for the message and deliver it to the doctor.

COPY AND SHREDDER MACHINES

Most nursing units have a **copy machine** available for making copies of written or typed materials. Photocopying of patient records is discussed in Chapter 6. The fax machine also can be used to make a minimal number of copies.

Patient forms that contain confidential information cannot be thrown into the wastebasket. **Shredder** machines or containers for materials to be picked up and taken to be shredded are placed on nursing units. Chart forms that have labels with patient name, patient account number, and health record identification number without documentation on them must be shredded.

FAX MACHINE

A **fax machine** is a telecommunication device that transmits copies of written material over a telephone wire from one site to another (Fig. 4-7). Reports and other documents are faxed to and from health care institutions and doctors' offices. Often, the HUC has the responsibility of faxing medical record/s requests, signed by the patient, to another health care facility and will receive faxed record/s at the nurses' station.

Many hospitals are moving toward a paperless system but have not yet implemented the electronic record. Physician order sheets are faxed to the pharmacy when paper charts

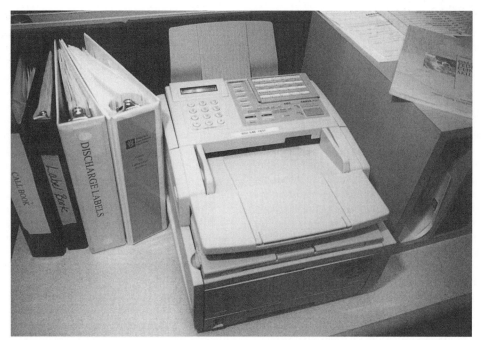

Figure 4-7 A facsimile (fax) machine.

are used. When faxing the physicians' orders, the HUC can use the fax machine to make a copy of the orders to give to the appropriate nurse. Fax machines have a re-dial option, allowing a document to be sent to the location last programmed into the machine. Many health care workers in the nurses' station use the fax machine. Therefore, it is important not to use the re-dial option that may send a document to the wrong location. Patient information is extremely confidential, and if it is sent to the wrong location, an employee may be disciplined or terminated. The fax machine is not for personal use, such as sending jokes to coworkers, entries in contests, etc.

✎ TAKE NOTE

Do not use the re-dial option when using the fax machine. It may result in confidential patient information being sent to the wrong location.

PNEUMATIC TUBE

The pneumatic tube is a system in which air pressure transports tubes carrying supplies, requisitions, or messages from one hospital unit or department to another (Fig. 4-8). These items are placed into a special carrying tube, which then is inserted into the **pneumatic tube system**; a keypad is used to enter the location to where the message is to be sent. Medications that do not break or spill are transported in this manner. Do *not* place specimens obtained by a painful or difficult procedure into the pneumatic tube. When a tube carrying supplies or other items arrives at the nursing unit, it is the responsibility of the HUC to remove the tube from the pneumatic tube system as soon as possible and disperse the items accordingly. Instructions for the operation of the hospital's pneumatic tube system will be provided during hospital orientation.

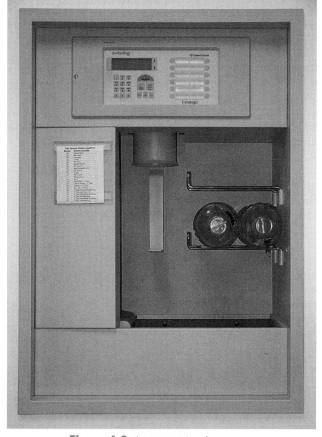

Figure 4-8 A pneumatic tube system.

Some health care facilities have a telelift system that is operated in much the same way and for the same purposes as the tube system. It consists of a small boxcar that is carried on a conveyor belt to designated locations. A keypad is used to program the car to go to a specific unit of a department.

COMPUTERS

The health care facility's computer system contains a great deal of information that is confidential and that must not be tampered with; therefore, a security system is used. When hired, each employee is assigned an identification code and a password. When the computer is used, a password is required to gain entry into the system. Employees are asked to sign a confidentiality statement. Never share the identification code and password with anyone. It is imperative for patient confidentiality and employee protection that employees sign off of the computer when leaving the nursing unit for a break, or when going home. When someone is signed onto the computer with their identification code, any misuse will be tracked back to that individual.

E-mail

E-mail (electronic mail) is used to send and receive messages and is frequently used for communication between the HUC and hospital personnel and departments within the hospital. Guidelines to be followed when using e-mail in the workplace include the following: (1) Do not use for personal messages, or to send inappropriate material such as jokes; and (2) send or respond to the necessary person or department only; refrain from "sending to all" or using "reply to all" unless necessary.

Computer Use in Hospitals with the Paper Patient Chart

Most hospitals provide several **computer terminals** on each nursing unit, so that doctors, residents, and nursing staff have easy access to patient information such as patient location, diagnostic test results, and physicians' orders. A computer terminal is usually made up of three components: the **keyboard**, the monitor (**viewing screen**), and the printer. The HUC usually has a separate terminal for ordering diagnostic tests, supplies, and equipment and for entering discharges, transfers, and admissions. At minimum, basic computer knowledge and typing skills are necessary to perform the ordering and data entry tasks required. A mouse is used to select information to be entered into the computer. The mouse is used to move the **cursor**, which is a flashing indicator that shows the user the area on the screen that will receive the information. The cursor may be moved to any area on the screen; once the cursor is at the desired location, the user will click the mouse.

Information typed on the keyboard is displayed on the computer screen. A **menu** can be brought up on the screen so that an item or a test to be ordered can be selected, or a menu can be recalled for informational purposes only, such as a census (list of room numbers with patients' names and their admitting physicians' names). Computers are connected to a printer, and at any given time, the user can give the computer a command to print any of the stored information. For instance, when the HUC uses the computer to order a patient's diet, the diet order prints out on the printer located in the nutritional care department. The HUC should be alert to printed material being sent via the printer and should remove the printed documents as soon as possible.

Many health care facilities have bedside computers available in each patient's room so nursing personnel can record care and treatments provided. These records generally are printed every 24 hours for placement on the patient's paper chart.

At times, the computer is shut down for scheduled routine servicing (usually at night) or because of mechanical failure. During these times, **downtime requisitions** are used to process information. When computer function returns, the information processed by the paper method must be entered into the computer.

Computer Use in Hospitals with the Electronic Medical Record

When the EMR system is implemented, multiple computers are made available on the nursing unit, including a desktop for the HUC to use, additional desktops for doctors, nurses, and authorized ancillary health care workers to use (Fig. 4-9), **computers on wheels (COWs)** (Fig. 4-10), and computer tablets, also called **pen tabs** (Fig. 4-11), for nurses and/or doctors to use. The doctor can enter orders directly into the patient's EMR, access computerized reports, access diagnostic images, access diagnostic test results, and access nurses' notes for review. Nurses can enter documentation and notes directly into the patient's medical record, access the doctor's orders, access diagnostic test results and diagnostic images for evaluation, and access computerized reports. (Many nurses use personal data processors, which are handheld computers that contain software that has been downloaded into them, such as a nurses drug reference, a medical dictionary, and other nursing reference books. Nurses use this information to calculate drug dosages and to research information.)

The HUC monitors the patient's EMRs for tasks that need to be performed. A telephone icon appears on the computer screen next to the patient's name when there is an HUC task that must be performed to complete the doctor's order. This could be a telephone call to schedule a consult, a call to obtain medical records from another facility, or other tasks to be discussed in future chapters. The HUC accesses doctors' telephone numbers and locates patients for visitors or doctors on the computer. If requested to do so, the HUC enters data into the computer and may access computerized reports.

Health care facilities use many different types of computer programs, and many have developed special programs to suit their individual needs. The CD included with the *Skills Practice Manual* will provide practice with the basic skills needed to function in a health care setting. Computer training usually is provided for new employees, and some facilities allow HUC students to sit in on these classes. Students will be instructed in the specifics of the hospital computer program by an experienced working HUC during their clinical experience. Application of computers for transcription of handwritten doctors' orders and management of the EMR will be introduced in their respective chapters.

DOCUMENT SCANNER

A **document scanner** is a device used to transmit images of documents/pictures into a computer system (or set of computer programs) used to track and store electronic documents and/or images of paper documents. This **document management system (DMS)** uses bar codes to identify types of documents. The scanner is used by the HUC to scan outside documents, handwritten progress notes, reports, and other documents into the patient's electronic record (Fig. 4-12). These documents are sent to the health information

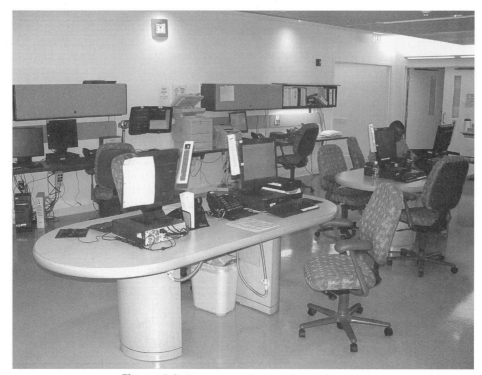

Figure 4-9 Computer stations on the nursing unit.

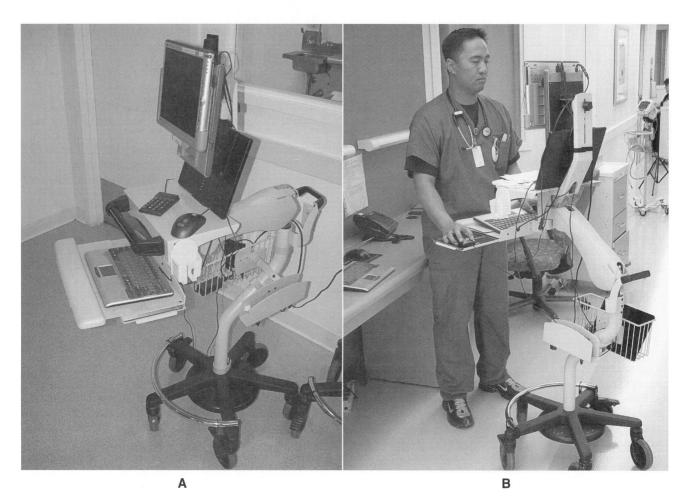

A   B

Figure 4-10 A, An example of a computer on wheels (COW). **B,** A nurse using a COW to enter documentation into a patient's electronic record

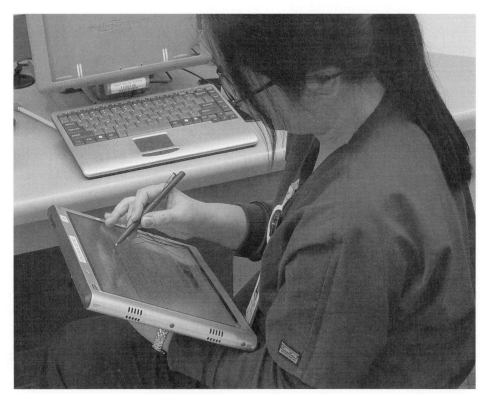

Figure 4-11 A nurse using a Pen Tab.

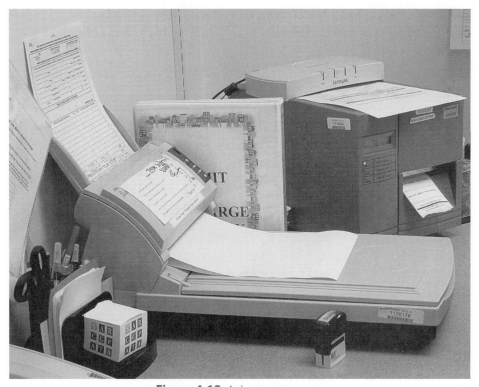

Figure 4-12 A document scanner.

management systems (HIMS) department and are certified by the health information technician before they become a part of the patient's permanent EMR.

Bundles of up to 14 documents may be placed in the scanner at a time; documents containing color (e.g., electrocardiograms) have to be scanned alone. After documents are scanned, the originals should be rubber-banded and placed in a bin to be picked up by someone from the HIMS department. Documents are then stored for a specified length of time prior to being shredded.

LABEL PRINTER

A label printer is a machine that prints patient labels from information entered into the computer. The **label printer** is located near the work area of the HUC. Patient labels usually contain the name of the patient, age, date of birth, the doctor's name, and patient identification numbers. When electronic records are implemented, labels with bar codes are used to identify types of documents. Labels are placed on forms or documents for identification purposes.

NURSING UNIT CENSUS BOARD

Many nursing units have small white boards in the nurses' station area on which to record census information. These boards show unit room numbers, admitting doctors' names, and the name of the nurse assigned to each patient. The patient's name intentionally may be omitted to maintain patient confidentiality. The HUC has the responsibility to remove the names of discharged or transferred patients while adding the names of newly admitted or transferred patients.

New HIPAA (Health Insurance Portability and Accountability Act) laws (see Chapter 6) may change the current usage of census boards.

NURSING UNIT BULLETIN BOARD

The HUC may be given the responsibility of maintaining the nursing unit bulletin board. This responsibility includes posting material in an attractive manner and keeping posted material current. The material to be posted on the bulletin board may be determined by the nurse manager or may be set forth by administration policy. Bulletins regarding changes that will take place in the facility, nursing policies, and schedules of staff development classes are examples of materials posted on the bulletin board.

If the date is not indicated on the bulletin, the HUC should indicate the date posted. Policy changes are very important. It may be requested that each person initial the notice after reading it so the nurse manager will know that all unit employees have read it. The HUC then would place the initialed notice on the nurse manager's desk when it is removed from the bulletin board. A neat board with up-to-date notices prompts unit personnel to read what is posted.

KEY CONCEPTS

The ability to use the computer, telephone, intercom, and other communication devices efficiently and effectively contributes to the smooth operation of the nursing unit. As technology advances, the need for the HUC to have enhanced computer skills is increasing. Accuracy in taking telephone messages and in communicating them to the appropriate person is a must for an efficiently run nursing unit.

REVIEW QUESTIONS

1. List four guidelines to follow when leaving a message on voice mail.

a. _____

b. _____

c. _____

d. _____

2. List eight rules of telephone etiquette.

a. _____

b. _____

c. _____

d. _____

e. _____

f. _____

g. _____

h. _____

3. List six items to be recorded when taking a telephone message.

a. _____

b. _____

c. _____

d. _____

e. _____

f. _____

4. Define the following terms/abbreviations.

a. menu

_____

b. computer terminal

_____

c. modem

_____

d. viewing screen

_____

e. doctors' roster

_____

f. downtime requisition

_____

g. shredder

_____

h. pneumatic tube system

_____

i. label printer

_____

j. document scanner

_____

k. COW

_____

l. DMS

_____

5. Three circumstances that require the use of the telephone hold button are

a. _____

b. _____

c. _____

6. Briefly describe how the HUC would plan a call to a doctor's office regarding a patient.

_____

_____

_____

7. Discuss the HUC's responsibility in maintaining the unit bulletin board.

_____

_____

_____

8. If you are an HUC working on 4 East, write out what you would say when answering the telephone.

_____

_____

9. A. You have received a telephone call from Dr. Johnson for Dr. Taylor, whom you need to locate. You would

a. say nothing, and place the telephone receiver on the desk because it is rude to put a doctor on hold.

b. say, "Hold for a minute and I will find her for you."

c. say, "Just a minute," and then place the caller on hold.

d. say, "May I place you on hold while I find her for you?" Wait for an answer.

B. When you find Dr. Taylor, she is talking to a patient and you can't interrupt her. You would

a. wait until Dr. Taylor is finished, and then notify her that she has a call.

b. return to the caller and tell him to be patient because it will be a few minutes.

c. return to the caller, explain the situation, and ask if he would prefer to remain on hold or leave a number for Dr. Taylor to return the call.

d. return to the caller and tell him to call back in a few minutes.

C. Now Dr. Taylor is available and the caller is still on hold. You would say,

a. "There is someone on line 1 for you."

b. "It's Doctor Johnson for you."

c. "Dr. Johnson is on line 1."

d. "Dr. Johnson is on line 1 regarding the consultation ordered on Mrs. White."

10. List three tasks that the HUC would perform on the computer terminal located on the nursing unit that is using the paper chart.

a. _____

b. _____

c. _____

11. List three tasks that each of the following health care personnel would perform on the computer terminals located on the nursing unit when the EMR system is implemented.

Doctor:

a. _____

b. _____

c. _____

Nurse:

a. _____

b. _____

c. _____

HUC:

a. _____

b. _____

c. _____

12. Explain the importance of signing off the computer when going on a break, leaving for lunch, or going home.

_____

_____

13. List two guidelines to follow when using e-mail in the workplace.

a. _____

b. _____

14. List two examples of misuse of e-mail.

a. _____

b. _____

15. Discuss a possible repercussion of using the re-dial option on the hospital fax machine.

_____

_____

16. List three items that may be scanned into the patient's EMR.

a. _____

b. _____

c. _____

17. List three uses of the locator system.

a. _____

b. _____

c. _____

18. List three methods of paging health care personnel within the health care facility.

a. _____

b. _____

c. _____

19. Discuss how the HUC would be notified when there is an HUC task that must be completed on a patient's record when the electronic record has been implemented.

_____

_____

THINK ABOUT...

1. Have you ever been placed on hold without your permission or been forgotten and left on hold until you finally hung up? Discuss how you felt when this happened.
2. Discuss telephone experiences that you have had with a person that was discourteous. How could the person have handled each situation in a courteous manner?
3. Discuss possible consequences of sending inappropriate material by e-mail in the workplace.

Communication and Interpersonal Skills

CHAPTER OBJECTIVES

Upon completion of this chapter, you will be able to

1. Define the terms in the vocabulary list.
2. Explain why implementation of the electronic medical record is requiring even better communication skills for the health unit coordinator (HUC).
3. Give instances that exemplify human needs, classify each according to Maslow's hierarchy of human needs, and give appropriate responses to meet the listed needs.
4. List four components of the communication process.
5. Interpret and apply the communication model.
6. List examples of verbal and nonverbal communication.
7. Discuss two types of nonverbal communication.
8. Identify causes of unsuccessful communication.
9. List nine ways to improve listening skills.
10. List five ways to improve feedback skills.
11. Describe the importance of culturally sensitive care in the health care setting.
12. List five guidelines to follow that could improve intercultural communication.
13. Identify assertive, nonassertive, and aggressive behaviors.
14. Respond to situations using assertiveness skills.

15. List six steps to follow when dealing with a person on the telephone who is angry.
16. Identify five ways that communication and interpersonal skills are used in the health care setting.
17. List twelve preceptor guidelines for training an HUC student or a new employee.
18. List ten student guidelines for completing their clinical experience.

VOCABULARY

Ageism Discrimination on grounds of age
Aggressive Behavioral style in which a person attempts to be the dominant force in an interaction
Assertive Behavioral style in which a person stands up for their own rights and feelings without violating the rights and feelings of others
Broken Record Assertive skill wherein a person repeats his stand over and over again
Communication The process of transmitting feelings, images, and ideas from the mind of one person to the mind of another person for the purpose of obtaining a response
Conflict Emotional disturbance; a person's striving for their own preferred outcome, which, if attained, prevents others from achieving their preferred outcomes

Cultural Differences Factors such as age, gender, race, socioeconomic status, etc.

Culturally Sensitive Care Care that involves understanding and being sensitive to a patient's cultural background

Culture A set of values, beliefs, and traditions that are held by a specific social group

Decoding Process of translating symbols received from the sender to determine the message

Elitism Discrimination based on social/economic class

Empathy One's ability to recognize, perceive, and directly feel the emotion of another, or the ability to "put one's self into another's shoes"

Encoding Translating mental images, feelings, and ideas into symbols to communicate them to the receiver

Esteem Needs A person's need for self-respect and for the respect of others

Ethnocentrism The inability to accept other cultures, or an assumption of cultural superiority

Feedback Response to a message

Fogging Assertive skill in which a person responds to a criticism by making noncommittal statements that cannot be argued against

HUC Clinical Experience The time the HUC student spends on a nursing unit (after completing the classroom portion of an educational program) with a working HUC to acquire hands-on work experience

HUC Preceptor An experienced working HUC who is selected to train/teach an HUC student or a new employee

Interpreter A person who facilitates oral communication between or among parties who are conversing in different languages

Love and Belonging Needs A person's need to have affectionate relationships with people and to have a place in a group

Message Images, feelings, and ideas transmitted from one person to another

Negative Assertion An assertive skill in which a person verbally accepts having made an error without letting it reflect on their worth as a human being

Negative Inquiry An assertive skill in which a person requests clarification of a criticism to get to the real issue

Nonassertive A behavioral style in which a person allows others to dictate her or his self-worth

Nonverbal Communication Communication that is not written or spoken but creates a message between two or more people through eye contact, body language, or symbolic and facial expression

Paraphrase Repeating a message in your own words to clarify meaning

Physiologic Needs A person's physical needs, such as the need for food and water

Precept To train or teach (a student or a new employee)

Receiver The person who receives the message

Self-Actualization Need The need to maximize one's potential

Self-Esteem Confidence and respect for oneself

Sender The person who transmits the message

Stereotyping The assumption that all members of a culture or ethnic group act in the same way (generalizations that may be inaccurate)

Subculture Subgroup within a culture; people with a distinct identity but who have specific ethnic, occupational, or physical characteristics found in a larger culture

Verbal Communication The use of language or actual spoken words

Workable Compromise Dealing with conflict in such a way that the solution is satisfactory to all parties

EXPANDING COMMUNICATION ROLE FOR THE HEALTH UNIT COORDINATOR

The health unit coordinator (HUC) is the liaison between the doctor, the nursing staff, ancillary departments, visitors, and patients. **Communication** is the main function of the HUC, and with the implementation of the electronic medical record(EMR), this role is expanding. Often, the HUC assists doctors, nurses, and ancillary personnel in entering and retrieving information regarding the patient's EMR. The HUC has a larger role in listening to visitor, patient, and nursing unit personnel complaints and in problem solving. Working in the health care environment can become extremely stressful at times. If communication breaks down and tempers become short, chaos most likely will result, and the risk of error will be increased. It is important for the HUC to know how to deal with and ease the tension to maintain the efficiency of the unit. Information in this chapter will assist the HUC student in acquiring the skills necessary to handle these responsibilities.

INTERPERSONAL BEHAVIOR

To develop effective communication and interpersonal skills, you must first attain an understanding of interpersonal behavior. *Interpersonal* refers to something that happens between persons. Behavior is how people act—what they say or do. Research indicates that in conversation, a person behaves according to who the other person is and how they behave. An understanding of interpersonal behavior assists us in understanding our own behavior and in understanding the behavior of others.

Although several models may be used to study interpersonal behavior, we have chosen Maslow's Hierarchy of Needs, developed by the late Abraham Maslow, a famous psychologist. Maslow's human needs model emphasizes that all people have the same basic needs, and that these needs motivate and influence a person's behavior, consciously or unconsciously. The needs are arranged in a pyramid, with the most basic or immediate needs at the bottom of the pyramid and less critical needs at the top of the pyramid (Fig. 5-1). Needs that are lower in the pyramid have the greatest influence on a person's behavior. For instance, a person works harder to meet the need for water to drink than to meet the need for **self-esteem**.

As lower level needs are satisfied to an adequate degree, we become increasingly concerned about satisfying the next or a higher level need. Most people find that all their needs are both partially satisfied and partially unsatisfied at the same time. Unsatisfied needs influence an individual's behavior in terms of motivation, priorities, or action taken. According to Maslow, the average person is satisfied

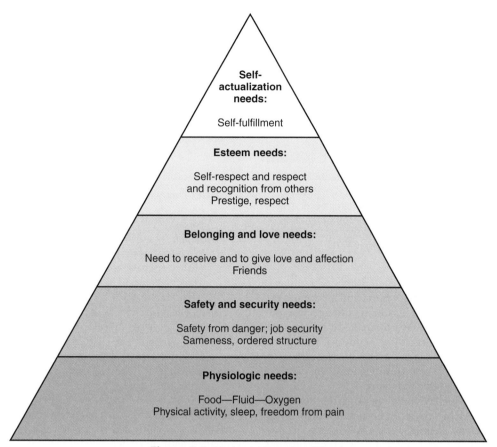

Figure 5-1 Maslow's Hierarchy of Needs.

perhaps 85% in their physical needs, 70% in their safety needs, 50% in their love needs, 40% in their self-esteem needs, and 10% in their self-actualization needs.

Maslow's Hierarchy of Needs
Physiologic Needs

Each person needs food, fluids, oxygen, physical activity, sleep, and freedom from pain. These needs are the most basic and the most dominant of all human needs. They are the first to develop in the human organism. The normal adult probably has satisfied their **physiologic needs**.

What about the person who is ill or hospitalized? The illness itself, diagnostic testing, or surgery may interrupt a person's normal eating and drinking habits. Diseases such as emphysema make it impossible for the body to receive the amount of oxygen needed to function normally. Physical activity is decreased on the patient's admission to the hospital, affecting the body's need for exercise.

Safety and Security Needs

Everyone has the need to be sheltered, to be clothed, to feel safe from danger, and to feel secure about their job and financial future. Each person has a need for a certain degree of sameness, familiarity, order, structure, and consistency in life. Freedom from fear, anxiety, and chaos is also important.

The normal healthy person probably has met these basic needs; however, illness or hospitalization may interrupt a person's ability to continue to satisfy them. What about the patient who is waiting for test results to learn a diagnosis, the unpredictable course of a lengthy illness, the fear of death, the cost of medical care, or the unfamiliarity of hospital routines and medical procedures? Many obstacles may interfere with efforts to meet the safety and security needs of a person who is ill or hospitalized.

Hospital employees who are new on the job may feel insecure, and they usually make more mistakes during this stressful time. Rumors about layoffs, true or not, can affect the security needs of employees and often send them scurrying to apply elsewhere for employment.

SCENARIO

Bill, a patient, has been fasting since midnight for an upper GI. It's now 11:00 A.M., the test is completed, and Bill is ready for his breakfast. When the HUC tells him that his tray will not arrive from the nutritional care department until 11:30 A.M., Bill becomes angry. Bill's behavior is influenced by his unsatisfied physiologic need.

SCENARIO

Donna, a patient, has just been told by her surgeon that the test results show she has a tumor that may be malignant. The surgeon has recommended she have surgery as soon as possible. Donna approaches the HUC and demands that she be able to speak to her family physician immediately. Donna's behavior is motivated by unsatisfied security needs.

Belonging and Love Needs

Once physiologic and safety needs are relatively well met, the **need for love and belonging** surfaces. Now, the person has a desire for affectionate relationships with others and is motivated to belong to or be a part of a group. Patients who are hospitalized, especially for a long time, may be cut off from their family, friends, or group.

> ## SCENARIO
>
> Sarah, a 76-year-old woman, has been hospitalized for 2 weeks. During this time, she has been visited only once by her daughter. In an attempt to meet her belonging needs, she has been turning on her call light hourly for minor requests.

Esteem Needs

As a person develops satisfying relationships with others, **esteem needs** and the need for self-respect and for the respect of others emerge. Esteem needs may be met by seeking special status within a group, owning a company, learning a skill very well, or developing a talent to be performed for others. Attainment of self-respect leads to feelings of adequacy, self-confidence, and strength. These qualities result in prestige, recognition, and dignity for the individual.

Hospitalization frequently interferes with the ability to meet esteem needs. Many aspects of hospitalization such as wearing hospital gowns, sharing a room with others, having side rails on the bed, and being referred to as a room number or a disease instead of by name serve to depersonalize the patient. Often, busy hospital personnel overlook a patient's past accomplishments and status.

> ## SCENARIO
>
> Tom has been hospitalized for longer than a week. He is walking past the nurses' station and stops to read the name tag of the HUC. "You are Jenny Mason. That's a nice name. You know, since I have been in the hospital, no one has called me by my name. I feel like I've lost my identity."

Self-Actualization Needs

Once a person feels basic satisfaction of the first four needs, the next step is for him or her to become "self-actualized." Self-actualization is the development of a personality to its full potential. Contentment, self-fulfillment, creativity, originality, independence, and acceptance of other people all characterize the self-actualized person. Self-actualization is growth motivated from within an individual. As Maslow expressed it, "What a man can be, he must be." Thus, self-actualization is the desire to become what one is capable of becoming. It is growing and changing because you feel it is important. A self-actualized person has taken steps to make this happen.

Examples of Different Needs in a Conversation

The human needs model can be used to demonstrate interpersonal behavior between HUCs and hospital personnel or between HUCs and patients or visitors.

> ## SCENARIO
>
> Mahatma Gandhi is an example of a self-actualized person. This Indian leader frequently sacrificed his physiologic and safety needs for the satisfaction of other needs when India was striving for independence from Great Britain. In his historic fasts, Gandhi went weeks without nourishment to protest governmental injustices. He was operating at the self-actualization level.

HUC: "Mary is in isolation. You will need to put this gown on before going into her room." *(No dominant need expressed.)*

Husband: "Mary is in isolation? What are you talking about? What for? I want to know exactly what is going on here!" *(Safety need expressed. The husband is concerned about Mary's safety and is also concerned that he may contract what Mary has.)*

HUC (defensively): "Look, if you don't want to wear the gown, don't go in. I don't make the rules here." *(Esteem need expressed. The HUC interprets the husband's request for information as an attack on her competence; self-esteem is at stake. Fighting back is used to try to satisfy self-esteem needs.)*

In this example, if the HUC had perceived that the husband's question was motivated by *safety* needs, she would have responded with understanding rather than with defensiveness and aggression.

EXERCISE 1

Match the level of need on "Maslow's Hierarchy of Human Needs" listed in Column 2 with the human needs listed in Column 1. Write the letter preceding the level in the space provided to indicate your answer.

Column 1	Column 2
1. The need for oxygen	a. Physiologic needs
2. The need for shelter	b. Safety and security needs
3. The need to be safe from danger	c. Belonging and love needs
4. The need to be loved	d. Esteem needs
5. The need for respect	e. Self-actualization needs
6. The need to feel self-confident	
7. The need for acceptance within a group	
8. The need to belong	
9. The need for exercise	
10. The need for the feeling of security	

COMMUNICATION SKILLS

Most of us spend much of our time communicating, but few of us communicate as effectively as we should. Many factors contribute to communication difficulties. For instance, the English language has grown considerably throughout its history, and the language now consists of approximately 750,000 words. It is impossible to know how many words an individual may have in their vocabulary, but it is believed that an average educated person comprehends about 20,000 words. How does the speaker know which of the 750,000 words are included in the receiver's 20,000-word vocabulary? The medical world also has a growing language of its own, which is made up of abbreviations and medical terms. "Remember now, Sidney is NPO," or "Your doctor feels that you may have diverticulitis, so she has scheduled you for a BE tomorrow" may have little meaning to those not familiar with the medical terms. Some words have more than one meaning. For instance, a *chip* in the computer world has a much different meaning than a *chip* used in a poker game.

Communication is 55% visual, including facial body language and symbolism; 38% vocal qualities, including tone, loudness, firmness, hesitations, and pauses; and 7% verbal, actual words (Fig. 5-2). There is often inconsistency between what a person is saying and how they appear. ("Of course I'm listening to you, Mother," says the 9-year-old boy as he sits glued to the television set, leaving the mother wondering whether the child is indeed listening to her.)

Another major weakness in the communication process involves poor listening skills. Often, we are thinking of something else while the speaker is talking to us; we are formulating a response or prejudging what is being said.

> *Daughter:* I have stopped eating breakfast meats.
> *Mother:* But breakfast is the most important meal of the day. You should not give it up.

Instead of listening to what is being said, the mother has prejudged that the daughter is skipping breakfast altogether rather than just breakfast meats.

Because the HUC is the communicator for the nursing unit, effective communication is vital for job success and for proficient operation of the nursing unit.

Communication takes place daily with nurses (Fig. 5-3, *A*), physicians (Fig. 5-3, *B*), allied health professionals, patients (Fig. 5-3, *C*), visitors, and administrators. The HUC is often the first person seen by the new patient and visitors. The words, gestures, facial expression, and body posture that is

used can suggest that one is opinionated, supportive, thoughtful, or insecure. The tone of voice, the words spoken, and the facial expressions used during the patient's or the visitor's initial contact with the nursing unit leaves a lasting impression.

Components of Communication

Communication is the process of transmitting images, feelings, and ideas from the mind of one person to the minds of one or more people for the purpose of obtaining a response. The communication process consists of four components:

> **Sender:** the person transmitting the message
> **Message:** the images, feelings, and ideas transmitted
> **Receiver:** the person receiving the message
> **Feedback:** the response to the message

Communication seems like a simple process; however, the act of communicating does not guarantee that effective communication has taken place, or that the message sent was the same as the message received. For example, a program was developed for a computer to translate one language into another. The computer translated the English phrase "out of sight, out of mind" into Russian, and then translated it back into English as "invisible idiot."

Communication Model

A model is a representation of a process—a map, for instance. We will use a model to take a closer look at the communication process, to identify why so many of us communicate poorly, and to find ways to improve our ability to communicate with others (Fig. 5-4).

Sender

The **sender** must translate mental images, feelings, and ideas into symbols to communicate them to the receiver. This process is called **encoding**. When encoding, the sender decides whether to send the message in verbal symbols or in nonverbal symbols (Fig. 5-5). What are the right words to use so the receiver will understand the message? Different words are used if you are speaking to a child, to an adult, or to another health care professional. Nonverbal symbols, such as facial expressions, may be used to communicate the message. Encoding occurs each time we communicate. A poor choice of words or an inconsistency between verbal and nonverbal messages may result in unsuccessful communication.

Message

Once the idea, feeling, or image is encoded, it is sent to the receiver. This step of the communication process is called the **message**.

Receiver

As the message reaches the **receiver**, the verbal and nonverbal symbols are decoded. **Decoding** is the process of translating symbols received from the sender to determine the message. Unsuccessful decoding can be caused by inconsistency in the verbal and nonverbal symbols received from the sender. For instance, "Of course I love you," said harshly

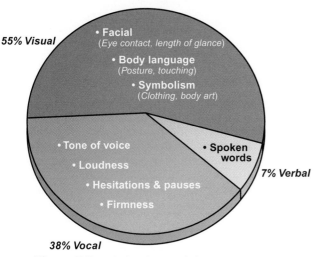

Figure 5-2 Verbal and nonverbal communication.

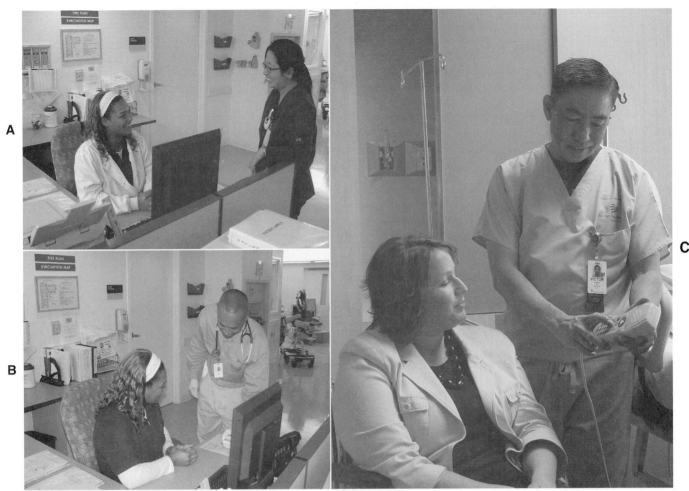

Figure 5-3 The HUC is the communicator for the nursing unit. **A,** Communicating with a nurse. **B,** Assisting a doctor. **C,** Answering a patient's questions regarding visiting hours, operation of call light, etc.

may be difficult to decode correctly. Lifestyle, age, cultural background, environment, and poor listening habits are other reasons for incorrect decoding. In successful communication, the ideas, feelings, and images of the sender match those of the receiver (Fig. 5-6, *A*). In unsuccessful communication, errors occur in encoding or in decoding the message (Fig. 5-6, *B*).

Verbal and Nonverbal Communication

Two methods of communication are verbal and nonverbal. **Verbal communication** is the use of language or the actual words spoken, whereas **nonverbal communication** is the use of eye contact, body language, facial expression, or symbolic expressions such as clothing that communicate a message. Sometimes our verbal and nonverbal communications contradict each other. For example, when a person is asked, "What is wrong?" and responds, "Oh nothing, I'm just fine" and shrugs his shoulders, frowns, and turns away, the dejected body language is more believable than the words spoken.

Types of Nonverbal Communication

Nonverbal communication can be separated further into two types: symbolic and body language.

Symbolic	Body Language
Clothing	Posture
Hair	Ambulation
Jewelry	Touching
Body art	Personal distance
Cosmetics	Eye contact
Automobile	Breathing
House	Hand gestures
Perfume or cologne	Facial expressions

Listening Skills

Listening is something we have done all our lives, but most of us have had little or no training in how to do it effectively. We take it for granted. Many of us think of communication as the sender giving us a message, but for successful communication to occur, the sender and the receiver both must participate actively in the communication process. Active participation for the receiver requires effective listening skills.

Five Levels of Listening

According to Dr. Stephen R. Covey in his best-selling book, *Seven Habits of Highly Effective People,* we listen at five different

Sender   Receiver

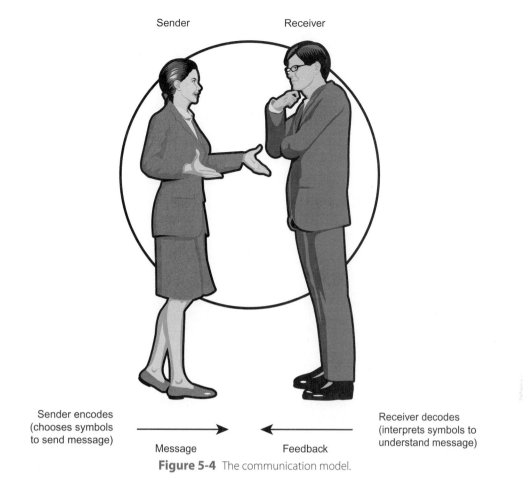

Sender encodes
(chooses symbols
to send message)

Receiver decodes
(interprets symbols to
understand message)

Message   Feedback

Figure 5-4 The communication model.

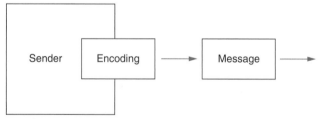

Figure 5-5 The communication process: message sending.

levels, depending on our interest in what is being said or what we might be doing while we are listening.

1. *Ignoring:* making no effort to listen
2. *Pretend listening:* giving the appearance that you are listening
3. *Selective listening:* hearing only the parts that interest you
4. *Attentive listening* (also called active listening): paying attention and focusing on what the speaker says and comparing it with your own experience
5. *Empathic listening:* listening and responding with both the heart and the mind to truly understand, realizing that all persons have the right to feel as they do

Guidelines for Improving Listening Skills

1. *Stop talking.* The first step toward improving listening skills is to stop talking. The adage that we have two ears and one mouth may indicate that we need to listen twice as much as we speak.
2. *Teach yourself to concentrate.* The average person speaks between 100 and 200 words a minute. The listener can process up to 400 words a minute. Often we find ourselves pretending to listen, listening selectively to the speaker, not listening for meaning in the message, or hearing only what interests us; in so doing, we miss important cues or even words. "We cannot send you any help" has a much different meaning from "We cannot send you any help *right now.*"
3. *Take time to listen.* When someone talks to you, stop what you are doing and look at the speaker. Practice attentive listening by focusing on the meaning of the words and watching for the nonverbal symbols. "I wish I were dead" spoken by an elderly patient may mean "I'm lonely."
4. *Listen with your eyes.* Practice empathetic listening by looking into the eyes of the sender. What is the sender saying? A visitor standing at the desk saying, "My mother is not back from surgery yet" may really be saying, "I'm frightened. She has been in surgery so long there must be complications."
5. *Listen to what is being said, not only to how it is being said.* Use both attentive and empathetic listening to fully understand what is being said. Avoid being distracted by a lisp, by how fast the sender is talking, or by what the sender is wearing, for instance. Concentrate on the verbal and nonverbal communication symbols used by the sender.

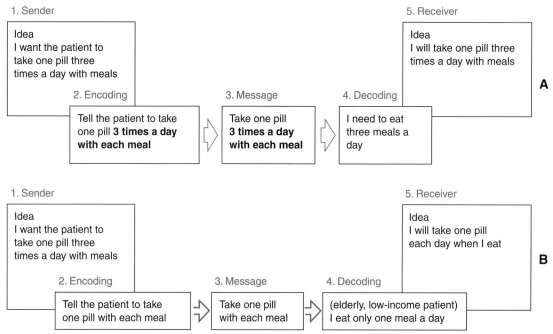

Figure 5-6 A, An example of successful communication. **B,** An example of unsuccessful communication.

6. *Suspend judgment.* Often, we react emotionally to what is said or what we think is being said. We prejudge what the speaker is saying and unconsciously tune out ideas or beliefs that do not match our own.

7. *Do not interrupt the speaker.* Interrupting the speaker or finishing the sentence discourages the sender and breaks down communication. To break this habit, try apologizing each time you interrupt the sender.

8. *Remove distractions.* Noise, a ringing telephone, and conversations of others are types of distractions that interfere with effective listening.

9. *Listen for both feeling and content* (seek to understand). Use empathetic listening by keeping in mind that all persons have the right to feel as they do.

Feedback

Feedback, the response to the message sent, is the final component in the communication process. Effective communication is virtually impossible without it. Feedback tells the sender how much of the message was understood, indicates whether the receiver agrees or disagrees with the message, and helps the sender correct confusing or vague language. Feedback can be as simple as a nod, it may be an answer to a question, or it may be used to encourage further communication and to assist the sender in developing ideas or sharing feelings.

Guidelines for Improving Feedback Skills

1. *Use paraphrasing* (repeat the message to the sender in your own words). Phrases such as "Let me see if I have this right…" and "This is what you want…" are acceptable as lines leading into paraphrasing. For example: "Let me repeat that to you. For the dressing change tomorrow, you want a dressing tray, size 7 gloves, and three packages of 4 × 4's."

2. *Repeat the last word or words of the message* (to allow the speaker to more fully develop the thought). Be careful not

to parrot the whole message, or the speaker may respond with "That's what I just said."

Patient: I'm not sure I want to have the myelogram.
Health Unit Coordinator: Myelogram?
Patient: Yes, I'm scheduled for one this afternoon, and frankly I'm scared stiff. My neighbor had one…

3. *Use specific rather than general feedback.* "Your idea has merit" is more meaningful than "You are so bright."

4. *Use constructive feedback rather than destructive feedback.* Do not use feedback that makes a person feel worse. "Moving your work station to the other counter may work" is better than saying, "That's a dumb idea, it won't work there!"

5. *Do not deny senders' feelings.* The use of statements such as: "Don't worry" or "You shouldn't feel that way" to someone who is frightened that they have cancer is of no help. Feedback that encourages the person to expound on their fears is much more helpful to the person.

Intercultural Communication Skills

The United States often is referred to as the "melting pot" because of its culturally diverse society. **Cultures** are developed when groups of people spend an extended time together. Each of us has values, beliefs, habits, and customs as a result of the backgrounds that make up our culture. **Subcultures** are smaller groups of people with certain ethnic, occupational, religious, or physical characteristics within the larger culture (e.g., elderly people, teens, nurses, Christians, athletes). It is essential for health care workers to understand and evaluate their own values, beliefs, and customs before working with and caring for people of varying cultures in health care. Many **conflicts** occur in the health care delivery system that are caused by cultural misunderstanding (e.g., verbal and nonverbal language, lack of courtesy, objectivity). **Culturally sensitive care** involves taking the time

Table 5-1 **Variations Among Selected Cultural Groups**

	African Americans	Asians	Hispanics	Native Americans
Verbal communication	Asking personal questions of someone met for the first time is seen as improper and intrusive.	High respect for others, especially those in positions of authority	Expression of negative feelings is considered impolite.	Speak in a low tone of voice and expect that the listener will be attentive.
Nonverbal communication	Direct eye contact in conversation often is considered rude.	Direct eye contact with superiors may be considered disrespectful.	Avoidance of eye contact usually is a sign of attentiveness and respect.	Direct eye contact often is considered disrespectful.
Touch	Touching another's hair often is considered offensive.	It is not customary to shake hands with persons of the opposite sex.	Touching often is observed between two persons in conversation.	A light touch of the person's hand instead of a firm handshake often is used when greeting a person.
Family organization	Usually have close, extended family networks. Women play key roles in health care decisions.	Usually have close, extended family ties. Emphasis may be on family needs rather than on individual needs.	Usually have close, extended family ties. All members of the family may be involved in health care decisions.	Usually have close, extended family ties. Emphasis tends to be on the family rather than on individual needs.
Time	Often present-oriented	Often present-oriented	Often present-oriented	Often present-oriented
Alternative healers	"Granny," "root doctor," voodoo priest, spiritualist	Acupuncturist, acupressurist, herbalist	Curandero, espiritualista, yerbo	Medicine man, shaman
Self-care practices	Poultices, herbs, oils, roots	Hot and cold foods, herbs, teas, soups, cupping, burning, rubbing, pinching	Hot and cold foods, herbs	Herbs, corn meal, medicine bundle

Data from Giger JN, Davidhizar, RE: *Transcultural nursing,* ed 3, St. Louis, 1999, Mosby; Spector RE: *Cultural diversity in health and illness,* ed 5, Upper Saddle River, NJ, 2000, Prentice Hall; Payne KT: In Taylor OL, editor: *Nature of communication disorders in culturally and linguistically diverse populations,* San Diego, 1986, College Hill Press.

to learn about the cultural backgrounds of patients and may require incorporating their beliefs and practices into their care plan. Refer to Table 5-1 to learn about the cultural backgrounds of African Americans, Asians, Hispanics, and Native Americans.

Often, people judge others by the standards of their own values and beliefs and find it difficult to accept other cultures. This is

referred to as *ethnocentrism.* HUCs may have attitudes regarding a patient's refusal of treatment because of religious beliefs, a patient who is admitted for sex change surgery, or a patient who is a former alcoholic who is receiving a liver transplant. These attitudes are based on ethnocentrism and must not affect the care given to these patients. It is also very important to avoid stereotyping and to refrain from making assumptions or drawing conclusions about a patient or a coworker on the basis of race or ethnicity. Patients and coworkers deserve to be treated and respected as unique individuals, regardless of their gender, age, economic status, religion, sexual status, education, occupation, physical makeup or limitations, or command of the English language.

Guidelines for Speaking to Someone Who Does Not Speak English Well

While working as an HUC, you may need to speak to someone from a different culture who does not speak English well.

Use the following guidelines in this process:

- Do not speak loudly.
- Talk distinctly and slowly.
- Emphasize key words.
- Let the listener read your lips.
- Use printed words (after determining the reading ability of the listener) and pictures.
- Do not use slang or jargon.
- Organize your thoughts.

✐ TAKE NOTE

Guidelines for Improving Intercultural Communication

- Understand and evaluate your own values, beliefs, and customs before working with and caring for people of varying cultures.
- Take the time to learn about the cultural backgrounds of patients; this may involve incorporating their beliefs and practices into their care.
- Do not judge others by the standards of your own values and beliefs.
- Avoid stereotyping or making assumptions about a patient or a coworker on the basis of race or ethnicity.
- Treat everyone with respect as unique individuals, regardless of their gender, age, economic status, religion, sexual status, education, occupation, physical makeup or limitations, or command of the English language.

- Choose your words carefully.
- Construct your sentences to say exactly what you want to say.
- Observe body language carefully.
- Try to pronounce names correctly.
- Ask for feedback to assess understanding.
- Ask how the person wishes to be addressed.
- Call for an **interpreter** if necessary and if available.
- Speak directly to the person, even if an interpreter is present.

✐ TAKE NOTE

Most hospitals provide a list of interpreters who speak and understand various languages and may be called when necessary to provide assistance in communicating with patients or visitors.

ASSERTIVENESS FOR THE HEALTH UNIT COORDINATOR

Have you ever said "Yes" to a request but really wanted to say "No," or left a conversation wishing you had "stood up for yourself"? If your answer is Yes, then you responded to the request in a **nonassertive** behavior style.

Have you ever allowed a situation to get out of control, then "blown up" and later wished you had handled the situation better? If your answer is *Yes,* then you responded to the situation in an **aggressive** behavioral style.

A third type of response is an **assertive** behavior style, in which an individual expresses her or his wants and desires in an honest and appropriate way, while respecting other people's rights.

As an HUC, you may have to ask patients or visitors to change their behavior to conform to safety regulations and hospital rules, or to allow for the comfort of others. For example, you may have to ask a patient's relative not to smoke

---

BILL OF ASSERTIVE RIGHTS

- You have the right to judge your own behavior, thoughts, and emotions, and to take responsibility upon yourself for their initiation and consequences.
- You have the right to offer no reasons or excuses to justify your behavior.
- You have the right to judge whether you are responsible for finding solutions to other people's problems.
- You have the right to change your mind.
- You have the right to make mistakes—and be responsible for them.
- You have the right to say "I don't know."
- You have the right to be independent of the goodwill of others before coping with them.
- You have the right to be illogical in making decisions.
- You have the right to say "I don't understand."
- You have the right to say "I don't care."
- **You have the right to say "No" without feeling guilty.**

From Smith MJ, *When I Say No, I Feel Guilty.* Copyright © 1975 by Manuel J. Smith. Used by permission of Doubleday, a division of Random House.

---

in the hospital, or you may have to ask a patient to turn down the television volume at the request of the patient's roommate. Asking another person to change their behavior can provoke a defensive reaction. Knowing you have a choice of behavior styles and choosing the best way to handle a given situation assists you in communicating more effectively.

As an HUC, you may have encounters that could lead to conflict each day that you are on the job. Using assertiveness, the art of expressing yourself clearly and concisely; being able to clarify when necessary; and being able to explain and communicate in an open, honest manner are techniques that enable you to cope effectively with problems and conflicts as they arise (see the Box *A Bill of Assertive Rights*).

Behavioral Styles
Nonassertive Behavioral Style

A nonassertive response is typically self-denying and does not express true feelings. The person does not stand up for his rights and allows others to choose for him. Because of inadequate response to the situation, the individual feels hurt and anxious. Nonassertive HUCs may have strong opinions about things that are going on at the nurses' station but may keep those feelings to themselves.

SCENARIO

Kim feels that she is scheduled to work more weekends and holidays than the other HUCs on the unit. Instead of saying anything to the nurse manager, she is upset every time she looks at the new work schedule.

A nonassertive choice avoids conflict; therefore, feelings of frustration or anger are not expressed to the person responsible.

SCENARIO

Robert spent 15 minutes in the unit lounge complaining to coworkers about how Betsy, a nurse, is condescending toward him and makes disparaging remarks in conversations with him. She expects him to leave what he is working on to run special errands for her. He is angry and frustrated but refuses to talk to her directly about these problems.

A nonassertive approach to requesting behavior change is to use general or apologetic statements, or to use words that minimize the message. This low-key approach allows others to easily ignore the request.

SCENARIO

Two visitors were relaxing in a visitors' lounge near the nursing station. They both lit cigarettes. A "No smoking" sign is posted nearby. Mary approaches the visitors and says, "I'm sorry, but I have to ask a little favor. This is not my rule, but smoking is not allowed here."

A nonassertive approach and response often result when one is intimidated by someone in a higher position.

> ### SCENARIO
>
> The EMR record has been implemented at the hospital where Tammy works, and she has been told that absolutely no handwritten physicians' orders should be accepted. Dr. Jamison has admitted a new patient and hands Tammy a sheet of handwritten orders. Tammy accepts the order sheet and says, "I was told that we were not to accept any handwritten orders, would you mind entering the orders into the computer for me?" Dr. Jameson replies, "You can enter them into the computer for me, can't you?" Tammy replies, "Yes, sir."

Aggressive Behavioral Style

An aggressive response is typically self-enhancing at the expense of others. The person may express feelings but hurts others in the process. Verbal attacks, disparaging remarks, and manipulations indicate aggressive behavior. An aggressive HUC uses "you" statements, often followed by personal judgments. Use of "you" statements provokes greater defensiveness than is aroused by the use of "I" statements.

> ### SCENARIO
>
> Kim feels that she is scheduled to work more weekends and holidays than the other HUCs. An aggressive Kim may approach the nurse manager and say, "You are simply unfair, and you don't care about me. I have to work more weekends and holidays than the others."

Statements that use *always* and *never* are often part of aggressive communications.

> ### SCENARIO
>
> Robert is upset with the nurse, Betsy, because she expects him to leave what he is doing to run errands for her. Robert responds aggressively, "You *always* expect me to stop my work for you; you think what you want is so important and you *never* think about anyone else."

An aggressive HUC makes demands instead of requests. Demanding does not elicit another's cooperation and generates defensiveness. Disparaging remarks cause the receiver to feel humiliated.

> ### SCENARIO
>
> An aggressive HUC asks the visitors to stop smoking by saying, "Put out your cigarettes. You can't smoke here. Can't you see the big 'No smoking' sign?"

An aggressive approach may result when one feels intimidated by someone in a higher position.

> ### SCENARIO
>
> Dr. Jamison has admitted a new patient and hands Tammy a sheet of handwritten orders. Tammy refuses the order sheet and says, "I know you and all doctors on staff have been told that all orders have to be entered into the computer. You need to enter them into the computer, and don't think about asking me to do it!"

Assertive Behavioral Style

An assertive response includes standing up for your rights without violating the rights of others. Assertive behavior is self-enhancing but not at the expense of others. It involves open, honest communication and the ability to express needs, expectations, and feelings. Being assertive also means being able to accept compliments with ease and to admit errors. It means taking responsibility for your actions. It is common for a person to assert himself or herself verbally only after frustration builds. At that point, it is too late to communicate assertively, and an aggressive response is used instead. It is useful to use assertiveness in all interactions before frustration builds. It is easy for the beginner to confuse assertive behavior with aggressive behavior. To distinguish the difference, remember that with assertive behavior, the rights of another are not violated.

An assertive HUC is able to use clear, direct, nonapologetic expressions of feelings and expectations. Descriptive rather than judgmental criticisms and "I" rather than "you" statements are used.

> ### SCENARIO
>
> Kim, as an assertive HUC, chooses to talk to the nurse manager about her feelings. "I feel that I am working more weekends and holidays than the other HUCs. I had to work 2½ weekends last month and I am scheduled to work Christmas and New Year's Day this year. I would like to share working weekends and holidays equally with the others. I would be glad to work every third weekend, and our family celebrates Christmas on Christmas Eve, so I would be happy to work Christmas Day and have New Year's off. It would allow me more time to spend with my family.

An assertive HUC uses concise statements and specific behavioral descriptions.

> ### SCENARIO
>
> Robert is assertive in dealing with Betsy when he chooses to talk to her. He begins by using an "I" statement, then describes the incident in which he felt Betsy was condescending. "I felt you were condescending toward me when you said, 'Even **you** should have been able to see that I needed help.'" He also mentions the specific remark that she made that he found disparaging. Depending on the discussion that follows, it also may be appropriate for him to ask Betsy for a behavior change. Robert also describes an incident in which Betsy asked him to interrupt his work to run errands for her. He describes how he could be more productive if he was allowed to do the task for her when it was convenient to his work schedule.

Table 5-2 Comparison of Nonassertive, Aggressive, and Assertive Behavioral Styles

Components	Nonassertive	Aggressive	Assertive
Rights	Does not stand up for rights	Stands up for rights but violates the rights of others	Stands up for rights without violating rights of others
Choice	Allows others to choose (to avoid conflict)	Chooses for others	Chooses for self
Belief	I'm not OK, you're OK; lose/win	I'm OK, you're not OK; win/lose	I'm OK, you're OK; win/win
Responsibility	Others responsible for behavior; blame themselves for poor results; may blame others for feelings	Responsible for others' behavior; blames others for poor results. Feelings are not important.	Responsible for own behavior; assumes responsibility for own errors; assumes responsibility for feelings
Traits	Self-denying, apologetic, timid, emotionally dishonest; difficult to say, "No"; guilty, whining, "poor me"	Dominates, humiliates, sarcasm; self-enhancing at the expense of others; opinionated	Expresses feelings, feels good about self; candid, diplomatic; listens; eye contact
Goals	Does not achieve goals	Achieves goals at the expense of others	May achieve goals
Word choices	Minimizing words such as "I'm sorry" "I believe" "I think" "Little," "sort of" General instead of specific statements; statement disguised as questions	"You statements" Always/never statements Demands instead of requests	"I understand…" "I feel…" "I apologize…" Neutral language Concise statements
Body language	Lack of eye contact; slumping, downtrodden posture; words and nonverbal messages that do not match	"Looking-through-you" eye contact; tense, impatient posture	Erect, relaxed posture; eye contact; verbal and nonverbal messages match

An assertive HUC uses requests instead of demands and personalizes statements of concern.

SCENARIO

Mary, an assertive HUC, approaches the visitors and says, "Please stop smoking in the hospital. Smoking is not allowed anywhere in the hospital, but there are designated smoking areas located outside the cafeteria on the back patio, where you can sit down and have a cigarette."

Assertive behavior is the most effective way to communicate no matter what an individual's status is in comparison with yours.

SCENARIO

Dr. Jamison has admitted a new patient and hands Tammy a sheet of handwritten orders. Tammy hands the order sheet back to him and says, "I know it is difficult to get used to the EMR; if you need any assistance in entering these orders into the computer, let me know."

Assertiveness is based on the belief that each individual has the same fundamental human rights; therefore, the doctor is not better than the HUC, and the teacher is not better than the students. In becoming assertive, you do not need to focus on changing your personality, but rather, on changing your behavior in specific situations. It is highly unlikely that anyone is always assertive; however, once assertiveness is learned, it can be one of your behavioral choices.

Table 5-2 compares nonassertive, aggressive, and assertive behavioral styles.

EXERCISE 2

Identify the behavioral style shown in each of the following statements by writing AG for aggressive, AS for assertive, and NA for nonassertive in the spaces provided.

1. "I would like to have Monday off." _____

2. "You should know how to order diets. You have been here long enough." _____

3. "I'm sorry. I'm so forgetful. I won't let it happen again." _____

4. "I would kind of like to go on my break now." _____

5. "The next NAHUC chapter meeting is tomorrow at 6:00 p.m. I am going. Would you like to go with me?" _____

6. "I know nothing about it. You were here yesterday—you should know." _____

7. "I would like to finish transcribing this set of orders before I take this specimen to the lab." _____

8. "I wish somebody else around here would answer the phone once in a while." _____

9. "Your chart is right here, Dr. James. I would think you could find it on your own." _____

10. "I apologize; I did not order the liver scan. I will order it immediately." _____

11. "You are always late. You never care that I have to stay over and cover for you." _____

12. "I really hate to ask you this, and you don't have to do it, but would you work for me on Saturday?" _____

13. "May I help you find your chart, Dr. McLean?" _____

14. "I don't know what the nurse manager thinks I am, a machine or something. We need more help around here." _____

15. "You should know how to locate Mrs. Saulter's CT report without my help by now!" _____

16. "I know I'm not supposed to enter these orders into the computer for you, but if you don't tell anyone, I will enter them for you." _____

17. "Mrs. Smith, I would like you to turn your light off so Mrs. Jones can rest." _____

18. "Mary, I would like to switch days off with you." _____

Evaluating Your Assertiveness

Table 5-3 is an assertive inventory that has been developed by Alberti and Emmons. These authors state that the inventory "provides a list of questions which should be useful in increasing your awareness of your own behavior in situations which call for assertiveness. The inventory is not a standardized psychological test. There are no right answers. The only "score" is your own evaluation of how you measure up to what you would like to be able to do. Take time now to respond to the questions in the inventory.

Assertiveness Skills

The goal of using assertiveness in communication is to arrive at an "I win, you win" conclusion—in other words, a **workable compromise**. A workable compromise involves dealing with a conflict in such a way that the solution is satisfactory to all involved parties. Four assertiveness skills that may be used to reach a workable compromise are broken record, fogging, negative assertion, and negative inquiry.

Broken Record

The **broken record** is an assertiveness skill that allows you to say no over and over again without raising your voice or getting irritated or angry. You must be persistent and not give reasons, excuses, or explanations for not doing what the other person wants you to do. By doing this, you can ignore manipulative traps and argumentative baiting.

> *Jane:* "Let's go to lunch."
> *Sue:* "Thanks for asking; However, *I can't go, I just started a new diet.*"
> *Jane:* "So what! You start a new diet every week. It has never stopped you from going before."
> *Sue:* "Well, thanks anyway, but *I just started a new diet, I can't go to lunch.*"
> *Jane:* "Well, you don't have to eat anything fattening."
> *Sue:* "Thanks anyway. *I can't go. I just started a new diet.*"

Fogging

Fogging is an assertiveness skill that allows you to accept manipulative criticism and anxiety-producing statements by offering no resistance and by using a noncommittal reply, while calmly acknowledging that there may be some truth in what the critic is saying, yet retaining the right to remain your own judge. When you use fogging, it is hard for the other person to see exactly what you are saying.

> *John:* "You are really too slow to do this job!"
> *Bill:* "I can see it may appear that I am a slow worker; however, I have only been here a month. I will speed up once I know the procedures better."

Negative Assertion

Negative assertion is an assertiveness skill that allows you to accept your errors and faults without becoming defensive or resorting to anger. It is a technique of admitting errors without affecting your worth as a human being. It includes not using self-depreciation, such as "that was so stupid of me."

> *Dr. Smith:* "You didn't scan my progress notes from this morning into Mr. Jones's chart as I requested!"
> *Sue:* "You're right. I did not scan them, I apologize. I will scan them now."

Negative Inquiry

Negative inquiry is an assertiveness skill that allows you to actively prompt criticism to use the information or, if manipulative, to exhaust it. By doing this, you obtain clarification about the criticism and hopefully bring out possible hidden issues that may really be the point.

> *Nurse manager:* "Your work is not what I expect of an HUC. If you want to stay on this unit, you will have to improve."
> *Unit coordinator:* "When you say my work is not what you expect, what is it about my work that is not up to your expectations?"

Table 5-3 **The Assertiveness Inventory**

The following questions will be helpful in assessing your assertiveness. Be honest with your responses. All you have to do is draw a circle around the number that best describes you. For some questions, the assertive end of the scale is at 0; for others, it is at 3.

Key: 0 means *no* or *never;* 1 means *somewhat* or *sometimes;* 2 means *usually* or *a good deal;* and 3 means *practically always* or *entirely.*

1.	When a person is highly unfair, do you call it to their attention?	0	1	2	3
2.	Do you find it difficult to make decisions?	0	1	2	3
3.	Are you openly critical of others' ideas, opinions, or behaviors?	0	1	2	3
4.	Do you speak out in protest when someone takes your place in line?	0	1	2	3
5.	Do you often avoid people or situations for fear of embarrassment?	0	1	2	3
6.	Do you usually have confidence in your own judgment?	0	1	2	3
7.	Do you insist that your spouse or roommate take on a fair share of household chores?	0	1	2	3
8.	Are you prone to "flying off the handle"?	0	1	2	3
9.	When a salesperson makes an effort, do you find it hard to say "No," even though the merchandise is not really what you want?	0	1	2	3
10.	When a latecomer is waited on before you, do you call attention to the situation?	0	1	2	3
11.	Are you reluctant to speak up in a discussion or a debate?	0	1	2	3
12.	If a person has borrowed money (or a book, a garment, or something else of value) and is overdue in returning it, do you mention it?	0	1	2	3
13.	Do you continue to pursue an argument after the other person has had enough?	0	1	2	3
14.	Do you generally express what you feel?	0	1	2	3
15.	Are you disturbed if someone watches you at work?	0	1	2	3
16.	If someone keeps kicking or bumping your chair in a movie or at a lecture, do you ask the person to stop?	0	1	2	3
17.	Do you find it difficult to keep eye contact when talking to another person?	0	1	2	3
18.	In a good restaurant, when your meal is improperly prepared or served, do you ask the waiter or waitress to correct the situation?	0	1	2	3
19.	When you discover that merchandise is faulty, do you return it for an adjustment?	0	1	2	3
20.	Do you show your anger by name-calling or using obscenities?	0	1	2	3
21.	Do you try to be a wallflower or a piece of furniture in social situations?	0	1	2	3
22.	Do you insist that your property manager (mechanic, repairman, etc.) make repairs, adjustments, or replacements that are their responsibility?	0	1	2	3
23.	Do you often step in and make decisions for others?	0	1	2	3
24.	Are you able to express love and affection openly?	0	1	2	3
25.	Are you able to ask your friends for small favors or help?	0	1	2	3
26.	Do you think you always have the right answer?	0	1	2	3
27.	When you differ with a person you respect, are you able to speak up for your own viewpoint?	0	1	2	3
28.	Are you able to refuse unreasonable requests made by friends?	0	1	2	3
29.	Do you have difficulty complimenting or praising others?	0	1	2	3
30.	If you are disturbed by someone who is smoking near you, can you say so?	0	1	2	3
31.	Do you shout or use bullying tactics to get others to do as you wish?	0	1	2	3
32.	Do you finish other people's sentences for them?	0	1	2	3
33.	Do you get into physical fights with others, especially with strangers?	0	1	2	3
34.	At family meals, do you control the conversation?	0	1	2	3
35.	When you meet a stranger, are you the first to introduce yourself and begin a conversation?	0	1	2	3

EXERCISE 3

Practice writing verbal responses to the situations described in the following exercise. Use the behavioral style indicated. Practice using assertiveness skills when giving answers.

1. A coworker comes in at 3:00 P.M. and finds that no admission charts have been made up for the new admits. She throws a chart down in front of you and storms off. You did not have time to put the charts together.

Assertive:

_____

Nonassertive:

_____

Aggressive:

_____

2. You have been asked to float to the pediatric unit. You work on orthopedics. When you arrive on Peds, a nurse says to you: "It would really be nice to get someone who knows what they're doing."

Assertive:

_____

Nonassertive:

_____

Aggressive:

_____

3. You forgot to order a CBC this morning while transcribing Mr. Barrett's orders. When the error was discovered by the patient's nurse, she said, "You didn't order the CBC on Mr. Barrett this morning!"

Assertive:

_____

Nonassertive:

_____

Aggressive:

_____

4. A local celebrity is a patient on your unit. The doctor has left strict instructions that only relatives can visit the patient and for only short periods. A visitor has just approached the nursing station. He claims he is the local celebrity's manager and must see the patient about some financial matters today.

Assertive:

_____

Nonassertive:

_____

Aggressive:

_____

5. Your immediate supervisor has just told you that your work is just not acceptable and to improve it or else.

Assertive:

_____

Nonassertive:

_____

Aggressive:

_____

6. It is 9:00 A.M., and Dr. Frank has asked you to please locate the reports from an outside facility that she requested yesterday on one of her patients. You look in the computer, and cannot locate them, but you find them in the basket of documents to be scanned. When you tell this to Dr. Frank, she responds angrily, "What in the hell is going on here? Can't anybody do anything right on this unit?"

Assertive:

_____

Nonassertive:

_____

Aggressive:

_____

STEPS TO DEALING WITH AN ANGRY TELEPHONE CALLER

At times, the HUC is confronted with an angry or disgruntled telephone caller. Following the few helpful steps outlined here will assist you in handling the situation effectively.

1. *When answering the telephone, always identify yourself by nursing unit, name, and status* (Fig. 5-7). Doing this puts you on a more personal level with the caller. Also, callers may become even more upset if they need to ask questions to determine whom they are talking to.
2. *Avoid putting the person on hold.* Placing an angry person on hold may escalate their anger.

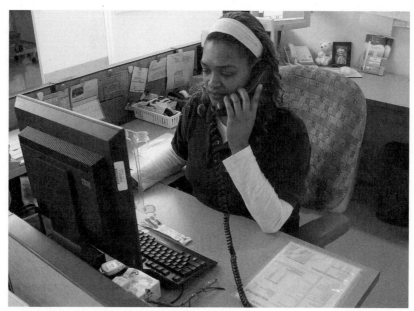

Figure 5-7 When you answer the telephone, always identify yourself by nursing unit, name, and status.

3. *Listen to what the caller is saying.* Do not become defensive. Keep in mind that the caller is not really angry with you.
4. *Write down what the caller is saying.* The notes may come in handy, and they help you control your own anger.
5. *Acknowledge the anger.* Use phrases such as, "I understand that you are angry" and "I hear your frustration."
6. *Do not allow the caller to become abusive.* Say, "I feel you are becoming abusive" or "Please call me back in a few minutes so we can talk about this calmly."

HOW COMMUNICATION AND INTERPERSONAL SKILLS ARE USED IN THE HEALTH CARE SETTING

Following are five major areas in which the HUC may use communication and interpersonal skills discussed in this chapter in the health care setting:

1. *Obtaining information.* Often, the HUC must obtain information to communicate a message in a correct and timely manner. Applying assertiveness skills to ask a question correctly, using appropriate listening skills when receiving the response and when the situation calls for it, and using the guidelines for speaking to a person who does not speak English well will be useful.
2. *Providing information.* The HUC will be providing information to visitors, doctors, nursing staff, and other hospital departments, as well as to institutions outside the hospital. Being aware of verbal and nonverbal use of language will be helpful in doing this.
3. *Developing trust.* Trust is vital to a healthy work environment, and assertive communication plays a big role in establishing and maintaining this trust.
4. *Showing understanding.* Understanding the needs of patients, families, and coworkers will foster successful communication in the work environment. Using Maslow's Hierarchy of Needs and intercultural communication skills will be helpful in this area.

5. *Relieving stress.* Stress in the workplace is a constant; how we manage it makes a difference. Recognizing the three behavioral types and using assertiveness skills can be helpful in this area. Using the communication model of selecting words carefully for communication and using effective listening skills may help avoid or alleviate stressful situations.

GUIDELINES FOR PRECEPTING A HEALTH UNIT COORDINATING STUDENT OR A NEW EMPLOYEE

When given the opportunity to **precept** (to train or instruct) a student or to orient a new employee to your nursing unit/hospital, keep in mind what it was like when you were new and inexperienced—were you made to feel welcome, or were you made to feel that you were in the way? How did it affect your clinical/orientation experience? When you are selected to be a **preceptor** (trainer or teacher), your nurse manager is indicating that she/he has confidence in your expertise and your knowledge and ability to teach the student or new employee what they need to know. To provide the best learning experience, it is important to make the new employee feel comfortable so she/he will ask questions, if necessary, to fully understand what you are teaching. Every person learns at a different pace; some will remember what you have told them the first time, some will need to write it down, and others will need to actually perform the task before mastering it. The following guidelines should assist you in becoming an efficient preceptor and in providing a successful **clinical experience** or orientation.

Guidelines for the Health Unit Coordinating Preceptor

- Provide a copy of dates and times the student or new employee is to be on the nursing unit to complete their clinical experience (provide a copy of your schedule to the student and the student's instructor or to the new employee).
- Obtain a list of objectives (provided by the hospital or by the school), so all are clear on what is to be accomplished by the end of the clinical experience.

- Take the student/new employee on a tour of the nursing unit and hospital, so that he/she can become aware of where restrooms, cafeteria, and hospital departments are located.
- Set a positive example—be on time each day, return on time from appropriate breaks, and maintain a positive attitude regarding your job, the hospital, the administration, and nursing unit personnel.
- If the student/new employee does not call prior to being late or absent, it is the preceptor's responsibility to notify the instructor or nurse manager.
- Notify the student and your nursing unit or the new employee and the nurse manager if you are going to be tardy, absent, or transferred to another unit (preferably an hour prior to the start of the shift).
- Stay with the student/new employee to monitor progress and check off objectives as completed with competence, as instructed in the clinical/orientation packet.
- Provide feedback to the student/new employee, and offer suggestions for improvement.
- Notify the student's instructor or the new employee's nurse manager if the student/new employee is not dressed according to hospital/school dress code (the student may have a more strict dress code), is not performing in an appropriate and professional manner, or is having difficulty completing objectives.
- Notify the student's instructor or the new employee's nurse manager if you have questions or concerns.
- Notify the student's instructor or the new employee's nurse manager immediately if you have serious concerns.
- Complete an evaluation form regarding the student's clinical experience.

Guidelines for the Health Unit Coordinating Student or New Employee

- Be sure you know when and where you are to complete your clinical experience, and know the name of your preceptor.
- If you are a student, provide your preceptor with a list of objectives and the instructor's telephone and/or pager number.

- The student/new employee should notify the nursing unit, the preceptor, and the instructor or nurse manager an hour prior to the start of the shift (unless emergency) if he or she is going to be tardy or absent.
- The student must notify the instructor if he or she leaves the hospital prior to the end of the shift.
- It is the student's responsibility to notify the instructor if the preceptor is going to be late, absent, or transferred to another unit.
- The student or new employee should arrive dressed appropriately and prepared to learn and work each day and should be accountable for their learning.
- The student needs to be flexible and should refrain from saying, "That's not the way we were taught in class" or "That's not the way we did it at Previous Community Hospital."
- The student or new employee should communicate openly with the preceptor and instructor or nurse manager regarding any problems with their clinical performance.
- The student/new employee should have the list of objectives/evaluation forms completed and signed off by the preceptor 2 days prior to the last clinical day.
- The student/new employee should complete an evaluation form regarding their clinical experience or orientation.

KEY CONCEPTS

Effective communication is essential in the health care setting. Quality patient care requires an efficient, professional, and culturally sensitive team. Health care can be extremely stressful, so it is vital that personnel remain calm, exercise assertiveness skills, and have empathy for patients and coworkers. Each member of a health care team is important and necessary, and it is imperative that staff members maintain a positive attitude regarding the job, hospital, administration, and nursing unit personnel. About one third of your time is spent at your job!

REVIEW QUESTIONS

1. Write an example of a hospitalized patient's situation that exemplifies each of the first four needs outlined in Maslow's Hierarchy of Needs.

   a. physiologic

   _____

   b. safety and security

   _____

   c. belonging and love

   _____

   d. esteem

   _____

2. Four components of the communication process are

a. _____

b. _____

c. _____

d. _____

3. Define the following terms:

a. encoding

_____

b. decoding

_____

4. Using the communication model, demonstrate a successful communication process and an unsuccessful communication process. Identify at which step of the process the errors occurred.

a. successful communication

_____

_____

_____

b. unsuccessful communication

_____

_____

_____

5. List two common errors in encoding a message.

a. _____

b. _____

6. List two common errors in decoding a message.

a. _____

b. _____

7. List three examples of *symbolic* nonverbal communication.

a. _____

b. _____

c. _____

8. List three examples of body language used in nonverbal communication.

a. _____

b. _____

c. _____

9. Fill in the percentage used of each of the following verbal and nonverbal types of communication during the process of communicating messages:

a. Facial expression and eye contact, including the length of glance _____%

b. Vocal qualities, including tone, loudness, firmness, _____% hesitations, and pauses

c. Verbal, actual words _____%

10. Identify the cause(s) of unsuccessful communication in each of the following situations:

a. A nurse interviewing an Asian patient sits on the side of his bed while making direct eye contact. The patient looks away, avoiding eye contact. The nurse thinks the patient is despondent or is being rude. (Refer to Table 5-1.)

_____

_____

b. Mrs. Fredrick, an elderly female patient who has never been ill before, is admitted to the hospital. Joe, a young male CNA, is assisting her into bed. Joe tells Mrs. Fredrick, "OK, honey, your doctor has ordered that you be NPO because you're going to have a UGI this morning." Mrs. Fredrick begins to cry.

_____

_____

c. Dr. James asks Sue, the HUC, to answer her calls while she is in the treatment room performing a procedure. Sue leaves the nurses' station for a short break and doesn't hear the operator paging Dr. James. When Dr. James returns to the nursing station and asks for her message, Sue says, "What message?" Dr. James angrily walks away.

_____

_____

d. Cindi, the registered nurse who is caring for Stan Potter, a homeless man, does not spend the usual amount of time with him on admission because he is dirty and doesn't have any social skills.

_____

_____

12. List nine listening skills that you feel would most help you improve your interpersonal communication.

a. _____

b. _____

c. _____

d. _____

e. _____

f. _____

g. _____

h. _____

i. _____

13. List the five feedback skills that you feel would help you improve your interpersonal communication.

a. _____

b. _____

c. _____

d. _____

e. _____

14. Explain "culturally sensitive care."

_____

_____

15. List five guidelines to follow that could improve intercultural communication.

a. _____

b. _____

c. _____

d. _____

e. _____

16. Label the following behaviors as assertive, nonassertive, or aggressive.

a. self-denying

_____

b. self-enhancing at the expense of others

_____

c. open, honest, and respectful of others' rights

_____

17. Explain the following assertiveness techniques.

a. Broken record

_____

_____

b. Fogging

_____

_____

c. Negative assertion

_____

_____

d. Negative inquiry

_____

_____

18. List six steps that you should follow when dealing with an angry caller.

a. _____

b. _____

c. _____

d. _____

e. _____

f. _____

19. Define the following terms:

a. ethnocentrism

_____

b. elitism

_____

c. subcultures

_____

d. culture

_____

e. stereotyping

_____

f. HUC preceptor

_____

20. List twelve preceptor guidelines for training an HUC student or a new employee.

a. _____

b. _____

c. _____

d. _____

e. _____

f. _____

g. _____

h. _____

i. _____

21. List ten student guidelines for completing the clinical experience.

a. _____

b. _____

c. _____

d. _____

e. _____

f. _____

g. _____

h. _____

i. _____

j. _____

22. Identify five ways that communication and interpersonal skills are used in the health care setting.

a. _____

b. _____

c. _____

d. _____

e. _____

23. Explain why the implementation of the EMR is requiring even greater communication skills of the HUC.

_____

_____

_____

THINK ABOUT...

1. Do you remember a misunderstanding that occurred because someone interpreted something you said differently from the way you intended it? Discuss how you could have worded the message differently. Discuss what you think caused the misinterpretation.

2. How do you feel when you meet people from other cultures? Does it make you uncomfortable when others are speaking a different language than yours? Discuss how you can communicate with individuals who do not understand your language.

3. Discuss what the term "culturally sensitive care" means to you.

4. Discuss the importance of effective interpersonal communication for the HUC.

5. Can you remember someone who trained or oriented you and caused you to feel welcome and nurtured? What did this person do that made you feel that way?

6. Can you remember someone who trained or oriented you and caused you to feel unwelcome and in the way? What did this person do that made you feel that way?

CHAPTER 6

Workplace Behavior
Ethics and Legal Concepts

OUTLINE

CHAPTER OBJECTIVES

Upon completion of this chapter, you will be able to

1. Define the terms in the vocabulary list.
2. Write the meaning of the abbreviations in the abbreviations list.
3. List four factors that influence a worker's behavior.
4. Explain how personal values could affect interactions in the health care setting.
5. List six behavior traits that make up one's work ethics.
6. List four guidelines to follow in maintaining the confidentiality of the contents of a patient's chart.

7. Explain the purpose of the Privacy Rule contained in the Health Insurance Portability and Accountability Act.
8. Explain what is meant by "protected health information."
9. Explain the purpose of the Security Rule contained in the Health Insurance Portability and Accountability Act
10. Explain the term "electronic protected health information."
11. List six responsibilities of the health unit coordinator (HUC) in maintaining confidentiality of patient protected health information.

12. Explain why it is important for the HUC to be professional in their appearance.
13. List nine guidelines to follow when completing a job application.
14. List eleven guidelines to follow when writing a resumé.
15. Explain the importance of dressing appropriately when going for an interview.
16. Explain why the HUC should not accept or place calls or text messages when working on the nursing unit.
17. List five Joint Commission annual and pre-clinical/preemployment requirements.
18. List four additional/pre-clinical and preemployment requirements.
19. Identify two types of sexual harassment.
20. Discuss the first step to take when encountering sexual harassment.
21. Discuss immediate action to take when witnessing violence or potential for violence.
22. Discuss two purposes of an employee performance evaluation.
23. List two purposes of a patient's bill of rights.
24. Explain what the standard of care is for an HUC.
25. Identify six preventive measures that can be taken to minimize the risk of malpractice within the HUC practice.

VOCABULARY

Accountability Taking responsibility for ones actions; being answerable to someone for something one has done

Attitude A manner of thought or feeling expressed in a person's behavior

Autonomy Independence, personal liberty

Behavior What people do and say

Cardiopulmonary Resuscitation The basic life-saving procedure of artificial ventilation and chest compressions done in the event of a cardiac arrest (all health care workers are required to be certified in CPR)

Code of Ethics A set of standards for behavior that is based on values

Confidentiality Protecting the privacy of any confidential information, spoken or written

Damages Monetary compensation awarded by a court for an injury caused by the act of another

Defendant The person against whom a civil or criminal action is brought

Deposition Pretrial statement of a witness under oath, taken in question-and-answer form, as it would be in court, with opportunity given to the adversary to be present to cross-examine

Discrimination Seeing a difference; prejudicial treatment of a person

Ethics Behavior that is based on values (beliefs); how we make judgments in regard to right and wrong

Evidence All the means by which any alleged matter of fact, the truth of which is submitted to investigation at trial, is established or disproved; evidence includes the testimony of witnesses and the introduction of records, documents, exhibits, objects, or any other substantiating matter offered for the purpose of inducing belief in the party's contention by the judge or jury

Expert Witness A person who has special knowledge of the subject about which they are to testify; this knowledge must generally be such as is not normally possessed by the average person

Fidelity Doing what one promises

Hostile Environment A threatening or sexually oriented atmosphere or pattern of behavior that is determined to be a form of harassment

Implied Contract A nonexplicit agreement that affects some aspect of the employment relationship

Informed Consent Doctrine that states that before patients are asked to consent to a risky or invasive diagnostic or treatment procedure, they are entitled to receive certain information: (1) a description of the procedure, (2) any alternatives to it and their risks, (3) risks of death or serious bodily disability from the procedure, (4) probable results of the procedure, including any problems with recuperation and anticipated time of recuperation, and (5) anything else that is generally disclosed to patients who are asked to consent to a procedure

Liability Condition of being responsible for damages resulting from an injurious act or from discharging an obligation or debt

Medical Malpractice Professional negligence of a health care professional; failure to meet a professional standard of care, resulting in harm to another, for example, failure to provide "good and accepted medical care"

Negligence Failure to satisfactorily perform one's legal duty, such that another person incurs some injury

Philosophy Principles; underlying conduct

Plaintiff Person who brings a lawsuit against another

Principles Basic truths; moral code of conduct

Quid Pro Quo (Latin) Involves making conditions of employment (hiring, promotion, retention) contingent on the victim's providing sexual or other favors

Respect Holding a person in esteem or honor; having appreciation and regard for another

Respondeat Superior (Latin) "Let the master answer." Legal doctrine that imposes liability upon the employer as a result of the action of an employee. *Note:* The employee is also liable for their own actions

Retaliation Revenge; payback

Scope of Practice Legal description of what a specific health professional may and may not do

Sexual Harassment Unwanted, unwelcome behavior; sexual in nature

Standard of Care The legal duty one owes to another according to the circumstances of a particular case; it is the care that a reasonable and prudent person would have exercised in the given situation

Statute Law passed by the legislature and signed by the governor at the state level and the president at the federal level

Statute of Limitations Time within which a plaintiff must bring a civil suit; this limit varies with the type of suit, and it is set by the various state legislatures

Tact Use of discretion regarding the feelings of others

Tort A wrong against another person or his property that is not a crime but for which the law provides a remedy

Values Personal beliefs about the worth of a principle, standard, or quality; what one holds as most important

Values Clarification Examination of our value system

Work Ethics Moral values regarding work

ABBREVIATIONS

Abbreviation	Meaning
APS	Adult Protective Services
CE	covered entity
CPR	cardiopulmonary resuscitation
CPS	Child Protective Services
EPHI	electronic protected health information
HIPAA	Health Insurance Portability and Accountability Act
IIHI	individually identifiable health information
NINP	no information, no publication
PHI	protected health information
SNAT	suspected nonaccidental trauma

EXERCISE 1

Write the abbreviation for each term listed below.

1. Adult Protective Services _____

2. Child Protective Services _____

3. No information, no publication _____

4. Suspected nonaccidental trauma _____

5. Health Insurance Portability and Accountability Act _____

6. Protected health information _____

7. Covered entity _____

8. Cardiopulmonary resuscitation _____

9. Electronic protected health information _____

10. Individually identifiable health information _____

EXERCISE 2

Write the meaning of each abbreviation listed below.

1. APS

   _____

2. CPS

   _____

3. NINP

   _____

4. SNAT

   _____

5. HIPAA

   _____

6. PHI

   _____

7. CE

   _____

8. CPR

   _____

9. EPHI

   _____

10. IIHI

   _____

WORKPLACE BEHAVIOR

Many factors may influence a person's workplace **behavior**. What is most important to a person or what each needs or gets from the work affects a person's behavior.

Factors That Influence Workplace Behavior

The following are factors that influence a person's behavior in the workplace:

1. Philosophy and standards of the organization
2. Leadership style of supervisors
3. How meaningful or important the work is to the person
4. How challenging the work is for the person
5. How the person fits in with coworkers
6. Personal characteristics of a worker, such as abilities, interests, aptitudes, values, and expectations

Many job options exist for a health unit coordinator (HUC) in the health care field. Choose a position that will best satisfy personal needs. If one loves to be around children, pediatrics may be ideal, or if an individual wants to be challenged, the emergency room or an intensive care unit may be the best choice. If a job that will provide solitude is wanted, the recovery room may be an option, or if a more social setting is preferred, a medical-surgical unit may be a better choice. Consider options carefully.

Personal values may have a significant impact on interactions with others on the job. The HUC position requires communication that is provided in a nonjudgmental way. Examining one's value system is important when one is preparing to work in the health care setting.

How Values Influence Interactions in the Health Care Setting

A person's values are formed by the age of 6 and are influenced by parents, siblings, extended family, friends, peers, teachers, and work supervisors. Significant emotional events in our lives and other life experiences may change our values. For example, losing a loved one may cause one to treasure family and to value life in a way one had not before. Life experiences can change what we view as most important and also can help us gain **empathy** for others. Our values can have a major impact on how we relate to others and on the choices and decisions that we make. Diane Uustal, a well-known nurse and ethicist, describes values as being "a basis for what a person thinks about, chooses, feels for, and acts on" (Uustal, 1992). The personal values of an HUC may cause problems in their interactions.

SCENARIO

Joan, an HUC, has a father who was an abusive alcoholic. Joan is adamant about her feelings regarding alcoholics and is very much against drinking. Mr. Thomas is admitted because he was in a car accident that was caused by his drunkenness. Whenever Mr. Thomas approaches the desk to talk to Joan, she is very rude to him. Joan is allowing her personal values to influence her behavior. It is important to remain nonjudgmental when dealing with patients and their families, and to ensure that personal values do not affect communication with others. At times, this may be difficult, especially when one is communicating with a person who has been identified as an abuser of a child, a spouse, or an elderly person.

A patient's values can also influence our behavior when they conflict with our own values.

SCENARIO

A patient is admitted with internal bleeding; his religion prohibits him from receiving a blood transfusion. Janet, an HUC, states that she cannot understand how anyone could risk his or her life because of a silly religious belief. The patient has a right to his own values and the right to refuse treatment.

Conversation and statements made at the nursing station or anywhere in the hospital may be overheard. Health care professionals must be aware of what they say and judgments that they make.

SCENARIO

Susan, an HUC working in the pediatric intensive care unit, says to John, a registered nurse (RN) who is taking care of a 5-year-old little girl on life support after a near drowning, "Why don't her parents take her off of life support, she is like a vegetable!" The little girl's father overhears the comment, approaches Susan, and says, "Young lady, I hope you never have to make that decision." Susan is devastated.

VALUES CLARIFICATION

Values clarification is an important tool for HUCs to use in their preparation to become competent professionals. Examining one's values and committing to a virtuous value system will assist

one in making ethical decisions. It is essential for HUCs to understand and be aware of their values and to remain nonjudgmental of the values others hold that differ from their own. Value conflicts include cultural, spiritual, social, and ethnic differences.

EXERCISE 3

This exercise is intended to guide you in examining your feelings and values related to future employment in health care. Complete the following sentences:

1. A patient has the right to

   _____

2. The health care team works best when

   _____

3. I fail to show respect for others' values when

   _____

4. The most difficult situation to deal with would be

   _____

5. When communicating with patients and families, it is important to

   _____

WORK ETHICS

Work ethics refers to a person's moral values regarding work. It is essential that the HUC have the following work ethic traits.

Behavior Traits That Make Up a Person's Work Ethics

Dependability: Patients and members of the health care team rely on you to report to work when scheduled and to be on time. You are also depended upon to perform duties and tasks as assigned and to keep obligations and promises. Adequate sleep and abstinence from drugs are essential to maintain your dependability. Lack of sleep, use of illegal drugs, or misuse of prescription drugs would clearly endanger patients.

Accountability: Part of being dependable is being accountable. Accountability is taking responsibility for your actions (i.e., being answerable to someone for something you have done). HUCs must be aware of and never exceed their **scope of practice**. If you are unable to report to work or to do your job, it is your responsibility to communicate this to the staffing office at least 2 hours before your scheduled shift.

Consideration: Be considerate of the physical condition and emotional state of the patients and your coworkers.

Cheerfulness: Greet and converse with patients and others in a pleasant manner. HUCs cannot bring personal problems to work. Sarcasm, moodiness, and bad tempers are inappropriate in the workplace.

Empathy: Make every attempt to see things from the viewpoint of patients, families, and coworkers. Keep in mind that stress and worry can affect people's behavior, so refrain from treating a display of anger or frustration as a personal attack.

Trustworthiness: Your employer, patients, and coworkers have placed their confidence in you to keep patient information confidential. HUCs have access to a lot of information and must not engage in gossip regarding patients, coworkers, physicians, or the hospital.

Respectfulness: Respect is a primary value in health care and can be shown in many ways, including tone of voice, body language, **attitude** toward others, and attitude about work. All life is worthy of respect. We all have a right to our own value system and must respect that others have a right to theirs. Make every attempt to understand the values and beliefs of your patients and coworkers that may differ from your own.

Courtesy: Be polite and courteous to patients, families, visitors, coworkers, and supervisors. Address people by name (e.g., Mrs. Johnson, Dr. Smith). Other courteous acts include saying "please" and "thank you" and not interrupting when others are speaking.

Tactfulness: Be sensitive to the problems and needs of others. Be aware of what you say and how you say it.

Conscientiousness: Be careful, alert, and accurate in following orders and instructions. Never attempt to perform a procedure or a task that you have not been trained or licensed to perform.

Honesty: Be sincere, truthful, and genuine, and show a true interest in your relationships with patients, families, visitors, and coworkers. If you make an error, bring it to the attention of the appropriate person(s). Never attempt to cover up an error!

Cooperation: Be willing to work with others, especially in the team-oriented climate of health care. When coworkers work as a team, everyone involved benefits.

Attitude: Attitude is a manner of thought or feeling that can be seen by others when they are observing your behavior. The tone of your voice and your body language can change the message you are trying to send. Your attitude will be reflected in your work. Be positive about your job and the contribution that you are making.

AN OVERVIEW OF THE HEALTH INSURANCE PORTABILITY AND ACCOUNTABILITY ACT OF 1996 (HIPAA)

The American Health Insurance Portability and Accountability Act of 1996 (HIPAA) is a set of rules to be followed by doctors, hospitals, and other health care providers. The purpose of this law is to protect private individual health information from being disclosed to anyone without the consent of the individual. Except under unusual circumstances, consent must be given in writing. Private information can be used in research studies if it is "de-individualized," so that the identity of the individual cannot be ascertained from the information disclosed.

Under HIPAA, individuals have the right to:

- notice of the health provider's privacy practices
- request restrictions on who is allowed to access their health information

- access, inspect, or copy their personal health information
- request an accounting of all disclosures of their health information
- request corrections or amendments to their health information

Health care providers are required to:

- provide security for both paper and electronic individual health information
- institute a complaint process to investigate complaints
- train staff regarding the law

HIPAA Patient Privacy Rule

The HIPAA Patient Privacy Rule contained in the Health Insurance Portability and Accountability Act was implemented on April 14, 2003. The Patient Privacy Rule establishes regulations for the use and disclosure of *protected health information (PHI)* and mandates that all patients be provided a copy of privacy policies when treated in a doctor's office or when admitted to any health care facility. When admitted to the hospital, patients will be given a facility directory opt-out form to sign that indicates whether they wish to be listed in the hospital directory (Fig. 6-1). If the patient chooses not to be listed, their chart is labeled *no information/no publication (NINP)*, meaning that no information will be provided to anyone who calls, including stating that the patient is in the hospital.

HIPAA Security Rule

The Security Rule is a key part of HIPAA that became effective as of April 21, 2003. This rule applies to electronic protected health information (EPHI), which is individually identifiable heath information (IIHI) in electronic form. IIHI relates to (1) an individual's past, present, or future physical or mental health or condition, (2) an individual's provision of health care, and (3) past, present, or future payment provided for provision of health care to an individual. The primary objective of the Security Rule is to protect the **confidentiality**, integrity, and availability of EPHI when it is stored, maintained, or transmitted. Covered entities (CEs) must comply with the Security Rule. These include health plans (e.g., health maintenance organizations [HMOs], group health plans), health care clearinghouses (e.g., billing and repricing companies), and health care providers (e.g., doctors, dentists, hospitals) who transmit any EPHI.

The HUC has access to a great deal of PHI and IIHI because of the very nature of the job; this information must be treated with absolute confidentiality by all health personnel. All health care personnel are required to sign a confidentiality agreement upon initiation of employment.

A HUC has two responsibilities in ensuring the confidentiality of patient information: (1) to avoid verbally repeating confidential information, and (2) to control the patient's paper chart or manage the patient's electronic record in a manner that ensures confidentiality of its contents.

Following are basic guidelines that will help you establish discipline regarding confidentiality of patient information.

FACILITY DIRECTORY OPT OUT FORM

☐ I hereby request that my name, location, general condition, and religious affiliation NOT BE INCLUDED in the facility directory. By invoking this right, I understand that people inquiring by phone or in person will be told, "*I have no information about this patient.*" No deliveries, except U.S. Mail, will be forwarded to me (e.g., flowers).

- -

☐ I hereby request that my name, location, and general condition be released ONLY to those persons listed below. No deliveries, except U.S. Mail, will be forwarded to me (e.g., flowers). (Religious affiliation, if any, will only be provided to clergy.)

_____   _____

_____   _____

- -

☐ I hereby request that my name, location, and general condition be released to anyone EXCEPT those persons listed below. No deliveries, except U.S. Mail, will be forwarded to me (e.g., flowers). (Religious affiliation, if any, will only be provided to clergy.)

_____   _____

_____   _____

- -

☐ I hereby request that my name, location, general condition and religious affiliation BE PLACED in the facility directory.

PRINT PATIENT NAME: _____ DATE: _____

PATIENT SIGNATURE: _____ DATE: _____

WITNESS SIGNATURE: _____

Form to be forwarded or faxed to Admitting Department.

File original in permanent medical record.

Figure 6-1 Facility directory opt-out form.

Guidelines for Maintaining Patient Confidentiality

Do not discuss patient information (other than what is necessary to care for the patient). All patient information is confidential. Some information, such as that about sexual preferences or sexually transmitted diseases, is so confidential that it is obvious to treat it as such; however, other information, such as the patient's age, weight, or test results, may be more difficult to identify as confidential material. Remember: Never discuss any patient information except when necessary for treatment reasons.

Conduct conversations with other health care personnel outside of the hearing distance of patients and visitors. Do not hold conversations about patient information in the hallways or cafeteria, or away from the hospital. Be aware of the identity of others who are at the nurses' station during discussions regarding patients. Often, overheard bits of information may be misconstrued by patients or visitors, and this could result in unnecessary concern. Even if the medical information is factual, it can produce unnecessary worry, anxiety, or even panic in a patient, family member, or visitor.

Do not discuss medical treatment with the patient or relatives (unless specifically instructed to do so by the doctor or the nurse).

Do not discuss general patient information. Often, hospital personnel, other patients, visitors, or your own friends, relatives, or neighbors may ask you questions regarding a specific patient (especially if the patient is a celebrity) out of curiosity. Politely refuse to give out the information, and then quickly change the discussion to another subject.

Do not discuss hospital incidents away from the nursing unit. Discussing code arrest procedures, unexpected death, and similar information with persons other than health professionals or within hearing distance of others may instill fear in them regarding health care; such apprehension may even cause them to delay necessary health treatment in the future.

Refer all telephone calls from reporters, police personnel, legal agencies, and other investigative sources to the nurse manager. If in doubt about the authenticity of a telephone caller, obtain information from the caller so the call may be returned. After the caller's identity has been confirmed, the person may be called back.

Guidelines for Maintaining Confidentiality of the Patient's Paper Chart

Follow the hospital policy for duplicating portions of the patient's chart. Duplication of the patient's chart forms may be the responsibility of the HUC or the health records department of the hospital. (Read the hospital policy and procedure manual to determine policy regarding copying a patient's chart.)

Control access to the patient's chart. Only authorized persons, such as doctors and hospital personnel, should have access to the chart. Always know the status of the person who is using the chart at the nurses' station. Do not give a chart to someone on request because they "look like a doctor." Should relatives or friends of a patient request to see the chart, do not give it to them under any circumstance. If a patient requests to see their chart, advise the patient that you will notify the nurse and/or doctor. A patient has a legal right to see their own chart, but the doctor may need to write an order, and the doctor or the nurse will go over the information in the chart with the patient.

Ask outside agency personnel for picture identification. Reviewers for insurance companies have the responsibility of examining patient charts to ensure that tests, procedures, and hospital days will be paid for by the patients' insurance. Social workers from protective services also need to review patient charts when investigating possible abuse. It is the responsibility of outside agency personnel to show the HUC picture identification; if they fail to do this, the HUC must ask to see identification.

Control transportation of the patient's chart. Never send the patient's chart to another department through the pneumatic tube system. Do not give patients their charts to hold while they are being transported from one area of the hospital to another.

Managing the Patient's Electronic Medical Record

Access to the patient's EMR may be limited. The HUC is privy to demographic protected patient information and will be responsible for scanning reports, hand written progress notes, etc. It is the responsibility of the HUC to protect and maintain the patient's confidentiality by being aware of who is in the nursing station looking over their shoulder and/or eavesdropping on conversations.

WORKPLACE APPEARANCE

Professional appearance will earn the trust, respect, and confidence of one's employer, coworkers, patients, and others. A professional appearance also demonstrates self-confidence and sends a message that one respects himself and his position. Follow the dress code outlined in the policy and procedure manual of the facility where you work. All employees represent the facility for which they work; patients and visitors gain their first impressions of a facility through the appearance of its employees (Fig. 6-2).

Guidelines for Workplace Appearance

Female: Clothes or uniforms should fit well, should be modest in length and style, and above all should be clean, mended, and wrinkle free. Color and design of undergarments should not be visible through your clothes or uniform. When business dress is called for, slacks or skirts are appropriate with a blouse or sweater. Denim is usually not acceptable.

Male: Slacks and shirt or sweater should fit well, and they should be clean and pressed.

Female and Male: Shoes should be clean and appropriate, as defined in the dress code. Most facilities do not allow open-toe or open-heel shoes. Most nursing personnel wear white tennis shoes (not hightops) for comfort.

Female: Socks/stockings should be worn, especially with a skirt or dress.

Male: Socks should be worn.

Female and Male: Jewelry worn should be modest. Body piercing may or may not be acceptable in your chosen place of employment. Some earrings will interfere with talking on the telephone. Good taste is the key.

Female and Male: *Tattoos may or may not be acceptable in your chosen place of employment. Again, good* taste is called for.

Female and Male: Hair should be clean and well groomed. Control long hair to keep it out of your face and off of your collar.

Female: Sculptured nails and nail polish are not acceptable for health care workers. Sculptured nails and chipped nail polish provide a place for microorganisms to grow.

Female: Makeup should be modest in amount and color.

Female: Perfumes, colognes, and hair spray should be very light or not worn at all.

Male: Aftershave, colognes, and hair spray should be very light or not worn at all. Patients with respiratory problems, allergies, or nausea could experience ill effects from the aroma.

EMPLOYMENT ISSUES

Pre-Clinical/Employment Requirements

Drug Testing

A urine drug test is required for all students and employees prior to starting a clinical experience or employment in the hospital. Notify the testing agency if you are taking any prescribed medication for pain or sleep that may be detected on the drug screen. Do not drink an excessive amount of water prior to the urine drug test because when the urine is diluted, you may need to repeat the test at your expense.

Fingerprinting and Background Checks

Most health care agencies require a fingerprinting card and a background check prior to a clinical experience and/or employment. Always be honest about any convictions because these will be discovered in the background check, and not disclosing would be viewed as dishonest. If there is a problem in one's background, one may add, "will discuss during the interview."

Immunizations

Immunizations are required prior to a clinical experience or employment; these usually include an MMR (measles, mumps, and rubella), a tuberculosis (TB) skin test, and a hepatitis screen.

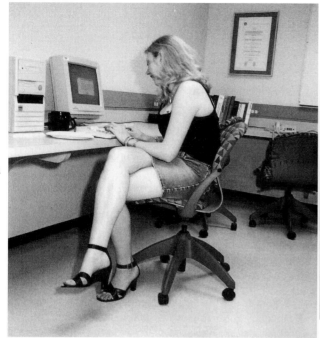

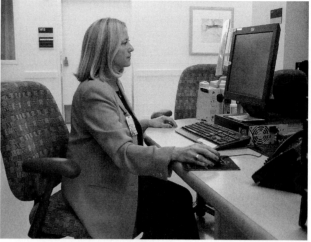

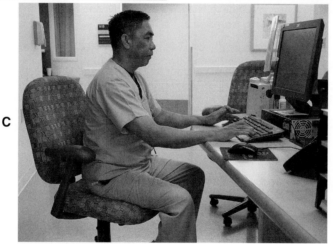

Figure 6-2 **A,** This HUC is inappropriately dressed. **B,** This HUC is appropriately dressed in business attire. **C,** This HUC is appropriately dressed in scrubs.

If you have a positive TB skin test, a chest x-ray will be required. A TB skin test is required annually while one is employed at a health care facility.

Signed HIPAA Confidentiality Statement

In compliance with the HIPAA law of 1996, all health care students and employees are required to sign a confidentiality statement prior to beginning a clinical experience or employment. By signing this statement, the student or employee agrees not to discuss or review any information regarding a patient unless the discussion or review is part of the assignment. Students or employees also state that they understand that they are obligated to know and adhere to the privacy policies and procedures of the health care facility. Signing the confidentiality statement is an acknowledgment that medical records, accounting information, patient information, and conversations between or among health care professionals about patients are confidential under law and this agreement.

TJC (The Joint Commission) Required Pre-Clinical/ Employment and Annual In-services

Prior to a clinical experience or employment, TJC requires the following:

CPR (cardiopulmonary resuscitation) training
Fire and safety in-service
Infectious disease in-service
HIPAA in-service

Health care facilities provide classes, handouts, or videos with posttests for the in-services.

Drug Test for Cause

If the smell of alcohol is detected on a student's/employee's breath, or if inappropriate behavior is observed, a drug test may be requested by the supervisor or the instructor. If the student or employee refuses the drug test, she will be sent home and most likely will be terminated from the HUC program or employment.

Cell Phone Use

Almost everyone owns a cell phone; some find it difficult to be without their cell phone. Everyone has encountered the rudeness of those cell phone users who talk loudly while standing in the middle of the walkway at the mall, blocking doorways while talking on the phone, talking loudly in restaurants while others are trying to have a quiet meal, or talking while driving, thereby slowing traffic down and not paying attention. Cell phones are heard ringing in hospitals, movie theaters, school classes, airplanes, and even at funerals. Some often forget about others' personal space, boundaries, and apologies. Cell phones are banned for personal use on hospital units. Ringing cell phones and conversations are annoying and distracting to nursing unit personnel, as well as to patients in nearby rooms.

Cell phones should be turned off while one is working on the nursing unit. Calls recorded on voice mail may be listened to during breaks. If an important call is expected, phones may be placed on vibrate and taken off of the nursing unit. Text messaging is also banned while one is working on the nursing unit. Full attention is expected and should be given to your work responsibilities.

General Guidelines for Using a Cell Phone

- Respect people in close proximity (speak softer, turn cell phone off when appropriate to do so, and pay attention to your surroundings).
- When in a public place, keep conversations brief. Remember you are a professional.
- Spend time with family and friends, not with a phone.
- Follow rules for cell phone use in hospitals, schools, and airplanes, and while pumping gas.
- Do not drive while using a cell phone.

Elevator Etiquette

Hospital elevators are very busy places, and it is important to know appropriate elevator etiquette. When the elevator button light is lit, it is not necessary to continue to push the button; this may be causing the door to close on someone on another floor who is trying to enter or exit the elevator. When the elevator does arrive, stand aside and allow people to exit before you try to enter. When you are riding on an elevator and are going to a higher floor in the building, stand to the side or in the back, so others may exit on their floors. Patients who are being transported on stretchers and personnel who are pushing hospital equipment have priority for using elevators.

Attendance, Punctuality, and Appropriate Breaks

Guidelines regarding attendance, punctuality, and breaks are provided by the employer in an employment packet during orientation. It is essential that nursing unit personnel work as a team, and that each member of the team is reliable and acts in a responsible, professional manner. When a student is completing their clinical experience on a nursing unit, this should be viewed as an extended evaluation or appraisal period. A student's preceptor and the other nursing unit personnel will be continually appraising the student's knowledge, attendance, punctuality, and professionalism. A student can also evaluate the health care facility while making an employment decision.

Sexual Harassment

Sexual harassment is defined as unwanted and unwelcome behavior that is sexual in nature. There are two forms of sexual harassment: (1) *quid pro quo*, which involves making conditions of employment (e.g., hiring, promotion, retention) contingent on the victim's providing sexual favors, and (2) a hostile working environment, which is an environment that a *reasonable person* would find hostile and abusive.

Victims of harassment may feel intimidated, anxious, angry, ashamed, and/or helpless. Often, sexual harassment is not reported because the victim believes "no action would be taken" against the perpetrator, fears **retaliation**, or has concern for the abuser.

If feeling harassed, health care workers should (1) advise the person to stop, that they do not like or welcome this behavior, (2) document the comments and behavior of the person, and (3) file a complaint with the supervisor or with management.

Violence in the Workplace

Violence has increased in our society and in the workplace—perhaps, in part, because of overcrowding, political and social differences, and other issues. Workplace violence may be defined as violent acts (including physical assaults and threats of assault) directed toward persons at work or on duty. Physical assaults include attacks ranging from slapping and beating to the use of weapons. Threats are expressions of intent to cause harm; these include verbal threats, threatening body language, and written threats.

When a patient is admitted to the hospital as a victim of gang-related or domestic violence, a restraining order is often put in place to prohibit individuals responsible for the violence from having any contact with the patient. Often, the patient has an "NINP" (no information, no publication) order written on the chart. This would require the HUC or anyone who answers the phone to deny any information about that patient, including the patient's presence in the hospital. The patient's name would not be listed on the census board, would not be posted outside the room, and would not be written on the outside of the chart. Usually, an alias would be used to avoid visitor suspicion. A code word or phrase is given to the patient's family, so the health care worker can know that a person is authorized to visit the patient. All telephone calls from reporters, police personnel, legal agencies, and other investigative sources should be referred to the nurse manager.

The HUC is able to see most of what is happening on the nursing unit from their location at the nurses' station. The HUC must be alert to signals that may be associated with impending violence. Signals of impending violence may include the following:

- Verbally expressed anger and frustration
- Body language, such as threatening gestures
- Signs of drug or alcohol use
- Presence of a weapon

- The presence of someone who has a restraining order that prohibits them from being there

The HUC should not approach the threatening person but should present a calm attitude and should call security immediately.

Agencies That Investigate Abuse

All states have mandatory reporting laws for suspected child or elder abuse. Some states have mandatory reporting laws for domestic abuse. Child Protective Services (CPS) will be called to investigate suspected child abuse (SNAT, suspected nonaccidental trauma). Adult Protective Services (APS) will be called in to investigate elder or domestic abuse. Social workers from these agencies must show picture identification to the HUC before looking at a patient's chart. If the social worker fails to do this, it is the responsibility of the HUC to ask for identification. It is important to keep this information strictly confidential and to remain nonjudgmental when interacting with family members.

Employee Performance Evaluations

After an employee is hired, during and after training, they must be evaluated. The performance evaluation (also called a performance appraisal) is the ongoing process of evaluating the employee's job performance. This process should provide both positive feedback and suggestions on how to improve in areas where improvement is needed. The basic purposes of the evaluation process are to provide feedback and to make compensation decisions (concerning salary increases). It would be helpful to the HUC and to the nurse manager for the employee to keep a record of accomplishments, classes taken, and in-services attended during the evaluation period.

Often, supervisors ask their employees to complete an evaluation form to assess their own performance. This provides an opportunity for you to let your supervisors know how valuable you are to the organization. Do not be modest, but do be honest regarding your contributions and accomplishments. Performance evaluations are placed in the employee's file.

JOB APPLICATIONS, RESUMÉS, AND INTERVIEWS

Job Applications

Prior to completing a job application, assemble information and make a fact sheet, or take a resumé with you that can be used as a reference. A resumé may also be provided to the employer, if requested. It is important for you to enter accurate information, including correct dates. Have a list of work-related references (check with references to make sure they are comfortable with being called) with you in case you are asked to provide them.

General guidelines for completing a job application include the following:

- Follow directions carefully.
- Be neat, and be sure of dates and spelling (if possible, type or use black ink).
- When there are gaps in employment, explain (e.g., "raising children," "returned to school"). If you were doing anything for pay during this time, write "self-employed."

- When stating a reason for leaving your last job, make it sound positive (e.g., "returned to school," "decided on a career change").
- If you have little work experience, emphasize other strengths. List volunteer jobs.
- List the most recent work or educational experience first, not last.
- When asked the pay that you desire, do not identify a specific amount. It is often best to write "open" or "negotiable."
- If you did not graduate, write "attended" and list the institutions.
- Be honest.

Spaces left blank may cause concern. Always be honest regarding any convictions. Write, "Will discuss in interview." If a discrepancy is discovered, this will most likely result in your not being granted a job interview.

Resumés

The purpose of a resumé is to get an interview; it is hoped that the interview will result in your getting a job. The resumé is a marketing tool intended to create interest in one's abilities and potential. A resumé does its job successfully if it does not exclude one from consideration. Read time for a resumé (time spent by human resources when deciding to or not to interview) is about 10 seconds. A good resumé should be short, simple, and easy to read while gaining the reader's interest and revealing your value to the potential employer. Before writing a resumé, take time to do a self-assessment on paper. Outline skills and abilities, as well as work experiences and extracurricular activities. This will make it easier for you to prepare a thorough resumé.

General guidelines for creating a resumé include the following:

- Type using a simple font such as Times New Roman, 12 point (avoid using fancy type such as outline, shadow, script, or other difficult to read styles).
- Use standard 8.5 × 11″ paper in white, ivory, or gray (avoid flashy colors).
- Keep a 1-inch margin on all four sides.
- Limit resume to one page, if possible.
- Single space within sections.
- Double space between sections.
- Bold, underline, or capitalize section headings to make them stand out.
- Use everyday language; be specific. Give examples.
- Do a spelling and grammar check.
- Produce quality photocopies.

Your resumé should include the following:

- Name, address, telephone, e-mail address, website address
- Objective or summary (be specific about the job wanted. For example: "To obtain an HUC position within a health care facility to apply my organizational skills and medical knowledge").
- Education (new graduates without a lot of work experience should list their educational information first). List most recent education first. Add grade point average (GPA) if higher than 3.0. List NAHUC (National Association of Health Unit Coordinators) certification, if applicable.

- Work experience (briefly describe work experience, including specific duties performed). List most recent work experience first. Be accurate with dates of employment.
- Other information (may include special skills or competencies, such as being bilingual or leadership experience in volunteer organizations). Your instructor can advise you on other information to add to your resumé.
- References (ask people if they are willing to serve as references before giving their names to a potential employer). Do not include reference information on your resumé. Note at the bottom of resumé should read, "References furnished on request."

Interviews

An interview can be very stressful. Take three deep breaths prior to starting an interview to relax. Think positively about your skills and abilities, and imagine yourself working in the position. First impressions are lasting ones, so be sure your appearance and posture demonstrate professionalism. Do not give the interviewer a reason to rule you out because you didn't take the time to look your best.

Guidelines for successful interviews include the following:

- Arrive on time (at least one-half hour early).
- Stand until you are asked to sit down.
- Project a positive attitude and confidence (make eye contact with interviewer).
- Be aware of the job description for the position for which you are applying.
- Give a firm handshake.
- Listen attentively to questions.
- Keep answers brief and to the point.
- Use body language to show interest.
- Smile, nod, and give nonverbal feedback to the interviewer.
- Ask about the next step in the process.
- Thank the interviewer.
- Write a thank you letter to anyone you have spoken to.
- Follow up with a telephone call if you do not hear back from the interviewer in 3 days.

HEALTH CARE ETHICS

Ethics is that part of **philosophy** that deals with judgments about what is right or wrong in given situations. Each health

---

NAHUC CODE OF ETHICS

1. Members shall conduct themselves in such a manner as to gain the respect and confidence of patients, health care personnel, and the community, and shall respect the human dignity of each individual.
2. Members shall protect patients' rights, including their right to privacy.
3. Members shall strive to achieve and maintain a high level of competency.
4. Members shall strive to improve their knowledge and skills by participating in educational and professional activities and sharing the benefits of their attainments with their colleagues.
5. Unethical and illegal professional activities shall be reported to the appropriate authorities.

---

care profession has a **code of ethics** that has been derived from a set of basic **principles** that define the concepts of right or wrong for that profession. NAHUC has an established code of ethics (see the Box *NAHUC Code of Ethics*).

Patient Care Partnership/Patients' Bill of Rights

The American Hospital Association (AHA) approved the first patients' bill of rights in 1973. The expectation was that observance of these rights would result in more effective patient care and greater satisfaction for the patient, the patient's physician, and the health care organization. The AHA has since published the *The Patient Care Partnership*, which includes "Understanding Expectations and Rights and Responsibilities." In summary, patient expectations and rights include high-quality hospital care, a clean and safe environment, involvement in care, protection of privacy, help when leaving the hospital, and help with billing claims. The patients' bill of rights has been adopted and modified many times. In 1998, an Advisory Commission on Consumer Protection and Quality in the Health Care Industry appointed by the President of the United States issued a Patients' Bill of Rights (see the Box *Patients' Bill of Rights*). The Joint Commision now requires that all hospitals have a bill of rights and a notice of the facility's privacy practices. Copies must be given to each patient or parent of the patient on admission. Additionally, a copy of the bill of rights should be posted at entrances and in other prominent places throughout the hospital. The patients' bill of rights varies in wording among hospitals, but all are based on the following basic ethical principles.

Ethical Principles for Patient Care
Respect

This principle declares that the patient has the right to considerate and respectful care. Respect is to hold in esteem or honor and to show a feeling of appreciation and regard. Health care workers must provide services with respect for human dignity and the uniqueness of each patient, unrestricted by considerations of social or economic status, personal attributes, or the nature of health problems.

Autonomy

This principle means that an individual is free to choose and implement his own decisions. From this basic principle, we have derived the rule involved in **informed consent**.

The patients' bill of rights states that a patient has the right to refuse treatment to the extent permitted by law and to be informed of the medical consequences of that choice. This right does not judge the quality of a decision by a patient's decision to refuse treatment; it only states that the patient has the right to make the decision. This is the process of **autonomy** at work.

Veracity

The principle of veracity requires both the health care professional and the patient to tell the truth. The health care professional must disclose the truth so the patient can practice autonomy; the patient must be truthful so that appropriate care can be given. Although in some situations, health care professionals may feel justified in lying to a patient to avoid some greater harm, other alternatives must be sought. Lying will almost always harm patient autonomy and cause the potential loss of credibility of the provider.

Beneficence

This is the principle that any action a health care professional takes should benefit the patient. This principle creates an ethical dilemma for clinical practitioners more than it does for HUCs. The dilemma arises because of the advanced technology that is available to practitioners today. In cases where a patient is maintained on life support machines and is in a coma or a vegetative state, is it of benefit to maintain the patient on machines?

Nonmaleficence

This principle, which comes from the Hippocratic Oath, means that a health care professional will never inflict harm on the patient. Although similar to the principle of beneficence, it differs in that beneficence indicates a positive action promoting good. In nonmaleficence, the principle is to refrain from inflicting harm. HUCs should always be aware of the seriousness of transcribing doctors' orders because an error may result in harm to the patient.

Confidentiality

Principle 2 of the NAHUC Code of Ethics and the American Hospital Association's "A Patient's Bill of Rights" outline the individual's right to privacy in health care. HUCs who breach the confidentiality of a patient's medical record have not only violated ethical standards, but may well have violated the law.

Interconnection Between Ethical and Legal Issues

Ethical issues and legal issues often become intertwined in the health care context. An ethical dilemma is a situation that presents a conflicting moral claim—a situation that is at odds with one's personal system of values. Sometimes conflicts can occur between what is legal and what is ethical. For example, assume you are working in a gynecology clinic and a patient comes in for an abortion. You may believe that abortions should not be performed and are unethical. However, abortions are legal in our country.

To deal with these situations as an HUC, you must learn to examine your values and be aware of how they affect your work. All health care professionals must learn methods of reasoning through ethical dilemmas rather than reacting to them emotionally. Issues that may arise and cause conflict are usually situations involving the privacy rights of patients or the unprofessional conduct of a fellow health care worker.

In any of the potential problem areas you may encounter as an HUC, you must apply good judgment, honesty, and reasoning to come up with a moral and ethical way to resolve the conflict.

LEGAL CONCEPTS

The law is derived from three sources: (1) the constitution—both federal and state constitutions, (2) **statutes**—written laws drawn up by the legislature, and (3) common law—a case-by-case determination by a judge of what is fair under a given

---

PATIENTS' BILL OF RIGHTS

I Information Disclosure
You have the right to receive accurate and easily understood information about your health plan, health care professionals, and health care facilities. If you speak another language, have a physical or mental disability, or just do not understand something, assistance will be provided so you can make informed health care decisions.

II Choice of Providers and Plans
You have the right to a choice of health care providers that is sufficient to provide you with access to appropriate high-quality health care.

III Access to Emergency Services
If you have severe pain, an injury, or a sudden illness that convinces you that your health is in serious jeopardy, you have the right to receive screening and stabilization emergency services whenever and wherever needed, without prior authorization or financial penalty.

IV Participation in Treatment Decisions
You have the right to know all your treatment options and to participate in decisions about your care. Parents, guardians, family members, or other individuals that you designate can represent you if you cannot make your own decisions.

V Respect and Nondiscrimination
You have a right to considerate, respectful, and nondiscriminatory care from your doctors, health plan representatives, and other health care providers.

VI Confidentiality of Health Information
You have the right to talk in confidence with health care providers and to have your health care information protected. You also have the right to review and copy your own medical record and to request that your physician amend your record if it is not accurate, relevant, or complete.

VII Complaints and Appeals
You have the right to a fair, fast, and objective review of any complaint you may have against your health plan, doctors, hospitals, or other health care personnel. This includes complaints about waiting times, operating hours, the conduct of health care personnel, and the adequacy of health care facilities.

From the Advisory Commission on Consumer Protection and Quality in the Health Care Industry, 1998. Available at: http://www.consumer.gov/qualityhealth/rights.htm

set of facts. Laws are subject to change, but common law is especially changeable because each case presented to a judge is different. Judges look to cases that have been decided previously for guidance on how to rule in a particular situation. However, a judge is free to interpret the law in cases where no precedent exists, or to interpret against precedent. Most medical **negligence** or **medical malpractice** law is derived from common law. This means that medical negligence law, similar to other forms of common law, is constantly in a state of change.

Standard of Practice for the Health Unit Coordinator

While working as an HUC, one is responsible for performing at the level of competence of other HUCs who work under similar circumstances. This responsibility is one's legal duty as a health care professional and is the *standard of practice* to which this professional will be held. If one does not carry out this duty and a patient is injured as a result, the HUC may have been negligent of their duty and may be held liable for these actions (see the Box *Standards of Practice for Health Unit Coordinators*).

The standard of practice is established by **expert witness** testimony. For our purposes, an expert is a person who is trained in the HUC profession and who testifies at trial as to what a reasonably prudent HUC would have done under the circumstances in question. **Evidence** of the **standard of care** may also be found in textbooks, standards from NAHUC, policy and procedure manuals, or standards of the Joint Commision. This means that one must keep up with current practices in the profession, read current literature, be familiar with hospital policies and procedures that affect the HUC job, and know the current job description and the duties it details.

The standard of care for which the HUC is responsible becomes higher with increased experience and education. The actions of an HUC will be compared with those of a reasonably prudent HUC with the same experience and education under the same circumstances.

The role of the HUC has expanded broadly over the past 5 years. You are now recognized as an essential member of the health care team. Incidental to this greater recognition and expanding responsibility is an increased **accountability**. There is a **liability** dimension to accountability. The HUC may be held legally responsible for judgments exercised and actions taken in the course of practice.

MEDICAL MALPRACTICE

Medical malpractice is the professional negligence of a health care professional; the failure to meet a professional standard of care, resulting in harm to another; or the failure to provide, for example, "good and accepted medical care." According to the National Academy of Science, approximately 98,000 Americans die from "medical mistakes" each year. Each member of the nursing team is responsible for their actions. If the HUC is not sure about what the doctor has written because the handwriting is illegible, the doctor's orders must be clarified before they are transcribed. It may be necessary to call the doctor for clarification.

Negligence

Negligence is a legal term that means that someone failed to perform their legal duty satisfactorily, and another person was injured in some way because of that failure. This breach of duty is said to have occurred when something was done that should not have been done, or when something should have been done but was not. Either way, the person responsible for the duty is liable for whatever injury was suffered by the innocent party.

STANDARDS OF PRACTICE FOR HEALTH UNIT COORDINATORS

Standard 1: Education
Health unit coordinator personnel shall be prepared through appropriate education and training programs for their responsibility in the provision of nondirect patient care and non-clinical services.

Standard 2: Policy and Procedure
Written standards of HUCs' practice and related policies and procedures shall define and describe the scope and conduct of non-clinical services provided by the HUC. These standards, policies, and procedures shall be reviewed annually and revised as necessary. These revisions will be dated to indicate the last review, signed by the responsible authority, and will be implemented.

Standard 3: Standards of Performance
Written evaluation of HUCs shall be criteria based and related to the standards of performance as defined by the health care organization.

Standard 4: Communication
The HUC shall appropriately and effectively communicate with nursing and medical staff, all ancillary departments, visitors, guests, and patients.

Standard 5: Professionalism and Ethics
The HUC shall take all possible measures to ensure the optimal quality of nondirect, non-clinical patient care. Optimal professional and ethical conduct and practices of members of the National Association of Health Unit Coordinators shall be maintained at all times.

Standard 6: Leadership
The HUC shall be organized to meet and maintain established standards of non-clinical services.

For instance, one of the duties of an HUC is to transcribe doctors' orders accurately and promptly. If negligent in doing so—that is, if the orders are not transcribed properly or are not transcribed at all—the HUC may be responsible for a patient's injury that results from negligence.

Liability

Legally, each person is responsible for their own acts. When those acts are negligent and are performed during the course and scope of employment as an HUC, they have special ramifications.

The hospital is also liable for an employee's negligence on the job because of the legal doctrine *respondeat superior* (which means, "let the master respond"). This means that the employee and the hospital are held responsible for negligent acts of employees while on the job. Remember that the hospital is liable for the employee's actions only when they occur within the course and scope of employment. If the negligent act is a result of conduct outside the scope of employment (i.e., outside of the job description), the employee alone is held responsible.

The *respondeat superior* doctrine does not take away one's personal liability, but rather, creates an additional party for the injured person to hold responsible for the damages incurred.

PERMANENT LEGAL DOCUMENTS

A patient's chart contains their medical records and permanent legal documents on file at the hospital. All documentation is written in ink, and no erasures are allowed.

Because the medical record is the legal record of the patient's medical course, the HUC must treat it with special care and confidentiality. Only authorized persons may read patients' charts or have access to them. This protection of the legal record is part of one's duty as an HUC.

Informed Consent

An informed consent documents that the person signing it has been informed of the risks and characteristics of a planned procedure and understands them. The witness to signing of the consent by the patient or guardian must date and sign the consent. Telephone consents require that two health care personnel listen to the verbal consent given via the telephone, and that those personnel sign as witnesses. Preparation of informed consents and other types of consents is discussed in Chapter 8.

What the Health Unit Coodinator Can Do to Avoid Legal Problems

Following are some tips to help one avoid legal problems while working as an HUC:

Know the HUC job description. Do not engage in activities outside *the job description.*

Keep current with the facility's policies and procedures. If the policies and procedures are outdated, bring them to the employer's attention and participate in the revisions.

Keep current in the HUC practice. If called upon to do something that you are not qualified to do, get help and find out how to do it. Remember, a standard of care can be set by medical literature and periodicals. Continued education is a must for all health care workers. Of course, obtain proper training before assuming any professional position.

Do not assume anything. Question orders, policies, and procedures that do not seem appropriate. Do not do something unless you are sure you know how to do it. The biggest safeguard is to ask questions.

Do not perform nursing tasks, even as favors.

Be aware of relationships with patients. Patients who truly feel that you care and have tried to help them to the best of your abilities are less likely to see a lawyer if a problem arises.

KEY CONCEPTS

The modern health care professional is called upon to exercise professional behavior and judgment in many complex situations. By understanding confidentiality, legal duty, and ethical responsibility, one will be able to legally and morally fulfill his or her professional obligations.

REVIEW QUESTIONS

1. List four factors that influence a person's behavior.

a. _____

b. _____

c. _____

d. _____

2. Describe a situation in which a HUC's personal values could influence their interactions on the job.

_____

_____

3. List six behavior traits that make up one's work ethics.

a. _____

b. _____

c. _____

d. _____

e. _____

f. _____

4. Explain the purpose of the Privacy Rule contained in the HIPAA law.

_____

_____

5. Explain what is meant by "protected health information" contained in the HIPAA law.

_____

_____

6. Explain the purpose of the "Security Rule" contained in the HIPAA law.

_____

_____

7. Describe how the HUC may practice confidentiality in the following situations.

a. You are having dinner in the cafeteria with several other health care workers. A famous television star was admitted to your unit yesterday. The talk turns to the patient. You are asked, "Is she really only 35?" "What is her diagnosis?" and other personal questions. What is your response?

_____

_____

b. You are working at the nurses' station and you notice a patient's wife approaching your desk. At the same time, two other members of the hospital staff, unaware of the wife's presence, begin talking about her husband's condition. What do you do?

_____

_____

c. A patient approaches you at the nurses' station and says, "My roommate hasn't eaten anything today. I'm really worried about her. What is she in the hospital for?" How do you answer?

_____

_____

d. A telephone caller says that he is a reporter from the local newspaper and wants to know if a car accident victim was admitted to your nursing unit. What do you tell him?

_____

_____

e. You answer the telephone on the nursing unit. The caller states that he is a relative of the patient and then asks for personal patient information. The patient is hospitalized for a gunshot wound received during a fight and has "NINP" written in his chart. You are somewhat doubtful about the identity of the caller. How do you handle the situation?

_____

_____

f. You are riding home on the bus after work. Another hospital employee sits down beside you and states, "That was quite a code you had on your unit today. What all happened anyway?" How do you respond?

_____

_____

g. You are out in your yard and your neighbor stops to chat with you. During the conversation, your neighbor tells you her friend is in the hospital where you work, on the same nursing unit. The neighbor asks you what is wrong with her friend and how long she will be in the hospital. What do you tell her?

_____

_____

8. Six HUC responsibilities for maintaining confidentiality of patient information are

a. _____

b. _____

c. _____

d. _____

e. _____

f. _____

9. Four guidelines to follow to maintain confidentiality of the contents of a patient's chart are as follows:

a. _____

b. _____

c. _____

d. _____

10. Explain why it is important for the HUC to be professional in their appearance.

_____

_____

11. Identify two types of sexual harassment.

a. _____

b. _____

12. What is the first step to take if you feel someone is making inappropriate, sexually oriented remarks to you?

_____

_____

13. Explain the action you would take if you witnessed a visitor becoming angry and loud with a nurse on the nursing unit.

_____

_____

14. List two purposes of an employee performance evaluation.

a. _____

b. _____

15. What can you do to prepare for a performance evaluation?

_____

_____

16. List four TJC pre-clinical/employment and annual in-service requirements.

a. _____

b. _____

c. _____

d. _____

17. List four additional pre-clinical and preemployment requirements.

a. _____

b. _____

c. _____

d. _____

18. Match the terms in Column 1 with the appropriate phrases in Column 2.

Column 1

_____ 1. accountability
_____ 2. defendant
_____ 3. ethics
_____ 4. expert witness
_____ 5. statute
_____ 6. tort

Column 2

a. judgments of right or wrong
b. having the responsibility to answer for what you have done
c. a wrong that is not a crime
d. a law
e. a person against whom action is brought
f. a witness who has special knowledge
g. a person who brings a lawsuit against another
h. professional negligence
i. responsibility for damages resulting from an injurious act

19. Match the terms in Column 1 with the appropriate phrases in Column 2.

Column 1

_____ 1. statute of limitations
_____ 2. damages
_____ 3. *respondeat superior*
_____ 4. deposition
_____ 5. medical malpractice

_____ 6. standard of care
_____ 7. evidence
_____ 8. informed consent

Column 2

a. testimony of a witness
b. values and rules of conduct
c. pretrial statement of a witness under oath
d. time within which a plaintiff must bring a suit
e. information a patient is entitled to before consenting to an invasive treatment
f. failure to provide "good and accepted medical care"
g. "let the master answer"
h. care that a reasonable and prudent person would have given in a similar situation
i. monetary compensation

20. Indicate whether each statement is true or false.

a. _____ You, as a practicing HUC, are not held legally responsible for your errors in transcription because you are not licensed.

b. _____ It is acceptable to allow all medical personnel to read patients' charts because they understand the confidential nature of their contents.

c. _____ It is acceptable to help a patient to the restroom if you check first to make sure that the patient does not have an order for complete bed rest.

d. _____ You may use your cell phone on the nursing unit if you talk softly.

e. _____ You may use your cell phone on the nursing unit if you text message.

f. _____ A patient who is being transported on a stretcher and hospital personnel who are transporting hospital equipment always have priority for using an elevator.

21. For each of the following, identify the universal principle of medical ethics that is being applied.

a. The HUC safeguards the patient's right to privacy by judiciously protecting confidential information.

Principle involved: _____

b. The HUC maintains competence in Health Unit Coordinating.

Principle involved: _____

c. The HUC provides services with respect for the patient's right to be informed about their medical care.

Principle involved: _____

d. The HUC reports unethical or illegal professional activities that may harm the patient.

Principle involved: _____

e. The HUC participates in the profession's efforts to protect patients from misinformation.

Principle involved: _____

22. Write the two purposes of "A Patient's Bill of Rights."

a. _____

b. _____

23. Identify six preventive measures that you can take to minimize the risk of malpractice within your own practice.

a. _____

b. _____

c. _____

d. _____

e. _____

f. _____

24. List nine guidelines for completing a job application.

a. _____

b. _____

c. _____

d. _____

e. _____

f. _____

g. _____

h. _____

i. _____

25. List 11 guidelines for preparing a resumé.

a. _____

b. _____

c. _____

d. _____

e. _____

f. _____

g. _____

h. _____

i. _____

j. _____

k. _____

26. Explain the importance of dressing appropriately when going for an interview.

_____

_____

_____

27. Explain what the standard of care is for an HUC.

_____

_____

_____

28. Make a list of what is inappropriate in terms of the appearance of the HUC pictured in Figure 6-2, _A._

_____

_____

_____

THINK ABOUT...

1. Discuss what you are looking for in a job, and what you think the employer would be looking for in an employee.
2. Discuss why you chose a career in health care, and why you should be hired into a health care position.
3. Discuss the personal values that guide your daily interactions.
4. Have you experienced a situation that you considered to be sexual harassment? Discuss the action you took and the end result.
5. Discuss possible consequences of a health care worker's discussing a patient's protected health information outside the hospital.

Websites of Interest

http://www.acf.dhhs.gov

http://www.crisisinc.com

http://www.hipaa.org

http://www.jointcommission.org/

http://www.jobweb.com/resumes_interviews

CHAPTER 7

Management Techniques and Problem-Solving Skills for Health Unit Coordinating

CHAPTER OBJECTIVES

Upon completion of this chapter, you will be able to

1. Define the terms in the vocabulary list.
2. Write the meaning of the abbreviations in the abbreviations list.
3. List five areas of management.
4. List the purpose of each of the four reference books and manuals that are available on the nursing unit.
5. Briefly explain a method to record the location of patients and patients' charts, and discuss why it is necessary to keep a record of this information.
6. Describe the responsibilities of the health unit coordinator (HUC) regarding faxing and receiving faxed medical records and reports (with the use of paper charts and with CPOE).
7. List three types of documents that would need to be scanned into a patient's electronic medical record (EMR).
8. Explain why the HUC would need to closely monitor the patient's EMR.
9. List items that may be recorded on the nursing unit census worksheet.

10. List seven steps to follow when dealing with visitors' complaints.
11. Given a list of several HUC tasks, identify those that would have a higher priority and those that would be of lower priority.
12. Explain the importance of the change-of-shift report.
13. List eight time management tips for the health unit coordinator.
14. Define two types of stress, and provide an example of each.
15. List five techniques for dealing with stress on the job.
16. List five additional management tasks that may be assigned to the HUC with the implementation of CPOE.
17. Discuss the purpose of continuous quality improvement.
18. Identify and apply the five-step problem-solving model.
19. Identify two common work-related injuries.
20. Explain five guidelines that could prevent workplace injuries.
21. List four items that should be within reaching distance of the HUC's desk area.

VOCABULARY

Admission, Discharge, and Transfer Log Book (ADT Log Book) Book used to record all admissions, discharges, and transfers on a nursing unit for future reference

Admission, Discharge, and Transfer Sheet (ADT Sheet) Form used to record daily admissions, discharges, and transfers for quick reference and to assist in tracking empty beds

Brainstorming Structured group activity that allows three to ten people to tap into the creativity of the group to identify new ideas. Typically in quality improvement, the technique is used to identify probable causes and possible solutions for quality problems

Census Sheet List of patients' names, room and bed numbers, ages, acuity (level of care), and physicians' names located on a nursing unit (may be printed from a computer menu)

Census Worksheet Form used on a nursing unit that includes a list of each patient's name, room number, and bed number, with blank spaces next to each name. This may be used by the HUC to record patient activities (May also be called a Patient Information Sheet or a Patient Activity Sheet)

Central Service Department Charge Slip Form that is initiated to charge a discharged patient for any items used during their hospital stay that were not charged to the patient at the time of use

Central Service Department Credit Slip Form that is used to credit a patient for items found in the room unused after the patient's discharge, or if a patient was mistakenly charged for an item that was not used

Central Service Department Discrepancy Report List of items that are missing from the nursing unit patient supply cupboard or closet that were not charged to a patient. A discrepancy report is sent to the nursing unit each day from the central service department.

Change-of-Shift Report The communication process between shifts, in which nursing personnel who are going "off duty" report nursing unit activities to personnel coming "on duty" (HUCs may give the report to each other or may listen to the nurse's report)

Continuous Quality Improvement (CQI) The practice of continuously improving quality of each function at each level of every department of the health care organization (also called *total quality management*—or *TQM)*

Crisis Stress A profound effect experienced by individuals and resulting from common, uncontrollable, often unpredictable life experiences (death, divorce, illness, and others)

Ergonomics Branch of ecology that is concerned with human factors in the design and operation of machines and the physical environment

Patient Label Book Book used to store labels for patients when CPOE has been implemented; it is also used to store labels for discharged patients for a short time after the time of their discharge

Perennial Stress The wear and tear of day-to-day living, with the feeling that one is a square peg trying to fit into a round hole

Proactive To take action prior to an event; to use power, freedom, and ability to choose responses to whatever happens to us, on the basis of our values (circumstances do not control us; we control them)

Reactive To take action or respond after an event happens; circumstances are often in control of us

Standard Supply List A computerized or written record of the quantity of each item that the nursing unit currently needs to last until the next supply order date (separate lists are found inside cabinet doors, in supply drawers, and on the code or crash cart)

Stress A physical, chemical, or emotional factor that causes bodily or mental tension and may cause disease

Supply Needs Sheet A sheet of paper used by all nursing unit personnel to jot down items that need reordering

ABBREVIATIONS

Abbreviation	Meaning
ADT Log Book	book used to record all admissions, discharges, and transfers on a nursing unit
ADT Sheet	form used to record admissions, discharges, and transfers on a nursing unit on a daily basis
CQI	continuous quality improvement

EXERCISE 1

Write the correct abbreviation for each term listed below.

1. Admission, Discharge, Transfer Log Book

   _____

2. Admission, Discharge, Transfer Sheet

   _____

3. Continuous Quality Improvement

   _____

EXERCISE 2

Write the meaning of each abbreviation listed below.

1. ADT Log Book

   _____

2. ADT Sheet

   _____

3. CQI

   _____

INTRODUCTION

Webster's Dictionary defines *manage* as "to control or guide." The health unit coordinator (HUC) who learns to "manage or guide" certain facets within the job is able to realize the full potential of health unit coordinating.

To implement the management techniques discussed in this chapter, it is important to (1) understand the philosophy of the health care facility, and (2) know and understand the health unit coordinating job description for the nursing unit. Upon employment, study these areas carefully. Implementation of the electronic medical record (EMR) and computer physician order entry has resulted in increased managerial responsibilities for the HUC. It is important to remember that the nursing unit will function more efficiently when unit personnel work as a team. The HUC is an important member of the health care team who has great influence on how efficiently the nursing unit functions.

Although the HUC position does not include the direct management of people, how the HUC manages certain aspects of the job indirectly affects the other nursing unit personnel and the patients. Management can be divided into the following five areas:

1. Management of nursing unit supplies and equipment
2. Management of activities at the nurses' station
3. Management related to the performance of tasks
4. Management of time
5. Management of stress

MANAGEMENT OF NURSING UNIT SUPPLIES AND EQUIPMENT

Responsibility for control of equipment and supplies used on the nursing unit varies greatly among hospitals. However, this function definitely falls into the non-clinical category of tasks and may very well be part of the HUC job description.

Proper management of nursing unit supplies and equipment greatly enhances the delivery of patient care. Improper management can result in minor annoyances, such as the doctor's discovering that the batteries are burned out when attempting to use the unit's ophthalmoscope to examine a patient's eyes. Serious hindrances in the delivery of health care can also occur, such as failure to locate emergency equipment during a code blue. Management of nursing unit supplies and equipment involves all areas of the nursing unit. Besides the nurses' station and patients' rooms, the nursing unit may include the following areas:

Unit kitchen or galley: Used to store food items and to prepare beverages and snacks for patients
Linen room or cart: Used to store linens
Employee lounge: Used by nursing unit personnel for conferences, breaks, and other activities
Report room: Room used by nursing personnel who are going off duty to give a change-of-shift report to personnel who are coming on duty (report may be provided in person or may be tape-recorded)
Medication room: Used to store and to prepare medications for administration by nursing personnel
Treatment room: Room used to perform invasive procedures such as lumbar puncture
Utility room: Used for the storage and care of equipment and supplies. Some hospitals have two utility rooms. One is referred to as a contaminated or dirty utility room. This is an area where used equipment is stored until "pickup" by the supply department to be cleaned, sterilized, and repackaged for distribution as needed. The other storage room is an area where unused supplies and equipment, such as IV poles, are stored.
Visitor waiting room: Used as a visiting area for patients' relatives and friends
Conference room: Used for patient care conferences or as a place where a doctor or a pastor can speak to family members in private

Nursing Unit Supplies

Ordering of nursing unit supplies is discussed in Chapter 21. The management responsibilities of the HUC regarding supplies relate to the quantities of supplies needed and their location on the nursing unit. Supplies that the HUC may be directly responsible for maintaining include chart forms. In many hospitals, all patient chart forms are computerized, so they may be printed as needed. Other supplies include office supplies, batteries, nutritional care supplies, and other miscellaneous items. Supplies stocked on a unit will vary depending on the unit specialty, for example, a pediatric unit will stock diapers, bottles, and similar items, but an orthopedic unit will stock slings, sandbags, and other orthopedic items.

Only the needed quantity of supplies should be maintained on the nursing unit. Overstocking may result in waste because some items become outdated and are no longer useful. Understocking may result in wasted time and energy; in the long run, this may be costly. Most hospitals use a **standard supply list** (Fig. 7-1)—a computerized or written record of the quantity of each item currently needed by the nursing unit to last until the next supply order date.

Standard supply lists are sometimes located inside cupboard doors or at the bottom of drawers where supplies are stored. To determine and order the number of supplies needed, simply compare the quantity on the standard supply list with the quantity

Standard Supply List	
Form	Amount
Doctors' order forms	10 pks
CABG orders	5 pks
Doctors' progress notes	10 pks
Nurses' admission notes	10 pks
Allergy adverse reaction documentations	10 pks
Patient valuables check list	10 pks
Patient care documentation records	10 pks
Kardexes	5 pks
Medication administration records	5 pks
Graphic records	5 pks
Surgical consents	8 pks
Blood transfusion consents	8 pks
Reviewer communication records	5 pks
IV therapy records	5 pks
Home instructions	10 pks
Coding summary forms	10 pks
Health information checklist	10 pks
Anticoagulant therapy records	8 pks
Diabetic records	5 pks

Figure 7-1 An example of a standard supply list. Patient chart forms would be included, if not computerized.

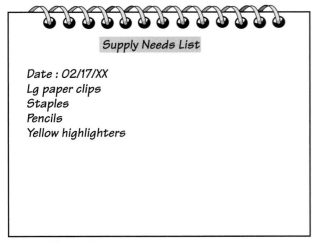

Figure 7-2 An example of a supply needs list.

of the item on the shelf, and requisition the difference. Keep in mind that the standard supply for many items may change; therefore, the standard supply list must be updated accordingly.

Another suggestion is to maintain a supply needs list for items (other than those maintained by the central service department) on the nursing unit bulletin board and ask all nursing unit personnel to record supplies that are running low (Fig. 7-2). This list may be used as a reference for items needed when you are ordering supplies for the nursing unit.

Efficient placement of supplies on the nursing unit facilitates the effective delivery of nursing care. Are supplies stored in a convenient location? Are frequently used items placed in the most accessible area? Is it easy to place storeroom items on the shelf? Ideas for a more efficient location of supplies on the nursing unit should be discussed with the nurse manager.

The HUC also may take inventory of nutritional care supplies such as crackers, juices, milk, coffee, and tea and order appropriate quantities for the nursing unit.

The HUC may be given the responsibility of retrieving items not charged to a patient that are also missing from the central service closet or locker. A common routine is for a technician from the central service department to take an inventory of the items stocked in the nursing unit central service closet or locker, and to replace used items each morning. A central service discrepancy report is a report that lists items that are missing from the supply closet or locker that were not charged to a patient. This discrepancy report and a list of items charged to patients from the previous day will be sent to the unit each afternoon from the central service department. The HUC, using the discrepancy report and the list of items charged to patients, will attempt to locate the missing items. A central service department charge slip is initiated to charge a discharged patient for any items that were not charged to him at the time of use. A central service department credit slip is used to credit a patient for unused items mistakenly charged to him. The cost of items that cannot be accounted for is charged to the nursing unit budget.

Equipment Stored at the Nurses' Station

Each nursing unit has standard equipment—flashlights, ophthalmoscopes, otoscopes, thermometers with disposable covers, bedside blood glucose monitors, and other items—that is used by doctors and nurses to examine patients. Check this equipment for working order near the beginning of the shift. If flashlights or

ophthalmoscopes need new bulbs or batteries, make sure these are replaced before the equipment is used again.

Computer terminals are used by nursing unit personnel as well as by physicians. Because overall management of their use is the responsibility of the HUC, notify hospital information systems if any repair is needed. Each authorized user is issued a code to operate the computer system. To avoid being held responsible for someone else's computer usage, always sign off the computer when leaving the nursing station.

Pneumatic tube systems are also used to transport information. Directions regarding use of the tube system are usually posted near it and are easy to understand. This is vital information, especially for students and new employees. Even small errors, such as inserting an item into the pneumatic tube system the wrong way, can interfere with the functioning of the system throughout the hospital. It is important to use caution and common sense when using the pneumatic tube system. Keep in mind that the tube system occasionally breaks down, so it may be very risky to use the pneumatic tube system to send records that are urgently needed or specimens that have been collected by invasive procedures.

Check the printer, label printer, copier, scanner, and fax machine frequently to replenish paper levels and to see that they are reproducing copies and labels clearly. Call hospital information systems as needed.

Nursing Unit Reference Materials

A small library of reference books is kept on the nursing unit. These may include such sources as (1) *Physician's Desk Reference* (PDR), (2) the *Hospital Formulary*, which is used to define drugs and their uses and to check on dosages and on adverse effects, (3) the institutional policies and procedures manual, which is used to reference hospital policies and procedures, (4) a disaster manual, which is used to provide direction and to outline responsibilities in case of a disaster, (5) a laboratory manual, which is used to define laboratory tests, specimen amounts, and collections required to perform tests, and (6) a diagnostic imaging manual, which is used to define diagnostic procedures and the preparations required to perform them. Make sure that textbooks and manuals are returned to their appropriate location after use. Keep hospital manuals up-to-date by periodically inserting revised material and discarding outdated material. Indexes of frequently used hospital extension numbers, in-hospital office numbers, and pager numbers are kept on the nursing unit and are kept up-to-date by the HUC.

A communication book may be used to preserve organizational information between shifts (Fig. 7-3). Keeping coworkers informed helps tie the work group together as a team.

General Maintenance of Nursing Unit Equipment

General nursing unit equipment includes furniture, electrical fixtures, bathroom items, and other equipment. Equipment requires maintenance, and the old saying, "An ounce of prevention is worth a pound of cure," applies here. Ideas for more efficient location of supplies offer an improvement opportunity and should be discussed with nursing management. Most hospital units have equipment lists that show when items are due for replacement.

Preventive management of nursing unit equipment may require that the HUC make rounds of the entire unit (i.e., kitchen, utility rooms, patient rooms, waiting rooms, linen room, and staff lounge) perhaps once or twice a week to check on the functioning of equipment located in these areas. Leaky

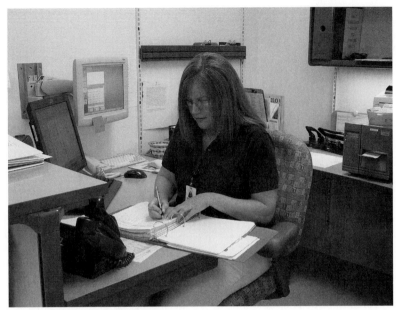

Figure 7-3 The HUC using a nursing unit communication book.

faucets, frayed electrical cords, and broken hinges are a few examples of the things to look for. Make a list of all items on the nursing unit that need to be checked. Then, make rounds; check each item on the list for its working order. Make a note of the items that need repair. Also, request that nursing unit staff note needed repairs in the unit communication book. The hospital information systems (HIS) department would be responsible for the repair of communication equipment, such as computers and telephones; other repairs would be handled by the maintenance department.

Preventive management does not take care of all maintenance needs for nursing unit equipment. Burned-out electric light bulbs, an overflowing toilet, and other unpredictable problems need immediate attention. For immediate repair service, notify the maintenance department by telephone or pocket pager and, if necessary, complete the appropriate requisition. Frequently, patients bring electrical devices such as electrical shavers, hair dryers, radios, and other items to the hospital for use during their stay. Prior to their use, these items must be examined for electrical shorts by the hospital maintenance department. The HUC places the call to initiate this process. When a patient reports that the telephone or call light is not functioning properly or is missing, or when a computer is not functioning properly, the HUC must notify the HIS department. When a patient or a nurse reports that a room or the nurses' station is too hot or cold, the HUC calls the maintenance department to address the problem.

Patient Rental Equipment

Reusable equipment used by an individual patient, such as an intravenous pump, is usually charged to the patient's bill on a daily basis. When the doctor discontinues the treatment that requires the rental equipment, nursing personnel usually place the equipment in a dirty utility room, where it is kept until it is returned to the proper department for cleaning. This equipment is picked up on a regular basis throughout the day. Personnel in the central service department will check the number printed on a label attached to the equipment to remove the daily charge to the patient. Often, the HUC will receive a call from the central services department to check in the "dirty utility room" for intravenous pumps; shortages are frequent because so many are in use.

Nursing Unit Emergency Equipment

The **code or crash cart** (discussed in Chapter 22) is usually stored on each nursing unit or in an area between nursing units. The code or crash cart is a cart stocked by the central service department and pharmacy staff with advanced breathing supplies, intravenous solutions and appropriate tubing, needles, a heart monitor, a defibrillator, an oxygen tank, and emergency medication (used when a patient stops breathing or the heart stops beating, or both). The cart is kept locked with a plastic lock (see Figure 22-X). It is a requirement of the Joint Commission (TJC) that the cart be unlocked and the contents checked according to hospital policy when the cart is not in use, to ensure that all equipment and supplies are accounted for and in working order, and that medications are not outdated. The nurse who checks the cart will request that the HUC order supplies or medication as needed. When the code or crash cart is completely checked and restocked, the nurse will again lock the cart after documenting the date and signing the form attached to the cart. When the cart is used for a code, it is vital that the cart be restocked and replaced per hospital policy.

TAKE NOTE

Emergencies, code procedures, disaster procedures, fire and electrical safety, and disaster procedures are discussed in Chapter 22.

Other emergency equipment includes fire extinguishers and fire doors. Because of the importance of emergency equipment, it must be checked frequently and immediately after use and should be restored as soon as possible to be readied for future emergencies.

The HUC must know the following information regarding emergencies:

1. Emergency equipment and supplies that are stored on the nursing unit and where they are located
2. How to call a code and what the responsibilities of the HUC are during a code (discussed in Chapter 22)
3. The location of the nursing unit fire extinguishers
4. Emergency procedures for the nursing unit (discussed in Chapter 22)
5. Signal codes and procedures for fire, behavioral alarms, disaster codes, and evacuation procedures (discussed in Chapter 22)
6. Procedures for dealing with a hazardous materials spill; although the HUC may not be directly responsible, knowing the procedures allows timely and safe removal of hazardous materials (discussed in Chapter 22)

During a crisis, hospital personnel often approach the nurses' station and ask the HUC to locate emergency equipment and initiate emergency procedures. Frequent fire and disaster drills are conducted in hospitals to prepare personnel for these disaster situations. The HUC and all hospital personnel must know what to do in the event of a fire or a disaster; these drills must be taken seriously.

Ignorance of code procedure or of the location of nursing unit emergency equipment may cause a delay in the delivery of emergency treatment, possibly resulting in serious consequences for patients.

MANAGEMENT OF ACTIVITIES AT THE NURSING STATION

In Chapter 1, we stated that the HUC coordinates activities involving the doctor, the nursing staff, the other hospital departments, patients, and visitors to the nursing unit. Good management techniques are necessary to coordinate these activities effectively.

The following guidelines may be of assistance in managing activities at the nurses' station.

Patient Activity and Information

The most efficient method for tracking patients and their activities is to use a **census worksheet**. A census worksheet is a list of the names, rooms, and bed numbers of patients located on a nursing unit, with blank spaces next to each name. A census worksheet may be printed from a computer menu. Print or prepare the sheet at the beginning of each shift. Use information on the patients' Kardex forms (see Chapter 10) or the

change-of-shift report to record each patient's information next to their name.

Record only patient activities pertinent to responsibilities of the HUC, including scheduled diagnostic procedures, surgeries, planned discharges, transfers, and so forth. Record the time (if known) of each activity (Fig. 7-4).

Record other data that may have to be referred to during the shift, such as (1) DNR (do not resuscitate) or no code, (2) NINP (no information, no publication), (3) no visitors allowed, (4) no phone calls to the patient's room, (5) the patient is in respiratory isolation, (6) the patient is out on a temporary pass, (7) the nurse who is assigned to the patient, and (8) the resident or attending physician who is assigned to the patient.

Keep the census worksheet next to the telephone and near the computer for quick reference. During the shift, update the information as changes occur.

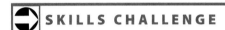

SKILLS CHALLENGE

To practice preparing a unit census worksheet, complete Activity 7-1 in the *Skills Practice Manual.*

The HUC is also responsible for maintaining the unit census board (as discussed in Chapter 4), which indicates patient names and their room numbers, and the names of doctors and nurses assigned to each patient. This board may not be in plain sight to visitors, in order to protect patient confidentiality.

Admission, Discharge, and Transfer Log Book

When patients are admitted to the nursing unit, the HUC places their labels in the **Admission, Discharge, and Transfer (ADT) Log Book** and writes the date of admission next to the label. If a patient is transferred to another unit within the hospital, the date of transfer and the destination are written next to the patient's label in the ADT book. If the patient is discharged to another facility or to home, the date and location (if not to home) are written next to the patient label.

Admission, Discharge, and Transfer Sheet

The HUC records all admissions, discharges, and transfers on the **ADT sheet** each day for quick reference regarding nursing unit activity for that day, and to determine the number of empty beds on the unit.

Patient Label Book

Patient labels are stored in each patient's chart when paper charts are used, and discharged patient labels are often kept in a **"patient label book"** in case additional charges or credits have to be made to the discharged patient's account. When computer physician order entry (CPOE) has been implemented, all patient labels may be stored in a "patient label book."

Patients and Patients' Charts That Leave the Unit

Record the time and destination next to the patient's name on the census worksheet when they leave the nursing unit for surgery, a diagnostic study, to visit the cafeteria with a relative, or for any other reason. When the patient returns to the nursing unit, draw a line through this recording. Keeping track of and

Room #	Patient Name	Activities
301	Breath, Les	DC Today
302	Pickens, Slim	Surg 11^{00} x ray to be sent $\bar{c}$ patient
303-1	Katt, Kitty	
303-2		
304	Bee, Mae	~~Call Dr. James $\bar{c}$ ABG results~~ Called Sue 9^{00}
305	Honey, Mai	NPO for heart cath @ 9^{00}
306-1		
306-2		
307	Pack, Fanny	No calls to room
308	Bugg, June	DC today
309	~~Kynde, Bee~~	Trans to ICU 11^{30}
310-1	Cider, Ida	DNR
310-2	Soo, Ah	~~Surg 8^{00}~~ Back @ 1^{30}
311-1	Bear, Harry	Resp isolation
311-2	Bread, Thad	
312-1	Kream, Kris	NINP
312-2	Pat, Peggy	~~Surg 9^{30}~~ Back @ 2^{00}

Figure 7-4 A census worksheet.

locating misplaced charts is essential for ensuring efficient use of time by doctors, nurses, and other professionals.

Health care personnel, doctors, and visitors look to the HUC to know the whereabouts of patients and/or patients' charts. When the census worksheet is maintained, the answer can be found quickly.

✐ TAKE NOTE

Many nursing units average 25 to 40 patients, and so it would be impossible to mentally log the whereabouts of each patient.

Faxing and Receiving Faxed Medical Records and Reports

When an order is written to obtain a patient's medical records or reports from another health care facility or doctor's office, the HUC prepares a medical record release form for the patient to sign. Usually, it is the nurse or doctor who asks the patient to sign the release form. The HUC then notifies the facility or doctor's office of the request, obtains the appropriate fax number, and provides the return fax number as needed; the release form is then sent, and the requested records or reports are faxed to the nursing unit. If paper charts are in use, the HUC places the signed release form and the faxed documents into the patient's chart. If the EMR is in use, the signed release and faxed documents are scanned into the patient's EMR, and hard copies of the release and faxed documents are placed in a receptacle to be sent to health information management.

Scanning Documents Into the Patient's Electronic Medical Record

The HUC is responsible for scanning electrocardiogram reports, telemetry strips, medical records, reports from outside facilities (when requested), handwritten physician progress notes, and any other relevant documents related to the patient's medical record. After these documents have been scanned, they are certified by a health information specialist and are entered into the patient's EMR.

Addressing Visitors' Requests, Questions, and Complaints

The HUC has more contact with visitors than do any other nursing unit personnel, because visitors usually stop at the nurses' station for information or other types of communication regarding a patient's hospitalization. As a visitor approaches the nurses' station, immediately acknowledge that person's presence, and provide assistance as soon as possible. At this moment, the HUC represents the entire nursing unit, and the manner in which the visitor is responded to helps shape their attitude about the care the patient is receiving, and about the hospital as a whole. It is the responsibility of the HUC to (1) communicate pertinent information to visitors, (2) respond to visitors' questions and requests, (3) initially handle visitors' complaints, and (4) locate the patient's nurse when necessary.

Pertinent information that is communicated to visitors includes the time for visiting hours, the number of visitors that may be in a patient's room at one time, isolation restrictions, and what items may or may not be taken into the patient's room. Examples of restricted items in the intensive care unit include flowers and plants. Latex balloons are banned in most hospitals because of latex allergies and the risk that children may aspirate broken pieces of the balloon. Refer to the hospital's policy manual for visitor regulations.

Visitors may ask the HUC such questions as, "May I take the patient to the cafeteria?" or "Can the patient have a milkshake?" or "When can the patient go home?" Many questions may be answered by checking information on the patient's Kardex form or computerized record. However, if there is any doubt about the answer, check with the nurse.

Never discuss aspects of the patient's medical condition with the patient's visitors. Refer all of these questions to the doctor or the nurse. If the answer to a question is not known, or the question should be referred to the nurse, respond to the visitor by saying, "I'll ask the nurse to come talk with you," or something similar, rather than saying, "I don't know," or "I'm not allowed to give out that information."

The HUC is often the first person to hear visitors' complaints, justified and unjustified. Visitors, especially the relatives of a critically ill patient, are under a great deal of **stress**. The uncertainty of the course of the illness, unfamiliarity with the hospital routine, and many other factors contribute to their feelings of uneasiness and insecurity. Also, they are often dealing with emotions such as guilt and/or anger. Often, these feelings are expressed in the form of complaints regarding the patient's care. The type of response that is given to the visitor's initial remarks may make the difference in whether the problem is solved at the nursing unit level, or whether it escalates up through the nursing administration to the chief executive officer. Follow these steps when dealing with visitor complaints.

> ✎ *TAKE NOTE*
>
> Check with the patient's nurse before giving permission for a patient to leave the nursing unit, to go outside, or to go to the cafeteria.

1. Listen carefully and attentively to what the person is saying. If the person's voice is raised or is angry in tone, remember that this hostility is not being directed to you personally. It is important to understand that the person is upset, and that listening carefully to what they are saying is the first step toward dealing with a challenging situation.
2. Ask pertinent, objective questions, and gather as many facts as possible. Demonstrate a caring attitude when gathering information. Whether or not the complaint is justified is not important at this time.
3. Respond to the complaint appropriately. Respond verbally with such phrases as, "I understand what you are telling me" or "I understand how you feel." Do not respond defensively with statements such as, "I wasn't here yesterday" or "That's not my job." If the complaint needs the attention of the nurse, say, "Please wait here; I will get the nurse to talk with you about this matter." If visitors appear even the least bit anxious or angry, refer them to the nurse immediately, because time often causes a situation to be exaggerated. Anger may be acknowledged by saying, "I can see you're angry" or something similar prior to referring the person to the nurse. Doing this demonstrates a caring attitude.
4. Refrain from eating or chewing gum when communicating with visitors; it may send an "I don't care" message.
5. Try to avoid answering the phone, but if it must be answered, ask the person on the phone to hold; then return to handling the complaint.
6. Document the complaint and your response after the conversation has ended, and relay the information to the patient's nurse as soon as possible.
7. If necessary, locate the patient's nurse and ask him or her to speak to the visitor after briefing the nurse regarding the complaint.

MANAGEMENT RELATED TO THE PERFORMANCE OF HEALTH UNIT COORDINATOR TASKS

Prioritizing Tasks

For an HUC, situations often occur in which several tasks have to be performed at the same time. Management involves being able to determine which task takes priority over another. Awareness and experience are necessary for one to develop skill in determining priorities. A task that is normally of lower priority sometimes becomes a high-priority task; for example, filing or scanning a report into a patient's chart may become a high priority if that patient is scheduled for surgery in a short time. Some of these tasks can be performed simultaneously, as when an HUC orders stat laboratory tests while conveying a message to the nurse regarding a patient's return from surgery.

Below is a list of the usual priority order of tasks:

1. Orders involving a patient in a medical crisis (take priority over all other tasks)
2. Transcribing stat orders
3. Answering the nursing unit telephone (preferably prior to third ring)
4. Communicating a telephoned message to the nurse that a patient has to be prepared to go to surgery, is now out of surgery and in the recovery room, or is returning from surgery back to their room

5. Notifying the patient's nurse and doctor of stat laboratory results
6. Transcribing preop and postop orders
7. Transcribing new admission orders and daily routine orders
8. Transcribing discharge and transfer orders, so that clerical work can be processed by the time the patient is ready to leave or be transferred
9. Performing additional and routine tasks

✐ TAKE NOTE

When computer physician order entry (CPOE) has been implemented, the HUC will not be transcribing the patient's orders. Monitoring the EMR for HUC tasks will be a high priority. A telephone icon is usually used to indicate an HUC task on the computer unit screen that contains the list of patients (census). HUC tasks may include scheduling procedures, placing phone calls, obtaining medical records from another facility, printing discharge instructions and prescriptions, scanning documents into the patient's EMR, and so forth. Otherwise, the priorities are the same.

It is important to constantly monitor the list of patients on the nursing unit for tasks. If tasks are missed or delayed, a patient's diagnostic tests and/or treatment could be delayed.

The following techniques may assist the HUC in managing the workload:

1. Ask for assistance when necessary.
2. Upon returning to the nursing unit from a break and finding several charts lying about, check each chart for new orders, place those that do not have new orders in the chart rack, read all new orders, notify the patient's nurse of any stats and provide the nurse with a copy of the orders, and fax or send copies to the pharmacy; then proceed to transcribe all other orders, one chart at a time. If CPOE has been implemented, check the computer for tasks.
3. Always finish transcribing a set of orders before you take a break.
4. Follow the ten steps of transcription (outlined in Chapter 9), and never sign off on orders before you ensure that each step has been completed.

Use of a Note Pad

Keep a note pad next to the telephone to record names and line numbers when more than one caller is placed on hold, and to list tasks that cannot be completed at the moment (Fig. 7-5). Information that is not urgent often must be communicated to a member of the nursing team. Consider the following two examples: (1) A telephone message is taken for Mary to call the pharmacy at her convenience. Rather than taking time to try to locate Mary, record this information on the note pad. When Mary returns to the nurses' station, communicate the message to her. Draw a line through the message on the memory sheet to indicate that the message has been communicated; (2) A call must be placed to a doctor's office, and the

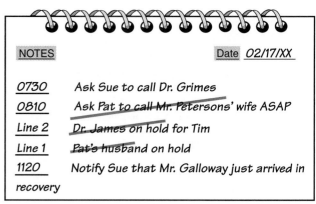

Figure 7-5 A note pad used as a memory sheet.

call cannot be completed because the line is busy. Record the task on the note pad, along with the doctor's telephone number and other pertinent data, so it will be available when the call can be placed. When the call is completed, cross it off on the note pad. During an 8- or 12-hour shift, countless items will be recorded on the note pad. Near the end of the shift, check that all listed items have been completed, and take care of any that remain.

Ergonomics for the Health Unit Coordinator

Ergonomics is the study of work for the purpose of making the workplace more comfortable, improving both health and productivity. Two types of common work-related injuries have been identified: (1) acute, which consist of fractures, crushing, and low back strain injuries, and (2) cumulative, which occur over time as the result of repetitive motion activity. Cumulative injuries include carpal tunnel syndrome, tendonitis, or low back pain. Discomfort and fatigue, whether personal or work related, can cause inefficiency, as well as cumulative injuries. A comprehensive approach to ergonomics addresses three areas of work: physical, environmental, and emotional.

The following guidelines in each area may be of assistance in reducing injury risks for the HUC.

Guidelines for the Prevention of Workplace Injuries

- The computer terminal should be located where it will reduce awkward head and neck postures; position the terminal so that you must look slightly downward to look at the middle of the screen. The preferred viewing distance is 18 to 24 inches (Fig. 7-6).
- Chairs should be adjusted so that one can sit straight yet in a relaxed position, with a backrest supporting the small of the back and feet flat on the floor.
- Adjust chair back to a slightly backward position and extend legs out slightly, so there are no sharp angles that result in pressure on hip or knee joints.
- Wrists should be straight while typing, with forearms level and elbows close to the body—reduce bending of the wrists by moving the entire arm.
- Use a computer wrist pad.
- Eliminate situations that would require constant bending over to complete tasks.
- Shift weight in the chair frequently.

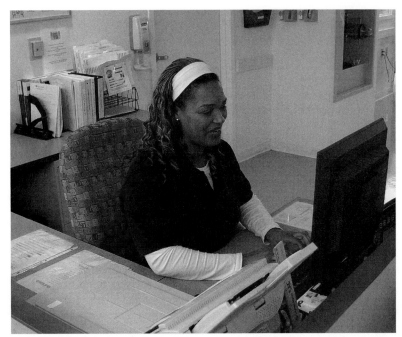

Figure 7-6 An HUC demonstrating proper body positioning when using a computer terminal.

- Use proper body mechanics when lifting—don't bend over with legs straight or twist while lifting, and avoid trying to lift above shoulder level.
- Take frequent mini-stretches of the neck (lean head down in each direction for a 5-second count).
- Stand, walk, and stretch back and legs at least every hour. These small breaks in position help avoid neuromuscular strain and alleviate the tension of job stress.

Organization of the Nurses' Station

A well-organized and neat nurses' station gives the appearance of a well-run nursing unit. First, use the Box *Organizing Items Within Reaching Distance* to check the work area at the nurses' station. Figure 7-7 shows the HUC with computer, telephone, scanner, label printer, and fax machine within close proximity.

Note: Before you initiate changes in the work area, discuss these changes with all coworkers and the nurse manager. Frequently take the time to stand back and observe the nurses' station area. Is it cluttered and disorganized in appearance? If

so, take a moment to restore all items to their original places. Return charts to the chart rack (if paper charts are being used).

Time Management

The ability to manage time may be the single most important factor in successful health unit coordinating. However, it is not easy to learn how to effectively use time. Experience, awareness, flexibility, and motivation are all necessary to achieve the goal of using time to its full potential.

William Rochti in *Leadership in the Office* (1963) tells a story that superbly demonstrates how the day tends to "go" when there is no plan for managing time:

A farmer told his wife, "I'll plow the south 40 tomorrow." The next morning, he went out to lubricate the tractor. But he needed oil; so he went to the shop to get it. On the way, he noticed that the pigs hadn't been fed. He started for the bin to get them some feed, but some sacks there reminded him that the potatoes needed sprouting. He walked over toward the potato bin. En route, he spotted the woodpile and remembered that he'd promised to

---

ORGANIZING ITEMS WITHIN REACHING DISTANCE

- Counter space should be sufficient that the room is not cramped and people do not have to lean over others to obtain charts, office supplies, or other items.
- The label printer should be in close proximity to the work space.
- Frequently used forms should be stored within reaching distance.
- Charts (if paper charts are being used) should be located in an area where they can be easily reached.
- The telephone should be within easy reach.
- The fax machine should be in close proximity to the work space.
- The unit scanner should be in close proximity to the work space (if the EMR and CPOE are utilized).
- The unit shredder or receptacle for paper to be shredded should be in close proximity.
- The unit reference books and manuals should be kept within reaching distance.

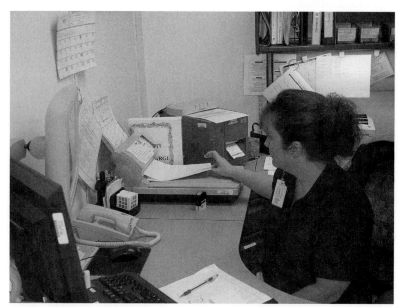

Figure 7-7 The HUC with the computer, telephone, scanner, label printer, and fax machine within close proximity.

carry some wood to the house. But he had to chop it first, and he'd left his ax behind the chicken coop. As he went for the ax, he met his wife, who was feeding the chickens. With surprise, she asked, "Have you finished the south 40 already?" "Finished!" the farmer bellowed. "I haven't even started."

Similar to the farmer, the HUC who is engaged in one part of the job is constantly seeing other tasks that need to be done. Knowing how to plan the day to make the best use of time helps avoid the pitfalls of the farmer. The following time management techniques may be of assistance to the HUC.

Time Management Techniques

1. Plan for rush periods. Take time at the beginning of each day to prepare for anticipated rush periods. For example, because it is always busy in the morning while the doctors are making rounds, allow time to assist the doctors in locating their charts and other items they may need. If several surgery patients are scheduled to be admitted, a rush can be anticipated in the afternoon, when they arrive to the unit from the postanesthesia care unit (PACU); if there are several empty beds on the nursing unit in the morning, a rush during admitting time in the afternoon can be expected.

2. Plan a daily schedule for routine HUC tasks; schedule routine tasks to be done at the time of day that produces the best outcome. Plan to perform regular tasks, such as transcribing doctors' orders and placing telephone calls, according to demand between the scheduled routine tasks. Follow the plan while making changes as required to improve use of time.

3. Group activities. Save time by grouping activities together, such as delivering specimens to the laboratory on the way to lunch, or checking the patients' charts to see if new forms are needed at the same time that reports are filed.

4. Complete one task before beginning another. This is not always possible because a stat order always takes precedence over whatever else is being done. However, apply this principle as consistently as possible.

5. Know the job and perform it well. A nursing unit is made up of many people who work together to perform the overall function of caring for patients. For the nursing unit to function effectively, each person must first know their job description and must perform the tasks outlined in the job description. It is important to stay within the boundaries of the job and not drift over into performing tasks assigned to other health care personnel. For example, on a busy day, it may seem appropriate to "help out" the nursing staff by feeding a patient or passing out food trays. This practice is not acceptable for two reasons: First, HUCs are not educationally prepared to perform clinical tasks, and second, when the HUC leaves the desk, health unit coordinating tasks are left unattended.

6. Take the breaks assigned. Often on a busy day, the immediate solution to getting the job done may appear to be to skip lunch, coffee breaks, or both. Do not be tempted to do so. Often, a few minutes away from the pressure gives the HUC the opportunity to recoup and return to handle the situation with renewed vigor and speed.

7. Delegate tasks to volunteers. Determine which tasks volunteers have been trained in and are allowed to do. Filing records in the chart is a time-consuming task that can usually be performed by volunteer workers. Work out a plan to have volunteer assistance each day at the times that are most helpful. Remember that volunteer workers volunteer because they want to work.

8. Avoid unnecessary conversation. Often, many other health care professionals can be found within the nurses' station; thus, it is very easy to be drawn into unnecessary conversation. Be aware of this, and avoid it when possible.

✎ TAKE NOTE

As an HUC, your greatest contribution to the function of the nursing unit as a whole is to know the job and to perform it to the best of your ability. If asked by other health care personnel to perform tasks that are part of their job description, politely refuse to do so.

Stress Management

Stress is a physical, chemical, or emotional factor that causes bodily or mental tension and may be a factor in disease causation. There are two types of stress: (1) **perennial stress**—the wear and tear of day-to-day living with the feeling that one is a square peg trying to fit into a round hole, and (2) **crisis stress,** which results from common, uncontrollable, often unpredictable life experiences that have a profound effect on individuals (e.g., death, divorce, illness). Hospital units are often very stressful, and the personnel who deal with life-and-death situations often become extremely stressed. The HUC is at the center of all activity at the nursing station and is often said to be in the hot seat. The following stress management techniques may assist the HUC in dealing with stress.

Stress Management Techniques

1. Effective time management is the first step in managing stress.
2. Realize that nurses, doctors, and other health care workers may be working under a lot of stress, so do not take their expressions of frustration personally.
3. Say "no" tactfully when asked to do additional work if there truly is not time.
4. Ask for help when it is needed.
5. Keep a sense of humor. Humor is a great stress reliever as long as it is timely and appropriate. Ethel Barrymore said, "You grow up the first day you laugh at yourself."
6. Take scheduled breaks.

Remember, 10% of stress is what actually happens, and 90% is the reaction to it.

Additional Management Tasks with Implementation of the Electronic Medical Record and Computer Physician Order Entry

Tasks added to the duties of the HUC with the implementation of the EMR and CPOE may include assisting doctors, nurses, and ancillary personnel in use of the computer system; scanning documents into the patient's EMR; tracking and maintaining mandatory TJC requirement records for nursing unit personnel, including cardiopulmonary resuscitation (CPR), infectious disease control, fire and safety training, universal (standard) precautions, tuberculosis skin testing, and HIPAA (Health Insurance Portability and Accountability Act) training; monitoring and maintaining records of certification and licenses for nursing unit personnel; preparing work schedules for nursing unit personnel; preparing various reports as requested by the nurse manager; and serving on various committees.

CONTINUOUS QUALITY IMPROVEMENT

Continuous quality improvement (CQI), a requirement of TJC, is the practice of continuously improving quality at every level of every department for every function of the health care organization. Most hospitals have CQI committees that oversee the assessment and improvement of work processes, while focusing on what patients want and need.

How does this translate to the HUC? Quality improvement remains an important part of the job. Learn the language of quality. The quality movement is global because CQI results in products and services of better quality. Competition to provide the best product and service in the most efficient manner has increased worldwide. Find out who has the "best practices" in health unit coordinating, and put those methods to work whenever possible. The HUC is often asked to serve on a committee to solve quality improvement problems involving nursing unit clerical processes. A committee that is focused on this process may use two techniques—application of the following problem-solving model, and **brainstorming**.

The Five-Step Problem-Solving Model

1. Identify and analyze the problem.
2. Identify alternative plans for the solution.
3. Choose the best plan.
4. Put the best plan for the solution into place.
5. Evaluate the plan after it has been in place for a given time.

Application of the Five-Step Problem-Solving Model and Brainstorming

The admitting department reports to the nursing department that when patients are discharged, there is a long delay before the HUC provides this information to them. This causes inconvenience for patients who are going home and for those who are waiting for beds. The nurse manager asks Cynthia, an HUC, to join a committee (consisting of two admitting personnel, one nurse manager, and two HUCs) that has been assigned to find the cause and a solution to this problem. The committee meets several times and uses the five-step problem-solving model and brainstorming, as outlined below:

1. *Identify and analyze the problem:* The problem was discussed, and it was determined that (a) discharged patients had to wait for their paperwork to be processed because the admitting department was not notified of the discharge in time, and (b) new admissions had to wait for beds before they could be admitted. The group identified possible causes of the problems and recorded them on slips of paper that Cynthia collected to share later with the entire group. It was determined that the probable cause of the problems was that nursing unit personnel wanted to get caught up with their work before receiving a new admission, so they asked the HUC to delay notifying the admitting department of discharges.
2. *Identify alternative plans for the solution:* The brainstorming technique was used to identify alternative solutions to resolve the problem. Cynthia again collected the papers to share with the group as a whole. Some suggested solutions that were listed on a white board were as follows: (a) Ask the doctor to notify Admitting when discharging a patient, (b) hold a mandatory meeting for all HUCs to discuss the problem again, and (c) create a policy requiring that a discharge order be sent to the Admitting department within 20 minutes after it is written.
3. *Choose the best plan:* The committee members chose (c) as the best solution and planned the next meeting to create the policy.
4. *Put the plan for the solution into place:* The policy was created, approved, and implemented. The committee agreed to meet again in 6 weeks to evaluate the solution.
5. *Evaluate the plan after it has been in place for a given time:* The committee met one last time to evaluate the plan and concluded that the discharge process had been greatly improved.

EXERCISE 3

Use the problem-solving model and the brainstorming technique to solve the following problem:

The hospital has implemented CPOE, and you have been instructed not to accept any handwritten physician orders, and to report any doctor who does not comply with the new mandate. Dr. Peterson, when told that he is now expected to enter his orders directly into the computer, says, "I have been bringing patients to this hospital for 27 years, and I will handwrite my orders as I always have!" You have a special relationship with Dr. Peterson and are afraid that reporting him would destroy your relationship.

1. Identify and analyze the problem.

   _____

   _____

2. Identify alternative plans for the solution.

   _____

   _____

3. Choose the best plan.

   _____

   _____

4. Put the plan for the solution into place.

   _____

   _____

5. Evaluate the plan after it has been in place for a given time.

   _____

   _____

KEY CONCEPTS

To meet the challenge of management requires greater effort and motivation on the part of the HUC than just "getting the job done"; however, the effort and motivation are rewarding. Job success is self-made. To develop your career to its potential, take the step beyond "getting the job done," and employ essential management techniques. Implementation of the EMR and CPOE will increase management responsibilities and will require flexibility and perhaps additional education. Following ergonomic suggestions and adhering to time and stress management techniques will help make this job a more pleasurable experience.

REVIEW QUESTIONS

1. List five areas of management.

   a. _____

   b. _____

   c. _____

   d. _____

   e. _____

2. Briefly discuss the management responsibilities of the HUC regarding

   a. nursing unit supplies

   _____

   b. equipment stored at the nurses' station

   _____

   c. nursing unit reference material

   _____

d. maintenance of the nursing unit

_____

e. the patient's rental equipment

_____

f. nursing unit emergency equipment

_____

3. List five items that would be recorded on the census worksheet for quick reference during a shift.

a. _____

b. _____

c. _____

d. _____

e. _____

4. Discuss how a record of patient names and patient charts that are temporarily away from the nursing unit would be kept.

_____

_____

5. Why is it necessary to keep a written record of the whereabouts of each patient and each patient chart?

_____

_____

6. List seven steps to follow when dealing with visitor complaints.

a. _____

b. _____

c. _____

d. _____

e. _____

f. _____

g. _____

7. List four reference books that would be found on the nursing unit.

a. _____

b. _____

c. _____

d. _____

8. List the five steps that make up the problem-solving model.

a. _____

b. _____

c. _____

d. _____

e. _____

9. Describe HUC responsibilities in sending and receiving faxed medical records and reports (with paper charts and with CPOE).

a. with paper charts

_____

b. with CPOE

_____

10. Describe possible consequences when the HUC does not monitor the patient's EMR for HUC tasks to be performed.

_____

_____

11. List three tasks that are usually the highest priority for the HUC.

a. _____

b. _____

c. _____

12. Upon arrival of the HUC on the nursing unit, the following tasks must be done. Indicate the order in which you would perform these tasks by numbering them in the spaces provided.

a. There are two discharge orders to be processed.

_____

b. A nurse comes out of a room and asks you to call a code arrest on a patient.

_____

c. The telephone is ringing.

_____

d. A doctor has placed an order for a chest x-ray to be performed today.

_____

e. The surgical patients' charts must be checked to see whether necessary reports are included in preparation for surgery.

_____

f. Two tubes have just arrived in the pneumatic tube system.

_____

13. List eight steps that may be followed to make the best use of an HUC's time:

a. _____

b. _____

c. _____

d. _____

e. _____

f. _____

g. _____

h. _____

14. Define the following terms:

a. standard supply list

_____

b. census worksheet

_____

c. change-of-shift report

_____

d. central service department credit slip

_____

e. central service department charge slip

_____

15. Describe how you would respond to the following situations:

a. Mrs. Robert Frances, whose husband has been hospitalized for 3 weeks with a cerebral hemorrhage, walks up to the nurses' station and in a loud, angry voice states, "No one is taking care of my husband. When I came in today, his lunch tray was just sitting there, cold, no one was feeding him, and his bed was wet."

_____

_____

b. The visiting hours policy for the hospital states that children may visit patients only on weekends. A female visitor with a small child and a baby asks what room Mr. Blair is in. It is Tuesday afternoon.

_____

_____

c. The patient, Mr. Christine in Room 365-1, complains that the other patient in his room has six people visiting him at this time, and he finds this very upsetting.

_____

_____

d. You have been employed for a month on a very busy surgical nursing unit. The scanner is located so far from the working area that each time you need to use it, you must get up from your chair and walk to where it is located.

_____

_____

e. It is a very busy day; the beds are all full, and two nursing personnel have called in sick and cannot be replaced. At the moment, you are all "caught up" with your tasks. A nurse approaches you and asks, "Would you please help Mr. Tiesen to the restroom for me? His room is close to the nurses' station, so you will be able to hear the telephone ring."

_____

_____

16. List five informational items that the HUC who is going off duty should communicate during shift report to the HUC who is coming on duty.

a. _____

b. _____

c. _____

d. _____

e. _____

17. Discuss four guidelines to assist the HUC in managing the workload.

a. _____

b. _____

c. _____

d. _____

18. Define the term _ergonomics_.

_____

19. Identify two types of work-related injuries.

a. _____

b. _____

20. List five guidelines that can be followed to avoid workplace injury.

a. _____

b. _____

c. _____

d. _____

e. _____

21. List two types of stress, and provide an example of each.

a. _____

b. _____

22. List five techniques for dealing with stress on the job.

a. _____

b. _____

c. _____

d. _____

e. _____

23. Explain the purpose of continuous quality improvement.

_____

_____

24. List four items that should be within reaching distance of the HUC's desk area.

a. _____

b. _____

c. _____

d. _____

25. List three management tasks that may be added to the responsibilities of the HUC with the implementation of CPOE.

a. _____

b. _____

c. _____

26. List three types of documents that would be scanned into the patient's electronic record.

a. _____

b. _____

c. _____

THINK ABOUT...

1. Have you or has someone you know had a workplace injury? Discuss how this injury could have been avoided.
2. Think of a time when you were upset regarding the way you or a family member was treated in a health care setting. How was it resolved? Discuss how it could have been handled in a more professional manner.
3. Discuss your most effective technique for relieving stress.

Website of Interest

http://www.osha.gov

CHAPTER **8**

The Patient's Chart or Electronic Medical Record

OUTLINE

CHAPTER OBJECTIVES

Upon completion of this chapter, you will be able to:

1. Define the terms in the vocabulary list.
2. Write the meaning of the abbreviations in the abbreviations list.
3. List six purposes of a patient's chart (paper or electronic).
4. List five guidelines to be followed by all personnel when writing on a patient's paper chart.
5. List five guidelines to be followed by all personnel when entering information into a patient's electronic medical record (EMR).

6. Identify four standard patient chart forms that are initiated in the admitting department.
7. Name eight patient standard chart forms included in the admission packet and describe the purpose of each form.
8. Name eight patient supplemental chart forms and describe the purpose of each form.
9. List eight health unit coordinator (HUC) duties in maintaining a patient's paper chart.
10. List six HUC duties in monitoring and maintaining the patient's EMR.

11. List five guidelines to follow in the preparation of a consent form.
12. List four types of permits or release forms that patients may be required to sign during their hospital stay.
13. Describe the methods for correcting a labeling error and a written entry error on a patient's paper chart form.
14. Read and write military times.

VOCABULARY

Admission Packet A preassembled packet of standard chart forms to be used on admission of a patient to the nursing unit

Allergy An acquired, abnormal immune response to a substance that does not normally cause a reaction; may include medications, food, tape, and many other items

Allergy Bracelet A plastic bracelet (usually red) that is worn by a patient that indicates allergies they may have

Allergy Labels Labels affixed to the front cover of a patient's paper chart that indicate a patient's allergies

Identification Labels Labels that contain individual patient information for identifying patient records or other personal items

Imprinter Cards Small plastic cards with individual patient information used to identify patient records (used in some hospitals in place of identification labels)

Imprinter Machine A machine used to imprint information from patient identification imprinter cards onto chart forms

Name Alert A method of alerting staff when two or more patients with the same or similarly spelled last names are located on a nursing unit

Old Record A patient's paper record from previous admissions stored in the health information management department that may be retrieved for review when a patient is admitted to the emergency room, nursing unit, or outpatient department; older microfilmed records also may be requested by the patient's doctor

"Split" or Thinned Chart Portions of the patient's current paper chart that are removed when the chart becomes so full that it is unmanageable

Standard Chart Forms Forms included in all inpatient paper charts that are used to regularly enter information about patients

Stuffing Charts Placing extra chart forms in patients' paper charts so they will be available when needed

Supplemental Chart Forms Patient chart forms used only when specific conditions or events dictate their use

WALLaroo A locked workstation that is located on the wall outside a patient's room; it stores the patient's paper chart or a laptop computer, and when unlocked, it forms a shelf to write upon

ABBREVIATIONS

Note: These abbreviations are listed as they are commonly written; however, they also may be seen in upper case or lower case letters and with or without periods.

Abbreviation	Meaning
H&P	history and physical
Hx	history
ID labels	identification labels
MAR	medication administration record
NKA	no known allergies
NKFA	no known food allergies
NKMA	no known medication allergies
NKDA	no known drug allergies

EXERCISE 1

Write the abbreviation for each term listed below.

1. history _____

2. no known allergies _____

3. identification labels _____

4. history and physical _____

5. medication administration record _____

6. no known medication allergies _____

7. no known drug allergies _____

8. no known food allergies _____

EXERCISE 2

Write the meaning of each abbreviation listed below.

1. ID labels

   _____

2. NKFA

   _____

3. MAR

   _____

4. NKA

   _____

5. NKDA

   _____

6. H&P

   _____

7. Hx

   _____

8. NKMA

   _____

PURPOSES OF A PATIENT'S CHART/RECORD (PAPER OR ELECTRONIC)

The patient's paper chart or electronic medical record (EMR) serves many purposes, but for a health unit coordinator (HUC), the chart/electronic record is seen mainly as a means of communication between the doctor and the hospital staff.

The chart/EMR is also used for planning patient care, for research, and for educational purposes. As a legal electronic record/document, the medical record protects the patient, the doctor, the staff, and the hospital or health care facility. Careful entries/notations by doctors and other personnel provide a written or electronic record of the patient's illness, care, treatment, and outcomes of hospitalization. If the patient is readmitted to the hospital or health care facility, the paper chart may be retrieved from health information services. The advantage of the EMR is that all previous health information is immediately available on the computer.

✐ TAKE NOTE

Purposes of a Patient's Chart/Record (Paper or Electronic)
Means of communication
Planning patient care
Research
Education
Legal record/document
History of patient illnesses, care, treatment, and outcomes

The Patient Chart or Electronic Medical Record as a Legal Document

When a patient is discharged, the paper chart must be sent to the health information management department as soon as possible. Health information management personnel analyze and check the chart for completeness. When records are not complete or signatures are missing, those chart forms are flagged, and the appropriate nurses and/or doctors are notified that they must come to the health information management department to complete or sign the chart forms. Health information management personnel also analyze and check EMRs for completeness and notify the appropriate nurses and/or doctors when they must go into the computer to complete the records. Completed paper charts are indexed and stored where they are available for retrieval as needed.

Older paper records are microfilmed (documents are placed on film in reduced scale) and stored. Upon request, health information management personnel may retrieve microfilmed records. The length of time that the record must be stored depends on the laws of the state. Unless a patient has been readmitted to the hospital, the service department will not send **old records** to nursing units. Doctors and nurses must go to the health information management department to see or complete old patient records if the patient has not been readmitted to the hospital. The patient's previous EMR will be available on computer to the patient's doctor, or if the patient is readmitted to the hospital. The Security Rule, a key

part of the Health Insurance Portability and Accountability Act (HIPAA), protects a patient's electronically stored information (see Chapter 6).

The record may be subpoenaed and may serve as evidence in a court of law. As a legal document, it must be maintained in an acceptable manner.

GUIDELINES TO FOLLOW WHEN WRITING IN A PATIENT'S PAPER CHART

All persons who write in the paper chart follow standard guidelines. The HUC has minor charting tasks but is responsible for patient charts, so should be aware of the following basic rules:

1. All paper chart form entries must be made in ink. This is to ensure permanence of the record. Black ink is preferred by many health care facilities because it produces a clearer picture when the record is microfilmed, faxed, or reproduced on a copier.
2. Written entries on paper chart forms must be legible and accurate. Entries may be made in script or printed. Diagnostic reports, history and physical examination reports, and surgery reports are usually typewritten or computer generated.
3. Recorded entries on the paper chart may not be obliterated or erased. The method for correcting errors is outlined later on in this chapter.
4. All written entries on paper chart forms must include the date and time (military or traditional) of the entry.
5. Abbreviations may be used in keeping with the health care facility's list of "approved abbreviations."

GUIDELINES TO FOLLOW WHEN ENTERING INFORMATION INTO THE PATIENT'S ELECTRONIC MEDICAL RECORD

1. All entries into the EMR must be accurate.
2. Handwritten progress notes, electrocardiograms, and outside records and reports must be scanned into the EMR.
3. Errors made in care or treatment must be documented and cannot be falsified.
4. All entries into the EMR must include the date and time (military or traditional) of the entry.
5. Abbreviations may be used in keeping with the health care facility's list of "approved abbreviations."

MILITARY TIME

Military time is a system that uses all 24 hours in a day (each hour has its own number) rather than repeating hours and using AM and PM. When using military time, there are always 4 digits, the first two digits representing hours and the second two representing minutes. For example, 1:45 AM is recorded as 0145, and 1:45 PM is recorded as 1345; the colon is not needed when military time is used (Table 8-1). The hours after midnight are recorded as 0100, 0200, and so forth. Thirty minutes after midnight is written as 2430 (may also be written as 0030). Twelve noon is recorded as 1200 and the hours that follow are arrived at by adding the hours after noon to 1200. Thus, 1:00 PM is 1200 + 100 = 1300, 2 PM is 1200 + 200 = 1400, and so forth. See Figure 8-1 for a comparison of standard and military times. The use of military time eliminates confusion because hours are not repeated, and AM or PM is unnecessary.

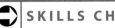 **SKILLS CHALLENGE**

To practice converting standard time to military time, complete Activity 8-1 in the *Skills Practice Manual.*

THE PATIENT'S PAPER CHART OR ELECTRONIC MEDICAL RECORD IS CONFIDENTIAL

As was discussed in Chapter 6, the paper chart/EMR confidential, and the HUC is a custodian of all patient medical records (paper or electronic) on the unit. Any information provided by the patient to the health care facility and the medical staff is confidential. All health care personnel are required to have a code and a password to gain access to a patient's EMRs. Portions of the patient's EMR may be available only to the patient's doctor and nurses.

Table 8-1	**Standard and Military Time Comparisons**		
12:15 AM	0015	1:00 PM	1300
12:30 AM	0030	1:15 PM	1315
12:45 AM	0045	1:30 PM	1330
1:00 AM	0100	1:45 PM	1345
2:00 AM	0200	2:00 PM	1400
3:00 AM	0300	3:00 PM	1500
4:00 AM	0400	4:00 PM	1600
5:00 AM	0500	5:00 PM	1700
6:00 AM	0600	6:00 PM	1800
7:00 AM	0700	7:00 PM	1900
8:00 AM	0800	8:00 PM	2000
9:00 AM	0900	9:00 PM	2100
10:00 AM	1000	10:00 PM	2200
11:00 AM	1100	11:00 PM	2300
12:00 Noon	1200	12:00 Midnight	2400

THE CHART BINDER

Forms that constitute the patient's paper chart are usually kept together in a three-ring binder. The binder may open from the bottom, or it may be a notebook that opens from the side, the top, or the bottom (Figure 8-2).

The chart forms in the binder are sectioned off by dividers placed in the chart according to the sequence set forth by the health care facility (Figure 8-3).

Paper charts are identified for each patient with a label that contains the patient's name and the doctor's name. The room and bed number may be written on the outside of the chart binder. Many health care facilities use colored tape on the outside of the chart to assist doctors in identifying their patients' charts. Labels or tape affixed to chart binders are often used to alert the hospital staff of special situations. For example, "name alert," a piece of tape with "name alert" recorded on it, may be placed on the chart binder to remind staff that more than one patient with the same or a similarly spelled last name is housed on the unit. When an order indicates that a patient's admission is not to be published, NINP (no information, no publication) is often recorded on the chart binder to remind staff members that no information is to be issued on a particular patient.

THE ELECTRONIC MEDICAL RECORD

The patient's EMR may be accessed by health care personnel after they enter a code and a password, by choosing the patient's name from the nursing unit census. A name alert flag may be placed on the patient's electronic medical record; if an order has been written stating that the patient's admission is not to be published, NINP is noted on the EMR.

THE CHART RACK FOR PAPER CHARTS

Many types of chart racks are available on the market. One type allows patient paper charts to be placed in a chart rack in which each slot on the rack holds one patient chart. Slots are labeled with the room and bed numbers; they usually are numbered in the same sequence as the rooms on the nursing unit (Figure 8-4). Another type of chart storage is a **WALLa-roo**, a locked workstation that is located on the wall outside the patient's room. It stores a patient's paper chart or a laptop

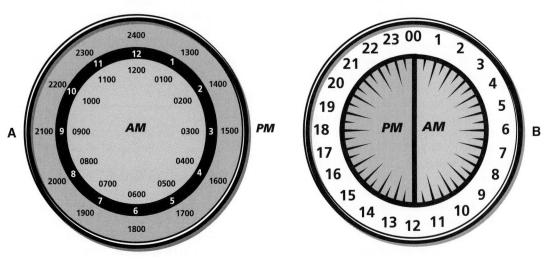

Figure 8-1 A, 24-hour clock showing military time. **B,** Military time.

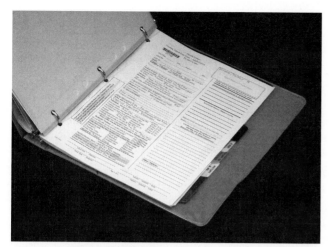

Figure 8-2 Patient's chart with dividers.

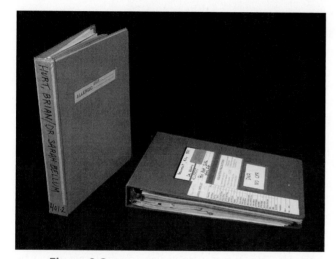

Figure 8-3 Patient chart binders properly labeled.

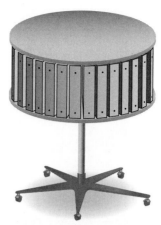

Figure 8-4 Chart rack.

computer and, when unlocked, forms a shelf to write upon (Figure 8-5).

PATIENT IDENTIFICATION LABELS

A packet of patient **identification labels** is printed from the computer when the patient is admitted and as needed during the hospital stay. Information on the identification labels usually includes the following: the patient's name, age, sex, account number, health record number, admission date, and attending physician's name; a bar code may be included for identification purposes (Figure 8-6). These identification labels are kept on the nursing unit in the patient's paper chart and are used to label chart forms, consents, requisitions, specimens, clothing, and other belongings. When the EMR is implemented, identification labels are kept in a "label book" and are used on consents, specimens, clothing, and other belongings. Labels may be generated from the computer and printed on a label printer.

STANDARD PATIENT CHART FORMS

Standard patient chart forms are included in all inpatient paper charts and may vary in different hospitals. When the EMR is implemented, information is entered into the computer on

similar electronic forms. The following **standard chart forms** are the most commonly used presently.

Standard Patient Chart Forms Initiated in the Admitting Department

1. Face Sheet or Information Form

The face sheet or information form (Figure 8-7) contains information about the patient, such as name, address, telephone number, name of employer, admission diagnosis, health care insurance policy information, and next of kin. In most health care facilities, the form originates in the admitting department and is then sent to the unit to be placed in the patient's chart. When the EMR is implemented, the information is entered directly into the patient's EMR. Several copies (at least five) should be maintained in the patient's paper chart to be taken by the attending physician and by consulting physicians to be used for billing purposes. Extra face sheets for each patient on the nursing unit should be kept in a notebook when the EMR is being used. The HUC can generate copies of the face sheet on the computer. The face sheet is also used on the nursing unit to locate information when staff must call the family or call consulting physicians.

2. Admission/Service Agreement Form (also may be called Conditions of Admission [COA])

The admission/service agreement form (Figure 8-8) is signed by the patient in the admitting department and then is sent to the unit to be placed in the patient's paper chart. When the EMR is implemented, the form is scanned into the patient's EMR. The form provides legal permission to the hospital/doctor to treat the patient and also serves as a financial agreement.

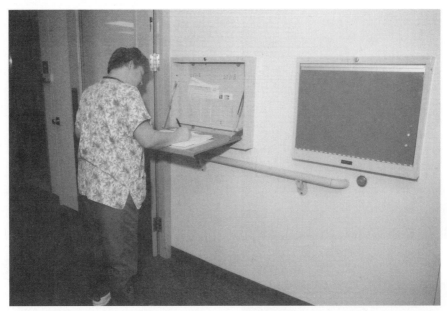

Figure 8-5 A workstation with storage for the patient's paper chart is called a WALLaroo.

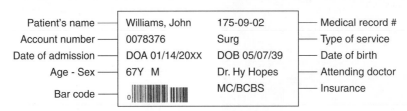

Figure 8-6 Patient identification label.

3. Patient's Rights

The Joint Commission now requires that all hospitals have a *bill of rights* and *a notice of the facilities privacy practices*. Copies must be given to each patient or parent of the patient on admission. Additionally, a copy of the bill of rights should be posted at entrances and other prominent places throughout the hospital. The patient's bill of rights varies in wording among hospitals, but all are based on following the basic ethical principles.

4. Advance Directive Checklist Form

An advance directive checklist form (Figure 8-9) documents that a patient was informed of their choice to declare health care decisions. Advance directives are discussed in Chapter 19. The Self Determination Act of 1990 mandates that all patients admitted to a health care facility must be asked whether they have or wish to have an advance directive. The patient or guardian signs the advance directive checklist, and it is placed in the patient's paper chart to document that the patient was advised of their choices. When the EMR is in use, the signed checklist is scanned into the patient's EMR.

Standard Patient Chart Forms Included in the Admission Packet

1. Physicians' Order Form

The physicians' order form, or doctors' order sheet (see the Evolve site), is the form on which the doctor requests care and treatment procedures for the patient. All orders should be dated and must be signed by the physician who is giving the order. This form may be available in duplicate or may be used as a single form. The duplicate of the original physician's order form may be sent to the pharmacy (commonly called the pharmacy copy), or the HUC may be required to fax a copy to the pharmacy to order the patient's medications. It is essential that the pharmacist see the original physician's orders to eliminate errors in the transcription process. A copy may be created on a fax machine and given to the appropriate nursing personnel.

When the EMR is implemented, the physician enters orders directly into the computer, and the orders are routed to the appropriate departments, including the pharmacy.

2. Physicians' Progress Record

The progress record is a form on which the physician records the patient's progress during the patient's hospitalization. Medical staff rules and regulations and the patient's condition dictate the interval allowed between notations (usually daily). The attending physician, residents, and consultants may write on this form (see the Evolve site).

When the EMR is implemented, the physician may enter progress notes directly into the computer or may handwrite them and request that the HUC scan them into the patient's EMR.

3. The Nurses' Admission Record

The nurse's admission record (Figure 8-10) usually precedes or leads into the nurse's notes. Upon admission to the

Opportunity Medical Center

Account #	Admit Date	Admit Time	Reg Init	Brought By	Info Provided By	MR Number
01149408	01/14/XX	1430	EG	Wife	Patient	30897811

Admitting Physician	Primary Care Phys.	Room #	Type	Service	Discharge Date	Time
John Bauer	John Bauer	406		Surg		

Patient Last Name First Middle	Former Name	Race	Rel Pref	Social Security #
Williams, John		C	do not	111-11-1111

Patient Address	Apt. No.	City	State	Zip Code	Patient Phone #
294 W Filmore St		Sinclaire	NJ	90376-9009	222-222-2222

Driver's License #	Age	Birth Date	Birthplace	Gender	MS	Occupation	Accident? Date/Time
N/A	67	05/07/39	Ohio	M	M	Teacher	N/A

Patient Employer	Employer Address	Employer Phone
Retired May 2005		

Spouse Name	Spouse Address	City	State	Spouse Phone
Elaine Ann	9030 W. 3 Ave	Peoria	Ohio	200-330-3333

Emergency Contact	Relationship	Home Phone	Cell Phone	Work Phone
Jean Sounders	daughter	102-202-2002	N/A	102-101-1001

Admitting Diagnosis	Admit Type	ICD9	Admit Source
MVA - diabetes	Surg		Clinic

Primary Insurance Plan	Primary Policy #	Authorization #	Primary Policy Holder
Medicare	111-11-1111A		

Insurance Plan #2	Secondary Policy #	Authorization #	Secondary Policy Holder
Pacific Care	22020111		

Insurance Plan #3	Tertiary Policy #	Authorization #	Tertiary Policy Holder

Guarantor Name	Rel to Pt	Mailing Address	Guarantor Phone

Guarantor Occupation	Employer	Employer Address	Employer Phone

Billing Remarks:

Principal Diagnosis:	MVA	Code:	050
Secondary Diagnosis:	Diabetes	Code:	268

Operations and Procedures:	Physician	Date	Code

Consulting Physician:

Final Disposition: ◯ Discharged ◯ Transferred ◯ Left AMA ◯ Expired   ◯ Autopsy ◯ Yes ◯ No

I certify that my identification of the principal and secondary diagnosis
and the procedures performed is accurate to the best of my knowledge.

Opportunity Medical Center _____

Attending Physician   Date

Figure 8-7 Face sheet or information form. (Copyright © 2004, Elsevier Inc. All Rights Reserved.)

Williams, John	175-09-02
0078376	Surg
DOA 01/14/20XX	DOB 05/07/39
67Y M	Dr. Hy Hopes
	MC/BCBS

MEDICAL TREATMENT AGREEMENT
(Conditions of Admission)

Patient or the patient's legal representative agrees to the following terms of hospital admission:

1. **MEDICAL TREATMENT :**

   The patient consents to the treatment, services and procedures which may be performed during this hospitalization or on an outpatient basis, which may include but are not limited to laboratory procedures, X-ray examinations, medical and surgical treatments or procedures, anesthesia, or hospital services rendered under the general or specific instructions of the responsible physicians or other health care providers. The hospital may establish certain criteria which will automatically trigger the performance of specific tests which the patient agrees may be performed without any further separate consent. This Medical Treatment Agreement covers E-ICU services and outpatient services provided by the hospital's extended treatment facilities, including services at other Banner facilities. Where the hospital routinely provides services for inpatients at an outpatient facility in close proximity to the hospital, the patient consents to transport to the outpatient facility for the requested services. This Medical Treatment Agreement is effective for this inpatient admission/outpatient visit and/or for recurring outpatient services of the same type for a period of one year following its execution. For obstetrical patients this Medical Treatment Agreement covers both outpatient and inpatient services and also covers and applies to both the obstetrical patient and the newborn(s). Photographs or videotapes may be made of diagnostic and surgical procedures for treatment and/or training purposes.

2. **LEGAL RELATIONSHIP BETWEEN HOSPITAL AND HEALTH CARE PROVIDERS:**

   The patients will be treated by his/her attending physician or health care providers and be under his/her care and supervision. Physicians and other health care providers furnishing services to the patient, including but not limited to the emergency room physician, hospitalist, radiologist, pathologist, and anesthesiologist, are generally not employees or agents of the hospital. These providers may bill separately for their services. Questions about whether a health care provider is an agent or employee of the hospital should be directed to Administration during normal business hours, and the Administrator On Call or the Chief Nursing Officer/Designee after hours, weekends, and holidays.

3. **MONEY AND VALUABLES:**

   VALUABLES AND MONEY SHOULD BE RETURNED TO YOUR RESIDENCE. The hospital has a safe in which to keep money or valuables. The hospital will not be responsible for loss of or damage to items not deposited in the safe (such as glasses, dentures, hearing aids, contact lenses, jewelry or money).

4. **TEACHING PROGRAM:**

   The hospital participates in training programs for physicians and heath care personnel. Some patient services may be provided by persons in training under the supervision and instruction of physicians or hospital employees. These persons in training may also observe care given to the patient by physicians and hospital employees.

5. **RELEASE OF INFORMATION:**

   The patient acknowledges and agrees that medical and/or financial records (INCLUDING INFORMATION REGARDING ALCOHOL OR DRUG ABUSE, HIV RELATED OR OTHER COMMUNICABLE DISEASE RELATED INFORMATION) may be released to the following.

   A. Health care providers who are providing or have provided health care to the patient or their agents; any individual or entity responsible for the payment of hospital's or other provider's charges; to health care providers or organizations accrediting the facility or conducting utilization reveiw, quality assurance, or peer review; and to the hospital's and provider's legal representatives and professional liability carriers.

   B. Individuals and organizations engaged in medical education and research, provided that information may only be released for use in medical studies and research without patient identifying information.

   C. Individuals and entities as specified by federal and state law and/or in the hospital's Notice of Privacy Practices.

   D. Patient records of services provided at any Banner facility or Banner Surgicenter may be exchanged among these facilities where necessary to provide appropriate patient care. This Release shall continue for so long as the medical and/or financial records are needed for any of the above-stated purposes.

6. **CONTRABAND:**

   Drugs, alcochol, weapons and other articles specified as contraband by the hospital may not be brought onto hospital premises. Any illegal substance will be confiscated and turned over to law enforcement authorities. If the presence of contraband is suspected, the patient's room and belongings may be searched, and visitors may be searched before visitation.

ACKNOWLEDGEMENTS

☐ I acknowledge receipt of the hospital's "Patient Rights and Responsibilities" brochure.

☐ I acknowledge receipt of the hospital's "Notice of Privacy Practices".

☐ I acknowledge receipt of either the "Important Message from Medicare" or the "Important from Tricare" (if applicable).

I have read and understand this Medical Treatment Agreement, have received a copy of this agreement, the hospital's "Notice of Privacy Practices," the hospital's "Patient Rights and Responsibilities" brochure, and where applicable the "Important Message from Medicare/Tricare." I am the patient, the parent of a minor child, or the legal representative of the patient and am authorized to act on the patient's behalf to sign this agreement.

Patient/Parent of Minor Child/Court-Appointed Guardian Patient-Appointed Agent/Statutory Surrogate Please circle the correct title	Witness
	Date: Time:

WHITE - Chart Copy, **CANARY** - Patient Services Copy, **PINK** - Patient Copy

Figure 8-8 Admission/Service Agreement.

Williams, John	175-09-02
0078376	Surg
DOA 01/14/20XX	DOB 05/07/39
67Y M	Dr. Hy Hopes
‖‖‖‖‖‖‖‖	MC/BCBS

MEDICAL TREATMENT AGREEMENT
(Conditions of Admission)

HEALTH CARE DIRECTIVES

If you have a Health Care Power of Attorney and/or Living Will you should provide it to the hospital to best assure that the hospital is aware of your wishes and that they are followed if you become unable to make or communicate your own health care decisions. If you do not have a Living Will or Health Care Power of Attorney and wish to have one, we can provide information and assistance.

I have completed a Health Care Power of Attorney

If Yes:
- ☐ Power of Attorney presented to hospital
- ☐ Power of Attorney requested from family

If No:
- ☐ "Making Decisions About Your Health Care" brochure provided
- ☐ Power of Attorney form provided
- ☐ Information declined

I have completed a Living Will

If Yes:
- ☐ Living Will presented to hospital
- ☐ Living Will requested from family

If No:
- ☐ "Making Decisions About Your Health Care" brochure provided
- ☐ Living Will form provided
- ☐ Information declined

Health Care Power of Attorney

To be completed by the **patient** only when a Health Care Power of Attorney has not been provided to the hospital.

Health Care Power of Attorney A.R.S. § 36-3224: I, as principal, designate:

_____
Name

_____
Address

_____
Phone

as my agent to act in all matters relating to my health care, including, without limitation, full power to give or refuse consent to all medical, surgical, hospital and related health care. This Health Care Power of Attorney is effective upon my inability to make or communicate health care decisions. All of my agent's actions under this power during any period when I am unable to make or communicate health care decisions, or when there is uncertainty whether I am dead or alive have the same effect on my heirs, devisees and personal representatives as if I were alive, competent, and acting for myself. This health care directive is authorized under A.R.S. § 36-3221 and continues in effect including for subsequent admissions, for all who may rely upon it except to those to whom I have given notice of its revocation.

_____   _____
Patient   Date   Time

I was present when the patient signed and dated this Health Care Power of Attorney. The Patient appears to be of sound mind and free from duress at the time he/she executed this Power of Attorney.

_____
*Witness

(*The witness may **not** be related to the patient by blood, marriage, or adoption; may **not** be the agent appointed as the Health Care Power of Attorney; may **not** be entitled to any portion of the patient's estate; and may **not** be directly involved in the patient's care.)

☐ **Unable to complete due to the need for immediate medical attention**
Additional attempts to complete

Date: _____   Time: _____   Initials: _____   Reasons: _____

Date: _____   Time: _____   Initials: _____   Reasons: _____

Date: _____   Time: _____   Initials: _____   Reasons: _____

WHITE - Chart Copy, **CANARY** - Patient Services Copy, **PINK** - Patient Copy

Figure 8-8 Cont'd

Williams, John	175-09-02
0078376	Surg
DOA 01/14/20XX	DOB 05/07/39
67Y M	Dr. Hy Hopes
[barcode] 0	MC/BCBS

FINANCIAL AGREEMENT

I agree that, in return for the services provided to the patient by the hospital or other health care providers, I will pay the account of the patient or make financial arrangements for payment prior to discharge satisfactory to the hospital and all other providers. I will pay the hospital's charges as set out in the hospital's chargemaster, which are the rates currently on file with the Arizona Department of Health Services. I understand that the chargemaster is available for inspection upon request. I understand that the rates charged for services rendered to the patient may differ from the amounts other patients are obligated to pay based upon each patient's private insurance coverage, Medicare/AHCCCS coverage, or lack of any such coverage. A delinquent account will be subject to interest at the legal rate of 10% per annum.

I request that payment of any authorized Medicare benefits be made on my behalf. I assign the benefits payable for physician services to the physician or organization furnishing the services or authorize such physician or organization to submit a claim to Medicare for payment.

If any signer (or the patient) is entitled to benefits of any type whatsoever, under any policy of health of liability insurance insuring patient, or any other party liable to patient, that benefit is hereby assigned to hospital and/or to the provider group rendering service, for application on patient's bill. HOWEVER, IT IS UNDERSTOOD THAT THE UNDERSIGNED AND PATIENT ARE PRIMARILY RESPONSIBLE FOR PAYMENT OF PATIENT'S BILL.

IN GRANTING ADMISSION OR RENDERING TREATMENT, THE HOSPITAL AND OTHER PROVIDERS ARE RELYING ON MY AGREEMENT TO PAY THE ACCOUNT. EMERGENCY CARE WILL BE PROVIDED WITHOUT REGARD TO THE ABILITY TO PAY.

X _____   _____
Patient or Other Party Agreeing to Pay   Relationship to Patient

_____   _____
Witness   Date & Time

WHITE-Medical Record Copy • **CANARY**-Patient Services Copy • **PINK**-Patient Copy

Figure 8-8 Cont'd

nursing unit, the patient answers printed questions on the form. A member of the nursing care team also compiles a short nursing history from the patient or family member regarding the patient's daily living activities, present illness, and medications the patient is taking. Also recorded on the nurse's admission history form are the patient's vital signs, height, weight, and any allergies to food or medications. The HUC enters this vital information, including height, weight, and allergies, into a patient profile screen on the computer. It is a responsibility of the HUC to label the front of the patient's chart with an **allergy** sticker and to place an insert into a plastic **allergy bracelet** for the patient to wear. It is standard practice in some facilities to use red ink to note the patient's allergies on chart forms. Some facilities also provide a separate allergy form that is included under the hard cover of the chart binder.

When the EMR is implemented, the nurse enters the admission information, including patient allergies, directly into the patient's EMR. The clinical decision support system then provides an allergy alert on the ordering screen if the doctor orders a medication for which a patient allergy has been documented.

4. Nurse's Progress Notes/Flow Sheet

The nurse's progress notes is a standard chart form that is used to outline the patient's care and treatment and to record the treatment, progress, and activities of the patient. The form is often located on a nurse's clipboard, in a separate chart at the foot of the patient's bed, or outside the room in a chart rack. The nurse's observations of the patient are recorded on the nurse's progress notes (see the Evolve site). Entries must be dated, timed, and signed by the nurse who is making the entry; the signature usually includes the nurse's first name, last name, and professional status (RN, LPN). These notes relate to the patient's behavior and reaction to treatment and other care ordered by the physician. The form serves as the written communication between the doctor and the nursing staff. Nursing students, as well as

ADVANCE DIRECTIVE CHECKLIST

Patient Name: _____

❏ Advance Directives Brochure Provided ❏ Advance Directives Brochure Refused

The Following Information Was Obtained From: ❏ Patient ❏ Other: _____

❏ **Patient HAS executed the following Advance Directive(s):**	COPY RECEIVED		COPY REQUESTED
	THIS ADMIT	PRIOR ADMIT	
❏ Declaration for Health Care Decisions (Living Will)	❏	❏	❏
❏ Medical Power of Attorney (MPOA)	❏	❏	❏
Name: _____			
Relationship: _____			
❏ Mental Healthcare Power of Attorney (MHPOA)	❏	❏	❏
Name: _____			
Relationship: _____			
❏ Combination Power of Attorney (that includes MPOA language)	❏	❏	❏
❏ Other: (specify)	❏	❏	❏

❏ Patient **HAS NOT** executed Advance Directive(s). (Check items below **ONLY** when talking with patient.)	**PATIENT Was Advised On** _____ . (date)
❏ **PATIENT** requests more information.	❏ of the *right to accept or refuse medical treatment.*
❏ Social Services notified.	❏ of the *right to formulate Advance Directives.*
❏ **PATIENT** chooses not to execute Advance Directives at this time.	❏ of the *right to receive medical treatment whether or not there is an Advance Directive.*

For Home Health/Hospice Use Only:

❏ Patient **HAS** EXECUTED Prehospital Medical Care (Arizona's Orange Card).

❏ Patient was advised of the *right to have Advance Directives followed by the health care facility and caregivers to the extent permitted by law.*

Signature of Facility Representative:	Department:	Date:

IF ADVANCED DIRECTIVE IS UNAVAILABLE, the patient indicates that the substance of the directive is as follows: (see reverse for script)

Living Will: _____

Medical Power of Attorney: _____

❏ Patient signature (legal representative if applicable): _____

❏ Witness signature (if patient physically unable to sign): _____ Reason: _____

Verification Upon Admit/Re-Admit or Transfer:

Verified with patient/legal representative that Advance Directives in medical record are current.	Verified with patient/legal representative that Advance Directives in medical record are current.	Verified with patient/legal representative that Advance Directives in medical record are current.
Signature:	Signature:	Signature:
Date:	Date:	Date:

PATIENT IDENTIFICATION

Williams, John	175-09-02
0078376	Surg
DOA 01/14/20XX	DOB 05/07/39
67Y M	Dr. Hy Hopes
‖‖‖‖‖‖	MC/BCBS

Figure 8-9 Advance directive checklist.

Directions for Completing the Advance Directive Checklist

A. Complete the first section as follows:

1. Write patient's name in the designated area and place patient label in lower right corner.
2. Offer a brochure. Check the appropriate box.
3. Indicate from whom the information was obtained: Patient or Other.
   If "Other", indicate the relationship to the patient.

B. Information for the second section may come from someone other than the patient.

1. Ask which (if any) advance directives the patient has executed and verify currency. Check all boxes that apply.
2. If a copy is provided check the box in the "Copy Received, This Admit" column across from the specific advance directive. If a copy was provided prior to this visit, check the appropriate box in the "Copy Received, Prior Admit" column. If neither, ask for a copy and check the "Copy Requested" column.

C. Information for the third section must be obtained from the patient.

1. If the patient has not executed advance directives, ask if the patient would like more information (in which case, Social Services should be notified) or if the patient chooses not to execute advance directives at this time. Check the corresponding box.
2. Advise the patient of his/her rights as listed on the form, check each box as you read each right, and list the date in the space provided.

D. Fourth section to be completed by Home Health/Hospice admitting RN.

E. Sign the form, indicate your department and date of signing. The patient, or if applicable, the patient's legal representative must sign the form. In the event the patient is mentally competent and able to communicate but physically unable to sign the form, a witness may sign the form. A reason must be indicated describing the physical ailment preventing the patient from signing. The original form is kept in the medical record.

To determine substance of the document, it is best to query the patient in this way:

"Mr./Mrs. _____ , I understand you have a Living Will/MPOA.......Can you tell me what it says?" (If the patient is unable to indicate this, offer to have them execute new documents and refer to Social Services.)

F. The final section should be completed by any PHCT member receiving the patient upon admit/re-admit or transfer. Verify with patient/legal representative that Advance Directives in medical record are current. Signature and date required.

*   **Refer to Advance Directives Policy, in the Patient Rights section of the Clinical Policy & Procedure Manual.**

Figure 8-9 Cont'd

registered nurses (RNs), licensed practical nurses (LPNs), and, in some facilities, certified nursing assistants (CNAs) may record on this form. Black ink is preferred for all shifts because colored ink, especially red and green, does not photocopy or microfilm well. The form is used during patient care conferences to evaluate patient progress and to plan discharge and future care.

When the EMR is implemented, the nurse's progress notes are entered directly into the patient's EMR. The nurse may use portable computers (discussed in Chapter 4) to enter information into the EMR at the patient's bedside.

5. Graphic Record Form

It is the task of the HUC or nursing personnel to graph the vital signs on the graphic record form (see the Evolve site). (Temperature may be calibrated in degrees Fahrenheit or degrees Celsius.) Other items recorded on the graphic record form by nursing personnel include intake and output, weight, and bowel movements.

When the EMR is implemented, the nurse may enter information directly into the patient's EMR or may use a device that automatically records the information into the EMR as it takes the vital signs.

6. Medication Administration Record (MAR)

All medications given by nursing personnel are recorded on a medication administration record (MAR) (see the Evolve site). As the doctor orders new medications, the date, drug, dosage, administration route, and time and frequency of administration of the medication are written on this form. This task is part of the transcription procedure and, therefore, is the responsibility of the HUC in many health care facilities. Some hospital pharmacies provide a computerized medication record for every patient each day. When a new medication is ordered, the nurse or HUC handwrites the name of the medication with administration instructions on the computerized form. Some hospitals have a computerized medication system by which the pharmacy will send an updated printed medication record to the nursing units for each patient every morning. New medications ordered during that day will be handwritten on the MAR by the patient's nurse or the HUC. Pharmacy personnel will add the new medications to the following day's printed MAR from the copy of the doctors' orders sent by the HUC.

When the EMR is implemented, medications are entered directly into the patient's computerized medication record when the doctor orders them. The nurse enters documentation regarding administration of those medications on the patient's computerized medication record.

7. Nurse's Discharge Planning Form

The nurse's discharge planning form (see the Evolve site) is used to prepare the patient for discharge from the health care facility. The nurse usually records information about the patient's health status at the time of discharge and provides instructions for the patient to follow after discharge from the health care facility.

When the EMR is implemented, the nurse enters information and instructions directly into the patient's EMR. When the patient is discharged, the HUC or nurse prints the discharge instructions from the computer to give to the patient.

8. Physician's Discharge Summary

The physician's discharge summary (see the Evolve site) is used by the physician to summarize the treatment and diagnosis the patient received while hospitalized, and it includes discharge information. A coding summary or diagnosis-related group (DRG) sheet may be part of the physician's discharge summary, or it may be a separate chart form.

When the EMR is implemented, the physician enters the discharge summary directly into the patient's EMR.

Standard Patient Chart Form Initiated by the Physician

History and Physical Form

The history and physical form is a chart form that is usually dictated by the patient's doctor, hospitalist, or resident. A medical transcriptionist in the health information management department types the dictated report and sends it to the nursing unit to be placed in the patient's chart. The history and physical (H&P) form may be completed after the patient is admitted to the hospital. Some doctors send a completed copy of the patient's history and physical with the patient, or they may send it to the hospital before the time of the patient's admission. The H&P form is used to record the medical history and the present symptomatic history of the patient. A review of all body systems or physical assessment of the patient is also recorded (see the Evolve site).

When the EMR is implemented, the doctor, hospitalist, or resident may enter information directly into the patient's EMR; alternatively, the health care provider may dictate the information, so the medical transcriptionist can enter it into the patient's EMR. The physician may bring the H&P from their office and request that the HUC scan the document into the patient's EMR.

PREPARING THE PATIENT'S PAPER CHART

Each health care facility has specific standard forms that are placed in all patients' paper charts. These forms are preassembled, clipped together (by the HUC or by volunteers), and filed in a drawer or on shelves near the HUC area. Some hospitals use computerized chart forms. These chart forms can be printed for individual patients with patient identification information printed on the forms. These assembled forms are often referred to as an **admission packet**.

Upon a patient admission, the HUC obtains an admission packet from the drawer or shelf and labels each form with the patient's identification (ID) labels. If the forms are computerized, the HUC chooses the patient's name on the computer and prints the forms with the patient's identification information printed on them. Forms that need dates and days of the week are filled in (see the Evolve site) and then are placed behind the proper chart divider in a chart binder.

Williams, John	175-09-02
0078376	Surg
DOA 01/14/20XX	DOB 05/07/39
67Y M	Dr. Hy Hopes
0 ‖‖‖‖‖‖‖‖	MC/BCBS

Nursing Admit Data Form - Adult Patient

PATIENT STORY

Pain /Comfort Evaluation: Check all that apply

Frequency: ☐ None ☒ Currently have ☐ Acute ☐ Chronic

Onset / Duration _____

Type: ☐ Constant ☒ Intermittent ☐ Sharp ☐ Dull ☐ Burning

☐ Crushing ☐ Stabbing ☒ Radiating ☐ Other _____

Pain Severity __3__ Location: *LOWER LEGS - RIBS*

Pain Scale: ☒ Numeric ☐ Wong-Baker ☐ Objective Sign/Symptom

If using OS/S, document values:_____

What makes it better? *MEDICATION*

What makes it worse? *MOVING*

Substance Use (per patient)   Info is Unknown or UTA☐

Tobacco: ☒ No ☐ Yes (answer the following) ☐ Smoke ☐ Chew

    Amt per day: _____ # of years _____ If quit, when _____

Alcohol: ☒ No ☐ Yes (answer the following) Last drink _____

    What kind: _____ Amt: _____ Frequency _____

Drugs: ☒ No ☐ Yes (answer the following) Last used_____

    What kind: _____ Frequency _____

Emotional / Spiritual / Religious   Info is Unknown or UTA☐

Religion / faith *DO NOT PUBLISH* ☐ None

Requesting Chaplain visit ☐ No ☐ Yes ☐ Chaplain notified (ext5437)

What spiritual /cultural practices/beliefs would you like supported while

being hospitalized _____ ☐ None

How can we support these _____ ☐ N/A

Are there any concerns that are troubling you while being hospitalized?

☐ Finances ☐ Job ☒ Insurance ☐ Housing ☐ Child care ☐ Pay for meds

☐ Homeless ☐ None ☐ Other _____

Educational   Info is Unknown or UTA ☐

Does the patient indicate he/she is motivated to learn? Yes ☒ No ☐

How does the patient best learn? ☐ Video ☐ Discussion ☒ Reading

☐ Audio tapes ☐ Pictures ☐ Demonstration ☐ Other_____

Based on the above, are there any barriers to learning ☒ No ☐ Yes

Describe_____

If yes, what alternatives to barriers are being suggested _____

Communication   Info is Unknown or UTA☐

Language at home: ☒ English ☐ Spanish ☐ Other (identify below)

    (don't forget sign language)

Able to speak: Ⓨ/N Write: Ⓨ/N Read Ⓨ/N

Visual Impairment? ☒ No ☐ Yes ( )R ( )L ( ) UTA

Hearing Impairment? ☒ No ☐ Yes ( )R ( )L ( ) UTA

Was an interpreter used ☒ N/A ☐ Yes Name _____

Language spoken *ENGLISH*

Outcomes Management   Info is Unknown or UTA ☐

Anticipate D/C to ☒ Home ☐ Nursing Home ☐ Rehab Facility ☐ Hospice

☐ Correctional Facility ☐ Foster Care ☐ Other_____

Who will care for patient at D/C ☒ Self ☐ Spouse /SO ☒ Family

☐ Attendant ☐ Other_____

May need: HomeHealth ☒ No ☐ Yes Community Resources ☐ No ☐ Yes

NOTIFICATIONS

Social Service Notified via STAR ☒ N/A ☐ Yes Date/ time _____

Rehab Services notified (0945) ☒ N/A ☐ Yes Date/time _____

Form faxed (5453) to Pharmacy ☐ Yes ☒ No, why? _____

[Vertical sidebar text:] If an area in blue has been checked, order a Social Service referral / If an area in green has been checked, order a Rehab referral / Do not forget to fax this page to the pharmacy / If an area in pink has been checked, initiate the Pneumococcal and influenza pre-printed order form

Prior Level of Function Info is Unknown or UTA☐

In the last 3 months pt was ☒ Independent

☐ Partial Care ☐ Total Care

In the last 3 months pt has needed help with

☒ NA ☐ Ambulation ☐ Bathing ☐ Eating ☐ Dressing

☐ Transferring ☐ Toileting ☐ Other _____

If any green area has been checked order a Rehab referral

Circle if a concern or deficit in an area seems to be

present   Info is Unknown or UTA ☐

Mobility   Balance   Ambulation

Upper Extremity   Lower Extremity   ADLs

Self Care   Cognition   Swallow

If any green area has been checked order a Rehab referral

Circle what medical equipment is used at home

Wheelchair   Ostomy   Walker

Cane   Crutches   Oxygen

Venous access device Glucose Meter   Feeding tube

Foley   Suprapubic   Ostomy

Other

Immunizations –   Info is Unknown or UTA ☐

If any pink highlighted area has been checked, the patient

should be offered pnuemo / flu vaccine. See Pneumococcal

and influenza pre-printed order form for details

Patient 65 or older? ☒ Yes ☐ No

Pnuemovac: ☐ Yes When? _____ ☒ No

Current diagnosis of Pneumonia ☐ Yes ☒ No

Influenza: ☐ Yes When? _____ ☒ No

Tetanus: ☒ Yes When? __2005__ ☐ No

Medical History: Info is Unknown or UTA ☐

Per: ☒ Patient ☐ Family ☐ Chart

Frequent admissions due to inability to meet the expense

of medication: ☐ Yes ☒ No

Dates of previous hospitalizations/surgeries: _____

__2005 – PNEUMONITIS__

# of ED visits or clinic visits in the last 6 months: ☒

Circle all that apply. If circled, you may provide additional

detail in narrative area below

Alzheimer's/Dementia: Psychiatric   Depression

GI Bleeds/Ulcer: Heart Disease   Hepatitis

Arthritis/Osteoporosis Asthma/COPD   HIV / AIDs

Blood Disorders   Emphysema   Diabetes

Sickle Cell   Chronic Alcohol   Cancer

Hepatitis / Cirrhosis   Spleenectomy   Stroke

Blood Transfusions   Kidney Problems   Thyroid

Current Pregnancy   Substance abuse Rehab TB

Chronic Immunosuppresion   Other _____

Is there anything else the patient or family thinks would be

helpful for us to know in order to plan the care for this patient?

☒ No ☐ Yes_____

Printed Name / Credentials   Signature / Credentials / Initials

printed Name / Credentials   Page 2 of 2   Signature / Credentials / Initials

Figure 8-10 Nurse's admission record.

Williams, John	175-09-02
0078376	Surg
DOA 01/14/20XX	DOB 05/07/39
67Y M	Dr. Hy Hopes
	MC/BCBS

Nursing Admit Data Form - Adult Patient
PATENT STORY

DT102

Date/Time 6/10 1800 Unit 3C Room # 306 Age 67

Admit Dx: _MVA – DIABETES_

Addl Dx: _HYPERTENSION_

Height _182_ cm (1 in /2.54 cm) Weight _89_ kg. (2.2lb/ kg.)
☐ Stated ☐ Bed scale ☐ Standing scale ☐ Other
Emergency Contact: Name / Phone / Relationship to patient

1. _JEAN SOUNDERS – DAUGHTER_

2. _102-202-2082_

Personal Property ☒ Taken by family ☐ In safe ☐ None _____
Property at bedside: ☐ Cane ☐ Walker ☐ WC ☒ Glasses /Contacts
☐ Hearing Aids ☒ Dentures: Upper / Lower / Partial
☐ Clothes _____ ☐ Prosthesis _____

Advance ☐ None ☒ In Chart ☐ Has Directive but not available
Directives: ☐ Refused info ☐ Info given to _____
Type: ☐ Advance directive ☐ Living will ☐ POA (medical)
What is the patient/family's intent if Advance Directive not available?

A Social Service referral may be needed to help pt / family (ext. 5321)
Social Services notified ☐ Yes Date/ time _____ ☐ N/A

Allergies: ☒ No known Info is Unknown or UTA ☐
☐ Iodine (reaction _____) ☐ Tape (reaction _____)
☐ Latex (reaction _____)
☐ Meds (List/reaction) _____
_____
☐ Food (List/reaction) _N/A_
☐ Other (List/reaction) _____

Allergy Band applied? ☐ Yes ☐ No, why?

Safety Alerts: ☐ Fall ☐ Skin ☐ Seizure ☐ Aspiration ☐ Flight ☐ None
☐ Harm to self ☐ Harm to others ☐ Isolation (type)

Nutrition: Diet at home: _DIABETIC_ Last ate at _1200_
Poor oral health ☐ Yes ☒ No Tube Feeding/TPN ☐ Yes ☐ No
Vomiting, nausea, clear liquids or NPO >3 days ☐ Yes ☐ No
Modified Diet (such as Low Sodium, Diabetic, Renal) ☐ Yes ☐ No
New Diabetic ☐ Yes ☒ No Breastfeeding ☐ Yes ☐ No
Pregnant ☐ Yes ☐ No Decubitis III / IV ☐ Yes ☐ No
Surgical patient and over 70 years ☐ Yes ☐ No
Difficulty with chewing or swallowing ☐ No ☐ Yes, why _____
Unplanned weight loss within last 3 months of 10+ lbs. ☐ Yes ☐ No
 If any yellow area has been checked order a Nutrition referral

Domestic Violence Do you feel safe in your home? ☒ Yes ☐ No ☐ None
Do you feel safe in your current relationship? ☒ Yes ☐ No ☐ None
Do your children feel safe in your current relationship ☒ Yes ☐ No ☐ None
If any blue area has been checked order a Social Service referral
Oriented to unit: ☒ Call light ☒ Bed Controls
☒ Phone/TV ☒ Mealtimes ☒ ID bands
☐ Smoking Policy ☒ Visiting Hours ☒ Side rails
☒ Pain Assessment Chart ☐ Isolation rules ☐ Hand washing
Info given to: ☐ Patient ☒ Family ☐ Unable to

NOTIFICATIONS
Nutrition Services faxed (1203) ☒ N/A ☐ Yes Date/time _____
Social Service Notified via STAR ☒ N/A ☐ Yes Date/time _____
Form faxed (5453) to Pharmacy ☒ Yes ☐ No. Why? _____
Infection Control Called (5276) ☒ N/A ☐ Yes Date/time _____

(sidebar, left margin)
If an area in yellow has been checked, order a Nutrition referral
If an area in blue has been checked, order a Social Service referral
Do not forget to fax this page to the pharmacy
If an area in pink has been checked notify Infection Control

Briefly describe the events that led to the admit

(Include where patient arrived from, ie: ED, PACU, home)

ADMITTED FROM ER STATUS POST MVA

Brief Social History / Support System

SEPARATED FROM WIFE FOR 5 YRS. HAS ADULT CHILDREN LIVES WITH DAUGHTER

Referred to Social Services ☒ N/A ☐ Yes Date/ time _____
Reason _____

**List the medications the patient is taking
including dose and frequency
Remember OTCs & Herbal supplements**

AVALIDE 300/12.5 mg ī PO QD.
LIPITOR 40 mg ī PO QD
GLYBURIDE 5mg ī QAM

Other / Updates:

Printed Name / Credentials _____

Signature / Credentials / Initials _____

2155 (07/04)

Figure 8-10 Cont'd

When the EMR is implemented, information details are directly entered or scanned into the patient's EMR. Patient identification labels are placed in a notebook that contains labels for all patients on that nursing unit, and extra face sheets are placed into another notebook that contains extra face sheets for all patients on that nursing unit.

✏️ TAKE NOTE

Thirteen Standard Chart Forms

Initiated in the Admitting Department
1. Face Sheet or Information Form
2. Admission/Service Agreement Form
3. Patient's Rights
4. Advance Directive Checklist

Initiated by the Physician
5. History and Physical Form (H&P)

Included in the Admission Packet
6. Physician's Order Form
7. Physician's Progress Record
8. Nurse's Admission Record
9. Nurse's Progress Notes/Flow Sheets
10. Graphic Record Form
11. Medication Administration Record (MAR)
12. Nurse's Discharge Planning Form
13. Physician's Discharge Summary

 SKILLS CHALLENGE

To practice preparing a patient's chart, complete Activity 8-2 in the *Skills Practice Manual.*

SUPPLEMENTAL PATIENT CHART FORMS

Supplemental patient chart forms are additional to the standard chart forms and are added to the patient's paper chart according to specific care and treatment provided. For example, if the patient has diabetes, is receiving medication, and is being monitored, the supplemental form (diabetic record) is added to the paper chart. This allows information to be recorded separately from other data, making interpretation easier. It is the responsibility of the HUC to obtain the needed forms, identify the appropriate forms by placing the patient's ID labels on them, and placing these forms behind the proper chart divider in the chart binder. If the hospital uses computerized **supplemental chart forms**, the HUC chooses the appropriate patient's name, prints the form with that patient's identification information on the form, and places the forms behind the proper chart divider in the chart binder.

When the EMR is implemented, information is entered into the patient's EMR on similar electronic forms.

Clinical Pathway Record Form

Most hospitals use clinical pathway record forms for particular diagnoses or conditions, such as coronary artery bypass graft or total hip or knee replacement. The clinical pathway record form is placed in the chart for those particular patients. The clinical pathway record form includes the surgeon's orders, a plan of care with treatment, and predicted outcomes (Figure 8-11).

When the EMR is implemented, the clinical pathway form is computerized or scanned into the patient's EMR.

Anticoagulant Therapy Record

The anticoagulant record (see the Evolve site) is used to document blood test results and the anticoagulant medication received by the patient who is undergoing anticoagulant therapy. A flow sheet allows the doctor to make a comparison of the patient's blood test results and the medications prescribed over time.

When the EMR is implemented, the information will be entered into a similar computerized form into the patient's EMR.

Diabetic Record

The diabetic record (see the Evolve site) is placed in the charts of patients who are receiving medication for diabetes. Results of the blood tests performed to monitor the effects of diabetic medications are also documented on the diabetic record.

When the EMR is implemented, the information is entered into a similar computerized form in the patient's EMR.

Consultation Form

The patient's attending physician may wish to obtain the opinion of another doctor. In this event, the physician requests a consultation by writing it on the doctors' order sheet. Most doctors dictate their report upon completion of the consultation. The hospital medical transcription department types the dictated report and sends it to the nursing unit to be filed in the patient's paper chart. Some doctors may prefer to write their findings on a consultation form. Additional information regarding consultations is found in Chapter 18.

When the EMR is implemented, the information is entered into the patient's EMR by the doctor or by the medical transcriptionist.

Operating Room Records

The number of forms required for maintaining a record of a patient's operation varies; these forms are usually assembled into a surgery packet. Such records are used by the anesthesiologist, operating room staff, and recovery room personnel (see Figure 19-X). Additional responsibilities regarding the surgery chart are discussed in Chapter 19.

When the EMR is implemented, the information is entered into a similar computerized form, or it is scanned by the HUC into the patient's EMR.

Therapy Records

Health care facilities use individual record sheets for recording treatments. It is possible to have record sheets for physical therapy, occupational therapy, respiratory care, diet therapy, radiation therapy, and others. These departments are discussed elsewhere in Section 3 (see the Evolve site).

When the EMR is implemented, the information is entered into a similar computerized form in the patient's EMR.

History: _____
IV: _____

Procedures: _____

A = achieved · N = not achieved

	Pre-hospital	Day of Surgery (Date)	Post-op day 1 (Date)	PO day 2	PO day 3	PO day 4 Discharge
Consult	Medical Clearance if necessary	PT consult in PM	PT therapy BID	PT BID Home Care and SS as appr	PT BID	PT
Tests	CXR, CBC, UA, PT, SMA20, EKG, Labs appropriate for age & health 72 hrs before	T & C 2 units (pre-op) (autologous when able) X-ray (in PACU)	H & H □ PT (if on coumadin) □	H & H □ PT □	H & H □ PT □	PT □
Mobility		dangle - stand prn	Knee exercises Chair BID (30 min) - up for dinner Stand/Amb	Cont exercises - Amb BID Chair BID (45 min) - up for lunch and dinner BRP	Continue mobility Chair (60 min) - up for all meals	Continue mobility Chair (60 min) - up for all meals
Treatments		Trapeze Drain IV therapy, incentive spir q2° DVT prophylaxes : (TED, foot compression device, coumadin, Lovenox) CPM 0 - 40° in PACU	Trapeze Drain Cap IV, incentive spir q2° DVT prophylaxes CPM 0 - 50°	Trapeze DC drain Cap IV, incentive spir q2° DVT proph Dressing change by physician CPM 0 - 60°	Trapeze Incentive spirometer DCIV DVT proph CPM 0 - 70°	CPM 0 - 80°
Meds		Pain Med (IV, IM) Pt states pain relief: A N Antibiotics	Pain Med (IV, IM) Pt states pain relief: A N DC Antibiotics	PO pain meds Pt states pain relief: A N	PO pain meds prn Pt states pain relief: A N	PO pain meds prn Pt states pain relief: A N
Nutrition Metabolic		DAT___	DAT___	DAT___	DAT___	DAT___
Elimination		Catheter of choice prn st cath foley after 3rd time	DC foley	Eval. bowel function (BCOC)	Bowel movement: A N	Bowel movement: A N
Health /Home Management			Screen for Home Care & Social Service needs	Prescription for home equipment identified by PT Order equipment	Complete transfer form	□ Home □ ECF
Health Perception	TKA pre-op teaching by Interdisciplinary Team	Review: □ TCDB, □ incentive spirometry, □ ankle pumps, □ ROM to arms, □ CPM, □ pain management	Instruct on: □ knee precautions	Instruct on: □ incisional care □ pain management	Discharge teaching: □ Medication □ review knee book	□ Written discharge instructions to patient and family
Signature						
Signature						
Signature						

Outcomes (Date met/initials)

1. In-out of bed □ indep or with min assist □ mod - max assist
2. On-off commode or chair □ indep or with min assist □ mod - max assist
3. Ambulates with assistive devices. □ 75 feet indep or with min asst □ 50 feet
4. AROM □ 0 - 70 - 90° □ 0 - 60°

Outcomes (Date met/initials)

5. Evidence of wound healing, no drainage
6. Performs total knee exercises without assistance
7. Re-establish elimination pattern.
8. Utilizes oral analgesics for pain control.

Figure 8-11 Clinical pathway (care plan with treatment and predicted outcomes) for total knee arthroscopy.

Parenteral Fluid or Infusion Record

A parenteral fluid record (see the Evolve site) is placed in the chart of a patient who receives an intravenous infusion. This form, when completed, is a written record of types and amounts of intravenous fluids administered to the patient. If bedside charting is in use, the parenteral fluid record or vital signs record may be initiated when the information is entered into the computer.

When the EMR is implemented, the information is entered into a similar computerized form in the patient's EMR.

Frequent Vital Signs Record

The frequent vital signs record (see the Evolve site) is used when vital signs are taken more often than every 4 hours.

When the EMR is implemented, the information is entered into a similar computerized form in the patient's EMR.

CONSENT FORMS

Surgery or Procedure Consent Form

A number of conditions require the patient or a responsible party to sign a special form granting permission for surgery or other invasive procedures to be performed upon the patient (Figure 8-12).

Patients who are hospitalized for surgery are required to sign a form permitting their doctor to perform the surgery named on the consent form. This form should not be signed until the physician has explained the surgery or invasive medical procedure and its risks, alternatives, and likely outcomes (informed consent). After receiving an explanation, a competent patient can give their informed consent.

Other invasive procedures that require the signing of consent forms by the patient or a responsible party are covered in chapters related to those specific procedures.

The HUC usually prepares the consent form for the physician or nurse to take to the patient for signature. If the surgery should be cancelled, the surgery permit is still valid unless the doctor or the surgical procedure has been changed.

Consent forms for surgery and other invasive medical procedures are legal agreements between the patient and the physician. In some health care facilities, it may be the physician's responsibility to write the name of the doctor who is to perform the surgery or invasive medical procedure, and to write the name of the procedure to be done.

Procedure for Preparing Consent Forms

In most facilities, the HUC prepares the consent form for the nurse or doctor to present to the patient for signature. The following steps assist the HUC in preparing the consent form:

1. Affix the patient's ID label to the consent form.
2. Write in black ink the first and last names of the doctor who is to perform the surgery or invasive medical procedure.
3. Write in black ink the surgery or invasive medical procedure to be performed exactly as the physician wrote it on the physician's order sheet, except that abbreviations must be spelled out. For instance, if the doctor's order reads: "amp of rt index finger," the consent form should read "amputation of the right index finger."

4. Spell correctly, and write all information legibly.
5. Do not record the date and time. The person who obtains the patient's signature will enter the date and time.

The patient may be required to sign other permit or release forms during hospitalization. Following are examples of situations that usually require a signature by the patient or by the patient's representative.

1. Release of side rails
2. Consent to receive blood transfusion (Figure 8-13)
3. Refusal to permit blood transfusion (Figure 8-14)
4. Consent form for human immunodeficiency virus (HIV) testing (Figure 8-15)

When paper charts are used, signed consent forms are filed in the patient's chart. When the EMR is implemented, all printed or handwritten signed consent forms are scanned into the patient's EMR by the HUC.

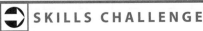

✐ TAKE NOTE

When paper charts are used, signed consent forms are filed in the patient's chart. When the EMR record is implemented, all printed or handwritten signed consent forms are scanned into the patient's EMR by the HUC.

➲ SKILLS CHALLENGE

To practice preparing a consent form for surgery, complete Activity 8-3 in the *Skills Practice Manual*.

Most health care facilities require that only licensed personnel witness the signing of consent forms. Personnel must follow these general rules when asking patients to sign consent forms.

1. The patient must not be under the influence of any "mind-clouding" medications.
2. The patient must be of legal age (18 years in most states).
3. The patient must be mentally competent.

METHODS OF ERROR CORRECTION

Because the patient's chart is considered a legal document, information recorded on a chart form must not be erased or obliterated by pen, by covering with a label, or by using liquid correction fluid. Only certain methods of correcting errors recorded on a patient's chart form are permitted.

Patient chart forms that are affixed with the wrong or incorrect ID label may be shredded if no notations have been made on them. If a chart form has notations on it, the chart form cannot be shredded. Draw an X with a black ink pen through the incorrect label and write "mistaken entry" with the date, time, and first initial, last name, and status (of the person correcting labeling error) above the incorrect label. Affix the correct patient ID label on the form next to the incorrect label (do not place the correct label over the incorrect label). It is also permissible to hand print the patient information in black ink next to the incorrect label that has an X drawn through it (Figure 8-16).

Williams, John	175-09-02
0078376	Surg
DOA 01/14/20XX	DOB 05/07/39
67Y M	Dr. Hy Hopes
	MC/BCBS

**CONSENT FOR
SURGERY/PROCEDURES/SEDATION/ANESTHESIA**

1. I authorize the following operation(s) or procedure(s) **(No Abbreviations)** _____

    _____

    to be performed by Dr. _____ and/or the associates or assistants of his/
    her choice, which may include medical or surgical residents. I understand a representative from a medical company, such as
    a sales representative, may be present during the surgical procedure to provide verbal technical advice to the surgeon,
    anesthesiologist, and/or staff.

2. During the course of the operation(s)/procedure(s), unforeseen conditions may arise, which may necessitate additional
    surgery or other therapeutic procedures to promote my well-being. I consent to other surgery / procedures as may be
    considered necessary or advisable by my physician(s) under the circumstances.

3. I consent to the use of sedation/anesthetics, as may be necessary and advisable,except _____
    I understand that sedation/anesthesia may involve serious risk, even though administered in a careful manner. I further
    understand that a patient should not drive, operate equipment, or drink alcoholic beverages for at least 24 hours after
    sedation/anesthesia.

4. To further medical and scientific learning, I consent to the photographing and/or video taping of the operation(s)/ procedure(s)
    that may reveal portions of my body, with the understanding that my identity is not to be revealed. To advance medical
    education, I give my permission for physicians, nurses, medical students, interns, residents, and other individuals who are
    participating in an educational process approved by the hospital to be present during the operation(s)/procedure(s).

5. I consent to the examination for anatomical purposes and disposal by the hospital of any tissue or body parts that may be
    removed during the operation(s)/procedure(s).

6. I understand that some physician(s) performing the operation(s)/procedure(s), administering sedation/anesthesia and
    those physicians providing services involving pathology and radiology, may not be the agents, servants, or employees of the
    hospital nor of one another and may be independent contractors.

7. I have been advised that prosthetic devices including, but not limited to, dentures, bridges, caps, crowns, fillings, dental
    implants, etc. are more easily damaged than normal teeth. I have been advised to remove all removable prosthetic devices
    prior to surgery, and I agree that responsibility for loss or damage will be mine if I fail to remove such dental or other
    prosthetic devices.

8. My physician has explained to me the nature, purpose, and possible consequences of the operation(s)/procedure(s) as
    well as significant risks involved, possible complications, expected postoperative functional level, expected alterations in
    lifestyle/health status and alternative methods of treatment. I further understand that the explanation I have received is not
    exhaustive and that there may be other, more remote risks and consequences. I have been advised that a more detailed
    explanation will be given to me if I so desire. I have received no guarantee or warranty concerning the results/outcome and
    cure and have been given an opportunity to ask questions, and have my questions answered to my satisfaction.

9. In the event a device is implanted during the operation(s)/procedure(s) and federal law requires the tracking of the device, I
    consent to the release of my social security number to the manufacturer of the device.

10. The patient is unable to sign for the following reason:

     ☐ The patient is a minor.

     ☐ The patient lacks the ability to make or communicate medical treatment decisions because of:

     _____

_____   _____   _____
Patient or Legally Authorized Representative   Date   Time

_____
Relationship to Patient

_____   _____   _____
Witness   Date   Time

Figure 8-12 Surgery consent form.

CONSENT FOR TRANSFUSION OF BLOOD OR BLOOD PRODUCTS

1. I HAVE BEEN INFORMED that I need or may need, during treatment, a transfusion of blood and/or one of its products in the interest of my health and proper medical care.

2. I HAVE BEEN INFORMED of the risks and benefits of receiving transfusion(s). These risks exist despite the fact that the blood has been carefully tested.

3. I HAVE BEEN INFORMED that the blood has been tested using all FDA-required, routine tests and that new, unlicensed, and experimental testing may or may not have been performed.

4. The alternatives to transfusion, including the risks and consequences of not receiving this therapy, have been explained to me.

5. I have read, or have had read to me, the Blood Transfusion Information regarding blood transfusions and have had the opportunity to ask questions.

6. I have been given the Paul Gann Safety Act Booklet (CA only).

7. I hereby consent to the transfusion(s).

This consent is valid for the following period of time(check one):

☐ One specific date only: _____

☐ Start Date: _____   End Date: _____

☐ This hospital admission

_____   _____   _____
Patient's Signature   Date   Time

_____
Signature of parent, legally appointed guardian or responsible person (for patients who cannot sign)

_____   _____   _____
Witness   Date   Time

Consent obtained under the direction of Dr. _____

_____   _____   _____
Physician Signature (if required by local policy)   Date   Time

NOTE:
Refusal form on reverse side
Chart Consent or Refusal Form

Separate "Blood Transfusion Information" sheet and give to patient, parent, or legal guardian.

Williams, John	175-09-02
0078376	Surg
DOA 01/14/20XX	DOB 05/07/39
67Y M	Dr. Hy Hopes
	MC/BCBS

Figure 8-13 Consent form for receiving blood transfusion.

To correct an error in a written entry made on a paper chart form, draw (in black ink) one single line through the error. Record the words, "mistaken entry," along with the date, time, and your first initial, last name, and status (of the person correcting the error) in a blank area near (directly above or next to the error) (Figure 8-17). Follow the facility policy for correction of erroneous computer entries. The procedure for correcting an error on the graphic sheet is covered in Chapter 21.

Mistaken entries are corrected in a similar manner when the EMR is used. Follow the facility policy for correction of erroneous computer entries. Errors in care or treatment must be documented on both the paper and the EMR, and an incident report must be completed, as discussed in Chapter 22.

The procedure for correcting an error on the graphic sheet is covered in Chapter 21.

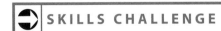 **SKILLS CHALLENGE**

To practice correcting labeling and written errors on a chart form, complete Activities 8-4 and 8-5 in the *Skills Practice Manual*.

REFUSAL TO PERMIT TRANSFUSION OF BLOOD OR BLOOD PRODUCTS

1. I request that no blood components be administered to _____
    during this hospitalization.   (patient name)

2. I hereby release the hospital, its personnel, and the attending physician from any responsibility whatsoever for unfavorable reactions or any untoward results due to my refusal to permit the use of blood or its components.

3. I fully understand the possible consequences of such refusal on my part.

    ☐ Physician aware of patient's refusal.   Physician notified: _____

Physician notified by:

| _____ | _____ | _____ |
| Signature | Date | Time |

| _____ | _____ | _____ |
| Patient's Signature | Date | Time |

Signature of parent, legally appointed guardian or responsible person (for patients who cannot sign)

| _____ | _____ | _____ |
| Witness | Date | Time |

| _____ | _____ | _____ |
| Witness | Date | Time |

REFUSAL

Williams, John	175-09-02
0078376	Surg
DOA 01/14/20XX	DOB 05/07/39
67Y M	Dr. Hy Hopes
	MC/BCBS

Figure 8-14 Form for refusal to permit blood transfusion.

MAINTAINING THE PATIENT'S PAPER CHART

As the person in charge of the clerical duties on the nursing unit, the HUC is responsible for maintaining the patient's chart.

Health Unit Coordinator Duties for Effective Maintenance of the Patient's Paper Chart

1. Place all charts in proper sequence (usually according to room number) in the chart rack when they are not in use.
2. Place new chart forms in each patient's chart before the immediate need arises. In many health care facilities, this is referred to as "stuffing the chart." Label each chart form with the patient's ID label before placing it in the chart. New chart forms are placed on top of old chart forms for easy access. The new forms may be folded in half to show that the old form has not been completely used.
3. Place diagnostic reports in the correct patient's chart behind the correct divider. Match the patient's name on the report with the patient's name within the chart (do not depend on room numbers because patients are often transferred to another room).
4. Review the patient's charts frequently for new orders (always check each chart for new orders before returning them to the chart rack).
5. Properly label the patient's chart so it can easily be located at all times.
6. Check each chart to be sure that all forms are labeled with the correct patient's name. Chart forms should be filed in the proper sequence.
7. Check the chart frequently for patient information forms or face sheets. Usually, five copies are maintained in the chart. Physicians may remove copies for billing purposes. The HUC may print additional copies of the face sheet from the computer or may order them from admitting.

CONSENT FOR HIV TESTING

1. My physician, _____, has recommended that I (my child) receive a blood test to detect the presence of antibodies to Human Immunodeficiency Virus (HIV), the virus that causes Acquired Immune Deficiency Syndrome (AIDS). I consent to this testing.

It has been explained to me that in some cases the tests may be positive when I have (my child has) not been infected with HIV. This is a false positive.

If the screening is positive, a second confirming test is done.

I understand that a negative result usually means that I have (my child has) not been exposed to HIV. However, there is a possibility of a false-negative result, especially in the time period immediately after exposure to the virus.

2. I have been advised by my physician and I understand the following:

- Positive test results could mean that I have (my child has) been exposed to the HIV; this would not necesarily mean that I have (my child has) AIDS, or will develop AIDS.
- That if I am (my child is) HIV positive, I (my child) can transmit the virus to other individuals by sexual contact, by sharing needles, or by the donation of organs, blood, and blood products.
- That if I am (my child is) HIV positive, I (my child) should not donate blood or blood products, or body organs because the virus can be transmitted to the recipient.

3. I understand that Arizona State Law and Regulations require the reporting of HIV cases to the Department of Health Services and that if my (my child's) test results are positive, they will be submitted to the Arizona Department of Health Services, and others whose authority is established by law, regulation, or court order.

4. I also understand that my request for the test and the test results will be part of my (my child's) hospital medical record and may therefore be requested by others, including insurers, third party payors or other individuals as outlined in the Conditions of Admission.

I have been given the opportunity to ask quesitons, I understand what is involved in HIV testing, and I freely consent to it.

_____   _____
DATE   SIGNATURE

_____   _____
LEGAL GUARDIAN   WITNESS SIGNATURE
(If patient cannot sign or under age)

Figure 8-15 Consent form for human immunodeficiency virus (HIV) testing.

8. Assist physicians or other professionals in locating the patient's chart.

Splitting or Thinning the Chart

The paper chart of a patient who remains in the health care facility for a long time becomes very full and eventually becomes unmanageable. When this occurs, the HUC may **"thin"** or **"split"** the chart. A doctor's order is not required to thin a patient's chart. In thinning the chart, some categories of chart forms may be removed and placed in an envelope for safekeeping on the unit. The following guidelines will assist the HUC in thinning a patient's chart:

1. Remove older graphics records, nurse's notes, medication forms, and other forms that are no longer needed in the chart binder. (Check the hospital policy and procedure manual to verify forms that may and may not be removed.)
2. Place the removed forms in an envelope.
3. Place the patient's ID label on the outside of the envelope.

4. Write "thinned chart" and record the date with your first initial and last name (of the person thinning the chart) on the outside of the envelope.
5. Place a label stating that the chart was thinned, along with the date, first initial, and last name (of the person thinning the chart) on the front of the patient's chart.
6. If the patient is transferred to another unit, transfer the thinned-out forms with the patient's chart.
7. When the patient is discharged, send all thinned-out forms with the patient's paper chart to the health information management department.

Reproduction of Chart Forms That Contain Patient Information

On some occasions, a copier is needed to reproduce portions of a patient's chart. For example, to ensure continuity of care when a patient is discharged to another health care facility. The patient's doctor must write an order specifying

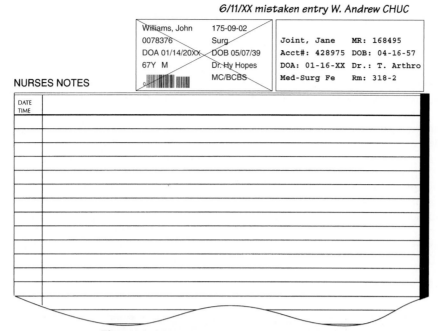

Figure 8-16 Method for correcting labeling error.

MEDICATION RECORD

Routine Medications

◯ - **CIRCLE ALL DOSES NOT GIVEN - STATE REASON IN NURSES NOTES**

DATE			6/10/XX	6/11/XX	6/12/XX	6/13/XX	6/14/XX
DAY OF WEEK			*Sun.*	*Mon.*	*Tues.*	*Wed.*	*Thurs.*
MEDICATION *11/6/XX mistaken entry* ~~prednisolone~~ *A. Hay. Chuc*			11-7				
			7-3				
DOSE *5 mg*	ROUTE	FREQUENCY	3-11				
MEDICATION *Prednisone*			11-7				
			7-3				
DOSE *5 mg*	ROUTE *p.o.*	FREQUENCY *Bid.*	3-11				
MEDICATION			11-7				
			7-3				
DOSE	ROUTE	FREQUENCY	3-11				
MEDICATION			11-7				
			7-3				
DOSE	ROUTE	FREQUENCY	3-11				
MEDICATION			11-7				
			7-3				
DOSE	ROUTE	FREQUENCY	3-11				
~ICATION			11-7				
	ROUTE	FREQUENCY					

Figure 8-17 Method for correcting a written error on the chart.

the specific chart forms to be copied, and the patient may or may not be required to sign a release form. Depending on hospital policy, the HUC may have the responsibility of copying the paper chart forms, or the patient's chart may be sent to the health information management department to be copied. After the forms are reproduced on the copier, original forms are replaced in the patient's chart and the copied records are sent to the receiving facility.

The patient's EMR is available on computer to other health care facilities, or the records may be printed from the computer. The patient may or may not be required to sign a release form for the records to be available or copied in this situation.

MONITORING AND MAINTAINING THE PATIENT'S ELECTRONIC MEDICAL RECORD

The HUC position has changed with the implementation of the EMR, but monitoring and maintaining the patient's records is still the responsibility of the HUC.

Health Unit Coordinator Duties for Monitoring and Maintaining the Patient's Electronic Medical Record

1. Monitor the patient's EMR consistently, and carry out HUC tasks as required and in a timely manner.
2. Assist nurses, doctors, and ancillary personnel as necessary in entering information and orders into the computer.
3. Report any necessary repairs regarding nursing unit computers and/or printers to the hospital information systems department.
4. Scan documents as required such as handwritten progress notes, electrocardiograms, outside medical records, and reports in a timely manner.
5. Place and maintain patient ID labels in a patient label book.
6. Place patient face sheets into a notebook to provide to physicians as requested.

KEY CONCEPTS

The patient's chart (paper or electronic) is a record of care rendered and the patient's response to care during hospitalization. When the EMR is implemented, all health care information is entered into or scanned into the patient's chart. When paper charts are in use, the nursing unit to which the patient is assigned adds forms to the patient's chart. The patient's medical information (paper or electronic) is a legal record and should be maintained as such.

Standard forms are placed on all patients' paper charts; supplemental forms may be added according to the need dictated by each patient's treatment and care. The purpose of the forms is the same for each hospital, but the sequence of forms in the chart and the placement of blank forms that are added may differ from hospital to hospital. When the EMR is implemented, information is entered into the computer on similar computerized forms. Information contained in the patient's paper chart or EMR must always be regarded as confidential.

REVIEW QUESTIONS

1. A group of patient chart forms preassembled to be used for new patients is usually called a(n) _____

2. List six purposes for keeping a paper chart or an EMR on each patient.

   a. _____

   b. _____

   c. _____

   d. _____

   e. _____

   f. _____

3. List five guidelines for writing on a patient's paper chart.

   a. _____

   b. _____

   c. _____

   d. _____

   e. _____

4. List five guidelines for entering information into a patient's EMR.

   a. _____

   b. _____

   c. _____

   d. _____

   e. _____

5. State the purpose of the following paper or electronic forms:

a. physician's order form

_____

b. graphic record form

_____

c. physician's progress record

_____

d. history and physical form

_____

e. nurse's progress notes

_____

f. medication administration record

_____

6. List four standard patient chart or electronic forms that are initiated in the admitting department, and describe the purpose of each.

a. _____

b. _____

c. _____

d. _____

7. Define what is meant by a supplemental patient chart form, and give two examples of supplemental forms.

a. Definition:

_____

b. 1st example:

_____

c. 2nd example:

_____

8. List five guidelines for preparing consent forms.

a. _____

b. _____

c. _____

d. _____

e. _____

9. List four types of permit or release forms that a patient may be required to sign during a hospital stay.

a. _____

b. _____

c. _____

d. _____

10. List eight duties that will assist the HUC in properly maintaining a patient's paper chart.

a. _____

b. _____

c. _____

d. _____

e. _____

f. _____

g. _____

h. _____

11. List six duties that will assist the HUC in properly maintaining and monitoring a patient's EMR.

a. _____

b. _____

c. _____

d. _____

e. _____

f. _____

12. Describe how to correct the following errors on a paper chart form.

a. Written entry error:

_____

b. Labeling error:

_____

13. 3:30 PM in military time is _____.

14. 2345 military time in standard time is _____.

15. Define the following terms:

a. stuffing charts:

_____

b. "split" or thinned chart:

_____

c. patient identification labels:

_____

d. name alert:

_____

e. allergy labels:

_____

f. old record:

_____

g. WALLaroo:

_____

THINK ABOUT...

1. Discuss possible consequences of allowing a stranger access to a patient's paper chart or EMR.
2. Discuss possible consequences of leaving a patient's side rails down without having them sign a release.
3. Discuss possible consequences of a patient's signing a consent form after being sedated, or of adding an additional procedure or changing the wording of a procedure after a patient has signed it.
4. Discuss what would happen if surgery personnel came to pick up the patient for surgery and it was discovered that the wording on the consent form was not exactly the same as that on the doctor's order.

Transcription of Doctors' Handwritten Orders

CHAPTER OBJECTIVES

Upon completion of this chapter, you will be able to:

1. Define the terms in the vocabulary list.
2. Describe the health unit coordinator's role in executing doctors' handwritten orders.
3. Name two criteria the health unit coordinator can use to recognize a new set of handwritten doctors' orders that need transcription.
4. List the four categories of doctors' orders and explain the characteristics of each.
5. Describe the purpose and process of kardexing.
6. List five areas commonly found on the Kardex form.
7. Describe the process of sending handwritten doctors' orders to the appropriate departments.
8. Name the symbols used in transcribing doctors' orders and describe the purpose for using each symbol.
9. Describe the purpose and process of signing off doctors' orders.
10. Explain why all entries on the doctor's order sheet are recorded in ink.
11. List in order the 10 steps of transcribing handwritten doctors' orders.
12. Discuss why accuracy is important in the transcription procedure.
13. Discuss the types of errors that may occur during the transcription procedure and the methods of avoidance that may be used.

VOCABULARY

Flagging A method used by the doctor to notify the nursing staff that a new set of orders has been written

Kardex File A portable file that contains and organizes the Kardex forms for each patient on the nursing unit

Kardex Form A form on which the health unit coordinator records doctors' orders; it is used by the nursing staff for a quick reference of the patient's current orders

Kardexing The process of recording and updating doctors' orders on the Kardex form (many hospitals have eliminated the paper Kardex form in favor of entering all patient orders into the computer)

One-Time or Short-Series Order A doctor's order that is executed according to the qualifying phrase, and then is automatically discontinued

Ordering The process of ordering diagnostic procedures, treatments, or supplies from hospital departments other than nursing

Requisition A paper form used to order diagnostic procedures, treatments, or supplies from hospital departments other than nursing when the computer is down (also called a downtime requisition)

Set of Doctor's Orders An entry of doctor's orders written on the doctor's order sheet, dated, notated for time, and signed by the doctor

Signing Off A process by which the health unit coordinator records data (date, time, name, and status) on the doctor's order sheet to indicate the completion of transcription of a handwritten set of doctor's orders

Standing Order A doctor's order that remains in effect and is executed as ordered until the doctor discontinues or changes it

Standing prn Order Similar to a standing order, except that it is executed according to the patient's needs

Stat Order A doctor's order that is to be executed immediately, then automatically discontinued

Symbols Notations written in black or red ink on the doctor's order sheet to indicate completion of a step of the transcription procedure

Telephoned Orders Orders for a patient that are called into a health care facility (usually to the patient's nurse) by the doctor

DOCTORS' ORDERS

It is predicted that the electronic medical record (EMR) will not be implemented nationwide for at least 5 years. When the EMR with computer physician order entry (CPOE) is not being used, the doctors' orders for a patient's care are handwritten or are preprinted on a doctors' order sheet. These orders include such items as diagnostic procedures, medications, surgical treatment, diet, patient activities, discharge, and so forth. As stated in Chapter 8, handwritten doctors' orders are legal documents that become a permanent record of the patient's chart.

The doctor writes all orders in ink, records the date and time, and signs each entry. The doctor may write one order or a series of orders; this is referred to as a **set of doctors' orders**. The doctor indicates to the nursing staff that a new set of orders is included by **flagging** the chart. Flagging techniques vary among health care facilities. New orders can be identified by the absence of symbols and by the absence of sign-off information. See Figure 9-1 for an example of a set of written doctors' orders. Sometimes, the doctor may write new orders and forget to flag the chart. Always check for new orders before returning a chart to the area where it is stored.

If the new orders are recorded at the top of the doctors' order sheet, check to see if the orders are a continuation from the previous sheet. When orders are recorded near the bottom of the doctor's order sheet instead of at the top, make diagonal lines across the remaining space so new orders will not be recorded there, and then continue on to the following page (Figure 9-2).

Categories of Doctors' Orders

Doctors' orders may be categorized according to when they are carried out and the length of time they are in effect. The transcription procedure varies according to the category of the order; therefore, it is necessary to recognize each category. The four categories include (1) standing, or continuing, orders, (2) standing, or continuing, prn orders, (3) **one-time, or short-series orders**, and (4) **stat orders**.

Standing (Continuing) Orders

Most doctors' orders fall into this group. **Standing orders** are in effect and are executed routinely as ordered until they are discontinued or changed by a new doctor's order. For example, in the order,

- BP lying, sitting, and standing tid

The doctor has ordered the patient's blood pressure (BP) to be taken with the patient lying, sitting, and standing and that it should be recorded three times a day (tid). A time sequence such as 0800, 1400, and 2000 is set up for the blood pressure to be taken daily. This routine continues until it is changed or discontinued by the doctor. Another example of a standing order includes the following:

- Regular diet

This order means that the patient receives a regular diet on each day of the hospital stay unless the order is changed or discontinued by the doctor.

```
Joint, Jane    MR: 168495
Acct#: 428975  DOB: 04-16-57
DOA: 01-16-XX  Dr.: T. Arthro
Med-Surg Fe    Rm: 318-2
```

Physicians' Order Sheet

Date	Symbol	Physicians' Orders
01/16/XX		Admit to med-surg
		CBR
		STAT CBC
		consultation with Dr. T.L. Payne
		HOB ↑ 30°
		Wt daily
		Rectal temp q 4°
		Intake and output
		Compazine 10 mg IM for nausea ana vomiting
		Dr. Thomas Arthro, M.D.

Figure 9-1 Example of a set of written doctors' orders. Interpretation of the abbreviations used in this figure and in subsequent figures in this chapter may be found in the Glossary and is explained in future chapters.

Physicians' Order Sheet

```
Joint, Jane    MR: 168495
Acct#: 428975  DOB: 04-16-57
DOA: 01-16-XX  Dr.: T. Arthro
Med-Surg Fe    Rm: 318-2
```

Date	Symbol	Physicians' Orders
01/16/XX	Ord K	May have reg diet
		Dr. Thomas Arthro, M.D.
01/16/XX	1000	Ellen Green CHUC
/////////////

Figure 9-2 Diagonal lines drawn at the bottom of a nearly filled doctors' order sheet.

Standing (Continuing) prn Orders

The Latin words *pro re nata*, meaning "as circumstances may require," are abbreviated as *prn* and are used by the doctor in a written order to indicate that the order is to be executed as needed. **Standing prn orders,** similar to standing orders, are in effect until they are changed or discontinued by the doctor. They differ from standing orders in that they are executed according to the patient's needs. For example, in the order,

- Acetaminophen 325 mg i or ii PO q4h prn H/A

The nurse may give 325 mg i or ii capsules as often as every 4 hours (q4h) as needed by the patient to relieve a headache. This does not mean that the medication is administered every 4 hours, because the patient may not have a headache at those times; therefore, it is impossible to set up a time sequence as discussed with the standing order.

In the order,

- Compazine 10 mg IM q6h for nausea or vomiting

The doctor uses a qualifying phrase, *for nausea or vomiting,* to indicate that it is a prn order.

Remember: A prn order may be recognized by the abbreviation *prn* or by the content of a qualifying phrase and is in effect until it is changed or discontinued by the doctor.

One-Time or Short-Series Order

The doctor may want a treatment or medication carried out once only or for a short period of time. This is indicated by a qualifying phrase, such as *give at 2:00* PM, or *give tonight and in* AM. Upon completion of the one-time or short-series order, the order is automatically discontinued. For example, in the following orders,

- Give patient Fleets enema this PM

The phrase "this PM" makes it a one-time order—thus, the order is discontinued after the enema is given.

- Blood pressure q2h until awake

The phrase "until awake" makes it a short-series order.

✐ TAKE NOTE

A one-time or short-series order may be recognized by the content of the qualifying phrase and is automatically discontinued after completion.

Stat Orders

Stat is the abbreviation for the Latin word *statim,* which means "at once." When included in a doctor's order, it indicates that the order is to be carried out immediately. Stat orders are usually written during an emergency or for patients who are critically ill. Because of the urgency of stat orders, they are communicated immediately to the nurse and/or department personnel responsible for carrying out the order. Stat orders are transcribed first when included in a set of orders. Stat orders are recognized by the word *stat* (meaning now) included in the order, as in the following examples,

- CBC stat
- CBC now (or CBC immediately)

The words *now* and *immediately* are usually considered to indicate stat orders that should receive urgent attention.

✐ TAKE NOTE

Categories of Doctors' Orders
Standing: In effect and given routinely until discontinued or changed by the doctor
Standing prn: In effect and given as needed by the patient until automatically discontinued or changed by the doctor
One-time or short-series: In effect for one time or a short period; automatically discontinued when the order has been completed
Stat: Given immediately, then automatically discontinued

The Kardex File and the Kardex Form

Each nursing unit may use a portable file that is referred to as the Kardex. This file contains one **Kardex form** for each patient on the unit. Approximately 15 to 20 individual patient Kardex forms can be included in one **Kardex file;** larger nursing units of 30 or more patients may need to use two Kardex files. Patient information such as room number, name, doctor's name, and diagnosis are recorded at the bottom of the Kardex form, so when filed in the Kardex file, the information remains visible (Figure 9-3).

Five main areas common to most Kardex forms are listed below.

1. Activity
2. Diet
3. Vital sign frequency
4. Treatment
5. Diagnostic studies

Other areas, such as intravenous therapy, intake and output, and weight, are also usually included on the form.

The Kardex form also may include an area for a patient care plan, which is completed by the nursing staff. The purpose of the Kardex is to maintain a current profile of a patient's information, current doctors' orders, and the patient's nursing needs. It provides a quick reference for the nursing staff, is used for planning and designating patient care, and is used for reporting patient information to the oncoming shift. The design of the Kardex form varies according to hospital and nursing unit needs, but the basic concept remains the same.

Kardexing

Kardexing is the process of recording all new doctors' orders onto each patient's Kardex form. The purpose of kardexing all the doctors' orders is to communicate new orders to the nursing staff and to update the patient's profile on the Kardex form. Kardexing is usually done in pencil because new doctors' orders may involve changing or discontinuing an existing order. However, information not subject to change, such as the patient's name, is usually recorded in black ink, and allergies are always recorded in red ink.

Accuracy in kardexing is absolutely essential. An error could result in the patient's receiving the wrong, and perhaps harmful, treatment. The patient's Kardex form is usually not considered a legal document, and in the past, it was usually discarded when the patient was discharged from the hospital. However, the present trend is toward filing the nursing care plan portion of the Kardex form with the patient's chart in the health information management department.

TAKE NOTE

Many hospitals that have not completely implemented the EMR are using a computerized kardexing system, eliminating the need for the Kardex form and the Kardex file. When the EMR is fully implemented, the Kardex is not used.

Ordering

Ordering is the process of inputting the handwritten doctors' orders into the computer or onto a paper **requisition**. Paper requisitions are seldom completed, even when paper charts are used because computer maintenance down time is usually scheduled at night when few orders are written. The procedure for using paper requisitions is included in this chapter to assist one in learning the tests/procedures performed in each of the various departments of the hospital. The purpose of the

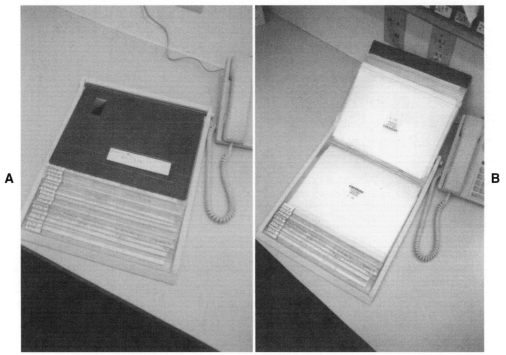

Figure 9-3 A portable file (a Kardex) as it appears closed **(A)** and open **(B).**

ordering step is to forward the doctors' orders to the hospital departments that will execute the orders.

Doctors' orders that involve diagnostic procedures, treatment, or supplies from hospital departments usually require the ordering step. Ordering by computer requires the HUC to select the patient's name from a computer screen and follow the steps to input the ordering information (according to the hospital computer program used). Ordering by requisition requires the HUC first to affix that patient's ID label on the requisition and, second, to copy or fill in all pertinent data from the doctors' orders.

✐ TAKE NOTE

If an imprinter and patient identification imprinter cards are used, the requisitions would be stamped with the patient information instead of using labels.

---

*In subsequent chapters, whenever instructions are to "label" a chart form or a requisition, if an imprinter with patient identification imprinter cards is used, substitute "label" with "imprint" or "stamp."

Symbols

As the HUC completes a part of the transcription procedure, a *symbol* is recorded on the doctors' order sheet to indicate completion of the task. The symbol may be written in black or red ink, depending on hospital policy, in front of the doctor's order (Figure 9-4).

By using symbols, the health unit coordinator provides a written record of the steps completed, which reduces the possibility of omitting or forgetting to complete a part of the transcription procedure. There are constant interruptions, and this could make it easy to forget where one left off when returning to transcribing a set of orders. Lack of order completion can cause delays in treatment, which may cause delays in or be harmful to the patient's recovery.

The following list of symbols is used in this textbook; however, symbols vary among hospitals. The instructor, therefore, may prefer that HUC students become familiar with symbols commonly used in hospitals in their area.

PC sent or faxed: Indicates that the pharmacy copy of the doctors' order sheet was forwarded to the pharmacy. Initial and record the time it was sent on the copy or original if faxed. *Note:* Some hospitals have a "faxed" stamp with an area in which to fill in initials and the time faxed.

Ord: Indicates that diagnostic tests, treatments, or supplies have been ordered by computer or by requisition. When using the computer method, record the computer order number above each ordered item.

K: Indicates that the order has been transcribed on the patient's Kardex form. It is also used to indicate that a discontinued order has been erased from the Kardex. Each order kardexed requires the date and its own line on the Kardex.

M: Indicates transcription of a medication order on the medication administration record (MAR) form.

Called (name and time): Indicates completion of a telephone call necessary to complete the doctor's order. Document the time of the call and the name of the person contacted above the order on the doctor's order sheet, and initial it.

```
Joint, Jane    MR: 168495
Acct#: 428975  DOB: 04-16-57
DOA: 01-16-XX  Dr.: T. Arthro
Med-Surg Fe    Rm: 318-2
```

Physicians' Order Sheet

Date	Symbol	Physicians' Orders
01/16/XX	K	Admit to med-surg
	K	CBR
	Ord K	STAT CBC called Pat 1450
	K	Consultation with Dr. T. L. Payne
	K	HOB ↑ 30°
	K	Wt daily
	K	Rectal temp q 4°
	K	Intake and output
	M	Compazine 10 mg IM for nausea and vomiting
		Dr. Thomas Arthro, M.D.
01/16/XX	1000	Ellen Green CHUC

Figure 9-4 Example of a transcribed set of doctor's orders, showing use of the symbols to indicate that the pharmacy copy has been faxed (step 2), the telephone call has been placed and documented (step 4), the test has been ordered (step 6), the orders have been Kardexed (step 7), and the medication has been written on the MAR (step 8). The set of orders has been signed off by the health unit coordinator, indicating completion of transcription (step 10).

Notified (name and time): Indicates that the appropriate health care team member has been notified of a *stat* order. Document the time of notification and the name of the person contacted above the order on the doctor's order sheet, and initial it.

Signing Off Doctors' Orders

Signing off is the process that is used to indicate completion of the transcription procedure of a set of doctors' orders. To sign off, the HUC records the date, time, full name, and status (may use the abbreviation *SHUC* if a student HUC, or *CHUC* if certified) on the line directly below the doctor's signature (see Figure 9-4). Once again, this is done in black or red ink because the doctor's order sheet is a legal document. In many hospitals, a registered nurse is required to cosign the transcribed orders. All hospitals require that registered nurses perform 24-hour chart checks, during which they will sign off on their assigned patients.

The sign-off procedure varies among health care facilities. For example, some health care facilities use black ink for the sign-off procedure. Some hospitals use red ink to distinguish the sign-off information from the written doctors' orders, and some require that the HUC draw a line to box off the orders when signing off.

TRANSCRIPTION OF DOCTORS' ORDERS

Transcription of doctors' handwritten orders is a process that is used to communicate doctors' orders to the nursing staff and other hospital departments. The transcription procedure includes kardexing, ordering, using symbols, the **signing-off** process, and sometimes other steps. How the HUC goes about performing this procedure varies among health care facilities and from individual to individual. See Figure 9-4 for a transcribed set of doctors' orders.

Doctor Ordering Hy Hopes   ☐ Stat   Joint, Jane   MR: 168495

Today's Date 01/16/XX   ☐ Routine   Acct#: 428975   DOB: 04-16-57

Collection Date 01/16/XX Time _____   DOA: 01-16-XX   Dr.: T. Arthro

Collected by _____   Med-Surg Fe   Rm: 318-2

Requested by J. Phoebe

Hematology	**Serology**	**Urinalysis/Urine Chemistry**
☐ Bleeding Time, Ivy	☐ ANA	☐ Routine UA
☐ CBC c̄ Diff	☐ ASO Titer	☐ Reflex UA
☐ CBC c̄ Manual Diff	☐ CEA	☐ Amylase (2 hr)
☐ Factor VIII	☐ CMV	☐ Bilirubin
☐ Fibrinogen	☐ IgG	☐ Calcium
☐ HCT	☐ IgM	☐ Chloride
☐ HGB	☐ Cocci Screen	☐ Creatinine Clearance
☐ H & H	☐ EBV Panel	☐ Glucose Tolerance
☐ Eosinophil Ct Absolute	☐ Enterovirus Ab Panel 1	☐ Nitrogen
☐ Eosinophil Smear	☐ Enterovirus Ab Panel 2	☐ Occult Blood
☐ ESR	☐ FTA	☐ Osmolality
☐ LE Cell Prep	☐ HbsAb	☐ Phosphorus
☐ Platelet Ct	☐ HbsAg	☐ Potassium
☐ PT	☐ Hepatitis Screen	☐ Pregnancy
☐ PTT (APTT)	☐ HIV	☐ Protein
☐ RBC	☐ Monospot	☐ Sodium
☐ RBC Indices	☐ PSA Screen	☐ Sp Gravity
☐ Reticulocyte Ct	☐ RA Factor	☐ Uric Acid
☐ Sickle Cell Prep	☐ RPR	
☐ WBC	☐ RSV	
☐ WBC c̄ Diff	☐ Rubella Screen	
☐ WBC c̄ Manual Diff	☐ Streptozyme	
☐ Other	☐ Other	

Write in Orders: _____

_____

Revised 3/12/XX

Figure 9-5 Completed downtime laboratory requisition.

Kardex Form

Activity 1/16 C(BR) HOB ↑30°	Date Ord	Treatments	Date Ord	Laboratory	Date Ord	Allergies	
	1/16	Consult Dr. T.L. Payne	1/16	stat CBC			
						Diagnostic Imaging	Date to be Done
Diet							
Vital signs 1/16 Rtemp q 4 h							
Weight 1/16 Daily							
IV		Respiratory Care		Pre OP Orders		Diagnostic Studies	
				Daily Lab			
I & O 1/16							
Retention Cath (Foley) ☐ Health Records _____		Physical Medicine					
Adm. Date 1/16		Consultations:		Surgery: Date:			
Name Joint, Jane		Doctor T.Arthro	Age 51	Diagnosis Osteoarthritis		Date of admission 1/16/xx	

Figure 9-6 Completed Kardex.

✎ TAKE NOTE

A panel of experienced nurses and HUCs developed ten steps of transcription to reduce the risk of errors. There will always be variances between what is done in the classroom, between hospitals, and even between nursing units within hospitals. Some of these differences may include the following: Symbols may be different or not be used at all, red ink or black ink only may be used to note orders (may be the policy), patient identification (ID) cards with imprinter machines may be used in place of labels, and different forms may be used. This and other chapters will assist the reader in coping with these variances. If the EMR is used, the HUC will not have the responsibility of transcribing doctors' orders.
FLEXIBILITY IS THE KEY!

Ten Steps for Transcription of Doctors' Handwritten Orders

Listed below are the 10 steps that make up the transcription procedure. It is important to note that each type of doctors' orders may require some or all of the steps to complete the transcription procedure. Always compare each order with the 10 steps of transcription when choosing the steps that are required for complete transcription of each order. This procedure is the simplest, yet most efficient method used for transcribing doctors' orders.

The following 10 steps of transcription will assist the HUC in transcribing doctors' handwritten orders efficiently and accurately:

1. Read the complete set of doctors' orders.
2. Order medications by sending or faxing the pharmacy copy of the doctors' order sheet to the pharmacy department.
3. Complete all stat orders.
4. Place telephone calls as necessary to complete the doctor's orders.
5. Select the patient's identifying information (i.e., name, account number, etc.) from the census on the computer screen, or collect all necessary forms.
6. Order diagnostic tests, treatments, and supplies (see Figure 9-5 for a completed downtime laboratory requisition).
7. Kardex all the doctors' orders except medication orders (see Figure 9-6 for a completed Kardex).
8. Complete medication orders by writing them on the **MAR.**
9. Recheck each step for accuracy and thoroughness.
10. Sign off the completed set of the doctor's orders.

Procedure 9-1 describes a method of carrying out the 10 steps of transcription.

Avoiding Transcription Errors

Throughout this chapter, the importance of accuracy during the transcription procedure has been emphasized, so errors that may cause serious harm to the patient can be avoided. Consider, for example, the consequences for the HUC who, during the transcription procedure, overlooks a doctor's order for the patient to have a stat medication, or orders a diet for a patient who has been ordered by the doctor to have nothing by mouth for a pending surgery or invasive medical procedure.

Table 9-1 outlines the types of errors that may occur during the transcription procedure and methods that may be used to avoid making these errors.

KEY CONCEPTS

Until the EMR with computer physician order entry is implemented, the transcription of doctors' orders is the single most responsible task that an HUC performs. An error may result

✐ TAKE NOTE

How to Avoid Errors of Transcription
Ask the doctor or nurse for assistance if a doctor's order cannot be read or understood.
Use information from the chart to correctly select the patient from the computer screen or to correctly label requisitions.
Record the sign-off information on the line directly below the doctor's signature.
Check the previous page for orders when the orders begin at the top of the page.

in a patient's being harmed or in their recovery time being extended. Completing the transcription procedure promptly, accurately, and thoroughly is always best practice in providing quality care for patients.

PROCEDURE 9-1

TRANSCRIPTION OF DOCTORS' ORDERS

STEP	TASK	NOTES
1.	Read the complete set of doctors' orders.	1. *Reading the complete set of orders gives an overview of the task at hand. Accurate reading and interpretation of each word of the doctors' handwritten orders are vital because each word and/or abbreviation carries a specific meaning.*
2.	Order medications. a. Remove and send the pharmacy copy of the doctors' order sheet, or fax original copy of doctors' order sheet to the pharmacy. b. Write PC sent or faxed, time, and initials on the doctors' order sheet (see Figure 9-4).	2. *Sending a copy or faxing the original doctor's order to the pharmacy helps avoid medication errors because no rewriting is involved. Completing this step first allows the patient to receive the medication as soon as possible.*
3.	Complete all stat orders.	3. *Stat orders are always transcribed first.*
4.	Place telephone calls as necessary to complete the doctors' orders. Upon completing this task, write the symbol *called* and the time *called* (be sure to include AM or PM, or use military time) and the name of the person receiving the call in ink in front of the doctor's order on the doctors' order sheet (see Figure 9–4).	4. *Doctors' orders may require a telephone call to be placed to another department or health agency to schedule appointments, procedures, etc. Recording the time of the call and the person's name who is receiving the call is helpful if follow-up is necessary.*
5.	Select the correct patient's name on the computer screen, and/or collect all necessary forms.	5. *This varies according to the type of doctors' orders included in the set. Collecting necessary forms at once saves time.*
6.	Order all diagnostic tests, treatments, and supplies. Using a computer with CD-ROM, which simulates a hospital computer system, do the following: a. Select the correct patient's name on the viewing screen. b. Select the department from the department menu on the viewing screen. c. Select the test, treatment, or supply from the menu on the viewing screen. d. Fill in required information. e. Order test, treatments, or supplies. f. Write the symbol *ord* or computer number in ink in front of the doctor's order on the doctors' order sheet (see Figure 9-4).	6. *This step includes ordering diagnostic procedures, treatments, and supplies from appropriate hospital departments.* *Check both the patient's name and the hospital number with the same information in the chart.*

Continued

PROCEDURE 9-1 —Cont'd

TRANSCRIPTION OF DOCTORS' ORDERS

STEP	TASK	NOTES
	Using handwritten requisitions: Although handwritten requisitions are seldom used, this process will assist the student in learning which departments would perform tests and procedures ordered. a. Affix the patient's identification (ID) label to the requisition (or imprint). b. Place a check mark on the requisition to indicate the test, treatment, or supply that is being requisitioned. c. Fill in today's date and the date the test or treatment is to be done in the appropriate spaces. d. Write in pertinent data, such as "patient blind" or "isolation." e. Sign name and status in the appropriate space on the requisition form. f. Write the symbol *ord* in ink in front of the doctor's order on the doctors' order sheet (see Figure 9-4).	*Selection of the correct patient when one is filling out requisitions is absolutely essential. The wrong selection could easily cause a patient to receive a diagnostic test or treatment intended for another patient. Always compare the name and hospital number on the requisition form with the same information in the chart. Remember: There may be more than one patient on the unit with the same last name. Label all requisitions for the patient whose orders are being processed at the same time.*
7.	Kardex all the doctors' orders. Begin with the first order, then proceed to the next until all the orders are completed (see Figure 9-6). Complete kardexing by doing the following: a. Write the date followed by the order in pencil under the correct column of the Kardex form. Carefully read what is already written in the column to evaluate whether the new order cancels an existing order. If this occurs, erase the existing order. If an order is discontinued, erase it from the Kardex. b. Write the symbol *K* in ink in front of the doctors' order on the doctors' order sheet (see Figure 9-4).	7. *Nursing orders that need to be implemented during the shift are often recorded on a clipboard in order to bring them to the immediate attention of the nurse.* **All doctors' orders are kardexed. Make sure the right patient's Kardex form is selected; many patients' Kardex forms are filed in a single Kardex file. To ensure accurate selection, check the name of the patient and the doctor on the Kardex form with the patient information in the chart.* **There may be more than one patient on the unit with the same last name.* Note: *Many hospitals are using a computerized kardexing system.*
8.	Complete medication orders by doing the following: a. Write the medication order on the medication administration record. b. Place the symbol *M* in ink in front of the doctor's order on the doctors' order sheet (see Figure 9-4).	8. *This procedure is covered in greater detail in Chapter 13.*
9.	Recheck the performance of each task for accuracy and thoroughness.	9. *This is an important step because it is easy to miss an order or a detail of an order.*
10.	Sign off the completed set of orders by writing the following in ink on the line directly below the doctor's signature: a. Date b. Time c. Full signature d. Status Figure 9-4 provides an example of this step.	10. *It is important to have completed all the tasks of transcription before signing off.* **Signing off is an indication that all the transcription steps necessary for the orders to be carried out as written have been performed.*

Table 9-1 Avoiding Transcription Errors

Types of Errors		Method of Avoidance
Errors of Omission	1.	Read and understand each word of the doctors' orders. If in doubt, check with a patient's nurse or the doctor.
	2.	Use symbols. It is especially important to write the symbol after each step of transcription has been completed.
	3.	When new orders are recorded at the top of the doctors' order sheet, check the previous order sheet to see whether these orders are continued from the previous page.
	4.	If the set of orders finishes near the bottom of the doctors' order sheet, cross through the remaining space with diagonal lines. This is done so that newly written orders will begin at the top of the new doctors' order form. When orders are recorded at the bottom of one page and are continued onto the next, it is easy to miss transcribing those recorded on the first page.
	5.	Record the signing-off information on the line directly below the doctor's signature to avoid leaving space in which future orders could be written and missed.
	6.	Check for new orders before returning a chart from the counter or elsewhere to the chart rack.
Errors of Interpretation	1.	When in doubt about the correct interpretation of doctors' orders, always check with the registered nurse or the doctor.
Errors in the Selection of the Patient's Identification (ID) Label or Errors in Selection of the Patient's Name on the Computer Screen	1.	Compare the patient's name and the hospital number on the order requisition form or on the computer screen with the same information in the patient's chart. Never select computer labels by the patient's room number only. *Note:* Other staff members frequently use the computer to retrieve information and may change screens while orders are being transcribed. Always double-check the patient information when entering orders into the computer.
Errors in Selection of the Patient's Kardex Form	1.	Compare the patient's name and the doctor's name on the Kardex form with the same information in the patient's chart. Never select by using room number alone. If the patient has been transferred, the room number imprinted on chart forms may no longer be correct. *Note:* Many nursing staff members use the Kardex for a quick reference and may flip to another patient's Kardex form while orders are being transcribed. Remove the Kardex form from the holder when transcribing orders and return it to its proper place in the Kardex holder when order transcription has been completed.
Errors in Reading the Doctor's Poor Handwriting	1.	When an order cannot be read because of the doctor's handwriting, refer to the progress record form in the patient's chart. The orders are often recorded on this form also, and using this information may assist in interpreting the orders on the physician's order form. If the order remains unclear, ask the doctor who wrote it or ask the patient's nurse for clarification. If a doctor has a reputation for poor handwriting, ask to go over the orders for clarification prior to their leaving the nursing unit.

REVIEW QUESTIONS

1. Why are symbols used as a part of the transcription procedure?

_____

_____

2. Demonstrate how the HUC would sign off on a set of doctors' orders.

_____

_____

3. List *in order* the 10 steps of transcribing handwritten doctors' orders.

a. _____

b. _____

c. _____

d. _____

e. _____

f. _____

g. _____

h. _____

i. _____

j. _____

4. Explain why doctors' orders, symbols, and sign-offs are recorded in ink on each doctors' order sheet.

_____

_____

5. Symbols are recorded on the doctors' order sheet (circle one):

a. after the step of transcription is completed

b. before the step of transcription is completed

c. at any time, as long as they are recorded accurately

d. after the patient's nurse has verified that the step of transcription is complete

6. List two ways that the HUC would recognize newly written doctors' orders that need transcription.

a. _____

b. _____

7. Why are doctors' orders recorded on the Kardex form?

_____

8. Why are doctors' orders written on the Kardex form in pencil?

_____

9. Define the following terms:

a. ordering:

_____

b. kardexing:

_____

c. requisition:

_____

d. flagging:

_____

10. Regarding the doctors' order sheet,

a. Which line is used for the signing-off procedure?

_____

b. Explain why:

_____

11. Why is accuracy essential for transcribing handwritten doctors' orders?

_____

12. Write in the symbol that is used to indicate completion of the following:

a. ordering

_____

b. writing of a medication order on the MAR

_____

c. kardexing

_____

d. telephone call

_____

e. pharmacy copy sent or faxed

_____

f. notification to appropriate person of a stat order

_____

13. When is it necessary to use the ordering step when transcribing doctors' orders?

_____

14. List five areas commonly found on a Kardex form.

a. _____

b. _____

c. _____

d. _____

e. _____

15. List the four categories of doctors' orders and write a brief description of each.

a. _____

b. _____

c. _____

d. _____

16. Identify each type (category) of order written below.

a. blood pressure q3h until alert

_____

b. morphine 8 to 12 mg IM q3-4h prn pain

_____

c. diazepam 10 mg PO now

_____

d. Premarin 1.25 mg PO daily

_____

e. regular diet

_____

f. Fleets enema this pm and repeat in am

_____

17. How would a stat order be identified?

_____

18. What would be the advantage of practicing ordering tests and procedures on seldom used paper requisitions?

_____

_____

19. Describe precautions that should be taken to avoid making the following transcription errors:

a. errors of omission (missing written doctors' orders)

_____

b. errors of interpretation (not understanding the written doctors' orders)

_____

c. errors in the selection of the wrong patient on the computer screen or in labeling requisitions

_____

d. errors in the selection of the patient's Kardex form

_____

e. errors in reading the doctor's poor handwriting

_____

THINK ABOUT...

1. Discuss the possible consequences if a medication is written on the wrong patient's medication administration record.
2. While transcribing a set of doctors' orders, the HUC places an "ord" symbol above an order for a chest x-ray before actually entering the order into the computer. The HUC is then distracted by a visitor requesting a patient's location, and someone borrows the chart that the HUC was working on before the orders were completed. Discuss what could happen when the chart is returned and the HUC finishes transcribing the orders.

CHAPTER 10

Patient Activity, Patient Positioning, and Nursing Observation Orders

CHAPTER OBJECTIVES

Upon completion of this chapter, you will be able to:

1. Define the terms in the vocabulary list.
2. Write the meaning of each abbreviation and write the abbreviation for each term in the abbreviation list.
3. Identify patient activity, patient positioning, and nursing observation orders.
4. Explain what is included in a patient's vital signs.
5. Explain how orthostatic vital signs are measured.
6. Identify the measurement that is referred to as the fifth vital sign.
7. Describe four methods of taking a patient's temperature.
8. Identify the nursing unit that would employ a cardiac monitor technician.
9. List two types of patients that may have an order for blood glucose monitoring.
10. List what is included in intake and output.

VOCABULARY

Activity Order A doctor's order that defines the type and amount of activity a hospitalized patient may have

Afebrile Without fever

Apical Rate Heart rate obtained from the apex of the heart

Axillary Temperature The temperature reading obtained by placing the thermometer in the patient's axilla (armpit)

Bedside Commode A chair or wheelchair with an open seat, used at the bedside by the patient for the passage of urine and stool

Blood Pressure The measurement of the pressure of blood against the artery walls

Cardiac Monitor Monitor of heart function, providing visual and audible record of heartbeat

Cardiac Monitor Technician A person who observes the cardiac monitors; health unit coordinators may be cross-trained to this position

Dangle The patient sits and dangles their feet over the edge of the bed

Diastolic Blood Pressure The minimum level of blood pressure measured between contractions of the heart; in blood pressure readings, it is the lowest, lower number of the two measurements

Emesis Vomit

Febrile Elevated body temperature (fever)

Fowler's Position A semi-sitting position

Intake and Output The measurement of the patient's fluid intake and output

Neurologic Vital Signs (Neurochecks) The measurement of the function of the body's neurologic system; includes checking pupils of the eyes, verbal response, and so forth

Nursing Observation Order A doctor's order that requests the nursing staff to observe and record certain patient signs and symptoms

Oral Temperature The temperature reading obtained by placing the thermometer in the patient's mouth under the tongue

Orthostatic Hypotension A temporary lowering of blood pressure (hypotension) usually due to suddenly standing up; also called postural hypotension

Orthostatic Vital Signs Measurement (Orthostatics) Recording the patient's blood pressure and pulse rate while the patient is supine (lying) and again while erect (sitting and/or standing)

Oxygen Saturation A noninvasive measurement of gas exchange and red blood cell oxygen-carrying capacity

Pedal Pulse The pulse rate obtained on the top of the foot

Positioning Order A doctor's order that requests that the patient be placed in a specified body position

Pulse Deficit The discrepancy between the ventricular rate detected at the apex of the heart and the arterial rate of the radial pulse

Pulse Oximeter A device that measures gas exchange and red blood cell oxygen-carrying capacity by attaching a probe to either the ear or the finger (also called an Oxygen Saturation Monitor)

Pulse Oximetry A noninvasive method of measuring gas exchange and red blood cell oxygen-carrying capacity (considered to be the fifth vital sign)

Pulse Rate The number of times per minute the heartbeat is felt through the walls of the artery

Radial Pulse Pulse rate obtained on the wrist

Rectal Temperature The temperature reading obtained by placing the thermometer in the patient's rectum

Respiration Rate The number of times a patient breathes per minute

Systolic Blood Pressure The blood pressure measured during the period of ventricular contraction; in blood pressure readings, it is the higher, upper number of the two measurements

Temperature The quantity of body heat, measured in degrees—Fahrenheit or Celsius

Trendelenburg Position A position in which the head is low and the body and legs are on an inclined plane (sometimes used in pelvic surgery to displace the abdominal organs upward, out of the pelvis, or to increase the blood flow to the brain in hypotension and shock)

Tympanic Temperature The temperature reading obtained by placing an aural (ear) thermometer in the patient's ear

Vital Signs Measurements of body functions, including temperature, pulse, respiration, and blood pressure

ABBREVIATIONS

Abbreviation	Meaning	Example of Usage on a Doctor's Order Sheet
A&O	alert and oriented	D/C to home when A&O
ABR	absolute bed rest	ABR × 12 hr
ad lib	as desired	up ad lib
Amb	ambulate	amb c̄ help
as tol	as tolerated	up as tol
Ax	axilla or axillary	ax temp tid
bid	two times per day	up in chair 20 min bid

Abbreviation	Meaning	Example of Usage on a Doctor's Order Sheet
BP	blood pressure	BP tid, call if systolic ↑ 150
BR	bed rest	BR until A&O
BRP	bathroom privileges	BRP only
BSC	bedside commode	may use BSC
c̄	with	up c̄ help
CBR	complete bed rest	CBR today
CMS	circulation, motion, sensation	check CMS fingers rt hand
CMT	cardiac monitor technician	HUC may be cross-trained as a CMT
CVP	central venous pressure	measure CVP q 4h
D/C or DC	discontinue or discharge	D/C BSC or DC to home today
HOB	head of bed	↑ HOB
h, hr, hrs	hour, hours	flat in bed for 8 h
I&O	intake and output	Strict I&O
lt, Ⓛ	left	↑ lt arm on pillow
min	minutes	up in chair for 5 min today
NVS or neuro ✓s	neurologic vital signs/checks	NVS q4h & record
°	degree or hour	elevate head of bed 30 degrees
OOB	out of bed	OOB ad lib
P	pulse	BP&P q4h
prn	as necessary	up prn
q	every	wt q day
q day	every day or daily	wt q day
qid	four times a day	VS qid
q other day	every other day	wt q other day
qh or q _h	every hour or every (fill in number) hour	check VS q2h
R	rectal	R temp
RR	respiratory rate	monitor RR q1h
rt, ®	right	↑ rt arm on pillow
Rout	routine	rout VS
SOB	shortness of breath	evaluate for SOB & notify physician
temp	temperature	rectal temp
tid	three times a day	up in chair tid
TPR	temperature, pulse, respiration	TPR&BP q4h
VS	vital signs	VS q4h
wt	weight	wt daily
↑	increase, above, or elevate	↑ arm on 2 pillows
↓	decrease, below, or lower	if BP ↓ 100/60, call me

THE JOINT COMMISSION'S LIST OF DISALLOWED ABBREVIATIONS

Table 10-1 The Joint Commission's Official "Do Not Use" List*

Do Not Use	Potential Problem	Use Instead
U (unit)	Mistaken for "0" (zero), the number "4" (four) or "cc"	Write "unit"
IU (International Unit)	Mistaken for IV (intravenous) or the number 10 (ten)	Write "International Unit"
Q.D., QD, q.d., qd (daily)	Mistaken for each other	Write "daily"
Q.O.D., QOD, q.o.d., qod (every other day)	Period after the Q mistaken for "I" and the "O" mistaken for "I"	Write "every other day"
Trailing zero (X.0 mg)†	Decimal point is missed	Write X mg
Lack of leading zero (.X mg)	Decimal point is missed	Write 0.X mg
MS MSO4	Can mean morphine sulfate or magnesium sulfate	Write "morphine sulfate"
MgSO4	Confused with morphine	Write "magnesium sulfate"

Additional Abbreviations, Acronyms, and Symbols (For Possible Future Inclusion in the Official "Do Not Use" List)		
> (greater than) and < (less than)	Misinterpreted as the number "7" (seven) or the letter "L"; confused for each other	Write "greater than" and "less than"
Abbreviations for drug names	Misinterpreted because of similar abbreviations for multiple drugs	Write drug names in full
Apothecary units	Unfamiliar to many practitioners; confused with metric units	Use metric units
@	Mistaken for the number "2" (two)	Write "at"
cc	Mistaken for U (units) when poorly written	Write "ml" or "milliliters"
μg	Mistaken for mg (milligrams) resulting in one thousand–fold overdose	Write "mcg" or "micrograms"

*Applies to all orders and all medication-related documentation that is handwritten (including free-text computer entry) or on preprinted forms.
†**Exception:** A "trailing zero" may be used only where required to demonstrate the level of precision of the value being reported, such as for laboratory results, imaging studies that report sizes of lesions, or catheter/tube sizes. It may not be used in medication orders or other medication-related documentation.
Courtesy of The Joint Commission, May 2005.

EXERCISE 1

Write the abbreviations for the following terms.

1. complete bed rest _____

2. with _____

3. alert and oriented _____

4. four times a day _____

5. degree or hour _____

6. blood pressure _____

7. every _____

8. ambulatory _____

9. absolute bed rest _____

10. increase or elevate _____

11. bathroom privileges _____

12. respiratory rate _____

13. as desired _____

14. every other day _____

15. two times a day _____

16. every day _____

17. three times a day _____

18. every hour _____

19. temperature _____

20. as tolerated _____

21. right _____

22. left _____

23. discontinue or discharge _____

24. vital signs _____

25. intake and output _____

26. out of bed _____

27. minutes _____

28. weight _____

29. bed rest _____

30. rectal _____

31. axilla or axillary _____

32. temperature, pulse, respiration _____

33. pulse _____

34. hour or hours _____

35. as necessary _____

36. neurologic vital signs or neurologic checks _____

37. decrease, below, or lower _____

38. head of bed _____

39. bedside commode _____

40. every 4 hours _____

41. circulation, motion, and sensation _____

42. shortness of breath _____

43. central venous pressure _____

44. routine _____

45. cardiac monitor technician _____

EXERCISE 2

Write the meaning of each abbreviation.

1. lt or Ⓛ

   _____

2. rt or ®

   _____

3. D/C or DC

   _____

4. VS

   _____

5. BP

   _____

6. tid

   _____

7. CBR

   _____

8. $\overline{c}$

   _____

9. TPR

   _____

10. BR

    _____

11. min

    _____

12. BRP

    _____

13. ad lib

    _____

14. ↑

    _____

15. OOB

    _____

16. A&O

    _____

17. wt

    _____

18. amb

_____

19. q other day

_____

20. q day

_____

21. bid

_____

22. qid

_____

23. qh

_____

24. ABR

_____

25. temp

_____

26. as tol

_____

27. I&O

_____

28. q

_____

29. P

_____

30. ax

_____

31. R

_____

32. prn

_____

33. RR

_____

34. q4h

_____

35. h, hr, or hrs

_____

36. NVS or neuro ✓s

_____

37. ↓

_____

38. rt

_____

39. SOB

_____

40. HOB

_____

41. BSC

_____

42. CMS

_____

43. CVP

_____

44. rout

_____

45. CMT

_____

PATIENT ACTIVITY ORDERS

Background Information

Patient activity refers to the amount of walking, sitting, and other motions that the patient may do in a given period during a hospital stay. The prescribed activity changes to coincide with the patient's stage of recovery. For example, after some major surgical procedures, the doctor may prefer that the patient remain in bed; as the patient recovers, the doctor increases the level of activity accordingly. The doctor indicates the degree of activity the patient should have by writing an **activity order** on the doctor's order sheet or by entering the order directly into the patient's electronic record when the electronic medical record (EMR) has been implemented. Common activity orders are listed here with interpretations.

✓ DOCTORS' ORDERS FOR PATIENT ACTIVITIES

CBR
The patient is to remain in bed at all times.

BR c̄ BRP
The patient may use the bathroom for the elimination of urine and stool but otherwise must remain in bed.

Dangle Tonight
The patient may sit and **dangle** his legs and feet over the edge of the bed. The doctor may specify the number of times per day the patient should dangle, such as *Dangle bid*, or may specify a period of time, such as *Dangle 5 min tid*.

Use Bedside Commode or Use BSC
The patient may use a portable commode at the bedside.

Note: The HUC may need to order the **bedside commode** from the central service department (depending on the type of nursing unit—a geriatrics or rehabilitation unit may have them available on the unit).

Up c̄ Help
The patient may be out of bed when assisted by a member of the nursing staff.

Up in Chair
The patient may sit in a chair. The doctor may specify the length of time and/or the number of times per day, especially if this activity is ordered after CBR. Example: *Up in chair 20 min tid.*

BRP When A&O
The patient may use the bathroom as desired when alert and oriented.

Up in Hall
The patient may walk in the hall.

Up as Tol
The patient may be out of bed as much as can be physically tolerated.

Up Ad Lib
The patient has no restriction on activity.

OOB
The patient may be out of bed. The doctor may qualify this order with another statement, such as *OOB bid*.

Amb
This is another way of saying that the patient may be up as desired.

May Shower
The patient may have a shower. A doctor's order is necessary for a hospitalized patient to have a shower or tub bath.

These orders are written in abbreviated form as the doctor would write them on the doctor's order sheet, *with one exception*: They are not written in a doctor's handwriting. Reading doctors' handwriting can be a difficult task. However, the repetitive reading of doctors' handwritten orders helps the HUC become more adept in this area. For assistance with abbreviations, refer to the Abbreviations list at the beginning of the chapter. ■

 SKILLS CHALLENGE

To practice transcribing an activity order, complete Activity 10-1 in the *Skills Practice Manual*.

PATIENT POSITIONING ORDERS

Background Information

Patient positioning is often determined by the nursing staff; however, the doctor may want the patient to remain in a special body position to maintain body alignment, promote comfort, and facilitate body functions. For example, the doctor may order the head of the bed to be elevated to ease the patient's breathing or may want the nurse to turn the patient to the unaffected side to promote healing. The doctor indicates a special position by writing the order on the doctor's order sheet. Because it would be impossible to discuss all patient **positioning orders**, only those that are most typical are described here. The following positioning orders are written in the same terms as are found on a doctor's handwritten order sheet. Refer to the Abbreviations list at the beginning of the chapter for assistance.

✓ DOCTORS' ORDERS FOR PATIENT POSITIONING

Elevate Head of Bed 30 Degrees or ↑ HOB 30 Degrees
The head of the bed is to be elevated 30 degrees. (The degree of elevation may vary according to the purpose of the order; for example, the doctor may write ↑ *head of bed 20 degrees.*)

Elevate Lt Arm on Two Pillows
The left arm is to be elevated on two pillows. Variations of this order include the degree of elevation and may involve other limbs; for example, *Elevate rt foot on pillow.*

Fowler's Position
The patient is placed in a semi-sitting position by elevating the head of the bed approximately 18 to 20 inches, or 45 degrees, with a slight elevation of the knees. The semi-**Fowler's position** is the same as Fowler's, but with the head of the bed elevated 30 degrees (Figure 10-1).

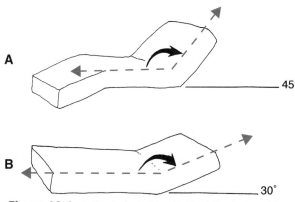

Figure 10-1 A, Fowler's position. **B,** Semi-Fowler's position.

Log Roll

The patient is turned from side to side or from side to back while keeping the back straight like a log, with a pillow between the knees.

Turn to Unaffected Side

The doctor wishes the patient to lie on the side that is free of injury.

Flat in Bed for 8 h No Pillow

The patient is to remain flat in bed for 8 hours, after which the standing activity order is resumed.

Turn q2h

The patient's position is changed every 2 hours to prevent skin breakdown (bedsores). ■

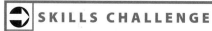 **SKILLS CHALLENGE**

To practice transcribing a patient positioning order, complete Activity 10-2 in the *Skills Practice Manual.*

NURSING OBSERVATION ORDERS

Background Information

The doctor may wish to have the nursing staff make periodic observations of the patient's condition; these observations are referred to as *signs and symptoms.* Some doctors may write "call" orders, if they want to be called in the event of certain circumstances. An example would be, *Call if P ↑ 110, R ↓ 10, T ↑ 101°, B/P systolic ↑ 160, diastolic ↑ 90.* The doctor may need this information to assist in diagnosing the patient's illness or interpreting the patient's progress. The doctor writes or electronically enters an order to request the information wanted. It is difficult to record all doctors' orders that may be encountered in this area. Outlined below are some of the more common ones as they might be written. For assistance with the interpretation of these abbreviations, refer to the Abbreviations list at the beginning of the chapter.

Orthostatic Vital Signs Measurement (Orthostatics)

When a doctor writes an order for **orthostatics**, the nurse will record the patient's **blood pressure** and **pulse rate** while the patient is supine (lying) and again while erect (sitting and/or standing). A significant change in vital signs may signify dehydration or **orthostatic hypotension,** which is a temporary lowering of blood pressure (hypotension) due usually to sudden standing up (orthostatic). Hypotension is more common in older people when they rise quickly from a chair, especially after a meal, and may be accompanied by a few seconds of disorientation. The change in position causes a temporary reduction in blood flow and therefore a shortage of oxygen to the brain. This leads to light-headedness and, sometimes, to a loss of consciousness. A positive test occurs if the patient becomes dizzy or has a pulse increase of 20 or more beats per minute or a systolic blood pressure decrease of 20 or more mm Hg (millimeters of mercury).

Blood Glucose Monitoring Orders

Blood glucose monitoring is routinely performed by the nursing staff (referred to as point-of-care testing [POCT]) for diabetic patients or patients who are receiving nutritional support (total parenteral nutrition). Different types of blood glucose monitoring devices are used to obtain capillary blood, usually from the patient's finger. One type of monitor is the ACCU-CHEK Advantage (referred to as ACCU-CHEK), in which a drop of blood is placed on a chemically treated strip. The strip is placed in a blood glucose monitor, and the patient's blood glucose results are displayed in numbers. The monitor is turned off by pressing the "O" button. Another type of blood glucose monitor is the One Touch, which can be used on the patient's arm rather than on the finger. The nurse uses the results of the blood glucose level test to administer or adjust insulin dosage according to the doctor's orders (see Chapter 13). The order for blood glucose monitoring is usually written on the Kardex form during the transcription procedures. The doctor may use the trade name of the device, such as ACCU-CHEK (Roche Diagnostics, Basel, Switzerland) or One Touch (LifeScan Inc., Milpitas, California, USA), when ordering blood glucose monitoring (Figure 10-2).

Note: Other POCT will be discussed in Chapter 14.

Oxygen Saturation (Pulse Oximetry) Orders

Pulse oximetry is a noninvasive measurement of gas exchange and red blood cell oxygen-carrying capacity. A probe is usually attached to the ear or the finger. A **pulse oximeter** (Figure 10-3) is often ordered to be applied continuously in the recovery room, an intensive care unit, or a pediatric unit. An alarm will sound when the **oxygen saturation** is too low. An order for pulse oximetry would be sent to the respiratory department and will be included in Chapter 16.

Cardiac Monitors and Cardiac Monitor Technicians

Health unit coordinators may be cross trained to be **cardiac monitoring technicians (CMTs)** who would work on a telemetry unit (see Figure 3-1). Cardiac monitoring technicians monitor patients' heart rhythms and inform nurses of important physiologic changes. They monitor up to 32 patients at a time and have direct and instant audio and visual contact with patients and nurses.

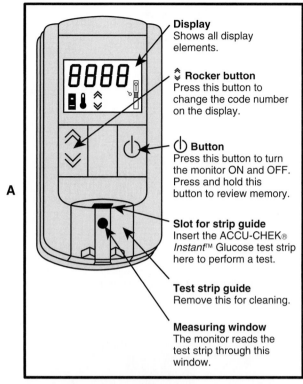

Display
Shows all display elements.

⌃⌄ Rocker button
Press this button to change the code number on the display.

⏻ Button
Press this button to turn the monitor ON and OFF. Press and hold this button to review memory.

Slot for strip guide
Insert the ACCU-CHEK® Instant™ Glucose test strip here to perform a test.

Test strip guide
Remove this for cleaning.

Measuring window
The monitor reads the test strip through this window.

A

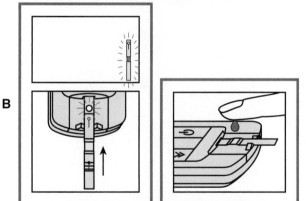

B

C

Figure 10-2 A, Example of a blood glucose monitor. **B,** The strip is placed on the monitor. **C,** Blood glucose results are displayed in numbers; the monitor is turned off by pressing the "O" button. (From Stepp CA, Woods MA: Laboratory procedures for medical office personnel. Philadelphia: Saunders; 1998.)

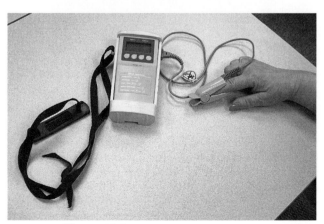

Figure 10-3 A handheld pulse oximeter.

✓ DOCTORS' ORDERS FOR NURSING OBSERVATION

VS q4h

The patient's vital signs are to be taken and recorded every 4 hours. **Vital signs** include **temperature, pulse rate, respiration rate,** and **blood pressure** reading. The temperature may be taken with a tympanic (aural) (Figure 10-4, *A*), oral, or rectal thermometer. Oral and rectal thermometers may be glass or electric (see Figure 10-4, *B, C*). Results of the temperature will indicate whether the patient is **febrile** or **afebrile**. The pulse is obtained from the radial artery in the wrist, unless otherwise indicated (see Figure 10-5 for locations of pulse points on the body). Variations of this type of order may include other time sequences and can read, for example, *VS q1h, VS q2h,* or may include a qualifying phrase, such as *VS q1h until stable then q4h.*

BP q h × 4

The blood pressure is to be taken and recorded every hour for 4 hours. Variations to this order may involve other time sequences, such as *BP q4h, BP tid,* and so forth, or a qualifying phrase, such as *BP q3h while awake* or *BP q4h if ↓ 100/60, call me.* Figure 10-6 shows a vital sign monitor stand with a screen that will register the vital signs.

VITAL SIGNS: ACCEPTABLE RANGES FOR ADULTS	

Temperature range:
    36°-38° Celsius
96.8°-100.4°
    Fahrenheit
	Average oral/tympanic:
	    37° C (98.6° F)
	Average rectal: 37.5° C
	    (99.5° F)
	Average axillary: 36.5° C
	    (97.7° F)

Pulse: 60-100 beats/min Respirations: 12-16 breaths/min Average blood pressure: 120/80 mm Hg	

*New recommendation for normal blood pressure is ↓ 120/80.

Observe for SOB and Notify Physician
The patient will be observed for shortness of breath (SOB) and, if severe, the nurse will notify the physician of the patient's condition.

Orthostatics q Shift
The nurse will take the patient's blood pressure and pulse rate while the patient is supine (lying) and again while erect (sitting and/or standing).

Apical Rate
The patient's heart rate is to be taken at the apex of the heart with a stethoscope.

Check Pedal Pulse R Foot q2h
Pulses are obtained from an artery (dorsalis pedis) on top of the foot.

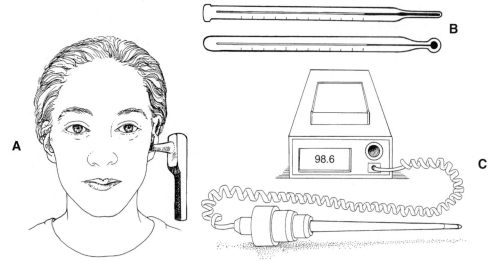

Figure 10-4 Types of thermometers. **A,** Aural—used to take tympanic membrane temperature in the ear. **B,** Glass—used to take oral, rectal, and axillary temperatures. **C,** Electric—used to take oral and rectal temperatures.

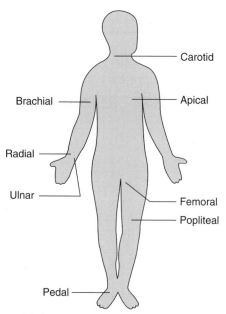

Figure 10-5 Location of the pulse points on the body.

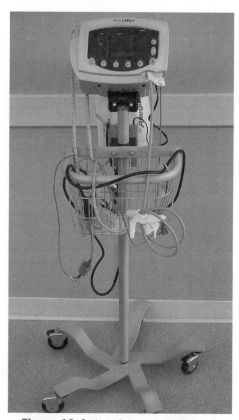

Figure 10-6 A vital signs monitor stand.

Neuro ✓s q2h

The patient's **neurologic vital signs** are taken and recorded every 2 hours.

I&O

The patient's fluid **intake and output** is measured and recorded at the completion of each shift. It is then calculated for 24-hour periods. Intake includes any oral liquid consumed or intravenous fluids infused; output consists of urine, **emesis,** wound drainage, or liquid stools. Figure 10-7 shows a typical intake and output form used by the nursing staff to calculate the patient's intake and output for an 8-hour shift.

Wt Daily

The patient is to be weighed daily and the weight recorded. A variation of this order may be *daily wt.*

Tympanic Temp q4h

The temperature is to be measured every 4 hours, with use of the tympanic (aural) thermometer (see Figure 10-4, *A*) as opposed to the oral method. A third method of measuring the body temperature is the axillary method. The doctor's order for this method may read, *axillary temp q4h.* A fourth is the rectal method. The doctor's order will read, *rectal temp q4h.*

24-Hour Intake and Output	Name _Mary Ryan_						
	Room _403A_						
	Date _9/10/XX_						

Shift	Fluid Intake			Fluid Output		Other	Stools
	Oral	I.V.	Piggy Back	Urine	Emesis	Suction ☐	
0700-1500	08³⁰ 100 cc 10⁰⁰ 30 cc 12⁰⁰ 320 cc 15⁰⁰ 500 cc 210	Credit _300_ Add _1000_ Add _____	50	07³⁰ 200 cc 11⁰⁰ 300 cc 13⁰⁰ 175 cc	200 cc		x1 lg amt
8 hr.	1160		50	675			
1500-2300		Credit _500_ Add _____ Add _____					
8 hr.							
2300-0700		Credit _____ Add _____ Add _____					
8 hr.							
24 hr.							

Iced Tea - 6 oz. (180 cc)
Water Glass - 6 oz. (180 cc)
Milk (carton) - 8 oz. (240 cc)
Fruit Juice - 4 oz. (120 cc)
Soup - 4 oz. (120 cc)
Ice Cream - 3 oz. (90 cc)
Jello - 3.5 oz. (105 cc)

Cup of Coffee or Tea - 7 oz. (210 cc)
Styrofoam Cup - 150 cc
Paper Cup - 150 cc
Coffee Creamer - 0.5 oz. (15 cc)
Cereal Creamer - 2 oz. (60 cc)
Coca Cola and Sprite - 12 oz. (360 cc)
H_2O Pitcher - 30 oz. (900 cc)

Figure 10-7 An intake and output form.

CVP q2h

A catheter is inserted, usually through the right or left subclavian vein, and is threaded through the vein until the tip reaches the right atrium of the heart (see Figure 11-11). The catheter is inserted by the doctor, and pressure readings are taken by the nurse.

Pulse Oximetry q4h

Oxygen saturation is to be measured every 4 hours. A portable pulse oximeter with a special sensor is used. The sensor is often left in place for continuous monitoring (see Figure 10-3).

Check CMS Fingers Rt Hand

The circulation, motion, and sensation (CMS) of the patient's right-hand fingers are to be checked as often as the nurse determines necessary. This type of order specifies observation of the patient's signs and symptoms relative to the patient's diagnosis and treatment. For example, this order was written after a cast was applied to the patient's right arm and hand.

ACCU-CHEK ac and hs

ACCU-CHEK is a type of commercial blood glucose monitor that is used to check the glucose level of blood. The doctor has ordered the test to be done four times a day (the order may be written as qid, which would be performed ac and hs).

Move Patient to Telemetry Unit, Place on Telemetry, and Notify Hospitalist of any Arrhythmias

The patient would be moved to the telemetry unit and placed on telemetry, and the CMT would monitor the patient's telemetry; if any abnormal heart rhythms are seen, the CMT would run a strip, notify the patient's nurse, and call the hospitalist if requested to do so.

Vs q shift

Vital signs are measured to detect changes in the patient's condition, assess response to treatment, and recognize life-threatening situations. Accurate recording of vital signs is essential.
Vital signs consist of the following:

Blood Pressure	Temperature	Pulse	Respiration Rate
	Oral	Apical	
	Tympanic (Aural)	Radial	
	Axillary	Pedal	
	Rectal	Femoral	
		Carotid	
		Popliteal	
		Brachial	

✐ TAKE NOTE

An order for pulse oximetry would be sent to the respiratory department. This will be discussed in greater detail in Chapter 16.

When paper charts are used, transcription of doctors' orders is a major responsibility of the health unit coordinator. This chapter has introduced doctors' orders for patient activity, patient positioning, and nursing observation. Refer back to this chapter as needed.

 SKILLS CHALLENGE

To practice transcribing a nursing observation order, complete Activity 10-3 in the *Skills Practice Manual.*

To practice transcribing a blood glucose monitor order, complete Activity 10-4 in the *Skills Practice Manual.*

To practice transcribing, automatically canceling, and discontinuing doctors' orders, complete Activity 10-5 in the *Skills Practice Manual.*

To practice transcribing a review set of doctors' orders, complete Activity 10-6 in the *Skills Practice Manual.*

To practice recording telephoned messages, complete Activity 10-7 in the *Skills Practice Manual.*

REVIEW QUESTIONS

1. Identify the following doctors' orders as nursing observation, activity, or positioning orders.

a. BRP

_____

b. log roll on lt side

_____

c. pulse oximetry

_____

d. TPR q4h

_____

e. CMS q2h

_____

f. wt 0700 q AM

_____

g. BSC prn

_____

h. HOB ↑ 30°

_____

   i. Up ad lib

      _____

   j. May dangle 20 min bid

      _____

   k. NVS q4h

      _____

   l. Fowler's position

      _____

  m. up in chair

      _____

   n. ACCU-CHEK ac & hs

      _____

2. Write out each doctor's order in the space provided.

   a. CBR

      _____

   b. BR $\overline{c}$ BRP when A&O

      _____

   c. wt q other day

      _____

   d. VS qid

      _____

   e. TPR&BP tid

      _____

   f. HOB 20°

      _____

   g. √ dressing for drainage q2h

      _____

   h. temp R or ax only

      _____

   i. neuro ✓s q4h

      _____

j. I&O q shift

_____

k. OOB ad lib

_____

l. up as tol

_____

m. TPR&BP q4h

_____

n. amb today

_____

o. DC VS

_____

p. ↑ HOB 30 degrees

_____

q. may use BSC

_____

r. CVP q hr

_____

s. check CMS toes lt foot

_____

t. ACCU-CHEK ac and hs

_____

u. call me if pt SOB

_____

3. Define the following terms.

a. dangle

_____

b. febrile

_____

c. afebrile

_____

d. emesis

_____

4. Vital signs consist of the following:

a. _____   c. _____

b. _____   d. _____

5. Explain how orthostatic vital signs are measured.

_____

_____

_____

6. Identify the measurement that is considered the "fifth vital sign."

_____

_____

_____

7. List four methods of taking a patient's temperature.

a. _____

b. _____

c. _____

d. _____

8. List the items that may be included in the measurement of a patient's I&O.

Intake	Output
a. _____	a. _____
b. _____	b. _____
	c. _____
	d. _____

9. Identify the nursing unit that would employ a CMT.

_____

_____

_____

10. List two types of patients who may receive an order for blood glucose monitoring.

a. _____

b. _____

THINK ABOUT...

1. Discuss errors that could occur because of misinterpretation of abbreviations.
2. Discuss possible consequences of a positioning or activity order being recorded incorrectly.
3. Discuss possible consequences of an order for NVS being overlooked or not carried out.

Nursing Intervention or Treatment Orders

CHAPTER OBJECTIVES

Upon completion of this chapter, you will be able to:

1. Define the terms in the vocabulary list.
2. Write the meaning of the abbreviations in the abbreviations list.
3. Describe the function of the central service department with regard to nursing treatment orders.
4. Explain why reusable equipment should be returned to the central service department as quickly as possible.
5. List the types of items stored in the central service department stock supply closet (C-locker or cart) on the nursing units.
6. List the types of items stored in the central service department.
7. List four types of enemas.
8. Explain two types of urinary catheterization procedures.
9. Describe two methods of administering intravenous therapy.
10. List three parts of an intravenous therapy order.
11. Identify three commercially prepared intravenous solutions.
12. Explain the importance of correct labeling of a blood specimen that is being sent for a type and crossmatch.

13. Explain the health unit coordinator's role in obtaining blood from the blood bank and the correct storage of blood.
14. Describe the use of each suction device from a provided list.
15. Describe the use of each heat therapy device from a provided list.
16. List the devices used for cold therapy
17. Explain additional health unit coordinator tasks that may be necessary when transcribing intravenous infusion orders.

VOCABULARY

Ace Wraps Elastic gauze used for temporary compression to various parts of the body to decrease swelling and reduce skin breakdown

Aquathermia Pad A waterproof plastic or rubber pad used to apply heat or cold that is connected by hoses to a bedside control unit that contains a temperature regulator, a motor for circulating the water, and a reservoir of distilled water (also called a K-pad or a water flow pad)

Arterial Line (art line) A catheter placed in an artery that measures the patient's blood pressure continuously

Autologous Blood The patient's own blood donated previously for transfusion as needed by the patient; also called *autotransfusion*

Binder A cloth or elastic bandage that is usually used for abdominal or chest support

Catheterization Insertion of a catheter into a body cavity or organ to inject or remove fluid

Central Line An IV catheter that is placed in a large vein, usually in the neck, chest, or groin

Compression Garment A tight-fitting, custom-made garment that is used to put constant pressure on healed wounds to keep down scarring

Donor-Specific or Donor-Directed Blood Blood donated by relatives or friends of the patient to be used for transfusion as needed

Egg-Crate Mattress A foam rubber mattress

Elevated Toilet Seat An elevated seat that fits over a toilet and has handrails; used for patients who have difficulty sitting on a lower seat

Enema The introduction of fluid and/or medication into the rectum and sigmoid colon

Extravasation The accidental administration of intravenously infused medicinal drugs into the surrounding tissue, by leakage (as with the brittle veins of elderly patients) or directly (by means of a puncture of the vein)

Foley Catheter A type of indwelling catheter (tube) that is inserted into the bladder for urine collection and measurement

Gastric Suction Used to remove gastric contents

Harris Flush or Return Flow Enema A mild colonic irrigation that helps expel flatus

Hemovac A disposable suction device (evacuator unit) connected to a drain that is inserted into or close to a surgical wound

Heparin Lock A vascular access device (also called *intermittent infusion device* or *saline lock*) that is placed on a peripheral intravenous catheter when used intermittently

Incontinence Inability of the body to control the elimination of urine and/or feces

Indwelling (Retention) Catheter A catheter that remains in the bladder for a longer period until a patient is able to void completely and voluntarily, or as long as hourly accurate measurements are needed

Infiltration The tip of the IV catheter comes out of the vein or pokes through the vein, and IV solution is released into surrounding tissue. This also could occur if the wall of the vein becomes permeable and leaks fluid

Infusion Pump A device used to regulate the flow or rate of intravenous fluid; more commonly called an *IV pump*

Intermittent (Straight) Catheter A single-use catheter that is introduced long enough to drain the bladder (5 to 10 minutes) and is then removed

Intravenous Infusion The administration of fluid through a vein

Irrigation Washing out of a body cavity, organ, or wound

Jackson-Pratt (JP) A disposable suction device (evacuator unit) that is connected to a drain that is inserted into or close to a surgical wound

Nasogastric Tube (NG tube) A tube that is inserted through the mouth or nose into the stomach and is used to feed the patient, or to drain stomach contents to prevent vomiting

Needleless IV Heplock A safe, sharp device that is placed on a peripheral intravenous catheter when used intermittently

Patent or Patency A term that indicates that there are no clots at the tip of the needle or catheter, and that the needle tip or catheter is not against the vein wall (open)

Penrose Drain A drain that is inserted into or close to a surgical wound; it may lie under a dressing, extend through a dressing, or be connected to a drainage bag or suction device

Peripheral Intravenous Catheter A catheter that begins and ends in the extremities of the body; used for the administration of intravenous therapy

Pneumatic Hose Stockings that promote circulation by sequentially compressing the legs from ankle upward, promoting venous return (also called *sequential compression devices*)

Rectal Tube A plastic or rubber tube designed for insertion into the rectum; when written as a doctor's order, *rectal tube* means the insertion of a rectal tube into the rectum to remove gas and relieve distention

Restraints Devices used to control patients who exhibit dangerous behavior or to protect the patient

Sheepskin A pad made out of lamb's wool or synthetic material; used to prevent pressure sores (used frequently in long-term care)

Sitz Bath Application of warm water to the pelvic area

Splinting Holding the incision area to provide support, promote a feeling of security; and reduce pain during coughing after surgery; a folded blanket or pillow is helpful for use as a splint

Swan-Ganz Catheter placed in the neck or the chest that measures pressures in the patient's heart and pulmonary artery

Ted Hose A brand name for an antiembolism (AE) hose

Urinary Catheter A tube that is used for removing urine or injecting fluids into the bladder

Urine Residual The amount of urine that is left in the bladder after voiding

Venipuncture Needle puncture of a vein

Void To empty, especially the urinary bladder

ABBREVIATIONS

Abbreviation	Meaning	Example of Usage on a Doctor's Order Sheet
@	at	Run @ 100 mL/hr
abd	abdominal	Up c̄ abd binder
ac	before meals	ACCU-CHEK ac and hs
ASAP	as soon as possible	Start IV ASAP
B/L	bilateral (both sides)	B/L Teds
cath	catheterize	Cath q 8 hr prn
CBI	continuous bladder irrigation	CBI c̄ NS 50 mL/hr
cm	centimeter	Chest tube 20 cm neg pressure
con't	continue, continuous	Foley cath to con't drainage
CVC	central venous catheter	Blood draws through CVC

Abbreviation	Meaning	Example of Usage on a Doctor's Order Sheet
D/LR	dextrose in lactated Ringer's	IV 1000 mL 5% D/LR at 125 mL/hr
D_5W	5% dextrose in water	1000 mL D_5W @ 125 mL/hr
$D_{10}W$	10% dextrose in water	1000 mL $D_{10}W$ @ 100 mL/hr
DW	distilled water	Irrig cath prn c̄ DW
ETS	elevated toilet seat	Order ETS for home use
gtt(s)	drop(s)	IV @ 60 gtts/min
HL or hep lock	heparin lock	Convert IV to Hep lock
H_2O_2	hydrogen peroxide	Irrigate wound c̄ H_2O_2 & NS equal strength
hs	bedtime, hour of sleep	Give TWE @ hs
irrig	irrigate	Irrig cath c̄ NS prn
IV	intravenous	Con't IVs as ordered
IVF	intravenous fluids	DC IVF at 1000 mL today
KO	keep open	KO IV c̄ 1000 mL 5% D/W
LR	lactated Ringer's	1000 mL LR 125 mL/hr
min, m	minute	Run @ 30 gtts/min
mL	milliliter	1000 D_5W @ 100 mL/hr
MR	may repeat	SSE now MR × 1
nec	necessary	SSE now MR if nec
NG	nasogastric	Insert NG tube
NS	normal saline	Give NS enema now
ORE	oil-retention enema	ORE today
p̄	after	Up p̄ breakfast
PICC	peripherally inserted central catheter	Insert PICC, follow protocol
SCD	sequential compression device	Apply SCD when in bed
sol'n	solution	Irrig cath c̄ NS sol'n
SSE	soap suds enema	SSE now
st	straight retention	Cath to st drain
TCDB	turn, cough, and deep breathe	TCDB q2h
TKO	to keep open	1000 mL D_5W TKO
TWE	tap water enema	Give TWE
VAD	vascular access device	Use VAD for blood draws
Δ	change	Δ catheter daily
/	per, by run	IV @ 150 mL/hr

EXERCISE 1

Write the abbreviation for each term.

1. soap suds enema _____

2. keep open _____

3. may repeat _____

4. solution _____

5. necessary _____

6. centimeter _____

7. tap water enema _____

8. nasogastric _____

9. normal saline _____

10. dextrose in lactated Ringer's _____

11. bedtime _____

12. distilled water _____

13. at _____

14. oil-retention enema _____

15. irrigate _____

16. intravenous _____

17. catheterize _____

18. lactated Ringer's _____

19. straight _____

20. sequential compression device _____

21. after _____

22. abdominal _____

23. turn, cough, and deep breathe _____

24. minute _____

25. drops _____

26. change _____

27. as soon as possible _____

28. per _____

29. hydrogen peroxide _____

30. before meals _____

31. continue _____

32. continuous bladder irrigation _____

33. to keep open _____

34. milliliter _____

35. intravenous fluids _____

36. elevated toilet seat _____

37. peripherally inserted central catheter   _____

38. vascular access device   _____

39. central venous catheter   _____

40. 5% dextrose in water   _____

41. 10% dextrose in water   _____

42. bilateral   _____

43. heparin lock   _____

EXERCISE 2

Write out each doctor's order in the space provided.

1. 1000 mL LR @ 125mL/hr, then DC

   _____

2. SSE HS MR $\times$ 1

   _____

3. Give ORE follow $\bar{c}$ TWE if nec

   _____

4. Irrig cath tid $\bar{c}$ NS sol'n

   _____

5. 1000 mL D_5W 0.9 NS @ TKO

   _____

6. Insert NG tube

   _____

7. TCDB q2h

   _____

8. IV tubing ASAP

   _____

9. Please obtain ETS for patient

   _____

10. Start IVF of $D_{10}W$ @ 120 mL/hr

    _____

11. Insert HL

    _____

12. Shave B/L inguinal groin area

    _____

13. Apply SCD when in bed

    _____

NURSING INTERVENTION OR TREATMENT ORDERS

Background Information

A nursing intervention is any act performed by a nurse that implements the nursing care plan or any specific objective of the clinical plan or pathway, such as turning a comatose patient to avoid the development of decubitus ulcers (bedsores), or teaching insulin injection technique to a diabetic patient before the time of discharge. Interventions may include support measures, activity limitations, administration of medications, or treatments given to relieve the current condition or to prevent the development of further stress. Currently, the emphasis is on a more holistic approach in nursing care. Holistic nursing or comprehensive care consists of total patient care that considers the physical, emotional, social, economic, and spiritual needs of the patient; the patient's response to illness; and the effects of the illness on the ability to meet self-care needs. Nursing interventions/treatment orders are discussed in this chapter.

✎ *TAKE NOTE*

When the electronic medical record (EMR) with computer physician order entry (CPOE) is implemented, physician orders are entered directly into the patient's electronic record, and the nurse can access these orders via computer. The health unit coordinator may have tasks to perform, such as ordering equipment from central services department (CSD). An icon may indicate a health unit coordinator (HUC) task, or it may be communicated as a nurse request.

COMMUNICATION WITH THE CENTRAL SERVICE DEPARTMENT

The CSD distributes the supplies that are used for nursing procedures. The supply purchasing department (SPD) is another name for the CSD. Although CSD supplies are frequently used when they are not mentioned in the doctor's orders, obtaining these supplies for the nursing staff may require a separate step in the transcription procedure for nursing treatment orders. For example, for the order *footboard to bed*, the HUC would order the footboard from the CSD. It is therefore necessary for the HUC to be familiar with frequently used CSD items and to learn the hospital's system for obtaining them.

The system for obtaining central service supplies varies among hospitals; thus, it is impossible to outline one procedure that would cover all hospital systems. Disposable or

Table 11-1 Items Obtained From the Central Service Department

Items That May Be Stored in the Nursing Unit CSD Closet or the C-Locker	Items That May Be Stored in the Central Service Department
Fleet enema	Alternating pressure pad
Rectal tube	Egg-crate mattress
Irrigation trays	Ted hose
Urinary catheter trays	Pneumatic hose
IV solutions*	Colostomy kit
IV catheters and needles	Stomal bags
IV tubing	Elastic abdominal binder
Suction catheters and tubing	Footboard
Sterile gloves	Foot cradle
Examination gloves	Feeding pump and tubing
Masks	IV infusion pump
Syringes and needles	Hypothermia machine
Disposable suture removal kits	K-pad
Dressings	Restraints
Abdominal pads	Adult disposable diapers
Telfa pads	Sitz bath, disposable
Gauze pads in various sizes	Sterile trays
Kling	Tracheostomy
Vaseline gauze	Bone marrow
Tape (various types)	Paracentesis
Alcohol pads	Lumbar puncture (spinal tap)
Glycerin swabs	Thoracentesis
Irrigation solutions, etc.	Central line, etc.

*Certain IV solutions are obtained from the pharmacy in some hospitals.

frequently used items are stored on each nursing unit (items will vary depending on the specialty of the nursing unit). That storage space is often referred to as the CSD closet or room, or the C-locker. When paper charts are used, a central service technician usually takes a daily inventory of the items stored in the closet or C-locker. Used items are replaced, and the patient's CSD current charge cards are collected. Some hospitals use a system with an exchange cart that is supplied with frequently used items and is exchanged every 24 hours. The unit receives another completely supplied cart while CSD replenishes the used cart. Reusable or infrequently used items are stored in the CSD. Refer to Table 11-1 for a comparison of items commonly stored on nursing units and items often stored in the CSD (note that items in each category may vary among hospitals).

In an effort to promote safety and to avoid needle sticks, several safety needles/sharps have been developed and are currently available, including the following: a **needleless intravenous (IV) heplock**/connector system, a safety lancet for finger sticks, a safety butterfly needle (Safety-Loc), and blunt suture needles (Ethicon, Somerville, NJ). These items may be stored on the nursing unit locker or closet or may need to be ordered from CSD.

The HUC, when transcribing an order for treatment, orders only those items stored in the CSD because the nursing staff can quickly obtain needed items from the CSD stock supply.

The nurse may ask the HUC to order items as needed. Items from CSD are usually ordered by computer or with the use of a downtime requisition (if the computer is down). Figure 11-1 shows a CSD downtime requisition.

> **✎ TAKE NOTE**
>
> Downtime requisitions are seldom used but are included in this and subsequent chapters. This will assist students in learning what supplies, tests, and procedures would be ordered from various hospital departments. The CD included in the HUC's *Skills Practice Manual* contains a simulated hospital computer program that may be used for this purpose as well.

It is important to remember that supplies used from the nursing unit supply closet or C-locker are also charged to the patient. The charging process is done by removing a bar code label from the item and placing it on the patient's CSD charge card. Figure 11-2, *A* shows a CSD card. The person who removes the supplies is responsible for placing the bar code label on the patient's CSD card. When the electronic record is implemented, the bar code labels are scanned into the appropriate patient's electronic record for charging purposes. Figure 11-2, *B* shows a computer used for this purpose located in a CSD closet.

> **✎ TAKE NOTE**
>
> When the hospital has implemented the EMR, items used from the CSD closet have bar code labels that are scanned into the appropriate patient's EMR for charging purposes.

Many items used for nursing treatments, such as enema bags or urinary catheterization trays, are *disposable*. This means that once the item has been used for the patient, it is discarded or is given to the patient for future use. The patient is charged for the disposable equipment.

Other items are *reusable*. They are cleaned or sterilized, if necessary, after use by a patient. These items are then available for another patient. The patient usually is charged a rental fee for the use of these items. Reusable items are numbered and tracked for charging or discontinuing the charge. When a reusable item, such as an IV infusion pump, is discontinued, it is placed in the dirty utility room. A central service technician usually picks up the item and returns it to the CSD. If a rental charge has been assessed, it is terminated, and the equipment is readied for use by other patients.

Equipment is discussed and illustrated throughout this chapter as it relates to nursing treatment orders. It is important that the HUC recognize the frequently used items that are required and must be requested during the ordering step of the transcription procedure. It is also important for the HUC to learn which items are stored on the unit and which are stored in the CSD. If information on size and/or weight is required for the ordering of an item, the HUC needs to check with the patient's nurse, and enter this information when ordering the item (e.g., **TED hose**).

Doctor ordering _____   ☐ Stat
Today's date _____   ☐ Routine
Requested by_____

CSD (Central Service Department)

☐ Adult disposable diapers
☐ Alternating pressure pad
☐ Colostomy kit
☐ Colostomy irrigation bag
☐ Egg-crate mattress
☐ Elastic abdominal binder   size_____
☐ Feeding pump with bag and tubing
☐ Feeding bag and tubing
☐ Footboard
☐ Foot cradle
☐ Hypothermia machine
☐ Isolation pack
☐ IV infusion pump with tubing
☐ K-pad with motor
☐ Nasal gastric tube   type_____   size_____
☐ Pleur-evac
☐ Pneumatic hose
☐ Restraints   type_____
☐ Sitz bath, disposable
☐ Stomal bags   type_____   size_____
☐ Suction canister and tubing
☐ Suction catheter   type_____   size_____
☐ TED hose   size_____
☐ Vaginal irrigation kit

Sterile Trays:

☐ Bone marrow
☐ Central line
☐ Lumbar puncture (spinal tap)
☐ Paracentesis
☐ Thoracentesis
☐ Tracheostomy

☐ Write in item _____

Figure 11-1 An example of a central service department (CSD) downtime requisition.

✐ TAKE NOTE

The HUC can best assist the nursing staff when transcribing nursing treatment orders by learning about equipment and supplies used on the nursing unit and ordering needed items.

INTESTINAL ELIMINATION ORDERS

Background Information

Enemas, rectal tubes, and colostomy irrigations are treatments used to remove stool and/or flatus (gas) from the large intestine.

An **enema** is the introduction of fluid into the rectum and sigmoid colon for the purpose of relieving distention (trapped gas) or constipation, or to prepare the patient for surgery and/or diagnostic tests. A doctor may order a *"high"* or a *"low"* cleansing enema. The terms *high* and *low* refer to the height from which the enema container is held; this determines the pressure with which the fluid is delivered. High enemas are given to cleanse the entire colon; low enemas cleanse only the rectum and the sigmoid colon. Common types of enemas include the following:

1. Oil-retention
2. Soap suds
3. Tap water
4. Normal saline

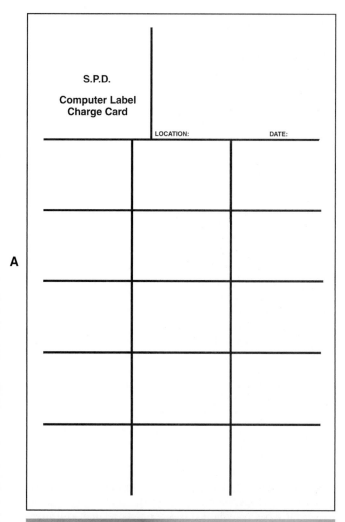

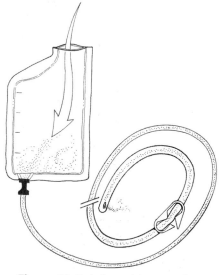

Figure 11-3 A disposable enema bag.

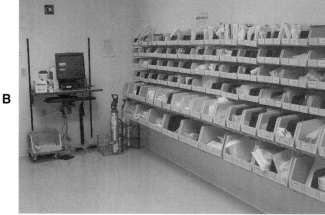

Figure 11-2 A, Central services department patient charge card.
B, Bar code labels are scanned into the patient's electronic medical
record via a computer located in the CSD closet.

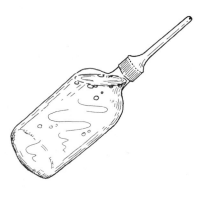

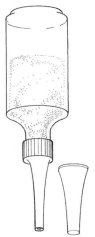

Figure 11-4 Commercially prepackaged enema.

Figure 11-3 is an example of a disposable enema bag used
to administer these types of enemas.

Fleet enema is a disposable, commercially prepackaged
sodium phosphate enema that is frequently used (Fig. 11-4).

The order for a *rectal tube* refers to the insertion of a disposable
plastic, latex-free, or rubber tube into the rectum for the purpose
of relieving distention or draining feces. The rectal tube may be
attached to a bag that captures the flatus and/or feces (Fig. 11-5).

Harris flush is a return-flow enema that is used to relieve
distention. A disposable enema bag is used to inject fluid into
the rectum. This fluid is allowed to return into the bag. The
process is repeated several times.

Colostomy (an artificial opening in the colon for passage of
stool) irrigation (the flushing of fluid resembling an enema)
is used to regulate the discharge of stool. Figure 11-6 shows a
disposable colostomy irrigation bag used for this treatment.

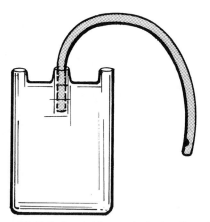

Figure 11-5 A disposable rectal tube in a flatus bag.

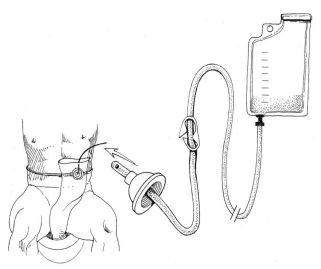

Figure 11-6 A disposable colostomy irrigation apparatus.

A doctor's order is required for the administration of an enema, rectal tube, or Harris flush. The order contains the name of the treatment, the type (when pertinent), and the frequency. If the frequency is not indicated (such as in the order, *tap water enema*), it is considered a one-time order.

Examples of intestinal elimination orders are listed below as they are usually written on the doctor's order sheet. Refer to the abbreviations list at the beginning of this chapter for assistance in interpreting the abbreviations.

✔ DOCTORS' ORDERS FOR INTESTINAL ELIMINATION

TWE now MR × 1 prn
Give ORE followed by NS enemas this A.M.
Harris flush for abdominal distention
NS enemas until clear
Give Fleet enema qd prn constipation
Rectal tube prn for distention ∎

URINARY CATHETERIZATION ORDERS

Background Information

Urinary catheterization is the insertion of a latex-free tube called a *catheter* through the urethral meatus into the bladder for the purpose of removing urine. The tube is usually made of plastic, and it varies in size. The doctor may order one of two types of catheterization procedures: retention or nonretention. Disposable sterile catheterization trays are used for both types, and each tray is marked with the size and type of catheter it contains.

An intermittent nonretention catheter, sometimes referred to as a ***straight catheter***, is used to empty the bladder, to collect a sterile urine specimen, or to check residual. *Residual* is the amount of urine that remains in the bladder after **voiding**. The **intermittent catheter** is removed from the bladder after completion of the procedure (5 to 10 minutes) (Fig. 11-7).

An indwelling retention catheter (also called a Foley catheter) remains in the bladder and is usually connected to a drainage system that allows continuous flow of urine from the bladder to the container. Doctors refer to this type of drainage system as a *straight drain* (Fig. 11-8).

The doctor may order the indwelling catheter to be irrigated on an intermittent or continuous basis to maintain patency (to keep the catheter open). This is referred to as a *closed system*, and it is usually used for those who have had surgery involving the urinary or reproductive system. The open irrigation system is used for irrigating the catheter at specific intervals. The open system requires the nurse to open a closed drainage system and insert an irrigation solution. A disposable irrigation tray is used for this procedure. The doctor indicates the solution to be used (normal saline, acetic acid, distilled water). For continuous and intermittent irrigation, special setups are used (Fig. 11-9).

Several types of typical doctor's orders related to urinary catheterizations are listed in the text that follows, recorded in abbreviated form as they would appear on the doctor's order sheet. Refer to the abbreviations list at the beginning of the chapter for assistance with these abbreviations.

✔ DOCTORS' ORDERS FOR CATHETERIZATION

Intermittent (straight) Catheter
May cath q8h prn
Straight cath prn
Cath in 8 hr if unable to void
Cath for residual

Indwelling (retention) Catheter
Insert Foley
Indwelling cath to st drain
Insert Foley cath for residual; if more than 200 mL, leave in
DC cath in A.M.; if unable to void in 6 hr, reinsert
DC cath this A.M.
Clamp cath 4 hr, then drain

Catheter Irrigation
CBI; use NS @ 50 mL/hr
Irrig Foley c̄ NS bid
Irrig cath prn patency
Intermittent CBI q4h × 6 ∎

Communication and Implementation of Nursing Treatment Orders

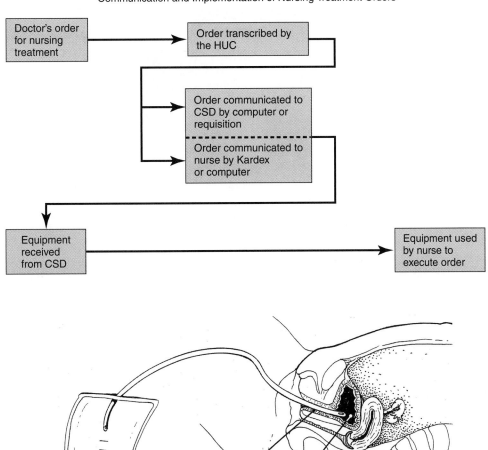

```
┌─────────────┐      ┌─────────────────┐
│ Doctor's order│────→│ Order transcribed by│
│ for nursing  │      │ the HUC          │
│ treatment    │      │                  │
└─────────────┘      └─────────────────┘

                     ┌─────────────────────┐
                     │ Order communicated to│
                     │ CSD by computer or   │
                     │ requisition          │
                     ├─────────────────────┤
                     │ Order communicated to│
                     │ nurse by Kardex      │
                     │ or computer          │
                     └─────────────────────┘

┌─────────────┐                              ┌─────────────────┐
│ Equipment   │                              │ Equipment used  │
│ received    │─────────────────────────────→│ by nurse to     │
│ from CSD    │                              │ execute order   │
└─────────────┘                              └─────────────────┘
```

Urethra

Urinary bladder

Figure 11-7 An intermittent (straight) catheter in place.

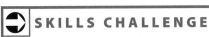

SKILLS CHALLENGE

To practice transcribing intestinal elimination and urinary catheterization orders, complete Activity 11-1 in the *Skills Practice Manual.*

INTRAVENOUS THERAPY ORDERS

Background Information

Until 1949, IV therapy consisted of the administration of simple solutions, such as water and normal saline, through peripheral veins. Equipment consisted of a glass bottle, a rubber tube, and a needle. Today, IV therapy includes the parenteral administration of fluids, medications, nutritional substances, and blood transfusions through peripheral veins and through central veins. The availability of sophisticated equipment allows IV therapy to be administered to the patient at home, as well as in the hospital. Fluids can be administered continuously or intermittently, and IV administration is done by the nurse, by the patient, or by the patient's family. Intravenous therapy is given to do the following:

* Administer nutritional support such as total parenteral nutrition (TPN) (covered in Chapters 12 and 13)
* Provide for intermittent or continuous administration of medication
* Transfuse blood or blood products
* Maintain or replace fluids and electrolytes

Intravenous Therapy Catheters and Devices
Peripheral Intravenous Therapy

In peripheral IV therapy, *peripheral* refers to blood flow in the extremities of the body. When therapy is administered, the cannula is inserted into a vein in the arm or hand or, on rare occasions, in the foot (adult). A vein in the scalp or foot is often used when peripheral IV therapy is administered to infants. The cannula is short (less than 2 inches), so it ends in the extremity. It is not threaded to the larger veins or to the heart as in central venous therapy (Fig. 11-10).

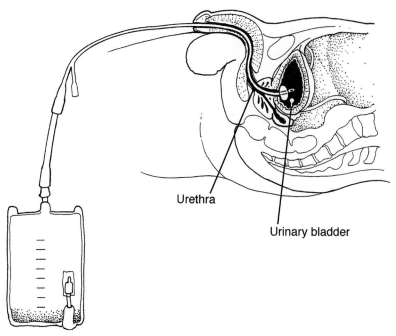

Figure 11-8 An indwelling (Foley) catheter in place and connected to a drainage bag (called *straight drainage*).

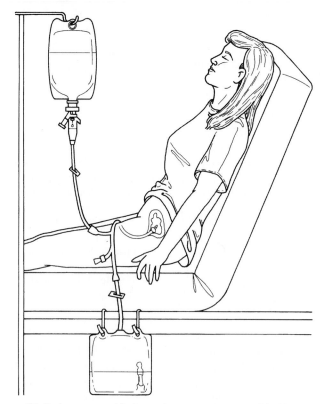

Figure 11-9 A setup used for intermittent or continuous bladder irrigation.

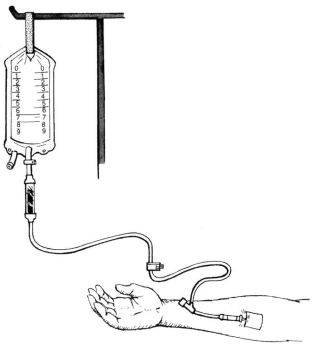

Figure 11-10 Peripheral IV therapy (venipuncture).

Peripheral IV therapy

- usually is initiated by the nurse at the bedside
- usually is started in a vein in the arm via **venipuncture**
- is used for short-term IV therapy (i.e., a week or less)
- is basic and easiest to initiate
- is used commonly in hospitals
- sometimes is given through a vascular access device (VAD)

Central Intravenous Therapy

In central IV therapy, *central* refers to the blood flow in the center of the body. To administer therapy, the catheter is inserted into the jugular or subclavian vein or a large vein in the arm and is threaded to the superior vena cava or the right atrium of the heart. A central venous catheter (CVC) is used. It is commonly referred to as a *central venous line* or a *subclavian line*. (Figure 11-11 shows various types of CVCs.) The HUC orders a **central line** tray and an infusion pump from the CSD and prepares a consent form.

Types of Central Venous Catheters

Peripherally inserted central catheters (PICC or PIC) generally are

- initiated by the doctor or by a nurse who is certified in the procedure at the bedside, and requires a consent form
- inserted into the arm and advanced until the tip lies in the superior vena cava
- x-rayed to verify placement
- used when therapy is needed for longer than 7 days
- used for antibiotic therapy, total parenteral nutrition, chemotherapy, cardiac drugs, or other drugs that are potentially harmful to peripheral veins
- sometimes used for blood draws

Percutaneous CVCs are

- sometimes referred to as subclavian lines
- initiated by the doctor at the bedside and require a consent form

- inserted through the skin directly into the subclavian (most common) or jugular vein and advanced until the tip lies in the superior vena cava or the right atrium of the heart
- x-rayed to verify placement
- used for short-term therapy (i.e., 7 days to several weeks)
- used for antibiotic therapy, TPN, or chemotherapy
- sometimes used for blood draws

Tunneled catheters are

- initiated by the doctor and are considered a surgical procedure; they require a consent form
- inserted through a small incision made near the subclavian vein
- inserted and advanced to the superior vena cava
- used with a device called a *tunneler*, which exits the catheter low in the patient's chest
- designed to allow the patient to administer his own therapy; the tips can be placed under clothing
- available in various types, including Hickman, Raaf, Groshong, and Broviac
- inserted for long-term IV therapy (i.e., longer than a month)
- used for home care, in long-term care facilities, and for self-administration
- sometimes used for blood draws (usually requires a doctor's order)

An implanted port is

- a surgical procedure that is performed by the doctor in a surgical setting
- inserted into the subclavian or jugular vein
- a container that is implanted under the skin in the chest wall
- inserted with the use of an incision; after insertion, the incision is closed, and the device cannot be seen but can be identified by a bulge
- different from other long-term catheters in that it has no external parts, is located under the skin, and does not require daily care
- used with a special needle that is inserted into the port to administer therapy
- available in different types, including Port-A-Cath, Med-I-Port, and Infus-A-Port
- used for long-term and or intermittent use; often, it is used for chemotherapy administration

Heparin Lock (heplock)

A **heplock**, or saline lock, is a venous access device (also called an *intermittent infusion device*) that is placed on a **peripheral IV catheter** when used intermittently. The heplock is used to maintain an intermittent line when IV fluids are no longer needed but IV entry is still required. It is commonly used for the administration of medication. It consists of a plastic needle with an attached injection cap. A needleless heplock is also available. The device is kept **patent** with heparin or saline flushes ordered by the doctor to be administered at specific intervals (flushes may require a doctor's order) (Fig. 11-12).

Intravenous Infusion Pump

An IV **infusion pump** is an electrical device that is used in the administration of intravenous fluid. It is used to measure a precise amount of fluid (regulates drips per hour) to be infused for a stated amount of time. The pump is ordered from CSD and is manufactured under several brand names (Fig. 11-13).

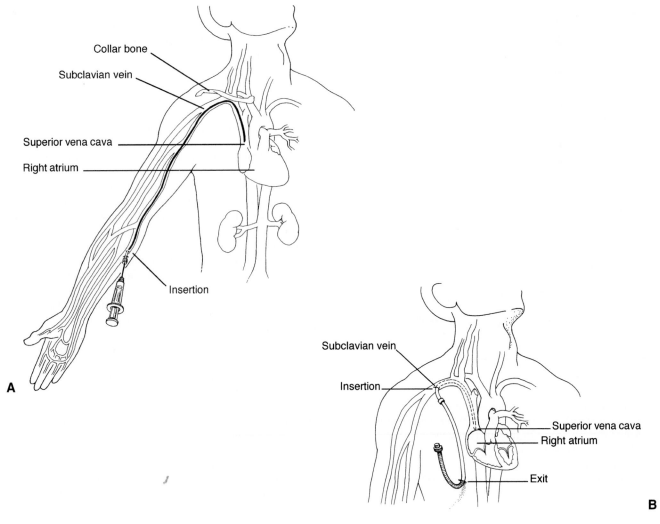

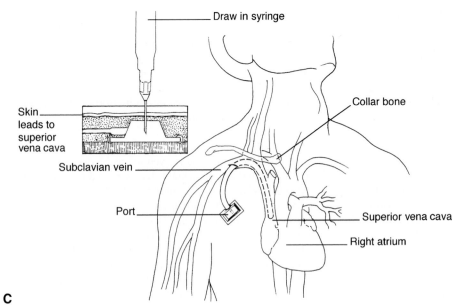

Figure 11-11 Types of CVCs. **A,** Peripherally inserted central catheter (PICC). **B,** Percutaneous CVC. **C,** Implanted port.

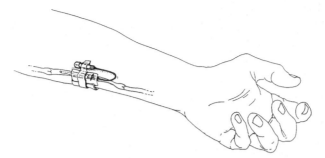

Figure 11-12 Intermittent infusion device (heparin lock).

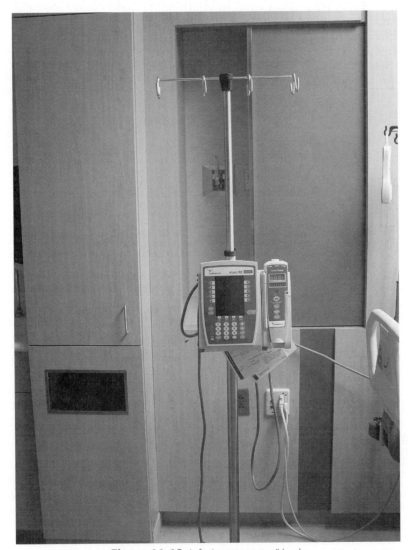

Figure 11-13 Infusion pump on IV pole.

FLUIDS AND ELECTROLYTES

The doctor orders the type, the amount, and the flow rate of solutions to be given. For example, in the IV order,

1000mL D$_5$W @ 125 mL/hr

D$_5$W is the type of solution. A large variety of solutions are available on the market, and the doctor must select the one that best meets the patient's needs.

Continuing this example, 1000 mL is the amount of solution the doctor wants the patient to have. Solutions are most commonly packaged in amounts of 1000 mL; however, 250 mL or 500 mL also may be ordered.

The notation "125 mL/hr" indicates the rate of flow per hour of the solution into the vein. Other examples of phrases used in stating the rate of flow are "60 gtts per min, to run for 8 hr" and "to keep open (usually 50 to 60 mL/hr)."

✏ TAKE NOTE

To determine the amount of time it will take for IV infusion to be completed, divide the number of milliliters in the IV bag by the rate of flow. In the doctor's order, 1000 mL 5% D/W @ 125 mL/hr, divide 1000 by 125. The answer is 8. The IV will run for 8 hours. Use this information to order the number of 1000-mL IV bags needed for a given amount of time.

Frequently, the HUC is required to order IV solutions at specific intervals; therefore, it is necessary to know the length of time it takes the IV to infuse. An IV of 1000 mL running at 125 mL/hr runs for 8 hours (1000 mL/125 mL = 8 hours). How many hours will an IV running at 100 mL/hr take to infuse?

Several one-time, continuous, and discontinuation IV orders, written in abbreviated form as commonly seen on the doctor's order sheet, follow. Use the abbreviations list at the beginning of this chapter for assistance in interpreting these, if necessary.

 ### DOCTORS' ORDERS FOR INTRAVENOUS THERAPY

1000 mL LR 125 mL/hr then DC
Con't IVs alternate 1000 mL/RL c̄ 1000 mL D₅W, each to run for 8 hr via CVC
KVO IV rate 30 mL/hr c D₅W
DC IV when present bottle is finished
D₅LR 100 mL/hr follow c̄ 1000 mL 5% Isolyte M at same rate
Alternate the following IVs
1000 mL D₁₀LR via Groshong cath
1000 mL 5% D/W plus 20 mEq KCl to run at 125 mL/hr
1000 mL D₅W 0.9 NS @ 100 mL/hr if pt not tol fluids
DC IV fluids, convert to hep lock c̄ rout saline flushes
Have IV team insert PICC
Use Port-A-Cath for blood draws ■

TRANSFUSION OF BLOOD, BLOOD COMPONENTS, AND PLASMA SUBSTITUTES

Background Information

An **IV infusion** of blood is called a *blood transfusion*. It usually is ordered for patients who have lost blood because of hemorrhage from trauma or surgery. Before the administration of blood and blood products, the patient must sign a specific consent form. A refusal form must be signed if the patient refuses to have a blood transfusion. Refer to Chapter 8, page 145 to see a blood transfusion refusal form.

The use of whole blood for transfusion is gradually lessening, and only parts or components of blood are being used. The following are commonly seen transfusion orders:

1. Packed cells (red blood cells) (frequently used)
2. Plasma
3. Platelet concentrate
4. Washed cells

COMMERCIALLY PREPARED IV SOLUTIONS THAT ARE COMMONLY USED

- Sodium chloride 0.45% (NaCl 0.45%, or half-strength NaCl)
- Sodium chloride 0.9% (NaCl 0.9%, or normal saline)
- 5% dextrose in water (5% D/W, or D₅W)
- 10% dextrose in water (10% D/W, or D₁₀W)
- 5% dextrose in 0.2% sodium chloride (5% D/0.2% NaCl)
- 5% dextrose in 0.45% sodium chloride (5% D/0.45% NaCl)
- 5% dextrose in 0.9% sodium chloride (5% D/0.9% NaCl)
- Lactated Ringer's solution with 5% dextrose (LR/ 5%D)
- 5% dextrose in 0.2% normal saline
- 5% dextrose in 0.45% normal saline
- Lactated Ringer's solution

Other IV solutions that contain essential body elements are sold under various trade names. For example, McGaw, a manufacturer of parenteral fluids, markets an IV solution with electrolytes under the trade name, Isolyte M. The same formula is sold by Abbott Laboratories as Ionosol T.

5. Fresh frozen plasma (FFP)
6. Cryoprecipitates
7. Gamma globulins
8. Albumin
9. Factor VIII

Transcribing Doctors' Orders for Blood Transfusions

A type and crossmatch is a laboratory study that is performed to determine the type and compatibility of blood; it must be done before the patient receives blood or certain blood components. A type and crossmatch is performed in the blood bank division of the hospital laboratory. It is essential that the HUC match the patient's name and information on the patient ID label affixed to the blood specimen with the patient name and information on the doctor's order sheet and with the name and information on the computer order screen. The specimen will be discarded if the specimen patient ID label and the patient name on the requisition are not the same. The patient then will need to have blood redrawn, causing additional discomfort, a delay in treatment, and additional charges.

The equipment used for infusion of blood is similar to that used for infusion of IV solutions. Blood is packaged in plastic containers and is ordered by the unit. The IV tubing used for blood contains a filter. Normal saline solution generally is used, along with blood administered via IV infusion pump. All containers and tubing must be disposed of after the blood is transfused.

The transfusion of blood is a potentially dangerous procedure. Special precautions are taken by the nursing staff to ensure the correct administration of blood. Proper storage of blood is essential to ensure safe administration. Blood is stored in the blood bank, in a special refrigerator designed to maintain constant temperature for safe storage of blood. It is often the HUC's responsibility to pick up the blood from the blood bank and bring it to the nursing unit. If blood for two different patients is to be obtained from the blood bank at the same time, two different health care personnel should pick up the blood. It is important for the HUC to know that if the blood is not used immediately, it must be returned to the blood bank for storage. Blood should be stored only in refrigerators designated for blood storage.

Planning for blood transfusions is becoming common practice because it greatly reduces the risk that blood-borne infection such as human immunodeficiency virus (HIV) or hepatitis B will be acquired. Patients, family, or friends may donate blood for a patient in advance. The patient's own blood transfusion is called *autologous* or an *autotransfusion*; the blood of relatives or friends is called *donor-directed*, or *donor-specific* blood. Blood also may be collected from the patient at the surgery site during surgery. This blood is then transfused back to the patient. The blood is collected in a device called a *cell-saver*, or *autotransfusion*, system.

Plasma extenders or plasma substitutes are ordered by the doctor to increase the level of circulating fluid in the body. These may be obtained from the pharmacy.

✓ DOCTORS' ORDERS FOR TRANSFUSION OF BLOOD, BLOOD COMPONENTS, AND PLASMA SUBSTITUTES

The nurse carries out the following orders for administration of blood, blood components, and plasma substitutes; however, the transcription procedure requires the ordering step of transcription. Blood bank ordering is described in Chapter 14, "Laboratory Orders."

Give 2 units of whole blood now

T & X-match 2 units PC & hold for surgery

Give 1 unit of packed cells tonight and one in the a.m.

Give 2 units of plasma stat

Give 1 unit PC now, draw stat H & H₂O $\bar{p}$ completion of transfusion

Give 2 units PCs $\bar{c}$ 20 mg Lasix $\bar{p}$ 1st unit

Transfuse 1 unit of **autologous blood** today

Autotransfusion per protocol

Doctors' orders for total parenteral nutrition and for intravenous medication are covered in Chapter 13. ∎

SUCTION ORDERS

Background Information

Suction may be ordered by the doctor to remove fluid or air from body cavities and surgical wounds. Suction may be ordered intermittently or continuously and may be accomplished manually or mechanically. The doctor may set up some types of suction apparatuses during surgery, and the nursing staff may initiate some other types, such as **gastric suction**. The doctor may write orders for the establishment, maintenance, or discontinuance of suction. Wall suction usually is installed at each patient's bedside. Usually, tubing and suction catheters used with wall suction are stored on the nursing unit supply closet or C-locker. The HUC may be asked by the nurse to

✎ *TAKE NOTE*

Ordering and Obtaining Blood

A mistake in labeling of a blood specimen that sent to the laboratory for a type and crossmatch will result in the specimen's being discarded; the patient will have to have blood drawn again. Avoid errors in labeling, which cause the patient additional discomfort and delays in treatment, by doing the following:

Matching the patient's name and information on the ID label affixed to the blood specimen to the patient name and information on the doctor's order sheet and the name and information on the computer order screen.

If two units of blood have to be picked up from the blood bank for two different patients on the nursing unit, avoid an error in identifying the units of blood by

* Having another person go to the blood bank to pick up the second unit

or

* Making two trips to pick up one unit at a time

When blood is brought to the unit and cannot be given immediately, return the blood to the blood bank for storage; here, the storage temperature will ensure the safety of the blood.

➲ SKILLS CHALLENGE

To practice transcribing IV therapy orders, complete Activity 11-2 in the *Skills Practice Manual*.

---

order additional tubing or a specific type and/or size of catheter for a patient.

Following are doctors' orders related to suctioning, along with a brief interpretation. Refer to the abbreviations list at the beginning of the chapter for assistance, if necessary.

✓ DOCTORS' ORDERS FOR SUCTIONING

Suction Throat prn to Clear Airway

When a patient is unable to clear respiratory tract secretions by coughing, the doctor may order manual (bulb suction device) or mechanical (wall suction) suctioning to clear the airways (Fig 11-14). Three pathways for suctioning respiratory tract secretions are through the nose, through the mouth, and through an artificial airway with the use of tubing connected to the wall suction.

Suction Tracheostomy prn

A tracheostomy is an artificial opening into the trachea (windpipe) that is performed to facilitate breathing. When the patient is unable to cough, suctioning is necessary to remove secretions. Usually, small catheters and tubing connected to wall suction are used to remove secretions (Fig. 11-15).

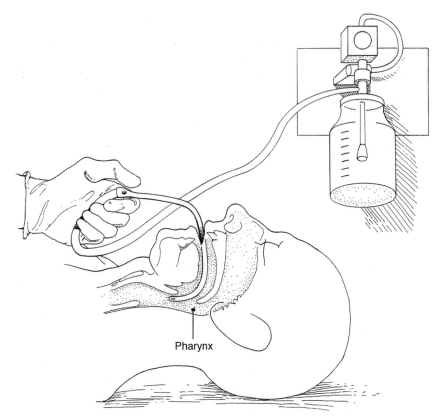

Figure 11-14 Throat-suctioning apparatus.

Assess Character of Penrose Drainage

Patients often return from surgery with a drain inserted into or close to the surgical wound if a large amount of drainage is expected. A drain such as a **Penrose drain** may lie under a dressing, extend through a dressing, or be connected to a drainage bag or a disposable wound suction device (also called *evacuator units*).

Keep Hemovac Compressed
Empty and Record JP Drainage q Shift

Hemovac and **Jackson-Pratt (JP)** are names of disposable wound suction devices (evacuator units) that are attached to an incisional drain during surgery. These devices exert a constant low pressure as long as the suction device is fully compressed. Figure 11-16 shows various surgical suction devices.

Insert NG Tube, Connect to Intermittent
Low Gastric Suction

The nurse or doctor inserts a **nasogastric (NG) tube** through the nose or mouth into the stomach. Correct placement of the NG tube is usually checked by inserting air into the tubing and listening to the stomach with a stethoscope. The tube then is connected to a wall-mounted suction unit, which provides intermittent removal of gastric contents and is usually set on low. (A high-pressure setting is never used without specific orders to do so.) Gastric suction often is ordered after gastrointestinal or other abdominal surgery, to prevent vomiting or for various other reasons.

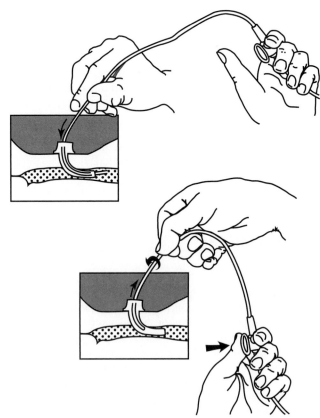

Figure 11-15 Suctioning of a tracheostomy with the use of a small catheter and tubing attached to wall suction.

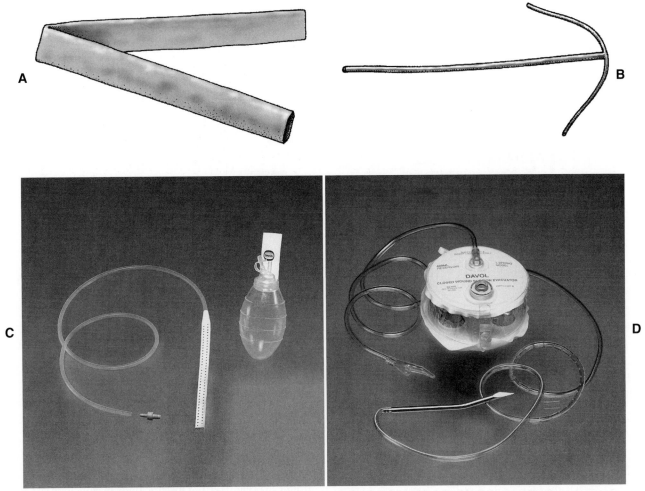

Figure 11-16 Types of surgical drains. **A,** Penrose. **B,** T tube. **C,** Jackson-Pratt. **D,** Hemovac. (From Ignatavicius D, Workman L: Medical-Surgical Nursing, 5th ed, Philadelphia, Saunders, 2006. **C** and **D** courtesy of C.R. Bard, Inc., Covington, Georgia.)

Irrig NG per Rout

The nurse irrigates the nasogastric tube per facility policy. An irrigation tray, usually disposable, is used for this procedure.

Clamp NG Tube Intermittently q1h

A clamp is applied to the NG tube or a plug is inserted into the distal end of the tube at 1-hour intervals and then is reconnected to the suction machine for 1-hour intervals.

Remove NG Tube and Gastric Suction

This is a typical example of an order to discontinue gastric suction.

Chest Tube 20 cm Neg Pressure

A chest tube is a catheter that is inserted through the thorax (chest) to reexpand the lungs by removing air or fluids that collect in the pleural cavity. Chest tubes are used after chest surgery and chest trauma. The chest tube is connected to a closed chest drainage system, such as Pleur-evac (Fig 11-17) or Thora-Sene III, which is connected to wall suction. The drainage system and chest tubes are disposable items. ■

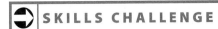
SKILLS CHALLENGE

To practice transcribing suction orders, complete Activity 11-3 in the *Skills Practice Manual.*

HEAT AND COLD APPLICATION ORDERS

Background Information

Heat and cold treatments are ordered for the patient by the doctor. Heat treatment is used to promote comfort, relaxation, and healing; to reduce pain and swelling; and to promote circulation. Cold treatment may be used to relieve pain, reduce inflammation, control hemorrhage, and decrease circulation.

Various methods for application of heat and cold are used; thus, a variety of doctors' orders are used to prescribe the methods intended. Typical doctors' orders for commonly used procedures for heat and cold applications follow, along with an explanation.

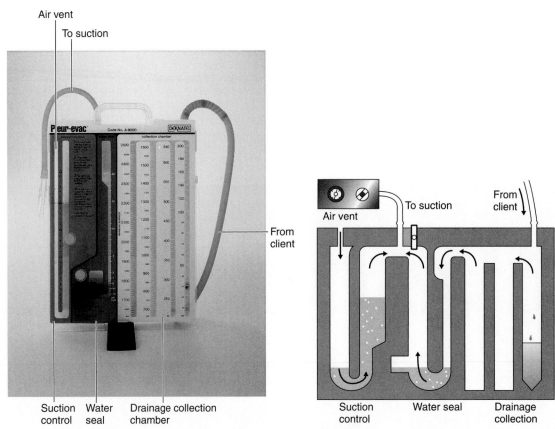

Figure 11-17 Pleur-evac—one of many available brands of chest draining systems. (From Ignatavicius D, Workman L: Medical-Surgical Nursing, 5th ed, Philadelphia, Saunders, 2006.)

✓ DOCTORS' ORDERS FOR HEAT APPLICATIONS

Aquathermia Pad With Heat to Lower lt Arm 20 min qid
An **aquathermia pad** (also called a K-pad or a water flow pad) is a device with a waterproof plastic or rubber pad that can be applied to various parts of the body. The pad contains channels through which heated or cooled water flows. The device includes hoses that are connected to a bedside control unit that consists of a temperature regulator, a motor for circulating the water, and a reservoir of distilled water. The pad and the patient's skin should be checked periodically to avoid the risk of accidental burns (Fig. 11-18).

Hot Compresses to Abscess on lt Ankle 10 min qh
Hot compresses are warm, wet gauze applied to a body part. They are used to treat small areas of the body. Usually, disposable items are used for this procedure.

Soak rt Hand 20 min in Warm NS Solution q4h While Awake
A soak is usually ordered to facilitate healing. For this order, the right hand is placed in a container of the prescribed solution to soak for 20 minutes every 4 hours while the patient is awake.

Sitz Bath 30 min tid
A **sitz bath** is used for the application of warm water to the pelvic area. Special tubs may be used for this procedure, or a disposable sitz bath that fits under a toilet seat may be ordered

from CSD (Fig. 11-19). Obstetric units may include sitz baths in patient bathrooms. ■

✓ DOCTORS' ORDERS FOR COLD APPLICATIONS

Alcohol Sponge for Temp Over 102°
An alcohol sponge is the bathing of a patient with a solution of alcohol and water for the purpose of reducing the patient's temperature.

Ice Bag to Scrotum as Tolerated for 24 hr
An ice bag may be a reusable plastic container, a commercially prepared disposable ice bag, or sometimes a disposable rubber glove filled with ice.

Hypothermia Machine prn if Temp ↑ 104°
The hypothermia machine circulates fluid through a network of tubing in a mattress-sized pad. It is used for prolonged cooling and to reduce body surface temperature. This is a reusable item that is returned to the CSD when discontinued by the doctor. ■

COMFORT, SAFETY, AND HEALING ORDERS

Background Information

The nursing staff selects and performs many tasks to promote the comfort, safety, and healing of the patient. However, doctors' orders are also written to address these needs.

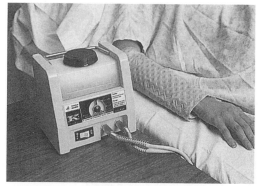

Figure 11-18 Aquathermia pad. (From Potter PA, Perry AG: Fundamentals of Nursing, 6th ed, St. Louis, Mosby, 2005.)

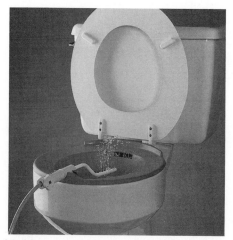

Figure 11-19 A disposable sitz bath. (Courtesy Andermac, Inc. From Mosby's Medical Dictionary, 7th ed, St. Louis, Mosby, 2006.)

Because such orders are varied, only typical examples with the interpretation of each are listed.

✔ DOCTORS' ORDERS FOR PATIENT COMFORT, SAFETY, AND HEALING

Specialty Beds

Many types of specialty beds are available to reduce the hazards of immobility to the skin and the musculoskeletal system; just a few are discussed here. The Hill-Rom air fluidized bed provides body support through the use of thousands of tiny soda-lime glass beads suspended by pressurized temperature–controlled air. The beads are covered with a polyester filter sheet. The bed is used to relieve pressure and to treat burn patients (Fig 11-20). KinAir III beds provide controlled air suspension to redistribute body weight away from bony prominences (see Evolve site), and FluidAir Elite beds use airflow and bead fluidization to achieve this. The Clinitron bed is filled with tiny sandlike pieces that are moving gently all the time. The Roto-Rest bed is specifically designed to support the trauma patient who is at risk for pulmonary complications. The critical care bed provides programmable kinetic therapy that administers lateral rotation to a range of 620 in both directions. The HUC must include the patient's height and weight when ordering these beds from CSD.

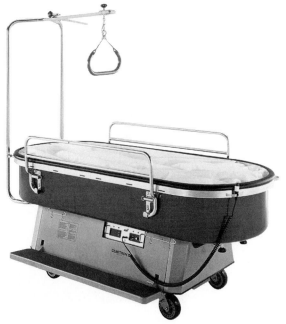

Figure 11-20 A Hill-Rom air fluidized bed. (©Hill-Rom Services, Inc. Used with permission. From Mosby's Medical Dictionary, 7th ed, St. Louis, Mosby, 2006.)

Egg-Crate Mattress

The **egg-crate mattress** is a foam rubber pad that resembles an egg crate or carton; it is used to distribute body weight evenly (Fig. 11-21). This is a disposable item that is used frequently in long-term care.

Other mattresses used to reduce the hazards of immobility to the skin and the musculoskeletal system include the Lotus Water Flotation Mattress, Bio Flote (an alternating air mattress), a static air mattress, and a foam mattress.

Sheepskin on Bed

A **sheepskin** is made of lamb's wool or of a synthetic material and usually measures about the same length and width as the patient's bed. The sheepskin is placed directly below the patient and is used to relieve pressure and prevent bedsores (decubitus ulcers). A sheepskin is usually considered a disposable item and is used frequently in long-term care.

Footboard on Bed

A footboard is placed at or near the foot of the bed so that the patient's feet, when placed against it, are at a right angle to the bed. It is used to prevent footdrop of patients who are in bed for long periods (Fig. 11-22). A footboard is a reusable item that would be ordered from CSD.

Foot Cradle to Bed

A foot cradle is a metal frame that is placed on the bed to prevent the top sheet from touching a specified part of the body. It is a reusable item that would be ordered from CSD.

ETS for Patient

An extended toilet seat (ETS) is ordered from CSD and is placed over the patient's toilet to make lowering and rising from a sitting position easier (Fig. 11-23).

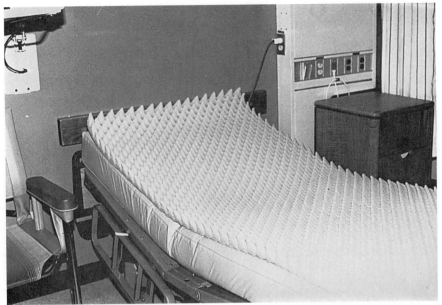

Figure 11-21 An egg-crate mattress.

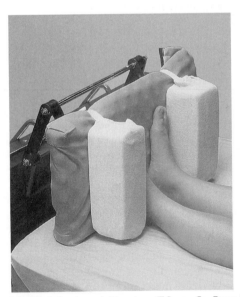

Figure 11-22 A footboard. (Courtesy JT Posey Co. From Mosby's Medical Dictionary, 7th ed, St. Louis, Mosby, 2006.)

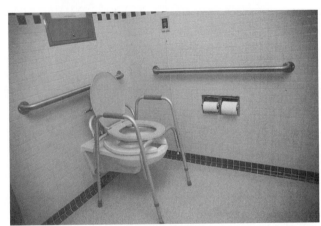

Figure 11-23 An extended toilet seat. (From Ignatavicius D, Workman L: Medical-Surgical Nursing, 5th ed, Philadelphia, Saunders, 2006.)

Immobilizer to lt Knee 20 Degrees Flexion
Immobilizers are used to keep a limb or body part in alignment (Fig. 11-24). They are reusable and are usually stored in the CSD closet or the C-locker on an ortho unit, but they are ordered from CSD if they are needed for a patient on another unit.

Sandbags to Immobilize lt Leg
Sandbags are placed on both sides of the leg to immobilize the leg. Sandbags are stored in the CSD closet or the C-locker on ortho units, but they would need to be ordered from CSD for other units.

Out of Bed With Elastic Abd Binder
An elastic abdominal **binder** is a disposable item that is often ordered after surgery to provide patient support (Fig. 11-25).

Measurements of the patient's waist and hips are usually required on the requisition to obtain the correctly sized binder. The doctor may also order an elastic binder for the chest after chest surgery.

Sling to rt Arm When Up
A sling is a disposable bandage that is used to support an arm. Slings may be stored in the CSD closet or the C-locker on an ortho unit, but they would need to be ordered from CSD if they are needed for a patient on another unit.

Thigh-High TED Hose to Both Legs
Teds, a brand name for antiembolism (AE) hose, are ordered to promote circulation to the lower extremities to help prevent blood clots. They are made in various sizes and may be ordered as thigh high or knee high, so the correct size and style information must be obtained from the patient's nurse. The patient takes the stockings home when discharged.

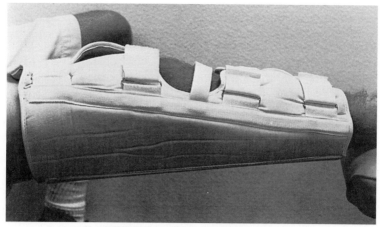

Figure 11-24 A knee immobilizer.

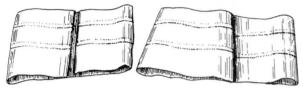

Figure 11-25 An elastic binder.

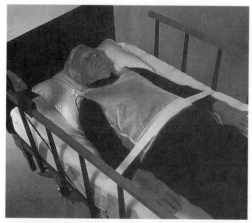

Figure 11-26 A jacket restraint. (Courtesy Medline Industries. From Mosby's Medical Dictionary, 7th ed, St. Louis, Mosby, 2006.)

Jacket Restraint for Agitation and Patient Safety

When restraint is absolutely necessary for patient safety, it requires a doctor's order. Various methods of restraint, including soft wrist, jacket **restraints**, and several types of commercial equipment, are available. The patient's mental and physical status must be assessed at close and regular intervals as prescribed by law and the agency's policies. Careful nursing documentation is essential when any type of restraint is applied. The HUC may have to place a restraint documentation form in the patient's chart. Figure 11-26 shows a patient in a jacket restraint.

May Shampoo Hair

Depending on the patient's condition, a doctor's order may be necessary for the hospitalized patient to have a shampoo. Appropriate equipment needed to do this for a bedridden patient usually is requisitioned from CSD and is reusable. Some hospitals may have a beauty shop located on the campus for the use of ambulatory patients.

Change Surgical Dressings bid

A bandage or other application over an external wound is called a *dressing*. Items used for this treatment are disposable and usually are stored in the nursing unit supply closet or the C-locker.

Pneumatic Compression to Left Calf

Pneumatic compression devices (also called *sequential compression devices [SCDs]*) are used to enhance venous blood flow by providing periods of compression. These devices prevent deep vein thrombosis (DVT) from forming in the legs as the result of inactivity. Different types of pneumatic compression devices may include boots, sleeves, or wraps to be placed on the patient's legs. Ted hose may be worn, in addition to the boots, to reduce some of the uncomfortable sensations produced by the boots, such as itching, sweating, and heat. Figure 11-27 shows various types of pneumatic compression devices.

TCDB q2h Splinting

The doctor may write an order for a postsurgical patient to turn, cough, and deep breathe every 2 hours after surgery to expel secretions, keep the lungs clear, and prevent pneumonia. **Splinting** or holding the incision area provides support and security and reduces pain during coughing. The doctor may also write an order for "do not cough" for patients who should avoid coughing.

Ostomy Nurse Referral

An ostomy nurse is trained to care for ostomy patients. The ostomy nurse is notified and will perform the care needed or will provide ostomy training to the patient. During the patient's stay in the hospital, the HUC will order supplies for ostomy care. Figure 11-28 displays stoma supplies used in the care of a colostomy.

Note: A colostomy is the creation of an artificial opening into a patient's colon. The patient then wears a bag over the opening (called a *stoma*) to catch stool.

Ask ostomy nurse to do ostomy teaching

Irrigate colostomy q A.M. ■

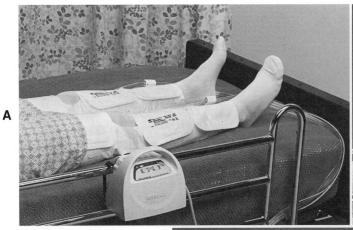

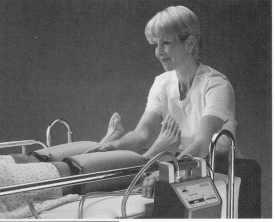

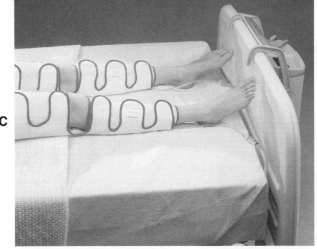

Figure 11-27 Types of pneumatic compression devices. **A,** Kendall SCD™ Compression System Controller, SCD™ Sleeves and T.E.D.™ Anti-Embolism Stockings. **B,** Venodyne pneumatic compression system. **C,** Flowtron DVT calf garments. (**A,** courtesy of The Kendall Healthcare Company, Mansfield, MA; **B,** courtesy of Venodyne, Inc., Norwood, MA; **C,** courtesy of Huntleigh Healthcare, Eatontown, NJ. From Ignatavicius D, Workman L: Medical-Surgical Nursing, 5th ed. Philadelphia, Saunders, 2006.)

 SKILLS CHALLENGE

To practice transcribing heat and cold applications and performing tasks related to comfort, safety, and healing orders, complete Activity 11-4 in the *Skills Practice Manual.*

✐ *TAKE NOTE*

Types of Nursing Treatment Orders
- Intestinal elimination orders
- Urinary catheterization orders
- IV therapy orders
- Blood transfusion orders
- Suction orders
- Heat and cold application orders
- Comfort, safety, and healing orders

COMPLEMENTARY AND ALTERNATIVE APPROACHES/THERAPIES

Background Information

During the past 20 years, a growing interest in complementary (additional treatment) and alternative (substitutions for traditional treatment) approaches/therapies has evolved. Many Americans are using complementary and/or alternative therapies. Most persons who receive complementary and alternative therapies pay for them out-of-pocket because most third party payers reimburse only for selected therapies such as chiropractic treatment and acupuncture. One of the reasons for the increase in these treatments is that individuals wish to be treated in a holistic fashion. Nurses believe in a holistic, caring philosophy; therefore, complementary and alternative therapies are consistent with nursing and nursing practice. It would not be common to see complementary or alternative therapies ordered in the hospital setting, but reference may be made to them, so a few are included here, along with a brief description of each.

Acupressure is a traditional Chinese medicine therapy that is used in nursing for a number of conditions such as

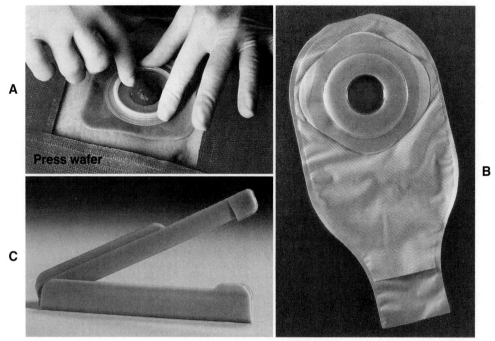

Figure 11-28 A, Stoma wafer that fits around a stoma on a patient with a colostomy. A drainable pouch is applied over the wafer and clamped **(B)** until the pouch is to be emptied **(C).** (Courtesy ConvaTec, Bristol-Myers Squibb, Princeton, New Jersey. From Mosby's Medical Dictionary, 7th ed, St. Louis, Mosby, 2006; and Ignatavicius D, Workman L: Medical-Surgical Nursing, 5th ed, Philadelphia, Saunders, 2006.)

the treatment of pain, nausea, and vomiting. Acupressure is similar to acupuncture, except that pressure is used in place of needles on one of 365 to 700 acupoints located throughout the body. Fingers press certain points on the body to stimulate the body's self-curative abilities.

Use of aromatherapy and herbal preparations is a fast growing area in complementary medicine. Use of essential oils can be traced back to ancient times. Essential oils may be applied in compresses, in baths, or topically on the skin. Essential oils are obtained from the flowers, leaves, bark, wood, roots, seeds, and peels of plants. Lavender and rose oils are used to promote relaxation and sleep. Peppermint has been used for stimulation and to promote concentration. Sandalwood and lavender have been used to ease depression. Essential oils are potent and are diluted before they are used.

Imagery has been used for many years in nursing. While performing painful procedures or treatments, the nurse may ask a patient to think about a pleasant event or a beautiful scene to ease anxiety. *Imagery* has been defined as the formation of a mental representation of an object, place, event, or situation that is perceived through the senses. Imagery has been used in a wide variety of situations such as reducing pain, nausea, and vomiting, decreasing anxiety, and promoting comfort during treatment for cancer.

Journaling is a reflective therapy; it is a tool that is used to record the process of one's life. Writing provides a vehicle by which a person can express feelings, gain new perspectives, and pay attention to what is in the unconscious. The writing is usually free flowing, and the patient writes whatever comes to mind without censoring any thoughts or feelings or correcting grammar or punctuation. The writing is done for oneself and need not be shared.

Magnets are used for a particular type of energy therapy. One of the primary reasons for using magnets is to relieve chronic pain, particularly back and joint pain. Magnets can be applied via wide belts and orthotics, or in mattresses and pillows.

Massage has a long history in nursing practice. Until recently, daily back rubs were a standard nursing procedure that was administered to all hospitalized patients. Massage involves the use of pressure and various strokes to manipulate soft tissues for therapeutic purposes. Hand massage can be used with persons with dementia to provide relaxation and to lessen aggressive behaviors. Patient permission must be obtained before massage is performed.

Music therapy is an established health care profession in which music is used to address physical, emotional, cognitive, and social needs of patients of all ages. It can improve the quality of life of persons who are well and can meet the needs of children and adults with disabilities or illnesses. Music therapy interventions are used to elevate patients' moods and to counteract depression; in conjunction with anesthesia or medication to alleviate pain; to promote movement for physical rehabilitation; to calm, sedate, or induce sleep; to help counteract apprehension or fear; and to lessen muscle tension in areas such as the autonomic nervous system for the purpose of achieving relaxation.

Tai chi is a traditional Chinese martial art that has been adapted to become a mind-body exercise. The goal of tai chi is to integrate body movements, mind concentration, muscle relaxation, and breathing to promote a flow of energy throughout the body.

Therapeutic touch is the use of hands on or near the body with the intention to heal. The practitioner directs her own interpersonal energy to help or heal another. Therapeutic touch has been used to reduce anxiety and pain, improve the immune system, and improve functional ability.

The procedure for nursing treatment orders is fairly simple after one has become familiar with the supplies and equipment necessary to implement each order. Ordering the wrong supplies and/or equipment may delay treatment but probably would not cause harm to the patient. When in doubt about the supplies or equipment needed, check with the nurse or with the CSD. Whether an EMR or paper charts are used, the HUC who is able to recognize supplies and equipment and their uses and to effectively use the CSD plays an invaluable role in helping the nursing staff to provide quality patient care.

REVIEW QUESTIONS

1. List five nursing treatment items that would be located in the nursing unit supply closet or the C-locker.

a. _____

b. _____

c. _____

d. _____

e. _____

2. List five nursing treatment items that would be stored in the CSD.

a. _____

b. _____

c. _____

d. _____

e. _____

3. List four types of enemas that a doctor may order.

a. _____

b. _____

c. _____

d. _____

4. List two types of urinary catheters and describe the function of each.

a. _____

b. _____

5. List three parts of an IV order.

a. _____

b. _____

c. _____

6. List two types of suction devices that could be inserted during surgery.

a. _____

b. _____

7. State two methods of administering IV therapy.

a. _____

b. _____

8. List three types of commonly used IV solutions.

a. _____

b. _____

c. _____

9. Explain what would happen if a patient's blood specimen sent for a type and crossmatch was labeled incorrectly (the patient's name on the ID label does not match the patient's name on the order requisition).

_____

10. List two devices used for heat application.

a. _____

b. _____

11. List two devices used for cold application.

a. _____

b. _____

12. Define the following terms.

a. heplock

_____

b. Hemovac

_____

c. Jackson-Pratt (JP)

_____

d. autologous blood

_____

e. donor-specific blood

_____

f. catheterization

_____

g. Penrose drain

_____

h. central venous catheter

_____

13. Define "urine residual."

_____

14. Rental equipment should be promptly returned to the CSD because

a. _____

b. _____

15. The patient's nurse asks the HUC to pick up a unit of packed cells from the blood bank. When the HUC returns to the nursing unit with the packed cells, the nurse states that the transfusion will not be started for hours. Explain what the HUC should do with the packed cells until the nurse can start the transfusion.

_____

_____

16. The HUC is asked to pick up two units of packed cells from the blood bank for two separate patients on the nursing unit. Explain what the HUC should do.

_____

_____

17. Briefly describe the function of the CSD as it relates to nursing treatment orders.

_____

_____

18. True or False

a. _____ Consent is required for insertion of a PICC.

b. _____ Consent is required for use of a peripheral intravenous catheter.

c. _____ Consent is required for insertion of a heplock.

d. _____ A Hemovac is connected to a drain in or near the surgical site and is inserted during surgery.

e. _____ A central line tray would have to be ordered for insertion of a PICC.

19. Rewrite the following doctors' orders using abbreviations.

  a. Have the IV team insert a peripherally inserted central catheter.

  _____

  b. Continuous intravenous fluids; alternate one thousand milliliters of lactated Ringer's with one thousand milliliters of five percent dextrose in water at one hundred twenty-five milliliters per hour via central venous catheter.

  _____

  c. Insert NG tube and connect to low gastric suction.

  _____

THINK ABOUT...

1. Discuss what some of the greatest fears might be for a hospitalized patient.
2. Discuss what patients have the right to expect of the nursing staff.
3. Discuss how the HUC can have a direct impact on the delivery of patient care.
4. Discuss why communication and teamwork between the HUC and the nursing staff are important.

Nutritional Care Orders

CHAPTER OBJECTIVES

Upon completion of this chapter, you will be able to:

1. Define the terms listed in the vocabulary list.
2. Write the meaning of the abbreviations in the abbreviations list.
3. Interpret the dietary orders included in this chapter.
4. Explain the importance of communicating patient food allergies to the nutritional care department.
5. List the diets that provide change in the consistency of food.
6. Identify two diets that may be requested by patients.
7. Identify five therapeutic diets.
8. List four diets that may be selected for the patient who is on a *diet as tolerated.*
9. List three types of formula or preparations used for tube feeding.
10. List three methods of administering tube feedings.
11. List three items a health unit coordinator may have to order when transcribing an order for tube feeding.

VOCABULARY

Anorexia Nervosa Intense fear of gaining weight or becoming fat, although underweight

Body Mass Index Body weight in kilograms divided by height in square meters; this is the usual measurement to define overweight and obesity

Bolus Rounded mass of food formed in the mouth and ready to be swallowed; also defined as a concentrated dose of medication or fluid, frequently given intravenously (discussed in Chapter 13)

Bulimia Nervosa Recurrent episodes of binge eating (rapid consumption of a large amount of food in a discrete period of time) and self-induced vomiting, along with use of laxatives or diuretics

Calorie A measurement of energy generated in the body by the heat produced after food is eaten

Diet Manual Hospitals are required to have available in the dietary office and on all nursing units an up-to-date diet manual that has been jointly approved by the medical and nutritional care staffs

Diet Order A doctor's order that states the type and quantity of food and liquids the patient may receive

Dietary Reference Intake (DRI) The framework of nutrient standards now in place in the United States; this provides reference values for use in planning and evaluating diets for healthy people

Dietary Supplements A product (other than tobacco) taken by mouth that contains a "dietary ingredient" intended to supplement the diet; dietary supplements come in many forms, including extracts, concentrates, tablets, capsules, gel caps, liquids, and powders

Dysphagia Difficulty eating and swallowing

Enteral Feeding Set Equipment needed to infuse tube feeding; includes plastic bag for feeding solution and may be ordered with or without pump

Enteral Nutrition The provision of liquid formulas into the gastrointestinal (GI) tract by tube or by mouth

Feeding Tube A small flexible plastic tube that is usually placed in the patient's nose and that goes down to the stomach or small intestine to provide and/or increase nutritional intake

Food Allergy A negative physical reaction to a particular food that involves the immune system (people with food allergies must avoid offending foods)

Food Intolerance A more common problem than food allergies, involving digestion (people with food intolerance can eat some of the offending foods without suffering symptoms)

Gastritis Inflammation of the stomach

Gastroenteritis Inflammation of the stomach and intestines

Gastrostomy Feeding Feeding by means of a tube inserted into the stomach through an artificial opening in the abdominal wall

Gavage Feeding by means of a tube inserted into the stomach, duodenum, or jejunum through the nose or an opening in the abdominal wall; also called *tube feeding*

Hydration Adequate water in the intracellular and extracellular compartments of the body

Ingestion The taking in of food by mouth

Kangaroo Pump A brand name of a feeding pump used to administer tube feeding

Kosher To adhere to the dietary laws of Judaism; the conventional meaning in Hebrew is "acceptable" or "approved"

Morbid Obesity An excess of body fat that threatens necessary body functions such as respiration

Nutrients Substances derived from food that are used by body cells, for example, carbohydrates, fats, proteins, vitamins, minerals, and water

Obesity An excess amount of body fat usually defined by body mass index

Parenteral Nutrition A mode of feeding that does not use the GI tract, instead providing nutrition by intravenous delivery of nutrient solutions

Percutaneous Endoscopic Gastrostomy Insertion of a tube through the abdominal wall into the stomach under endoscopic guidance

Recommended Dietary Allowance (RDA) The average daily intake of a nutrient that meets the requirements of nearly all (97% to 98%) healthy people of a given age and gender

Registered Dietitian One who has completed an educational program, served an internship, and passed an examination sponsored by the American Dietetic Association

Regular Diet A diet that consists of all foods and is designed to provide good nutrition

Rehydration Restoration of normal water balance in a patient through the administration of fluids orally or intravenously

Therapeutic Diet A regular diet with modifications or restrictions (also called a *special diet*) that must be ordered by the doctor

Total Parenteral Nutrition (TPN) The provision of all necessary nutrients via veins (discussed in detail in Chapter 13)

Tube Feeding Administration of liquids into the stomach, duodenum, or jejunum through a tube

ABBREVIATIONS

Abbreviation	Meaning	Example of Usage on a Doctor's Order Sheet
ADA	American Diabetic Association	1200 cal ADA diet
AHA	American Heart Association	Follow AHA diet
BMI	Body mass index	Calculate BMI
cal	calorie	1800 cal diet
CHO	carbohydrate	High-protein, low-CHO diet
chol	cholesterol	Low-chol diet
cl	clear	Cl liq diet
DAT	diet as tolerated	Advance DAT
FF	force fluids	Soft diet FF
FS	full strength	Δ Jevity FS @ 50 mL/hr
K or K+	potassium	High K+
Liq	liquid	Full liq diet
MN	midnight	NPO MN
Na or Na+	sodium	4000 mg Na diet (4000 mg/4 g)
NAS	no added salt	Reg diet, NAS
NPO	nothing by mouth	NPO after midnight
NSA	no salt added (same as NAS)	
PEG	percutaneous endoscopic gastrostomy	PEG in A.M.
RD	registered dietitian	RD consult requested
reg	regular	Reg diet

EXERCISE 1

Write the abbreviation for each term listed below.

1. sodium _____

2. midnight _____

3. nothing by mouth _____

4. regular _____

5. clear _____

6. calorie _____

7. American Diabetic Association _____

8. liquid _____

9. cholesterol _____

10. diet as tolerated _____

11. force fluids _____

12. carbohydrate _____

13. no salt added _____

14. full strength _____

15. percutaneous endoscopic gastrostomy _____

16. no added salt _____

17. registered dietitian   _____

18. potassium   _____

19. body mass index   _____

20. American Heart Association   _____

EXERCISE 2

Write the meaning of each abbreviation listed below.

1. Na or Na+

   _____

2. NPO

   _____

3. reg

   _____

4. MN

   _____

5. liq

   _____

6. cal

   _____

7. NSA

   _____

8. ADA

   _____

9. DAT

   _____

10. cl

   _____

11. chol

   _____

12. CHO

   _____

13. FF

   _____

14. FS

   _____

15. PEG

   _____

16. NAS

   _____

17. RD

   _____

18. K or K+

   _____

19. BMI

   _____

20. AHA

   _____

COMMUNICATION WITH THE NUTRITIONAL CARE DEPARTMENT

The procedure for ordering a new diet or a change/modification to an existing diet when paper charts are used requires the health unit coordinator (HUC) to communicate the order by computer to the nutritional care department. The HUC chooses the correct patient from the unit census screen on the computer, selects nutritional care department from the department ordering screen, then checks the box to order the specific diet from the options on the dietary screen, along with other items that apply (e.g., dietitian consult). The patient's food allergies and intolerances must be communicated to the nutritional care department (usually upon admission). Some food allergies or intolerances cause minor discomforts such as hives or upset stomach. True food allergies such as allergies to tree nuts, fish, shellfish, and peanuts can produce life-threatening changes in circulation and bronchioles called *anaphylactic shock*. NKFA indicates that the patient has no known food allergies.

A "write-in" option is provided for additional comments. The diet order would be sent to the nutritional care department by pressing "Enter" on the computer keyboard.

If the computer is shut down, order the diet from the nutritional care department by written requisition. The diet order is later entered into the computer to maintain a record (Fig. 12-1).

Most health care facilities provide each patient with the next day's menu of items that are allowed for the particular diet the doctor has ordered for the patient. The patient checks what foods they would like from the menu. The menu is then

```
Doctor ordering _____
Today's date _____
Requested by _____

┌─────────────────────────────┐
│ Nutritional Care Department │
└─────────────────────────────┘

☐ Bland                  ☐ Kosher              ☐ Restrict fluids to _____
☐ _____Calorie ADA       ☐ Low cholesterol     ☐ Snacks/supplements
☐ Clear liquid           ☐ Low sodium          ☐ _____Sodium
☐ Dysphagia _____      ☐ Mechanical soft     ☐ Soft
☐ Finger food            ☐ Modified fat _____  ☐ Vegetarian
☐ Force fluids           ☐ Pediatric           ☐ Calorie count
☐ Full liquid            ☐ Protein modified_____g  ☐ Dietitian consult
☐ Gluten free            ☐ Prudent cardiac     ☐ Early tray
                         ☐ Pureed              ☐ Guest tray
                         ☐ Regular             ☐ Hold tray
                         ☐ Renal               ☐ NPO _____
                                               ☐ Release from hold


☐ Other_____

Food allergies_____
Preferences_____
Comments_____
```

Figure 12-1 A nutritional care department requisition.

TAKE NOTE

When the electronic medical record (EMR) with computer physician order entry (CPOE) is implemented, the physician orders are entered directly into the patient's electronic record, and the dietary order is automatically sent to the nutritional care department. The HUC may have tasks to perform, such as ordering equipment from central services department (CSD). An icon may indicate a HUC task, or it may be submitted as a nurse request. The HUC must communicate with the nutritional care department (by e-mail or telephone) when ordering a diet for a patient who has completed a procedure or test that requires him to be NPO. *Some hospital nutritional care departments require that **all** diet orders be submitted in writing via computer.

TAKE NOTE

Patients' food allergies and intolerances must be communicated to the nutritional care department (usually on admission). Some food allergies and intolerances cause minor discomforts such as hives or upset stomach. True food allergies such as allergies to tree nuts, fish, shellfish, and peanuts can produce life-threatening changes in circulation and bronchioles called *anaphylactic shock.* "NKFA" indicates that the patient has no known food allergies.

the patient's trays are prepared. The dietitian also maintains a record (usually on computer) on each patient, which is updated with each order received.

TAKE NOTE

A downtime requisition is included for learning purposes. The CD included in the HUC's *Skills Practice Manual* is a simulated hospital computer program that may be used as well.

Background Information

During hospitalization, the doctor will order the type of diet the patient is to receive. The food is prepared by the nutritional care department and is designed to attain or maintain the health of the patient. Diets for the hospitalized patient can be divided into three groups: standard diets, therapeutic diets, and tube feedings (Table 12-1).

sent to the nutritional care department. Many facilities have initiated a system to better serve the patient and save the cost of printing menus. This requires the diet aide or technician to interview each patient upon admission to obtain and record food preferences and allergies. The diet aide may use a laptop computer to record the information. The doctor, nurse, diet aide, or diet technician may ask the dietitian to consult with the patient.

All dietary information, including orders for nothing by mouth, tube feedings, allergies, limit fluids, force fluids, and **calorie** count, must be sent to the nutritional care department, so necessary adjustments will be made when

Table 12-1 Description and Purpose of Common Hospital Diets

Type	Description	Purpose	Tray Condiments
Bland diet	May be used for patients who experience stomach irritation. Spicy foods containing black or red pepper and chili powder are omitted. Beverages that contain caffeine, cola, coffee, cocoa, and tea are omitted. Chocolate is also omitted. Any foods known to cause discomfort are omitted.	For patients with ulcers and other problems.	Salt, sugar
Prudent—low cholesterol/ reduced sodium	Controls the type of fat in the diet. Limits saturated fat and cholesterol found in foods from animal sources like eggs, dairy products, meat, and fish. Limits salt added to foods and on tray.	For patients who have high levels of blood cholesterol.	Pepper, sugar, salt substitute, or herbal seasoning mix
Sodium-controlled diet	Controls the amount of sodium in the diet. Salt and foods that contain salt are high in sodium and are limited. The sodium-controlled diet will vary according to the amount of sodium allowed.	For patients with heart disease, high blood pressure, kidney disease, or who are using certain drugs.	Sugar, pepper, salt substitute, if ordered
Diabetic diet	Total amount of food (calories) is carefully planned. Diabetic individuals cannot receive too much or too little food; therefore, portion sizes must be followed. Concentrated sweets like syrup, jelly, sweet desserts, and sugar are omitted. Snacks may be planned between meals to keep blood sugar levels balanced.	For patients who cannot produce enough insulin. Insulin is a substance that is important for helping sugar enter body cells. When insufficient insulin is made, sugar builds up in the blood.	Salt, pepper, sugar substitute
Renal	On the basis of individual needs, diet is controlled in terms of one or more of the following: protein, sodium, potassium, total fluid, and phosphorus.	For patients with renal disease.	Sugar, pepper, no salt substitutes
Neutropenic—no fresh fruits/vegetables, low bacteria	No fresh fruits or vegetables allowed.	Reduce the number of bacteria entering the stomach for patients on chemotherapy or those with immune deficiency diseases.	Sugar, no pepper or salt
Lactose controlled	Limits intake of milk and milk products.	For patients who experience stomach disturbances after drinking/ eating milk-containing foods.	Salt, pepper, sugar
NPO—nothing by mouth	Patient cannot receive fluids or solid foods.	Presurgery or as indicated for procedure or test	None
Clear liquid	Foods that are liquid or that become liquid at room or body temperature. Includes foods like tea, coffee, clear broth, gelatin, and carbonated beverages, as well as foods that can be seen through (e.g., apple, cranberry, grape juice).	For patients who are very sick and cannot eat anything else. For patients before or after surgery.	Sugar
Full liquid diet	This diet includes food from the clear liquid diet, with the addition of juices with pulp, such as orange. It also includes milk, ice cream, puddings, refined cooked cereals, strained cream soups, and egg nog.	For patients who cannot eat solid foods. For patients after surgery and after the clear liquid diet.	Salt, pepper, sugar
Regular diet/ DAT	All foods and beverages are allowed.	For patients who have no dietary restrictions.	Salt, pepper, sugar
Gastrointestinal soft diet	Limits raw, highly seasoned, and fried foods.	For patients with nausea and for distention in the postsurgical patient.	Salt, pepper, sugar

Table 12-1 Description and Purpose of Common Hospital Diets —Cont'd

Type	Description	Purpose	Tray Condiments
Mechanical soft diet	Any diet made soft with ground meats, soft canned fruits, and well-cooked vegetables.	For patients who have trouble chewing or swallowing.	Salt, pepper, sugar
Puree	Mechanically altered foods and full liquids allowed.	For patients with problems in chewing and swallowng.	Salt, pepper, sugar
No thin liquids/ thick liquids only	No milk (except milkshakes), juice (except nectars), broth soups (only cream soups), coffee, tea, or soda pop.	To prevent choking.	Salt, pepper, sugar

DAT, Diet as tolerated.

✐ TAKE NOTE

It is essential that all dietary information, including orders for nothing by mouth, tube feedings, allergies, limit fluids, force fluids, and calorie count, be sent to the nutritional care department, so necessary adjustments will be made when the patient's tray is prepared. All admitted patients require a diet order.

STANDARD DIETS

Standard hospital diets consist of a **regular diet** and diets that vary in consistency or texture (clear liquid–solid) of foods. A regular diet, also called *general, house, routine,* and *full,* is planned to provide good nutrition and consists of all items in the four basic food groups. This diet is ordered for hospitalized patients who do not require restrictions or modifications of their diets. Clear liquid, full liquid, soft, mechanical soft, and pureed are types of diets that vary in food texture or consistency.

 ## DOCTORS' ORDERS FOR STANDARD PROGRESSION DIETS

Clear Liquid
This diet is used for patients who cannot tolerate solid foods, including those in whom an acute illness has been diagnosed and patients who have just had surgery. It includes clear liquids only, such as broth, bouillon, coffee, tea, carbonated beverages, clear fruit juices, gelatin, and popsicles.

Full Liquid
Clear liquids with the addition of smooth-textured dairy products, custards, refined cooked cereals, vegetables, and all fruit juices. This diet is often ordered as a transitional step between a clear liquid diet and a soft diet.

Puréed
Full liquids with the addition of scrambled eggs, puréed meats, vegetables, fruits, mashed potatoes, and gravy.

Mechanical Soft
Includes the addition of ground or finely diced meats, flaked fish, cottage cheese, cheese, rice, potatoes, pancakes, light breads, cooked vegetables, cooked or canned fruits, bananas, soups, or peanut butter. This diet is prepared to meet the needs of patients who have difficulty chewing.

Soft
This diet is often used in the progression from a full liquid diet to a regular diet. It combines foods just described with nonirritating, easily digestible foods and modified fiber content, such as broiled chicken and boiled vegetables. It may be ordered postoperatively, for acute infections, or for gastrointestinal (GI) disorders.

Regular
No restrictions, unless specified.

Diet as Tolerated (DAT)
Usually, the doctor orders a diet such as clear liquid to progress diet as tolerated. The nurse can progress the patient's diet as the patient tolerates. The nurse can select a full liquid, soft, or regular diet for the patient, according to the patient's tolerance of food. For example, after the patient has tolerated clear liquids following a morning surgery, the nurse may order a full liquid diet for the evening meal. Usually, the patient is advanced from clear liquid to full liquid, to soft, and then to a regular diet, according to the current stage of recovery. ■

✐ TAKE NOTE

An order sent to nutritional care for a liquid diet must indicate *clear* or *full,* or nutritional care personnel will not know what to send to the patient.

✐ TAKE NOTE

When the doctor writes an order to advance diet as tolerated (DAT), the order usually includes the initial diet. The nurse may then select from standard (consistency) diets such as full liquid, soft, or regular to advance the diet. Variations may include mechanical soft or pureed, depending on the patient's ability to chew. *The HUC must ask the patient's nurse for the diet selection, then send this information to the nutritional care department. **The nutritional care department cannot determine what the patient can tolerate.**

Patient-Requested Diets

Many patients have food preferences or restrictions that are based on their culture or religion or religious holidays. This information is used to prepare food for those patients. Two examples of patient-requested diets include vegetarian diets and kosher diets.

Vegetarian diets are those in which the patient follows a plant-based diet and limits or excludes animal foods. Several types of vegetarian diets are available, such as the following:

- Ovolactovegetarian—includes all plant foods, dairy, and eggs
- Lactovegetarian—includes all plant foods and dairy
- Vegan—includes plant foods only
- Flexitarian—includes predominantly plant foods with non-vegetarian foods such as fish or poultry, on occasion

Kosher diets are those that adhere to the dietary laws of Judaism. A kosher diet involves the following:

- Species of animals—only healthy animals that have split hooves and chew their cud (hogs and pigs do not chew their cud) and only fish with scales and fins
- Manner in which food is processed—animals properly slaughtered and no mixing of milk and meat
- Time—leavened product properly disposed of before Passover and no food cooked on Sabbath
- All fresh fruits and vegetables are kosher
- Unprocessed grains and cereals are kosher
- Chicken eggs are kosher

See the Box *Other Religious Dietary Restrictions* for additional examples of dietary restrictions.

OTHER RELIGIOUS DIETARY RESTRICTIONS

Islam
- Pork
- Alcohol
- Caffeine
- Ramadan: fasting sunrise to sunset for a month
- Ritualized methods of animal slaughter required for meat ingestion

Christianity
- (Minimal or no) alcohol
- Holy day observances may restrict meat

Hinduism
- All meats

Church of Jesus Christ of Latter Day Saints (Mormons)
- Alcohol
- Tobacco
- Caffeine

Seventh-Day Adventists
- Pork
- Shellfish
- Alcohol
- Vegetarian diet encouraged

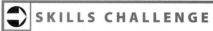

SKILLS CHALLENGE

To practice transcribing a standard hospital diet order, complete Activity 12-1 in the *Skills Practice Manual.*

THERAPEUTIC DIET ORDERS

Therapeutic diets, which must be ordered by a doctor, differ from the regular diet in that the foods served are modified to vary in caloric content, level of one or more **nutrients,** bulk, or flavor. The following list contains some common therapeutic diets and diets for specific conditions.

- Bland—This diet is designed to provide adequate nutrition during treatment of patients with inflammatory or ulcerative conditions of the esophagus, stomach, and intestines. It is mechanically, chemically, physiologically, and sometimes thermally nonirritating to the GI tract. A bland diet disallows caffeine, alcohol, black pepper, spices, or any other food that could be considered irritating.
- BRAT—This diet is commonly used as short-term dietary treatment for diarrhea, **gastroenteritis,** and some incidences of food poisoning. The name BRAT is an acronym for Bananas, Rice, Applesauce, and Toast. Oral **rehydration** solution or other liquids are usually given to the patient immediately. The diarrhea or gastroenteritis starts; a BRAT diet is usually administered after about 24 hours to prevent dehydration, once vomiting has stopped and the patient is able to eat.
- Soft/Low Residue—Addition of low-fiber, easily digested foods, such as pastas, casseroles, moist tender meats, and canned cooked fruits and vegetables. Desserts, cakes, and cookies without nuts or coconut are included.
- Low Cholesterol—300 mg/day cholesterol is in keeping with American Heart Association (AHA) guidelines for serum lipid reduction.
- Low Sodium—4-g (no added salt), 2-g, 1-g, or 500-mg sodium diet. These diets vary from no added salt to severe sodium restriction (500-mg sodium diet) that requires selective food purchases. Sodium intake is often restricted for patients with cardiovascular disease, hypertension, and kidney disease.
- Low Protein—Protein intake may be controlled in Parkinson's disease and in chronic kidney disease.
- High Fiber—Fresh uncooked fruits, steamed vegetables, bran, oatmeal, and dried fruits are added.
- Diabetic (American Diabetic Association [ADA])—Included food exchanges are recommended by the ADA. Usually, caloric recommendations are made for around 1800 calories. The exchange diet results in a balanced intake of carbohydrates, fats, and proteins. Total calories may vary to accommodate the client's metabolic demands, which may be affected by an exercise program, pregnancy, or, in some situations, another illness.
- Calorie Restricted—Diet may be limited to 1200 calories or 1400 calories.
- Renal—This diet is ordered for patients with renal disease. On the basis of individual needs, diet is controlled in terms of one or more of the following: protein, sodium, potassium, total fluid, and phosphorus.
- Cardiac Prudent—This diet is based on variations of diet recommendations of the AHA for low cholesterol and low sodium.

- Low Fat—Diets high in fat, especially saturated fat, are linked to high blood cholesterol levels and heart disease. High-fat diets can also increase risk for obesity and cancer. This is a diet low in fat, saturated fat, and cholesterol.
- High Potassium—A shortage of potassium in body fluids may cause a potentially fatal condition known as hypokalemia, which typically results from diarrhea, increased diuresis, and vomiting. Eating a variety of foods that contain potassium is the best way to get an adequate amount. Foods with high sources of potassium include orange juice, potatoes, bananas, avocados, apricots, parsnips, and turnips, although many other fruits, vegetables, and meats contain potassium. Diets high in potassium can reduce the risk of hypertension.
- Potassium Restricted—Some people with kidney disease are advised to avoid large quantities of dietary potassium. Patients with end-stage renal failure who are undergoing therapy by renal dialysis must observe strict dietary limits on potassium intake because the kidneys control potassium excretion, and buildup of blood concentrations of potassium may trigger fatal heart dysrhythmias.
- Hypoglycemic—The purpose of the hypoglycemic diet is to normalize blood sugar levels, thereby normalizing levels of stress hormones such as adrenaline and cortisol, which are thought to be responsible for the symptoms of mood swings, depression, anxiety, phobias, alcoholism, and drug addiction. This diet limits sugar, coffee, strong tea, nicotine if possible, refined carbohydrates, sugary drinks, candy bars, colas, cookies, and so forth. The diet consists of high levels of protein plus complex carbohydrate snacks every 3 hours or sooner, to provide a slow release of glucose and to prevent the hypoglycemic dip. A high-protein breakfast must be considered the most important meal of the day. Good sources of protein include eggs and white meat (e.g., chicken, fish). Eat plenty of green vegetables and fruits. The more varied the diet, the better it is.
- Low Carbohydrate—This diet involves restricted carbohydrate consumption, based on research that ties consumption of certain carbohydrates with increased blood insulin levels, and overexposure to insulin with metabolic syndrome (the most recognized symptom of which is obesity). Foods high in digestible carbohydrates (sugars and starches) are limited or are replaced by foods that contain a higher percentage of proteins, fats, and/or fiber.

Dysphagia diets include the following:

- Level I (most restricted): Severe dysphagia—Patients are just beginning to eat by mouth (unable to safely swallow chewable foods and unable to safely drink thin liquids). The diet consists of thick homogenous semiliquid textures and decreased fiber; no coarse textures, nuts, or raw fruits or vegetables are included.
- Level II: Moderate dysphagia—Patients can tolerate minimal easily chewed foods and cannot swallow thin liquids safely. The diet consists of thickened liquids with commercial thickener as needed, very thick juices and milk products, and decreased fiber; no coarse textures, nuts, or raw fruits or vegetables are included.
- Level III: Patients have difficulty chewing, manipulating, or swallowing foods. Patients are beginning to chew, and the diet is mechanically soft or edentulous. No tough skins,

nuts, or dry, crispy, raw, or stringy foods are included. Meats have to be minced or cut into small pieces; liquids are taken as tolerated.
- Level IV (least restricted): Persons can chew soft textures and swallow liquids safely. The diet includes soft textures that do not require grinding or chopping; no nuts or raw, crisp, or deep fried foods are included; liquids are taken as tolerated.

The postoperative diet for the gastric bypass procedure consists of the following:

- Stage 1: Clear liquids—1 ounce allowed at the beginning; continued for two to three meals
- Stage 2: Gastric bypass liquids—begun after clear liquids are tolerated; continued for 3 to 4 weeks
- Stage 3: Pureed—begun after postoperative week 4 (4-ounce meals, 6 to 8 times a day); continued for 1 to 2 weeks
- Stage 4: Soft, solids—begun after postoperative week 6; continued indefinitely

Gastric bypass liquids include nonfat milk, blenderized soups, 100% fruit juice (diluted ½ water, ½ juice), vegetable juice (e.g., V8, tomato), sugar-free Carnation Instant Breakfast powder mixed with nonfat milk, grits, oatmeal, cream of wheat, mashed potatoes (thinned down enough that it could go through a straw), nonfat sugar-free milkshakes, thinned baby food, and sugar-free drinks (e.g., sodas, tea).

> ### ✐ TAKE NOTE
>
> An order modifying a nutrient or number of calories would not change the consistency of a patient's diet.
>
> Example #1: If a patient is on a "soft diet" and the doctor writes an order for "low fat," the patient's diet would be "soft, low fat."
> Example #2: If a patient is on a "mechanical soft diet" and the doctor writes and order for "2 g Na," the patent's diet would be "mechanical soft, 2 g Na."

> **SKILLS CHALLENGE**
>
> To practice transcribing a therapeutic diet order, complete Activity 12-2 in the *Skills Practice Manual*.

TUBE FEEDINGS

Tube feeding, also called **gavage**, is the administration of liquefied nutrients into the stomach, duodenum, or jejunum through a tube inserted through the nose (a nasogastric or nasoenteral tube; Fig. 12-2) or through an opening in the abdominal wall (gastrostomy, duodenostomy, or jejunostomy; Fig. 12-3). Tube feedings are ordered for patients who have difficulty swallowing, who are unable to eat sufficient nutrients, or who cannot absorb nutrients from the foods they eat.

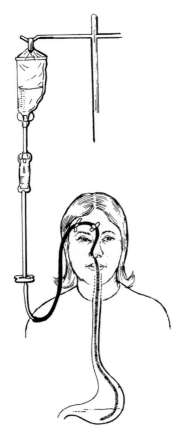

Figure 12-2 A nasogastric feeding tube. (Courtesy of Baxter Travenol Laboratories, Inc.)

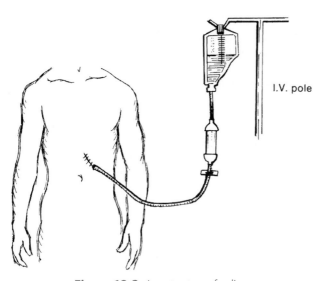

I.V. pole

Figure 12-3 A gastrostomy feeding.

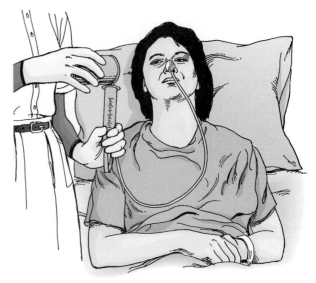

Figure 12-4 Administration of a bolus or intermittent feeding through a syringe. (From Potter PA, Perry AG: Fundamentals of Nursing, 6th ed, St. Louis, Mosby, 2005.)

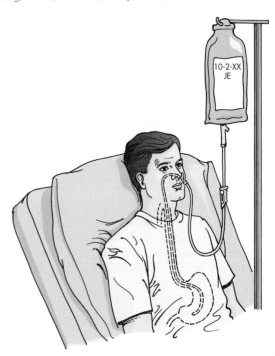

Figure 12-5 Administration of a bolus or intermittent feeding via an enteral feeding bag. (From Potter PA, Perry AG: Fundamentals of Nursing, 6th ed, St. Louis, Mosby, 2005.)

Tube feedings may be administered in a bolus, continuous, or cyclic manner:

- **Bolus** (intermittent) involves infusing 300 to 400 mL of formula over a short time (10 minutes) with a syringe (Fig. 12-4), or 300 to 400 mL every 3 to 6 hours over a 30- to 60-minute period with the use of an enteral feeding bag (Fig. 12-5).
- Continuous administration requires the use of a mechanical feeding infusion pump (called an enteral feeding pump or a **Kangaroo pump**) to control the rate of infusion (Fig. 12-6).

- With cyclic administration, feedings are infused over 8 to 16 hours during the day or night. Nighttime feedings allow greater freedom during the day. Daytime feedings are recommended for patients who have a greater chance of aspiration or tube dislodgment.

Types of nasogastric or nasoenteral tubes used for feedings include Entron, Dobbhoff, and Levin. Some of the commercially prepared formulas, including Isocal HN, Deliver 2.0, Ultracal HN Plus, Pulmocare, Jevity, Boost High Nitrogen, Boost Plus, Respalor, or Magnacal, may be ordered for tube

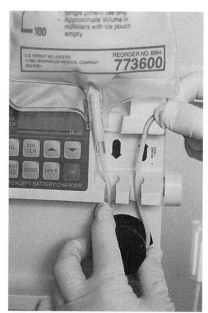

Figure 12-6 Connecting tubing through an enteral feeding pump to administer a continuous feeding by monitored drip. (From Potter PA, Perry AG: Fundamentals of Nursing, 6th ed, St. Louis, Mosby, 2005.)

feedings. To transcribe a tube feeding order, the HUC may have to order a nasogastric tube, formula, and a feeding infusion pump.

DOCTORS' ORDERS FOR TUBE FEEDING

Several types of formulas and other preparations are available to meet nutritional needs for different disease states. More than 50 medical food products are available, and changes are constantly made as new knowledge is acquired. Examples of a typical doctor's order for tube feeding are provided below.

Insert NG Feeding Tube, Verify Placement, and Begin Feeding of Isocal HN (1 cal/mL) @ FS 40 mL/hr. Progress by 10 mL/hr q2h as Tolerated to Final Rate of 90 mL/hr.
The nurse may verify tube placement by withdrawing a small amount of stomach contents or by injecting air with a syringe through the tube and listening with a stethoscope as air enters the stomach. The doctor has ordered that the prepared formula be started at full strength and the amount increased every 2 hours as tolerated to a final rate.

Tube Feeding of Boost Plus (1.5 cal/mL) FS Bolus by Syringe 45 mL q6h Given Over 20 min. Flush Tube 5 mL H₂O q2h.
The doctor is ordering the formula to be given full strength by bolus with the use of a syringe every 6 hours and to be given over 20 minutes. The nurse will flush the tube with water as ordered.

Magnacal FS @ 40 mL/hr Through Gastrostomy Tube. Insert Jejunostomy Tube. X-ray for Placement. When in Proper Position, Begin via Pump to Deliver 2.0 (2 cal/mL) @ 30 mL/hr for 8 hr, Then 40 mL/hr for 8 hr, Then Increase to Final Rate of 50 mL/hr.

> **SKILLS CHALLENGE**
>
> To practice transcribing a tube feeding order, complete Activity 12-3 in the *Skills Practice Manual*.

In this order for tube feedings, the doctor is requesting an x-ray to determine correct placement of the tube before formula is administered. ■

✓ DOCTORS' ORDERS: OTHER DIETARY ORDERS

The following orders pertain to the patient's intake of foods and liquids but are not orders for a specific type of diet.

Force Fluids
This order is probably written in addition to the patient's dietary order. The doctor wants the patient to drink more fluids. The HUC would send this order to the nutritional care department, so more fluids would be included on the patient's trays.

Limit Fluids to 1000 mL per Day
This order is also written in addition to the **diet order**. The patient's fluid intake is to be restricted to 1000 mL per day. Restriction of fluids is usually ordered for patients who are retaining fluids (a condition known as edema) because of a disease process. The nutritional care department should be notified of this order, so fluids would be limited on the patient's trays; the dietitian would also become involved.

NPO
This order means the patient is to have nothing by mouth. This is usually ordered after major surgery or during a critical illness. This information is sent to the nutritional care department to update the patient's dietary record, so a tray would not be prepared for the patient.

NPO Midnight
The patient is to have nothing by mouth after midnight. This is ordered to prepare a patient for surgery, treatment, or a diagnostic procedure. The nutritional care department is notified, so a tray would not be sent to the patient.

Sips and Chips
The patient may have only sips of water and ice chips. This order would also be sent to the nutritional care department to update the patient's dietary record.

Have Dietitian See Patient
The doctor is requesting that the dietitian discuss the diet with the patient or teach the patient about the diet. This order may require a phone call, in addition to sending a requisition to the nutritional care department.

Calorie Count Today and Tomorrow
This is usually ordered to document the quantities and types of food consumed by the patient for further nutritional evaluation by the dietitian. Send this information to the nutritional care department and notify the nurse who is caring for the patient. It may be required to prepare a form on which the patient's caloric intake will be recorded. ■

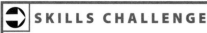

SKILLS CHALLENGE

To practice transcribing a review set of doctors' orders, complete Activity 12-4 in the *Skills Practice Manual.*
To practice recording telephone messages, complete Activity 12-5 in the *Skills Practice Manual.*

KEY CONCEPTS

Accuracy is essential in the transcription of dietary orders because an error could result in serious consequences. Imagine, for example, a patient who is NPO for surgery receiving breakfast, or a severely diabetic patient receiving a regular diet.

Hospitalized patients are dependent on hospital personnel to meet their dietary preferences and needs. The diet ordered by the doctor for the patient may be an integral part of the treatment plan, or it may be ordered to maintain health. In either case, mealtime is an important time for many patients, and for some, it may be the most positive experience of the day. The HUC is responsible for ordering late trays when a patient has missed a meal because of a test or procedure. It is important that the tray is ordered and delivered to the patient promptly. The nutritional care and nursing departments must work closely together to provide the patient with proper and pleasant meals. Thorough and prompt communication by the HUC facilitates this tremendously.

REVIEW QUESTIONS

1. Rewrite the following doctors' orders using symbols and/or abbreviations. Or, to practice writing doctors' orders, have someone read the orders while you record them. Practice using symbols and abbreviations.

a. nothing by mouth after midnight

_____

b. clear liquid breakfast, then nothing by mouth

_____

c. 1000-calorie American Diabetic Association diet

_____

d. low-cholesterol diet

_____

e. diet as tolerated

_____

f. regular diet

_____

g. low-sodium diet

_____

h. no salt added

_____

2. Define the terms listed below.

a. therapeutic, or special, diet

_____

b. regular diet

_____

c. tube feeding

_____

d. nothing by mouth

_____

3. List three methods of administering tube feedings.

a. _____

b. _____

c. _____

4. Below is a list of diets the doctor may order for the patient. Identify each diet as standard or therapeutic.

a. soft diet

_____

b. potassium-restricted diet

_____

c. 1200-cal diet

_____

d. full liquid diet

_____

e. 500-mg Na diet

_____

f. mechanical soft diet

_____

g. hypoglycemic diet

_____

h. low-triglyceride diet

_____

5. For the doctor's order "DAT," or "advance *diet as tolerated,*" list four diets that may be selected by the nurse for the patient.

a. _____

b. _____

c. _____

d. _____

6. Explain why a doctor's order for DAT requires the HUC to ask the nurse what diet to order from the nutritional care department.

_____

_____

7. List two reasons why a doctor would order the patient NPO MN.

a. _____

b. _____

8. List three commercially prepared formulas or preparations that may be ordered for tube feedings.

a. _____

b. _____

c. _____

9. List three items that may have to be ordered for a tube feeding.

a. _____

b. _____

c. _____

10. List two diets that may be requested by a patient.

a. _____

b. _____

11. Would a doctor's order for 2.5 g Na change a patient's previous order for a soft diet?

_____

12. Would a doctor's order for "limit fluids to 1200 mL/day" change a patient's previous order for a regular diet?

_____

13. Would an order for a patient to have sips and chips need to be sent to dietary?

_____

14. Why is it important to notify dietary of a patient's food allergy?

_____

_____

THINK ABOUT...

1. Discuss the possible consequences if a patient's food allergy is not communicated to the nutritional care department.
2. Discuss the importance of ordering a patient's diet as soon as possible when they return to the nursing unit after having undergone a procedure and is cleared to eat.

Medication Orders

CHAPTER OBJECTIVES

Upon completion of this chapter, you will be able to:

1. Define the terms in the vocabulary list.
2. Write the meaning of each abbreviation in the abbreviations list.
3. Recognize abbreviations that have been deemed unacceptable by the Joint Commission.
4. Explain the benefits of Computer Physician Order Entry regarding medication orders.
5. Define *standing, standing prn, stat, one-time,* and *short-series* medication orders.
6. List the five components of a medication order.

7. List four groups of drugs that usually have automatic "stop dates."
8. Name two reference books for medications.
9. List four routes by which medications are administered.
10. Demonstrate the procedure for using the *Physicians' Desk Reference* (PDR).
11. Describe the general purpose for selected drug groups.
12. Name three common skin tests performed and explain the purpose of each.
13. Recognize the most commonly used drugs, which are listed in italics in the "Drug Groups" section of the chapter, and name the drug group to which each belongs.

VOCABULARY

Admixture The result of adding a medication to a container of intravenous solution

Adverse Drug event injuries or harmful reactions that result from the use of a drug

Ampoule (Ampule) Small glass vial sealed to keep contents sterile; used for subcutaneous, intramuscular, and intravenous medications

Apothecary System Ancient system of weight and volume measurements used to measure drugs and solutions

Automatic Stop Date Date on which specific categories of medications must be discontinued unless renewed by the physician

Bolus Concentrated dose of medication or fluid, frequently given intravenously

Capsule Gelatinous, single-dose container in which a drug is enclosed to prevent the patient from tasting the drug

Central Line Catheter or Central Venous Catheter (CVC) Large catheter that provides access to the veins and/or to the heart to measure pressures

Computerized Medication Cart Storage cart that requires confidential user ID and a password to gain access to medications

Extravasation Leakage of fluid into tissue surrounding a vein

Food and Drug Administration (FDA) U.S. government agency whose purpose is to ensure that foods, drugs, cosmetics, and medical devices are safe and properly labeled

Heparin Lock (Heplock) An IV catheter with a small chamber covered with a rubber diaphragm or a specially designed cap to administer medications or to provide venous access in case of an emergency. Also called a *saline lock*

Hypnotics Drugs that reduce pain or induce sleep; can include sedatives, analgesics, and anesthetics

Infiltrate or Infiltration The process whereby a fluid passes into the tissues, such as when a local anesthetic is administered or an IV infiltrates (solution is not going into the vein, but into surrounding tissue)

Injectables Medications that are given by forcing a liquid into the body by means of a needle and syringe (intra-arterial, intradermal, intramuscular, intravenous, and subcutaneous)

Instillation To slowly introduce fluid into a cavity or a passage of the body to remain for a specific length of time before it is drained or withdrawn. (The purpose is to expose tissues of the area to the solution, to hot or cold, or to a drug or substance in the solution.)

Insufflate To blow a gas or powder into a tube, cavity, or organ to allow visual examination, to remove an obstruction, or to apply medication

Intramuscular Injection Injection of a medication into a muscle

Intravenous or Infusion Administered directly into a vein

Intravenous Hyperalimentation or Total Parenteral Nutrition Method used to administer calories, proteins, vitamins, and other nutrients into the bloodstream of a patient who is unable to eat. Must be infused into the superior vena cava through a central line catheter—not given through a peripheral IV catheter

IV Push Method of giving concentrated doses of medication directly into the vein

Lozenge Medicated tablet or disk that dissolves in the mouth

Medication Administration Record (MAR) List of medications that each individual patient is currently taking; it is used by the nurse to administer medications

Medication Nurse Registered nurse or licensed practical nurse who administers medications to patients

Metric System A system of weights and measures that is based on multiples of 10

Narcotic Controlled drug that relieves pain or produces sleep

Oral By mouth

Over-the-Counter Drugs The FDA defines OTC drugs as safe and effective for use by the general public without a doctor's prescription

Parenteral Routes Pertaining to a medication administered by a route that bypasses the gastrointestinal (GI) tract, such as a drug given by injection, intravenously, or by skin patch

Patient-Controlled Analgesia Medications administered intravenously by means of a special infusion pump controlled by the patient within order ranges written by the physician

Piggyback A method by which drugs are usually administered intravenously in 50 to 100 mL of fluid

Skin Tests Tests given to determine the reaction of the body to a substance injected intradermally or applied topically to the skin. Skin tests are used to detect allergens, to determine immunity, and to diagnose disease

Subcutaneous Injection Injection of a small amount of a medication under the skin into fatty or connective tissue

Suppository Medicated substance mixed in a solid base that melts when placed in a body opening; suppositories are commonly used in the rectum, vagina, or urethra

Suspension Fine-particle drug suspended in liquid

Tablet Solid dosage of a drug in disk form

Topical Direct application of medication to the skin, eye, ear, or other parts of the body

ABBREVIATIONS

Abbreviation	Meaning	Order Example
ac	ante cibum (before meals)	Sliding scale insulin ac
ADE	adverse drug event/s	ADEs are common and costly
amp	ampoule	Add 1 amp multi-vitamins to TPN bag q24h
ASA	acetylsalicylic acid aspirin	ASA 325 mg × 2 PO q4h prn
BCOC	bowel care of choice	BCOC as per patient request

Abbreviation	Meaning	Order Example
cap	capsule	amoxicillin 500 mg I cap q8h
CDSS	clinical decision support system(s)	CDSSs will reduce medication-related errors
dr or ℥	dram	phenobarb elixir 20 mg/5 mL ℥ PO tid
G, gm, or g	gram	cefadroxil 1 g IVPB q6h
gr	grain	chloral hydrate gr XV PO hs prn
IM	intramuscular	vitamin B_{12} 1000 mcg deep IM tomorrow
IV	intravenous	D/C IV if infiltrates
IVP	intravenous push	theophylline 5 mg/kg IVP now
IVPB	Intravenous piggyback	cephalothin 0.5 g IVPB q8h
KCl	potassium chloride	Add 40 mEq KCl to each IV
L	liter	1 L 5% D/W to run @ 125 mL/hr
LOC	laxative of choice	LOC prn constipation
mcg	microgram	vitamin B_{12} 1000 mcg IM
mEq	milliequivalent	Give 20 mEq KCl per open heart protocol
mg	milligram	ciprofloxacin 250 mg PO q12°
mL or ml	milliliter (same as cubic centimeter)	1000 mL 5% D/W @ KO rate
MOM	milk of magnesia	MOM 30 mL hs prn
noc	night	Ambien 10 mg po q noc
NTG	nitroglycerin	May leave NTG tablets @ bedside
N/V	nausea & vomiting	Compazine 10 mg IM q6h prn N/V
OTC	over the counter	The patient was not taking any OTC medications
oz	ounce	Add 8 oz of juice to Metamucil packet
pc	post cibum (after meals)	Maalox 15 mL tid pc
PCA	patient-controlled analgesia	PCA morphine sulfate 2 mg q15 min
PCN	penicillin	PCN 250 mg PO q6h
PO	per os (by mouth)	lorazepam 2 mg PO tid
pr	per rectum	bisacodyl supp 10 mg pr now
prn	pro re nata (as needed)	Maalox 30 mL prn GI discomfort
S/C, sq, or sub-q	subcutaneous	heparin 5000 unit Sub-q daily
stat	immediately	diazepam 10 mg IVP stat
subling, S/L	sublingual (under tongue)	nitroglycerin tab SL prn anginal pain
supp	suppository	acetaminophen supp prn for temp ↑ 100°(R)
syr	syrup	ipecac syr 15 mL now
tab	tablet	prednisone 25 mg PO tab bid
tinct or tr	tincture	Apply tinct of benzoin around operative site before applying tape
TPN	total parenteral nutrition	↑ TPN to 100 mL/hr
ung	unguent (ointment)	Neosporin ung tid to (R) elbow
WA	while awake	hydrocodone 5 mg PO q4h WA

See Table 10-1 for a list of incorrect and correct abbreviations, as approved by the Joint Commission (TJC). Additional abbreviations are seen in Table 13-1.

Table 13-1   Additional Abbreviations to Avoid

Abbreviation	Potential Problem	Preferred Term
IM	Because of poor writing, often misinterpreted as IV, causing the medication to be given via the wrong route	Write out "intramuscular"
D/C	Patient's medications may be prematurely discontinued when D/C means discharge and is followed by a list of medications	Write out "discontinue"
HS	May be misinterpreted as hour of sleep when written as meaning half-strength	Write out "half-strength"
IVP	When written to mean intravenous push, may be mistaken for intravenous piggyback (IVPB)	Write out "intravenous push"
S/C or S/Q	When poorly written, often mistaken for SL (sublingual)	Write out "subcutaneous"
Slash mark/	Misunderstood as the number "1" rather than the intended meaning "per"	Write out "per"

EXERCISE 1

Write the abbreviation for each term listed below.

1. liter _____

2. aspirin _____

3. immediately _____

4. capsule _____

5. tablet _____

6. milk of magnesia _____

7. adverse drug event _____

8. milligram _____

9. potassium chloride _____

10. gram _____

11. milliliter _____

12. milliequivalent _____

13. after meals _____

14. ointment _____

15. while awake _____

16. nausea and vomiting _____

17. grain _____

18. intramuscular _____

19. sublingual _____

20. tincture _____

21. by mouth _____

22. ounce _____

23. ampoule _____

24. dram _____

25. suppository _____

26. nitroglycerin _____

27. subcutaneous _____

28. microgram _____

29. night _____

30. syrup _____

31. intravenous piggyback _____

32. before meals _____

33. penicillin _____

34. per rectum _____

35. total parenteral nutrition _____

36. patient-controlled analgesia _____

37. clinical decision support system _____

38. intravenous push _____

39. laxative of choice _____

40. pro re nata (as needed) _____

41. over the counter _____

42. intravenous _____

43. bowel care of choice _____

EXERCISE 2

Write the meaning of each abbreviation listed below.

1. KCl

_____

2. ADE

_____

3. amp

_____

4. syr

_____

5. dr or ʒ

_____

6. noc

_____

7. mcg

_____

8. oz

_____

9. S/C, sq, or sub-q

_____

10. stat

_____

11. ac

_____

12. mEq

_____

13. pc

_____

14. ung

_____

15. mL

_____

16. PO

_____

17. tinct

_____

18. IM

_____

19. gr

_____

20. mg

_____

21. supp

_____

22. G, gm, or g

_____

23. CDSS

_____

24. N/V

_____

25. WA

_____

26. NTG

_____

27. ASA

_____

28. cap

_____

29. tab

_____

30. MOM

_____

31. L

_____

32. subling, S/L

_____

33. IVPB

_____

34. PCN

_____

35. TPN

_____

36. PCA

_____

37. pr

_____

38. prn

_____

39. LOC

_____

40. IVP

_____

41. OTC

_____

42. IV

_____

43. BCOC

_____

EXERCISE 3

The following is a list of medication orders typical of those that may be seen on the patient's chart. Write the meanings of the underlined abbreviations in the space provided.

1. morphine sulfate 14 mg <u>IM</u> q3h <u>prn</u> severe pain

_____

2. cephalothin 0.5 g <u>IVPB</u> q8h

_____

3. lorazepam 10 <u>mg</u> <u>PO</u> qid

_____

4. Neosporin ophthalmic 1 <u>gtt</u> in ea eye bid

_____

5. nitroglycerin 0.4 <u>mg</u> <u>subling</u> <u>prn</u> chest pain

_____

6. <u>MOM</u> 30 <u>mL</u> hs <u>prn</u> constipation

_____

7. Run <u>TPN</u> @ 120 <u>mL</u> per hr

_____

8. <u>ASA</u> 325 <u>mg</u> <u>PO</u> q4h prn for fever >101 <u>pr</u>

_____

9. Run <u>TPN</u> @ 50 <u>mL/hr</u> × 2 hr, then 125 <u>mL/hr</u>

_____

10. Check blood sugar <u>ac</u> & <u>hs</u>

_____

COMPUTER PHYSICIAN ORDER ENTRY AND CLINICAL DECISION SUPPORT SYSTEM

More than one million serious medication errors occur every year in U.S. hospitals. Two inpatient studies, one each in adults and in pediatrics, have found that about half of medication errors occur at the stage of drug ordering. **Adverse drug events (ADEs)** are injuries or harmful reactions that result from the use of a drug. It is estimated that 770,000 people are injured or die in hospitals from ADEs annually. One study of preventable inpatient ADEs in adults demonstrated that 56% occurred at the stage of ordering, 34% at administration, 6% at transcribing, and 4% at dispensing.

Medications are ordered automatically when computer physician order entry (CPOE) is implemented. The doctor enters orders directly into the computer, and they are automatically sent to the pharmacy. Eliminating handwritten orders will reduce errors of misinterpretation of medication orders caused by poor handwriting. Orders are integrated with patient information, including patient allergies, laboratory results, and prescription data. Clinical decision support systems (CDSSs) provide doctors with prompts that warn against the possibility of drug interaction, allergy, or overdose. The health unit coordinator will not have medication transcribing responsibilities but may be involved in ordering stock medications for the nursing unit. Some hospital pharmacies load stock medications into a **computerized medication cart** such as a Pyxis or an Accudose, which requires the nurse to enter a code to retrieve the medication.

✎ TAKE NOTE

Even though the health unit coordinator (HUC) does not have the responsibility of transcribing medications when CPOE is implemented, it is important to be familiar with commonly ordered medications. When a patient is discharged, the HUC may be required or asked to print the discharge instructions and medication prescriptions. If an error of omission or a discrepancy in the printouts occurs, the HUC can bring it to the nurses' attention. Knowledge of medications would be helpful in assessing the urgency when a patient calls on the intercom to request a medication by a name such as Dulcolax or oxycodone. Dulcolax would be a request for a laxative; a request for oxycodone would be a request for pain relief. Additional knowledge may be required for a future career choice or promotion.

TRANSCRIBING MEDICATION ORDERS WHEN COMPUTER PHYSICIAN ORDER ENTRY HAS NOT BEEN IMPLEMENTED

When medication orders are transcribed when CPOE has not been implemented, it is the HUC's responsibility to communicate the order to the pharmacy. This is done by faxing or sending the pharmacy copy of the doctors' orders. The pharmacist fills the medication orders by reading the copy of the original doctor's order sheet, thus reducing the possibility of an interpretation of handwriting error.

ADMINISTRATION OF MEDICATION

Medications are usually stored in medicine carts that are prepared by the pharmacy and sent to the units daily. Two types of medication carts are used. One is a **unit dose medicine cart** that contains "unit doses" in separate drawers or bins specifically labeled for each patient as ordered by the doctor(s). The pharmacist fills these orders by reading the computerized orders written by the physician, or by reading a hard or faxed copy of the physician's orders. The unit dose medication cart can be wheeled to the patient's bedside for administration of the medication (Fig. 13-1). The second type is a **computerized medication cart** that requires the nurse to enter a confidential user identification (ID) and password to unlock the cart. The nurse always verifies the name of the medication, the dose, and the patient's name before removing the medication. The computerized medication carts remain in the medication room and are not taken from room to room. Some hospitals lock IV solutions in a storage cabinet that is located next to the computerized medication cart, and both can be opened only when a nurse enters an assigned code (Fig. 13-2). All medications and/or IV solutions that are removed can be tracked on the computer by the code entered at the time of removal. When a computerized medication cart is used, the pharmacist enters the instructions for each patient's medications into the cart (usually for a 24-hour period).

When medication carts are not used, the pharmacist labels each medication with the patient's name, room number, and bed number, as well as the name, dosage, and frequency of administration, before sending to the nursing unit, where it is placed in a medicine room (med room).

A registered nurse or a licensed practical nurse who is caring for a number of specific patients will administer medications to those patients. Alternatively, a registered nurse or a licensed practical nurse may be assigned to serve as the "med nurse" and will administer medications to all patients on the nursing unit.

THE MEDICATION ADMINISTRATION RECORD

The **medication administration record (MAR)**, as described in Chapter 8, is a form on which nursing personnel record all medications given to the patient; it is a permanent part of the patient's chart (paper or electronic). Nurses use the MAR as a reference while preparing medications for administration (if medication carts are not used) and while administering medications. The nurse signs the MAR at the bottom of the form at the end of each shift to indicate that the patient received the medications as charted or did not receive any medications if none were ordered. Currently, three methods of completing MARs are used.

If an electronic medical record (EMR) is implemented in the facility, the registered or licensed practical nurse enters the medications administered into each patient's computerized MAR. The electronic MAR is a permanent part of the patient's EMR.

If the EMR is not being used, the pharmacy prepares a printed medication record for each patient, which is sent to the nursing unit each morning. The registered nurse

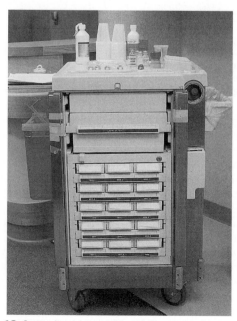

Figure 13-1 Medication cart. (From Lilley LL, Aucker RS: *Pharmacology and the nursing process*, ed 3, St. Louis, 2001, Mosby.)

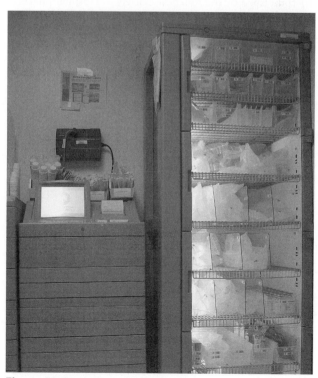

Figure 13-2 Computerized medication cart, including IV solutions.

or the HUC adds to the MAR any new medications ordered, along with any changes to medication orders made during the day. The pharmacist, after receiving the faxed physician orders, makes those changes, and the printed medication administration record sent the following morning reflects those changes. When the patient is discharged, the printed MARs become a permanent part of the patient's chart.

A handwritten MAR is used when CPOE or the printed MAR initiated by the pharmacy has not been implemented. Transcribing of medication orders may require the HUC to write the order on the MAR. In some hospitals, nurses are responsible for writing their assigned patient's medication orders on the MAR. Accuracy in copying the medication order from the physician's order sheet onto the MAR is absolutely essential. The HUC initiates the record on the patient's admission. The record varies in the number of days (3 to 10 days) that medications may be entered. When the last date of the dated period on the MAR is reached, a new record with new dates is prepared, and all medications still in use are copied onto the new form. Handwritten MARs are also a permanent part of the patient's chart. The MAR is a legal document, so entries are required to be written in ink (usually black) (Fig. 13-3). To discontinue medications on the MAR, indicate "DC" on the correct day and time, and draw a line through the days the medication will not be given. A yellow or pink highlight is usually drawn over the medication entry that is discontinued (see Fig. 13-3, A).

MEDICATION RESOURCES

Many nurses carry a personal digital assistant that may contain a nurse's drug reference, along with other electronic resource books. Reference books such as the *American Hospital Formulary* (published by the American Society of Hospital Pharmacists) or the *Physicians' Desk Reference* (PDR; published yearly by Medical Economics, Inc.) also may be kept on nursing units. Various nursing drug handbooks are frequently used on nursing units as well.

The individual hospital pharmacy frequently supplies each nursing unit with a listing of medications and dosage forms available in that particular pharmacy. The listing is the specific formulary compiled for that health care facility.

The PDR consists of different sections listed under the table of contents. Each section is printed on paper of a different color. The "Product Name" and the "Generic and Chemical Name Index" are the two sections that are most useful to the HUC.

Use of the *Physicians' Desk Reference*

The following exercises introduce use of the PDR. The instructor will assist, if necessary. It is recommended that during transcription of medication orders, the PDR or other drug resources should be used to check for spelling, drug category names, or other information that may be needed to transcribe the order accurately. (Other drug resources that may be used for this exercise include *Saunders Nursing Drug Handbook* [Saunders], *Gold Standard's Clinical Pharmacology,* and the Internet.)

EXERCISE 4

Using the PDR, in the section titled "Product Name Index," locate the following drugs in the "Product Information Section," and briefly state the purpose of each. (Read the paragraph titled "Indications and Usage" under the drug name to locate the purpose. Ignore entries listed in the "Product Identification" section. This section shows pictures of the drugs and dosages only.)

Example: Amoxil—an antibiotic

1. OxyContin

_____

2. Actos

_____

3. Paxil CR

_____

4. Coumadin

_____

5. Lipitor

_____

Using the "Generic and Chemical Names Index," locate the following and state the purpose of each.

6. ibuprofen

_____

7. levothyroxine

_____

NAMING MEDICATIONS

Most medications have several names. They are as follows:

1. *Generic name:* A generic drug is the same as a brand name drug in dosage, safety, strength, how it is taken, quality, performance, and intended use. The FDA bases evaluations of substitutability, or therapeutic equivalence, of generic drugs on scientific evaluations. By law, a generic drug product must contain identical amounts of the same active ingredients as the brand name product and must demonstrate the same effect. Generic names are not capitalized.
2. *Chemical name:* The exact designation of the chemical structure of a drug as determined by the rules of accepted systems of chemical nomenclature.
3. *Brand name, trade name, or proprietary name:* The general public often knows the drug best by this name. *The brand name is always capitalized and may have a trademark symbol* (™ *or* ®). Each company that manufactures a drug of the

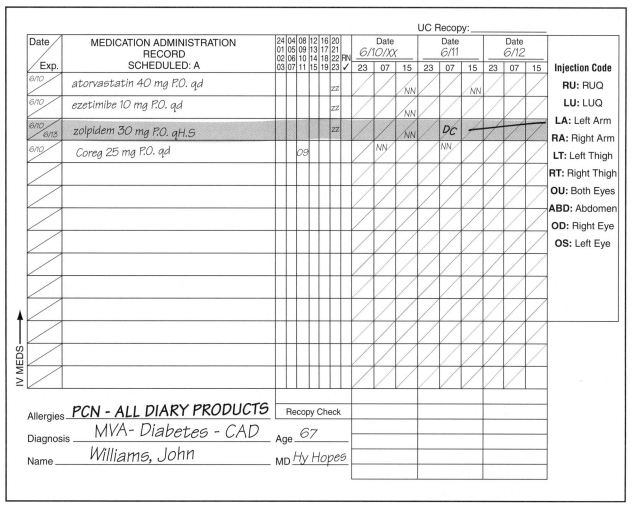

Date / Exp.	MEDICATION ADMINISTRATION RECORD SCHEDULED: A	24 01 02 03	04 05 06 07	08 09 10 11	12 13 14 15	16 17 18 19	20 21 22 23	RN ✓	Date 6/10/XX			Date 6/11			Date 6/12			Injection Code
									23	07	15	23	07	15	23	07	15	
6/10	atorvastatin 40 mg P.O. qd						zz						NN			NN		**RU:** RUQ
6/10	ezetimibe 10 mg P.O. qd						zz						NN					**LU:** LUQ
6/10 6/13	zolpidem 30 mg P.O. qH.S						zz						NN		DC			**LA:** Left Arm / **RA:** Right Arm
6/10	Coreg 25 mg P.O. qd		09							NN			NN					**LT:** Left Thigh

RT: Right Thigh
OU: Both Eyes
ABD: Abdomen
OD: Right Eye
OS: Left Eye

UC Recopy: _____

IV MEDS →

Allergies **PCN - ALL DIARY PRODUCTS**

Diagnosis MVA- Diabetes - CAD   Age 67

Name Williams, John   MD Hy Hopes

Recopy Check

PATIENT Williams, John   ALLERGIES **PCN- DAIRY PRODUCTS**

Date / Exp.	MEDICATION ADMINISTRATION RECORD PRN-ONE TIME & STAT: B	RN ✓	Date 6/10/XX			Date 6/11			Date 6/12		
			23	07	15	23	07	15	23	07	15
	temezepam; P.O. HS PRN										

PRN →

ONE-TIME ↑

Figure 13-3 A, Medication administration record (side A) shows a method of discontinuing a standing medication. **B,** Medication administration record (side B).

same chemical composition may assign it a brand name. For example, Tylenol, the brand name under which McNeil Laboratories manufactures acetaminophen (its generic name) is named Datril by Bristol Laboratories. *A drug has only one generic name but may have many trade names, depending on how many companies manufacture it.*

Some hospitals have a substitution rule. Under this rule, the pharmacist may substitute a different brand from the one that is prescribed, or the pharmacist may substitute the generic equivalent. It is good practice for the pharmacist to put an "equivalent" label on the container to decrease confusion on the nursing unit.

COMPONENTS OF A MEDICATION ORDER

Each medication order is written with specific components that include directions for the person who is giving the drug. These may be written in slightly different order, but the components remain the same.

Example:

Tylenol	325mg	PO	q4h	WA
1	2	3	4	5

The numbered portions of this drug order are:

1. Name of drug: Tylenol
2. Dose of drug (amount): 325 mg
3. Route of administration: PO (by mouth)
4. Time of administration (frequency): q4h (every 4 hours)
5. Qualifying phrase: WA (while awake)

Component 1: Name of the Drug

It is impossible to learn the names of all the drugs on the market; therefore, it may be helpful to keep a small notebook with an alphabetic index in which one can jot down the names of drugs that are encountered frequently. Periodic review will help one become more familiar with medication names.

Many medications are prepared in different forms, depending on their use (Fig. 13-4). The form is often included with the name of the drug, such as Neosporin *ointment*. For example, ointments are used on the skin or the mucous membranes of the body. Other medications may include a letter, as is shown in Components 2 and 3.

EXAMPLES OF DOCTORS' MEDICATION ORDERS THAT INDICATE A SPECIFIC FORM OF MEDICATION

- Neosporin ung ophthalmic right eye bid
Ophthalmic indicates that this ointment is to be used in the eye only.
- aspirin EC tab İ q3h prn
The *enteric-coated* (EC) aspirin dissolves only in the small intestine.
- aspirin T-R 650 mg PO q hs
Time-released (T-R) aspirin has a longer-lasting effect.
- aspirin supp 325 mg q3h for temp 101 (R)
Aspirin is contained in *suppository* (supp) form for insertion into the rectum.

COMMUNICATION AND IMPLEMENTATION OF MEDICATION ORDERS

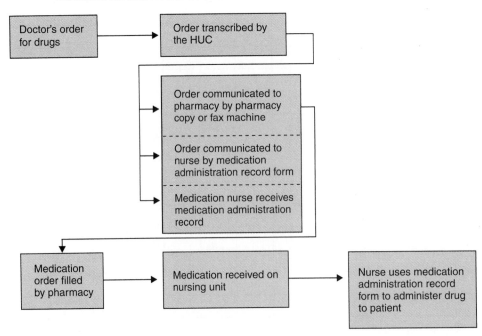

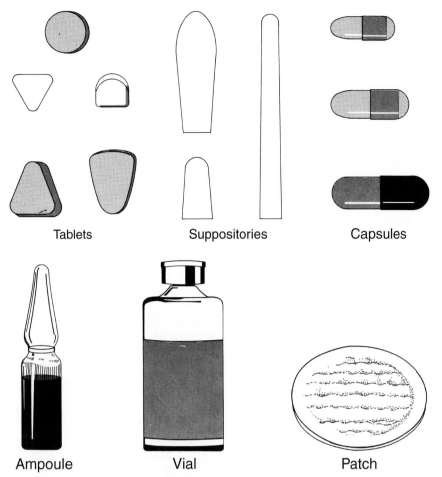

Figure 13-4 Common forms of medication.

Component 2: Dosage

The apothecary system and the metric system are the two methods of weights and measures in present-day hospital use. The metric system, which is based on multiples of 10, is the system of choice in scientific fields and is gradually replacing the apothecary system. However, until the apothecary system is completely phased out, the HUC must continue to be knowledgeable about both systems.

Apothecary System

The **apothecary system** for weighing and measuring drugs and solutions is an ancient system that was brought to the United States from England during the colonial period (see Table 10-1). Only those terms still used frequently today are listed. The terms are no longer used by many institutions because they are often mistaken for metric units.

Terms Related to Weight (Solid or Powder):
Grain (gr)
Dram (dr or ʒ)
Ounce (oz or ʒ)
Terms Related to Volume (Liquid):
Fluid dram (fl dr or ʒ)
Fluid ounce (fl oz or ʒ)

The abbreviation fl is not frequently used.

Measurements in this system are written in lowercase Roman numerals. These numerals have a line over them and may be dotted to avoid confusion with similar appearing letters or numerals. Also, the unit of measure precedes the numeral.

Examples: 1 grain—gr i̇
5 grains—gr v̄
A medication dosage that is less than 1 is written as a fraction.
Example: one-sixth grain—gr $\frac{1}{6}$.

Metric System

The **metric system** is used everywhere except in the United States. The weight, volume, and measurement units are used in hospital departments, as well as in the pharmacy. These basic units are as follows:

Weight = gram (g)
Volume = liter (L)
Length = meter (M)

Smaller and larger units in the metric system can be indicated by attaching prefixes to the basic units. This text does not cover all the prefixes used in the metric system because not all are used in doctors' orders.

To enlarge the basic unit 1000 times, the prefix *kilo* is added.

Example: kilogram (kg) = 1000 g.

To diminish the basic unit by 100, the prefix *centi* is added. The prefix *milli* diminishes the basic unit by 1000. A milligram (mg), milliliter (mL), and millimeter (mm) represent $\frac{1}{1000}$ of the basic unit. The symbol μ represents the prefix *micro*.

Example: 1 μ = 1 micrometer or 0.001 millimeter.

The terms *milliliter* (mL) and *cubic centimeter* (cc) are the same—the abbreviation "cc" is on TJC's "do not use" list.

Example: 1 L = 1000 mL.

The metric system uses the Arabic numerals that we all know—1, 2, 3, and so forth. Abbreviations are placed after the number, as in 50 mg or 500 mL.

Quantities less than 1 and fractions are written in decimal form (e.g., 0.25 mg, 1.25 mg, 1.5 g). See the Box *Conversion Information*.

Abbreviations used in medication dosages that *do not fall* within the apothecary or metric systems are as follows: gtt (drop), mEq (milliequivalent), and U (unit). *Note:* The abbreviation, U, is on the "do not use" list. Examples of their usage in doctors' orders are provided here:

Pilocarpine 1% gtts in each eye tid
Add 40 mEq KCl to each IV
Bicillin 600,000 U bid × 3 days

CONVERSION INFORMATION

Metric Conversions
Linear Measurements
    1 mm = 0.04 in
    1 in = 25.4 mm = 2.54 cm
    1 m = 39.4 in
    1 in = 0.025 m

Volume Measurements
    1 tsp = 5 mL
    1 tbsp = 15 mL
    1 fl oz = 2 tbsp = 30 mL
    8 fl oz = 240 mL
    1 liter = 1000 mL
    1 mL = 1000 microliters
    1 pint = 473 mL
    1 quart = 946 mL

Weight Measurements
    1 mg = 1000 mcg = 1,000,000 ng = 0.017 grain
    1 grain = 65 mg
    1 g = 1000 mg = 0.035 oz
    1 oz = 28.3 g
    1 kg = 1000 g = 2.2 lb
    1 lb = 0.45 kg = 454 g

Percentage Equivalents
    0.1% solution = 1 mg/mL
    1% solution = 10 mg/mL
    10% solution = 100 mg/mL

EXERCISE 5

Write the following doses in the correct form using the proper abbreviations. (Do not convert to different systems.)

1. Two grains   _____

2. Five milliliters   _____

3. Four drams   _____

4. One-half gram   _____

5. One and one-half grains   _____

6. Five hundred milligrams   _____

7. Fifteen grains   _____

8. One liter   _____

9. One thousand grams   _____

10. One-sixth grain   _____

11. One–one-hundred-fiftieth grain   _____

Component 3: Routes of Administration

Medications may be administered to patients via different routes of administration. Also, any one medication may be given by several different methods. The route of administration should always be included in a medication order; however, when in doubt, the route of administration should always be clarified. The following list contains the routes most frequently used in medication administration, with an example of each.

- Oral (mouth or PO)

The patient swallows the medication, which may be in the form of a **capsule**, pill, **tablet**, or liquid.

    Example: lorazepam 2 mg PO tid

- Sublingual

The tablet is placed under the tongue, where it is slowly absorbed.

    Example: Nitroglycerin gr $\frac{1}{150}$ subling prn anginal pain

- Inhalation

Liquid medications are most commonly administered by the respiratory care department as part of their treatment procedure.

    Examples: SVN c̄ unit dose albuterol tid
    1 PPB c̄ 3 mL saline qid

- Topical

Applied to skin or mucous membrane. Medications in this category may be available in the form of lotions, liniments, ointments, powders, sprays, solutions, suppositories, or transdermal preparations.

   a. Applied to skin

Example 1: Apply Neosporin ointment to rt leg ulcer bid.
   Example 2: Transderm-Nitro qd. (The medication is part of a flat disk that is applied to the body, usually the chest; the medication is released over a specified period.)

   b. Spraying onto skin or mucous membrane

Example 1: Spray lt ankle wound with Neosporin aerosol tid.
   Example 2: Rhinocort Aq nasal spray 1 spray ea nostril once daily.

   c. Instillation

These liquids are dropped into the eye, ear, or nose.
   Example: Instill metipranolol 0.3% 1 gtt ea eye bid.

   d. Insertions of drugs into body openings—suppositories

Example 1: prochlorperazine supp 5 mg q4h prn N/V.
   Example 2: clotrimazole vag supp 100 mg q A.M.

   • Injectable

Fluids or medications that are given by injection or intravenously (Fig 13-5).

   a. Intradermal: Injected between two skin layers. These injections are given principally for diagnostic testing.

Example: PPD intermediate today. PPD (purified protein derivative) is a tuberculin skin test order. The word "intermediate" indicates the strength of the drug.

   b. Subcutaneous (SC or SQ): The medication is injected with a syringe under the skin into the fat or connective tissue.

Example: heparin 5000 units SQ stat

   c. Intramuscular (IM): The medication is injected directly into the muscle.
   d. **Intravenous push (IV push or IVP):** A method of infusing a concentrated dose of medication over 1 to 5 minutes.
   e. Intravenous **piggyback** (IVPB): IVPB is a method of intermittent infusion of medication that has been diluted in 50 to 100 mL of a commercially prepared solution and is infused over 30 to 60 minutes through an established IV line. The medication concentration in the IVPB is lower than the medication concentration in the IV push and is administered over a longer time (Fig. 13-6).
   f. Volume control administration device: Another method of infusing IV medications through 5 to 10 mL of compatible IV fluids. The fluid is placed within a secondary fluid container separate from the primary fluid bag (see the Evolve site).

Heparin lock: A device used for intermittent intravenous infusion of medication, also used to maintain patent venous access for the infusion of medications in an emergency. A heparin lock or "hep-lock" also may be called a *saline lock* and is an IV catheter with a small chamber covered by a rubber diaphragm or a specially designed cap (see Fig. 11-12).

✎ TAKE NOTE

Between 600,000 and 1 million accidental needle sticks and sharps injuries occur annually in health care settings (American Nurses Association, 1999). The risk of exposure of health care workers to blood-borne pathogens has led to the development of "needleless devices" or special needle safety devices (Fig. 13-7). When "sharps" are used, they are placed in a "sharps disposal container" (Fig. 13-8).

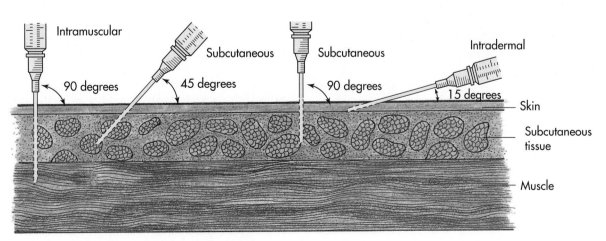

Figure 13-5 Angle of needle insertion for parenteral injections. (From Potter PA, Perry AG: *Fundamentals of nursing*, ed 6, St. Louis, 2005, Mosby.)

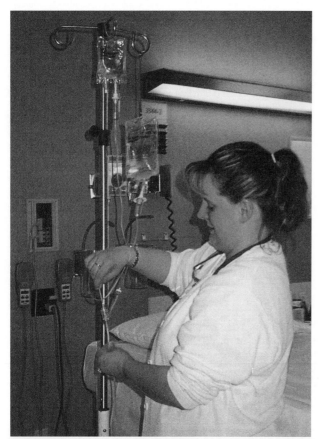

Figure 13-6 Piggyback setup. (From Potter PA, Perry AG: *Fundamentals of nursing*, ed 6, St. Louis, 2005, Mosby.)

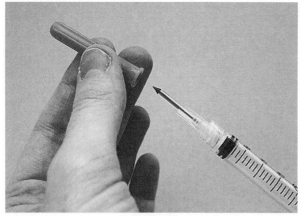

Figure 13-7 Syringe with needleless adapter. (From Potter PA, Perry AG: *Fundamentals of nursing*, ed 6, St. Louis, 2005, Mosby.)

Total Parenteral Nutrition

Total parenteral nutrition (TPN) or **intravenous hyperalimentation** is a common procedure that is used to provide nutrients to patients who are unable to receive food via the digestive tract. Nutrients, including carbohydrates, proteins, fats, water, electrolytes, vitamins, and minerals, are infused through a catheter that is placed directly into a large central vein and is advanced into the superior vena cava. The veins most often used are the jugular and the subclavian veins.

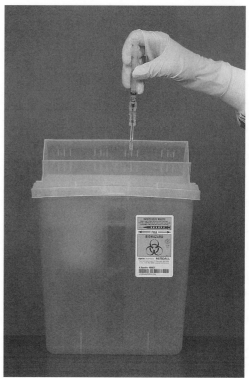

Figure 13-8 Sharps disposal using only one hand. (From Potter PA, Perry AG: *Fundamentals of nursing*, ed 6, St. Louis, 2005, Mosby.)

Some diseases that require TPN intervention are ileitis, bowel obstruction, massive burns, and severe anorexia. Patients who receive TPN require frequent (daily) blood tests for electrolyte and lipid levels (these laboratory tests are explained in Chapter 14).

TPN is usually a long-term therapy that is administered through **central venous catheters** designed for long-term use. Some common types of long-term central venous catheters are Hickman, Broviac, Groshong, and Port-A-Cath. The type of catheter used is dependent on the length of treatment. Insertion of a central catheter requires informed consent; the catheter is surgically inserted under local anesthesia and sterile conditions.

The complex composition of TPN solution requires a written doctor's order; it is prepared by the pharmacist under sterile conditions using a laminar flow hood. The solution is kept refrigerated until 30 to 40 minutes before the time of infusion. The infusion rate is controlled by an infusion pump (see Fig. 11-13). The infusion of TPN is closely monitored by the nurse because fluid overload is a serious complication for the patient who receives fluids via central venous access. Other complications that may develop include infection, phlebitis, thrombosis, electrolyte imbalance, and hyperglycemia. The nurse assesses the patient for change in status, and uses strict aseptic technique when changing dressings and when handling administration equipment and solutions.

The order for TPN is a preprinted form that is filled in by the doctor (Fig. 13-9). This form takes the place of the regular doctor's order form, and a copy is sent to the pharmacy. Because of the length and complexity of the TPN order, many hospitals transcribe only the date and TPN with rate and check the chart on the MAR. When the TPN solution is delivered from the pharmacy, the registered nurse checks it against the doctor's

ADULT TPN ORDER FORM

	Custom	Standard Central	Standard Peripheral
BASE SOLUTION			
g AA (60-120/d : 4 cal/g : 10 g/100 ml)	_____g	50 g/L	30 g/L
g Dextrose (200-700/d : 3.4 cal/g : 70 g/100 ml)	_____g	200 g/L	75 g/L
g Lipid (0-100/d : 9 cal/g : 20 g/100 ml)	_____g		40 g/L
ADDITIVES			
meq NaCl (60-150/d)	_____/bag	35/L or ____/L	35/L or ____/L
meq NaAcetate	_____/bag	_____/L	_____/L
meq KCl (30-100/d)	_____/bag	_____/L	_____/L
meq KAcetate	_____/bag	20/L or ____/L	20/L or ____/L
meq KPO4 (15-40/d)	_____/bag	15/L or ____/L	15/L or ____/L
meq NaPO4	_____/bag	_____/L	_____/L
meq CaGluconate (9-18/d)	_____/bag	4.5/L or ____/L	4.5/L or ____/L
meq MgSO4 (5-15/d)	_____/bag	5/L or ____/L	5/L or ____/L
mg ZnSO4	_____/bag	_____/L	_____/L
Multivitamin-12	_____/bag	Standard	Standard
Trace Elements (Zn, Cu, Mn, Cr)	_____/bag	Standard	Standard
Human Insulin R	_____/bag	_____/L	_____/L
Other: _____	_____	_____/L	_____/L
Other: _____	_____	_____/L	_____/L
Other: _____	_____	_____/L	_____/L
FINAL VOLUME to be infused over 24 hours	_____	_____	_____
RATE ml/hr	_____	_____	_____

_____ ml Iron Dextran/wk (0.5 ml = 25 mg Fe+ + q wk; incompatible with lipid-containing solutions. Lipids will be omitted from solution on the day iron is administered.)
_____ mg Vitamin K/wk (5 mg q wk)

IVPB Lipids _____ ml _____% Lipid q _____ . Run over _____ hrs.

LABORATORY
Daily: _____ Electrolytes _____ BUN _____ Creat _____ Glucose _____ CBC
Q Mon & Thurs: _____ SMA-20 _____Mg+ + _____ CBC
Q Week: _____ Protime _____Platelets
Other: _____
Other: _____
Other: _____

_____ Fingerstick glucose q _____ hrs.   Weight q _____

SLIDING SCALE:
Glucose	Sub Q Human Insulin R
Less than 80 mg%	Call M.D.
80 - 150 mg%	_____ units
151 - 200 mg%	_____ units
201 - 250 mg%	_____ units
251 - 300 mg%	_____ units
301 - 350 mg%	_____ units
Greater than 350 mg%	Call M.D.

Sign. _____

Date _____ Time _____

Phone or pager _____

IV Pharmacy Phone: X4557

ADULT TPN ORDER FORM

Figure 13-9 Total parenteral nutrition order form.

Table 13-2 Medication Time Schedule

Time Symbols	Meaning	Time Schedule	Military Time
qd	Once a day	9:00 A.M.	0900
		(5:00 P.M. [daily] for antico-agulants—to allow for results of prothrombin time)	1700
		(7:30 A.M. [daily] for insulin, which must be administered before breakfast)	0730
bid	Two times a day during waking hours	9:00 A.M. and 5:00 P.M. (9-5)	0900-1700
tid	Three times a day during waking hours	9:00 A.M.-1:00 P.M.-5:00 P.M. (9-1-5)	0900-1300-1700
qid	Four times a day during waking hours	9:00 A.M.-1:00 P.M.-5:00 P.M.-9:00 P.M. (9-1-5-9)	0900-1300-1700-2100
ac	One-half hour before meals. This varies according to when food cart arrives on unit.		
pc	One-half hour after meals. This varies according to when food cart arrives on unit.		
q3h	Every 3 hours	9:00 A.M.-12:00 Noon-3:00 P.M.-6:00 P.M.-9:00 P.M.-12:00 Mid-3:00 A.M.-6:00 A.M. (9-12-3-6-9-12-3-6)	0900-1200-1500-1800-2100-2400-0300-0600
q4h	Every 4 hours	9:00 A.M.-1:00 P.M.-5:00 P.M.-9:00 P.M.-1:00 A.M.-5:00 A.M. (9-1-5-9-1-5)	0900-1300-1700-2100-0100-0500
q6h	Every 6 hours	9:00 A.M.-3:00 P.M.-9:00 P.M.-3:00 A.M. (9-3-9-3)	0900-1500 2100-0300
q8h	Every 8 hours	9:00 A.M.-5:00 P.M.-1:00 A.M. (9-5-1)	0900-1700-0100
q12h	Every 12 hours	9:00 A.M.-9:00 P.M. (9-9)	0900-2100

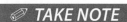

TAKE NOTE

Any change in the TPN order must be immediately sent to the pharmacy. The TPN solution is very expensive and is wasted if any change is ordered in the formula after it has been prepared.

order on the preprinted form. Many times, the doctor uses the regular doctor's order form to make small changes in the composition of the original order. The original order on the MAR must be discontinued and the changed order rewritten.

Peripheral Parenteral Nutrition

Peripheral parenteral nutrition (PPN) is one route of administration for nutrition provided as short-term therapy that usually lasts for less than 2 weeks. PPN is used for patients who need temporary nutritional supplements and who can tolerate a higher fluid infusion amount. The dextrose or sugar content of the formula is lower than in the TPN that is given through a central line. PPN is administered via a peripheral catheter that is inserted into a large vein in the arm. The worst adverse effect of PPN is phlebitis, which is severe inflammation of the vein.

Component 4: Frequency of Administration

Each hospital maintains a schedule of hours for administration of medications. These schedules are set up by the hospital nursing service, and it is important to learn the hours that are standard in the facility.

Table 13-2 lists examples of time frequencies used to administer medication, but these may vary among hospitals. Also, military time usually is used in place of standard time.

Note: Standard prn orders are never assigned a time because the drugs are administered as they are needed by the patient.

Component 5: Qualifying Phrases

At times, the doctor may wish to order administration of a drug only for specific conditions. A phrase to this effect may be included as the fifth part of the medication order. Not all orders contain qualifying phrases, but when included, they are an important part of the order. Some phrases commonly used are listed here:

- For severe pain
- For stomach spasms
- For N/V
- While awake
- For insomnia

Examples of Doctors' Orders With a Qualifying Phrase:
- hydromorphone 2 mg IM q4h prn <u>severe pain</u>
- ondansetron 4 mg PO <u>30 min before chemotherapy</u>
- may give Maalox 30 mL <u>for upset stomach</u>

EXERCISE 6

It is necessary for the HUC to identify the parts of a medication order quickly so as to recognize whether the order is complete, and to transcribe it correctly. The following exercise provides practice for this task.

Following the example below and using the numbers provided to indicate each part of a medication order, complete the following exercise.

Example:

Codeine	30 mg	PO	q4h prn	for severe pain
1	2	3	4	5

1. List the five parts of a medication order in consecutive order as used in the example above.
   a. _____
   b. _____
   c. _____
   d. _____
   e. _____

2. Identify each component of the medication orders below by writing the number of the component below the component part, as shown in the preceding example.

   a. prochlorperazine 5 mg suppository pr stat
   b. hydroxyzine 25 mg IM q6h prn anxiety
   c. levofloxacin 500 mg IV q day
   d. zolpidem 5 mg PO hs prn
   e. loperamide hydrochloride 2 mg PO after each unformed stool
   f. oxycodone 15 mg tab PO q4h prn severe pain
   g. Lente Insulin 25 units sq q day
   h. amoxicillin 500 mg PO q8h
   i. warfarin sodium 3 mg PO q day
   j. benazepril 20 mg PO q day

EXERCISE 7

Test knowledge of material covered thus far by completing the following exercise. A list of doctors' orders is provided for medications written, as they would be spoken. Rewrite the orders as they would be written, using abbreviations where needed (keep in mind abbreviations that are not allowed), and use the correct form for the apothecary and metric systems.

Example: morphine sulfate eight milligrams intramuscularly every four hours whenever necessary for severe pain

Answer: morphine sulfate 8 mg IM q4h prn severe pain

1. Tylenol five hundred milligrams every four hours by mouth for pain

   _____

2. ciprofloxacin hydrochloride four hundred milligrams intravenously every twelve hours

   _____

3. doxycycline two hundred milligrams by mouth now, then one hundred milligrams at bedtime, then one hundred milligrams twice a day for three days

   _____

4. Donnatal elixir five milliliters by mouth three times a day before meals

   _____

5. Timoptic ophthalmic 0.25% solution drops two in right eye twice a day

   _____

6. Benadryl fifty milligrams intramuscularly immediately

   _____

7. Coreg twenty-five milligrams one tablet by mouth in the morning and at bedtime

   _____

8. Coumadin five milligrams by mouth daily

   _____

THE FIVE RIGHTS OF MEDICATION ADMINISTRATION

It is vital that the HUC is accurate when reading and transcribing medication orders. Use the five rights listed below as a guide when transcribing medications.

1. *Right Drug:* It is important that close attention be paid to the drug order when one is transcribing medications. Many drugs have similar names and spellings.
2. *Right Dose:* Once again, accuracy in transcribing the medication dose is vital to patient safety.
3. *Right Time:* Pay special attention to stat or one-time orders, and let the nurse know if a stat or now medication is ordered.
4. *Right Route:* Never assume the route for a medication; always check if the order is not clear.
5. *Right Patient:* It is critical that medication orders are transcribed on the correct patient's chart or MAR. Always double-check the name on the chart when transcribing medication orders. If an error is made, make the correction immediately and notify the nurse of the correction.

CATEGORIES OF DOCTORS' ORDERS RELATED TO MEDICATION ORDERS

Categories of doctors' orders are especially relevant to medication orders. For example, a standing medication order must have times assigned on the MAR or medication Kardex form, whereas the standing prn order does not have times assigned. To review, read "Categories of Doctors' Orders," Chapter 9, then read and complete the following unit.

Standing Orders

Fill in the definition below.

A standing order is _____.

Examples of Standing Medication Orders

Humalog Insulin units 40 q day

This medication is administered one time each day, such as 0800, until discontinued.

penicillin VK 500,000 units IM q6h

This medication is administered every 6 hours, such as 0900, 1500, 2100, 0300, until discontinued.

hydroxocobalamin 1000 mcg IM twice a week

This medication is to be administered twice a week, such as on Monday and Thursday at 0900, until discontinued.

 SKILLS CHALLENGE

To practice transcribing standing medication orders, complete Activity 13-1 in the *Skills Practice Manual*.

Standing prn Orders

Fill in the definition below.

A prn order is _____.

Examples of Standing prn Orders

morphine sulfate 10 mg IM q4h prn severe pain

The morphine sulfate may not be given to the patient more often than every 4 hours and then only if needed. In a prn order, it is impossible to set up a time sequence.

MOM 30 mL hs prn constipation

Milk of magnesia, a laxative, is given as needed, usually when the patient communicates to the nurse that they are constipated. This order is in effect until discontinued by the doctor. Laxatives are usually administered at bedtime.

lorazepam 0.5 mg po @ hs prn for insomnia due to anxiety

Lorazepam may not be given other than at bedtime, and only if the patient exhibits an inability to sleep because of anxiety.

 SKILLS CHALLENGE

To practice transcribing standing medication orders, complete Activity 13-2 in the *Skills Practice Manual*.

One-Time or Short-Series Orders

Fill in the definition below.

A one-time or short-series order is _____.

Examples of One-Time or Short-Series Order Medication Orders

ciprofloxacin hydrochloride 400 mg IV @ 6 P.M. today and at 6 A.M. tomorrow

This medication is given at the two times ordered and then is discontinued.

prochlorperazine 10 mg IM to be given 1 hr before therapy tomorrow

This medication is to be administered 1 hour before the patient is sent for therapy tomorrow, and then the order is discontinued.

Give bisacodyl supp tonight

This medication is to be administered on the evening the order was written; then it is discontinued.

 SKILLS CHALLENGE

To practice transcribing one-time medication orders, complete Activity 13-3 in the *Skills Practice Manual*. To practice transcribing short-series order medication orders, complete Activity 13-4.

Stat Orders

Fill in the definition below.

A stat order is _____.

Examples of Stat Orders

heparin 20,000 units IV push stat

This order indicates that the heparin should be given immediately. The order then is to be discontinued.

tetracycline hydrochloride 500 mg PO now and then q6h

This medication order consists of two parts. The first part calls for the antibiotic tetracycline hydrochloride to be given immediately. Part 2 of this order contains a standing order for the medication to be given four times a day, such as 0900, 1500, 2100, and 0300. The standing order remains in effect until the doctor discontinues it.

Communication of Stat Medication Orders

The medication must be ordered immediately from the pharmacy via phone, fax, or pharmacy copy. Immediately communicate the medication order to the nurse verbally. The nurse who is giving the medication then must review the order directly from the doctor's order sheet.

 SKILLS CHALLENGE

To practice transcribing and communicating stat medication orders, complete Activity 13-5 in the *Skills Practice Manual*.

CONTROLLED SUBSTANCES

In 1971, the Controlled Substances Act updated previous laws that regulated the manufacture, sale, and dispensing of **narcotics** and drugs with the potential for abuse. These drugs are referred to as *controlled drugs* or *controlled substances*. Controlled substances are divided into five classes, or schedules. Each of these classes differs according to its potential for abuse; therefore, each is controlled to a different degree. The U.S. Attorney General has the authority to reschedule the class in which a drug is placed, remove a substance from the controlled list, or assign an unscheduled drug to a controlled category. Therefore, the drugs in particular classes are subject to change. Examples of scheduled drugs follow.

Schedule I

This group has such a high potential for abuse that the drugs usually are nonexistent in a health care setting except for specific, approved research. Examples are heroin, marijuana, lysergic acid diethylamide (LSD), peyote, mescaline, psilocybin, methaqualone, dihydromorphine, and others.

Schedule II

This group has a high potential for abuse, and use may lead to severe physical or psychological dependence. A written prescription signed by the physician is required for Schedule II drugs. In an emergency situation, oral prescriptions for limited quantities may be filled; however, the physician must provide a signed prescription within 72 hours. Prescriptions cannot be refilled. Examples include morphine, codeine, hydromorphone, methadone, meperidine, cocaine, oxycodone, fentanyl, etorphine hydrochloride, anileridine, and oxymorphone. Also in Schedule II are amphetamines and methamphetamines, phenmetrazine, methylphenidate, glutethimide, amobarbital, pentobarbital, secobarbital, and phencyclidine.

Schedule III

This group has less of an abuse potential than is seen in Schedules I and II and includes compounds that contain limited quantities of certain narcotic drugs and non-narcotic drugs such as derivatives of barbituric acid, except those listed in another schedule, methyprylon, nalorphine, benzphetamine, chlorphentermine, clortermine, phendimetrazine, anabolic steroids, and paregoric. Any suppository dosage form that contains amobarbital, secobarbital, or pentobarbital is included in this schedule.

Schedule IV

The controlled substances in this schedule have less of an abuse potential than is seen in agents listed in Schedule III; included are such drugs as barbital, phenobarbital, mephobarbital, chloral hydrate, ethchlorvynol, ethinamate, meprobamate, paraldehyde, methohexital, fenfluramine, diethylpropion, phentermine, chlordiazepoxide, diazepam, oxazepam, clorazepate, flurazepam, clonazepam, prazepam, lorazepam, alprazolam, halazepam, triazolam, mebutamate, dextropropoxyphene, and pentazocine.

Schedule V

The controlled substances in this schedule have less of an abuse potential than those listed in Schedule IV and consist of preparations that contain limited quantities of certain narcotic drugs, generally given for antitussive and antidiarrheal purposes.

As dispensers of controlled substances for medicinal purposes, hospital pharmacies are required to be registered with the Drug Enforcement Administration, which mandates that records be maintained on certain drugs (see the Evolve site).

Controlled drugs must be kept in a double-locked cupboard, a medication cart, or a computerized medication-dispensing system on the nursing unit. This is necessary because of the potential for theft and because the law requires it. A nurse carries the key to the locked cupboard or medication cart. If the medications are kept in a computerized medication system, an ID number and password and/or fingerprint identification may be required to access the medication drawers.

Each time a medication from the locked cupboard or cart is given, the nurse who administers the medication is responsible for writing the required information on the disposition sheet. Each drug and each dosage of the drug requires the use of a separate disposition sheet. When the disposition sheet is completed, it is returned to the pharmacy. If a computerized system is used, the nurse must verify the count of the medications left in the drawer after the drug has been removed. The count then is maintained on a computerized log.

Replacement of drugs in the cupboard or cart is usually performed under the direction and supervision of pharmacy personnel, who deliver the drugs in person to the nursing unit and in return receive a signed delivery slip from the nurse who accepts the drugs. The computerized cart keeps track of the number of medications given, to whom they were given, and the name of the nurse who removed the drug.

The computerized medicine cart allows controlled, regularly scheduled, and prn medications to be computer dispensed. Each nurse has a password that allows access to the system. The nurse must input the patient's name and the drug name, along with the dosage. The patient's medical record number also may be used. Dispensing medication by the computer method significantly decreases medication errors because the system will not dispense the drug if there is a discrepancy between the patient's orders and the drug requisitioned by the nurse.

Two advantages of using the computer-dispensing method are a decreased number of errors in medication administration and increased accuracy in accounting and billing procedures. One disadvantage of the computerized system is that all new and changed medication orders written after the system has been loaded will have to be handled in the regular fashion. The computer system works best on nursing units where changes in orders are infrequent.

Medications that fall into the category of controlled drugs have an automatic stop date. An automatic stop date means that after a certain period, for example, 72 hours, the drug may no longer be given to the patient unless it is renewed by a written order. Controlled substances usually have a 72-hour limit. Each health care facility develops its own list of drugs that have automatic stop dates.

Although other types of drugs are included under the heading "controlled substances," narcotics and hypnotics are the most frequently used.

DRUG GROUPS

Drugs are categorized into specific groups according to their primary function or use. Many drugs have more than one function or use, so they may be included on more than one list. Physicians may order drugs by their brand name or their generic name. Generic drugs frequently are ordered because they are less costly. Short lists of commonly ordered medications from several drug categories are listed here by their generic names, with brand names in parentheses. Many more drug groups are available than can be addressed in this brief introduction to drug categories. The following identifies the major groups of drugs and provides a brief description of each. Drugs listed are a few of the most commonly prescribed drugs. A list of the 200 most commonly prescribed drugs may be found on the Evolve website. Recognition of the drugs that have asterisks next to them (a total list is included on the Evolve website) is required to meet Chapter Objective #13. Drugs have one generic name and may have several brand names. Generic names for drugs are not capitalized, and brand names (appearing in parenthesis) are capitalized.

Drugs That Affect the Nervous System

Analgesics, Narcotic, and Analgesics, Non-Narcotic

Narcotics or opioid analgesics and non-narcotic analgesics are drugs that are ordered to relieve pain; they also may be called *painkillers*. Narcotic analgesics usually are ordered to relieve moderate to severe pain, have an automatic stop date, and commonly are administered orally, intramuscularly, or intravenously.

Examples of Narcotic Analgesics and Non-Narcotic Analgesics:

Examples of Analgesics, Narcotic	Examples of Analgesics, Non-Narcotic
*acetaminophen with codeine (Tylenol 1, 2, 3, or 4)	*acetaminophen (Tylenol)
acetaminophen with propoxyphene-N (Darvocet N)	*acetylsalicylic acid—aspirin (Ascriptin)
*codeine (Contin) hydrocodone with acetaminophen (Lortab, Vicodin)	flurbiprofen (Ansaid)
*meperidine (Demerol)	*ibuprofen (Advil, Motrin)
	naproxen (Anaprox, Naproxen)
*morphine sulfate (Roxanol)	
*oxycodone (OxyFAST, OxyContin)	

Patient-Controlled Analgesia

Patient-controlled analgesia (PCA) allows the patient to self-administer small doses of narcotics intravenously. A special IV infusion pump is used. The physician orders the number of individual doses, the frequency of delivery, and the total dose permitted within certain time periods called *lockout intervals*. The nurse receives the narcotic from the pharmacy in a syringe form or in a small cassette that fits into the PCA (Fig. 13-10).

✎ TAKE NOTE

Numbers that are assigned to analgesics that contain codeine differentiate the amount of codeine found in the medications. The numbers represent the following:
  #1 contains gr $\frac{1}{8}$ (8 mg) codeine
  #2 contains gr $\frac{1}{4}$ (15 mg) codeine
  #3 contains gr $\frac{1}{2}$ (30 mg) codeine
  #4 contains gr 1 (60 mg) codeine

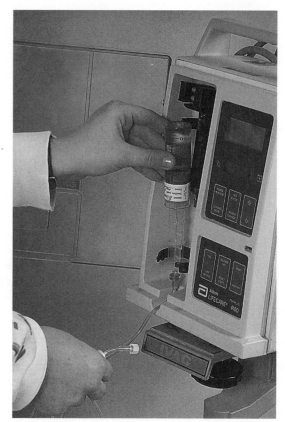

Figure 13-10 Patient-controlled analgesia (PCA) pump with syringe chamber. (From Potter PA, Perry AG: *Fundamentals of nursing,* ed 6, St. Louis, 2005, Mosby.)

An internal system within the PCA unit is programmed and does not permit the patient to overdose or self-administer the medication too frequently. The most common narcotics used in PCA systems are meperidine and morphine. Some conditions associated with patients who use a PCA include severe postoperative pain and the chronic pain of a terminal illness.

Sedatives and Hypnotics

Sedatives are drugs that cause relaxation and reduce restlessness without causing sleep. A sedative given in higher doses also may be called a hypnotic. A **hypnotic** is stronger than a sedative and is commonly used to induce sleep. Drugs also may be classified as sedative-hypnotics, and most have automatic stop dates. Adverse effects of these drugs include dizziness and excessive tiredness, so patients must be closely watched after sedatives and hypnotics are administered.

Examples of Sedative-Hypnotics:
  estazolam (Prosom)
  *flurazepam (Dalmane)
  *temazepam (Restoril)
  *zolpidem (Ambien)

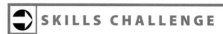

SKILLS CHALLENGE

To practice transcribing orders for medications with automatic stop dates, go to Activity 13-6 in the *Skills Practice Manual.*

Psychotherapeutic Drugs

Psychotherapeutic drugs are used to treat anxiety, depression, emotional disorders, and mental illnesses. Drugs included in this broad category are among the most commonly prescribed medications in the United States.

Examples of Psychotherapeutic Drugs:

Examples of Antianxiety Medications	**Examples of Anti-depression Medications**
*alprazolam (Xanax)	amitriptyline (Elavil)
*diazepam (Valium)	citalopram (Celexa)
*lorazepam (Ativan)	fluoxetine (Prozac)
	sertraline (Zoloft)

> ✎ **TAKE NOTE**
>
> Drugs that are used to treat patients with emotional and mental disorders vary according to the diagnosis. The patient may have to try several to find the one that works best for a specific condition.

Anticonvulsants

Anticonvulsants are drugs that prevent or relieve convulsions caused by epilepsy or other disorders.

Examples of Anticonvulsants:

clonazepam (Klonopin)	*phenobarbital (Luminal)
divalproex (Depakote)	*phenytoin (Dilantin)
*gabapentin (Neurontin)	

Drugs That Affect the Respiratory System

Drugs affect the respiratory system by assisting in drying secretions (**antihistamines**), relieving nasal stuffiness (**decongestants**), decreasing the cough reflex (**antitussives**), or assisting with increasing the flow of fluid in the respiratory tract, enabling secretions to be removed by the cough reflex (**expectorants**). Specific drugs given orally, via the IV route, or by inhalation are **bronchodilators** and are used to treat asthma and related conditions. Nasal decongestants can be administered orally, through an inhaler, or topically.

Examples of Respiratory Drugs:

Examples of Antihistamines	**Examples of Nasal Spray Decongestants**
cetirizine (Zyrtec)	budesonide (Rhinocort AQ)
*desloratadine (Clarinex)	fluticasone (Flonase)
*fexofenadine (Allegra)	oxymetazoline (Afrin)
loratadine	triamcinolone acetonide (Nasacort AQ)

Examples of Antitussive Drugs Non-Narcotic Form	**Examples of Drugs Used to in Treat Asthma and Related Conditions**
benzonatate (Tessalon Perles)	*albuterol (Proventil, Ventolin)
guaifenesin (Benylin E, Robitussin)	*aminophylline
	*fluticasone; salmeterol (Advair)
	montelukast (Singulair)
	methylprednisolone (Solu-Medrol)
	*theophylline (SloBid, Theo-Dur)

> ✎ **TAKE NOTE**
>
> Antitussives may or may not include a narcotic or an opiod.
> Codeine frequently is added to antitussive formulas, making them narcotic antitussive drugs, available by prescription only.

Drugs That Treat Infections

A huge category of medications is used to treat a variety of infections; these include antibiotic, antifungal, and antiviral drugs. **Antibiotics** are commonly prescribed for bacterial infection. For the doctor to order the "right drug for the right bug," to give the patient the best treatment possible, a culture of the wound is obtained, or blood cultures often are drawn before antibiotic therapy is initiated. Many different classifications and combinations of antibiotics are available; penicillin is the oldest form of antibiotic. Antibiotics usually have automatic stop dates. (*Note:* Many antibiotic names end in -*cillin*, -*oxacin*, or -*mycin*; this makes identification easier.)

Examples of Antibiotics:

*amoxicillin (Amoxil, Polymox)	*doxycycline (Vibramycin)
*azithromycin (Zithromax)	*erythromycin base (E-Mycin, Erythrotab)
cephalexin (Keftab)	levofloxacin (EES, Levaquin)
*ciprofloxacin (Cipro, Ciloxan)	*penicillin VK (Apo-Pen K, Pen Vee K)
*clindamycin (Cleocin, HCL, Dalacin)	tetracycline (Pontocaine)

Antifungals are drugs that are used to treat fungal infections. They are administered topically, orally, or through an intravenous piggyback (IVPB). Antifungals also are commonly used topically to treat oral fungal infections and vaginally to treat vaginal candidiasis.

Examples of Antifungals:
amphotericin B (Amphotec, Fungizone)
fluconazole (Diflucan)
nystatin (Mycostatin, Nilstat)

Antivirals are used to treat viral infections. Viral infections are difficult to treat because by the time viral symptoms begin to appear, the virus has completed the replication process in the body. Antiviral drugs are effective only during the replication stage of the viral illness, so by the time the person knows that they are ill, it is often too late for the drugs to be effective. Antiviral drugs may be prescribed orally, intravenously, or as a nasal spray. Many new antiviral drugs are being tested to fight diseases such as acquired immunodeficiency syndrome (AIDS), human immunodeficiency virus (HIV), influenza A, cytomegalovirus (CMV), herpes simplex, and respiratory syncytial virus (RSV).

Examples of Antivirals:
acyclovir (Zovirax)
ribavirin (Virazole)
zidovudine (Relenza)

Drugs That Affect the Endocrine System

Drugs Used to Treat Diabetes: Antidiabetics

Antidiabetics are given to lower blood sugar and are ordered for the diabetic or hyperglycemic patient.

Standing Order for Insulin. A standing order for insulin once a day states that it is scheduled to be given ½ hr ac breakfast. Also, if the doctor is normalizing the amount of insulin required by the patient, the doctor may order insulin to be given on a sliding scale.

Sliding Scale Insulin Orders. The amount of sliding scale insulin that is given is dependent on results obtained through blood glucose monitoring. This insulin may be given in addition to the daily insulin as ordered and prescribed by the doctor.

Example:
Sliding scale order (using bedside blood glucose monitoring)

Blood Sugar Level	Dosage or Action
200-249	5 U regular insulin
250-299	10 U regular insulin
300-349	15 U regular insulin
>350	Call the doctor

Not all diabetic patients have sliding scale orders or take insulin. Many diabetic patients control their illness through diet and exercise or use an oral medication to assist in controlling their blood glucose levels.

Examples of Diabetes Drugs:

Examples of Oral Antidiabetic Drugs	Examples of Subcutaneous Insulin
glimepiride (Amaryl)	insulin aspart (Novolog)
glipizide (Glucotrol)	*insulin glargine (Lantus)
*metformin (Glucophage)	*insulin lispro (Humalog)
*pioglitazone (Actos)	*NPH (Pork NPH Iletin II, Humulin N, Novolin N)
	*regular insulin

Hormones

Hormones are medications that replace or regulate glandular secretions from glands such as the thyroid, pituitary, and adrenals, and the male and female sexual organs. When these medications are ordered, the patient will be closely watched, and the medication dosages may have to be changed several times until the right level is found for each patient. Laboratory tests also are done to determine blood levels.

Examples of Hormone Medications:
estrogen (Premarin)
hydrocortisone (Cortef)
levothyroxine (Levoxyl, Synthroid)
medroxyprogesterone (Depo-Provera, Provera)
testosterone (Andronaq, Histerone)

Drugs That Affect the Cardiovascular System

This is another large category of drugs that affect the heart and the vascular system in various ways. Many of these drugs also have effects on the kidneys or renal system. Subcategories of drugs in this section include antiarrhythmic agents, antianginal drugs, antihypertensive medications, diuretic drugs, potassium replacements, anticoagulant agents, antilipidemic agents, and other medications that affect the cardiovascular system.

Antiarrhythmic Agents

Antiarrhythmic medications correct abnormal cardiac beats by several functions. This group of drugs is divided into classes that are identified by how they affect the cardiac cells. These drugs may be called cardiotonics, beta blockers, or calcium channel blockers, depending on which drugs are ordered.

Examples of Antiarrhythmics:

*digoxin (Lanoxin)	esmolol (Brevibloc)
*diltiazem (Cardizem)	lidocaine (Xylocaine, Zilactin)
disopyramide (Norpace, Rythmodan)	propranolol (Inderal)

Vasopressors

Vasopressors are medications that are given to treat shock, low blood pressure, and other related conditions. Vasopressors cause constriction of the smooth muscle of arteries and arterioles, which increases resistance to the flow of blood and thus elevates blood pressure.

Examples of Vasopressors:
dopamine (Intropin)
norepinephrine (Levophed)

Antianginal Agents

The heart must pump blood to all organs and tissues of the body, 24 hours a day, 7 days a week—an enormous job! Antianginal drugs are medications that are used to treat pain that results when the heart muscle does not get enough oxygen and nutrients to meet this demand. When enough blood does not reach the heart muscle (myocardium), the chest pain that results from this is called *angina pectoris.* Lack of blood supply to the heart, which is called *ischemic heart disease,* is one of the primary causes of death in the United States.

Antianginal drugs include three primary categories of medications: nitrates or nitrites, beta blockers, and calcium channel blockers. These are commonly listed as antiarrhythmics and antianginals because of the effects that they have on the heart.

Examples of Antianginal Drugs in the Nitrate Category:
isosorbide (Isordil, Sorbitrate)
nitroglycerin (Nitro-Bid, Nitro-Dur, Nitrostat, Transderm-Nitro)

It is common to see an order for "Nitroglycerin tabs to be left at bedside." If a patient begins to experience chest pain, the nurse then has the medication right at the bedside for the patient to place under the tongue.

Examples of Other Antianginal Medications:

*atenolol (Tenormin)	nifedipine (Procardia)
*diltiazem (Cardizem)	nitroglycerin (Nitro-Bid, Nitro-Dur, Nitrostat, Transderm-Nitro)
*metoprolol (Lopressor)	*propranolol (Inderal)

TAKE NOTE

Antiarrhythmics that may be ordered *stat* for a patient in a cardiac emergency include amiodarone, bretylium, and, possibly, lidocaine. These would be transcribed as a stat, one-time order, or they might be included under the emergency standing orders for the patient. An example of this type of order follows:

amiodarone 300 mg IV push now. May repeat once at 150 mg in 3-5 min.

Antihypertensive Agents

Antihypertensive drugs are medications that are used to lower high blood pressure. It is not uncommon for patients to try several antihypertensive medications or combinations of various antihypertensives before they find what works best for them. It is important for patients to manage their hypertension because it is the number one risk factor for stroke, congestive heart failure, and peripheral vascular disease (PVD).

Antihypertensive medications also include several subcategories of drugs that work in some way to lower blood pressure. These drugs may be ordered alone or in combination, depending on the needs of the patient. Categories include vasodilators, adrenergic agents, ganglionic blockers, angiotensin-converting enzyme (ACE) inhibitors, and calcium channel blockers.

Examples of Antihypertensives:

amlodipine (Norvasc)	*irbesartan (Avalide)
*atenolol (Tenormin)	*lisinopril (Prinivil, Zestril)
benazepril (Lotensin)	*nitroprusside (Nipride, Nitropress)
*carvedilol (Coreg)	(hypertensive emergency agent)
enalapril (Vasotec)	propranolol (Inderal LA)
*fosinopril (Monopril)	ramipril (Altace)

Diuretic Agents

These drugs sometimes are called "water pills." Diuretics are among the first drugs that often are prescribed to assist in the treatment of hypertension because they cause a quick decrease in circulating fluid volume, resulting in a decrease in pressure demand on the heart.

TAKE NOTE

Diuretic orders may be written as a one-time order or a continuing order, but the dosages are frequently changed on the basis of laboratory results and patient response.

Examples of Diuretics:

*bumetanide (Bumex)	quinapril (Accupril)
*furosemide (Lasix)	spironolactone (Aldactone)
*hydrochlorothiazide (Esidrix, HydroDIURIL)	

Potassium Replacements

Potassium replacements replace potassium that has been lost through the use of certain diuretics. Potassium may be given diluted in an IV medication, orally, or sprinkled on food or in fluid in granule form.

Examples of Potassium Replacements:

potassium chloride (Kaochlor, K-Lor, K-Lyte, Micro K, Slow-K)

Antihyperlipidemic Agents (Cholesterol-lowering Drugs)

Many studies have demonstrated that lowering cholesterol can greatly reduce the risks of heart attack and death in people at high risk for a heart attack. Antihyperlipidemic medications can lower cholesterol. They may be taken alone or may be used in combination.

Examples of Antihyperlipidemics:

*atorvastatin (Lipitor)	*lovastatin (Mevacor)
*ezetimibe (Zetia)	pravastatin (Pravachol)
fenofibrate (Tricor)	*simvastatin (Zocor)
*gemfibrozil (Lopid)	

TAKE NOTE

The antilipidemic drugs known as "statins" are indicated in italics. It is important to note that a patient who is taking these medications should not eat grapefruit or drink grapefruit juice. Grapefruit interacts with statins, causing the blood level of the medications to rise, increasing the risk of adverse effects from the medications.

Anticoagulant Agents

Anticoagulants are drugs that thin the blood and prevent clots from forming in the blood. Anticoagulants may have stop dates.

Examples of Anticoagulants:

acetylsalicylic acid (Aspirin)—an antiplatelet	*enoxaparin (Lovenox)—a form of heparin
*clopidogrel (Plavix)—an antiplatelet	*heparin (Hepalean)
dalteparin (Fragmin)—a form of heparin	*warfarin (Coumadin)
dipyridamole (Persantine)—an antiplatelet	

Laboratory tests are usually ordered if a patient is on anticoagulation therapy. These include prothrombin time (PT) or the international normalized ratio (INR) if a patient is on warfarin (Coumadin). If a patient is on heparin, different tests may be ordered, such as aPTT (activated partial thromboplastin time) and activated clotting time (ACT). The timing of these tests is critical because the patient's next dose or immediate action that needs to be taken is dependent on the outcome of these tests.

Also considered anticoagulants, acetylsalicylic acid (Aspirin), clopidogrel (Plavix), and dipyridamole (Persantine) are drugs that actually work on the platelets in the blood to prevent them from sticking together and forming a clot.

✎ TAKE NOTE

In the acute care setting, warfarin (Coumadin) is most frequently ordered for maintenance once patients have graduated from taking intravenous heparin.

Drugs That Affect the Gastrointestinal System

Antacids

Too much acid in the stomach produces an often painful condition called *gastric hyperacidity,* or GERD (gastroesophageal reflux disease). The category of both **over-the-counter (OTC)** and prescribed medications that is ordered for this condition is antacids. Many antacids are ordered as a prn order (e.g., May give Maalox 30 mL 3-4 ×/day as needed for upset stomach).

Examples of Antacids:
  *esomeprazole (Nexium)
  *lansoprazole (Prevacid)
  *omeprazole (Prilosec)

Antisecretory and Antiulcer Drugs

Antisecretory and antiulcer drugs decrease acid production by blocking the cells that help create acid or by inhibiting the proton pump, which pumps the acid.

Examples of Antisecretory Drugs:
  *cimetidine (Tagamet)
  *famotidine (Maalox H$_2$, Mylanta AR, Pepcid)
  *ranitidine (Zantac)

✎ TAKE NOTE

Sucralfate (Carafate) is a common antiulcer drug. This drug is unique because it actually forms an inside "patch" over a stomach ulcer, protecting the stomach lining and allowing it to heal.

Antidiarrheals and Laxatives

Antidiarrheals are drugs that lessen or stop diarrhea. They consist of both OTC and prescription medications.

Examples of Antidiarrheals:
  *diphenoxylate (Lomotil)
  loperamide (Imodium)

Laxatives are the medications that are used to treat constipation. They can stimulate a bowel movement, soften the stool for easier passage, or serve as a fiber supplement given to increase and maintain normal bowel function. Laxatives are frequently ordered as a prn medication and may be given orally, as a suppository, or as an enema.

Examples of Laxatives:
  *bisacodyl (Dulcolax)
  *magnesium citrate (Citrate of Magnesia)
  *phosphates (Fleet Phosphosoda, Fleets enema)
  *polyethylene glycol (GoLYTELY, Colyte)
  psyllium (Metamucil)

Antiemetic or Antinauseant Drugs

Nausea and vomiting are conditions that must be treated promptly because they can lead to serious complications for patients. Vomiting is also known as emesis; therefore, this category of drugs is often referred to as antiemetics. Drugs may be administered orally, intravenously, intramuscularly, or via suppository.

Examples of Antiemetics:
*chlorpromazine
   (Thorazine)
*dimenhydrinate   *prochlorperazine (Compazine)
   (Dramamine)
*hydroxyzine (Vistaril)   trimethobenzamide (Tigan)
metoclopramide (Reglan)

Drugs That Affect the Musculoskeletal System

Anti-inflammatory Drugs

Anti-inflammatory drugs are used to reduce inflammation and relieve pain. They are most commonly used in arthritis and arthritis-like conditions. These drugs are divided into two groups: steroidal and nonsteroidal anti-inflammatory drugs (NSAIDs).

Examples of Steroid Anti-inflammatory Drugs:
dexamethasone   *prednisolone (Pred Mild)
   (Decadron)
*hydrocortisone   triamcinolone
   (Cort-Dome, Hytone)   (Aristocort, Kenalog)
*prednisone (Deltasone)

Examples of Nonsteroidal Anti-inflammatory Drugs (NSAIDs):
diclofenac (Voltaren)   indomethacin (Indocin)
*flurbiprofen (Ansaid)   *naproxen (Anaprox, Naprosyn)
*ibuprofen (Motrin)   piroxicam (Feldene)
                          sulindac (Clinoril)

Muscle Relaxants

Muscle relaxants reduce spasms in the muscles.

Examples of Muscle Relaxants:
  *carisoprodol (Soma)
  *cyclobenzaprine (Flexeril)
  *orphenadrine citrate (Norflex)

Antineoplastics (Chemotherapy)

Antineoplastic drugs make up a large group of drugs that are used in the treatment of cancer. The uses and dosages vary widely, depending on the type of cancer that the patient has. Some chemotherapy drugs require special handling of the drug itself, or the patient receiving the drugs may need to follow special isolation precautions.

Examples of Antineoplastics:
cisplatin (Platinol-AQ)   *methotrexate (Folex, Mexate)
*cyclophosphamide   tamoxifen (Nolvadex, Tamofen)
   (Cytoxan)
doxorubicin (Adriamycin)   vincristine (Oncovin)
*interferon alfa (Intron A)

Vitamins

Vitamins are organic substances that are found in food. Occasionally, the body becomes deficient in vitamins, especially during illness.

Common Drug Dosages
The following list contains some frequently ordered medications and their usual adult dosages.

codeine (Contin)	15-60 mg
warfarin (Coumadin)	1-10 mg
meperidine (Demerol)	50-100 mg
heparin (Hepalean)	5000 U
digoxin (Lanoxin)	0.125-0.25 mg
morphine sulfate (Ethmozine)	10-15 mg

Examples of Vitamins:
*cyanocobalamin—vitamin B_{12} (Hydro-Cobex)
*multivitamin (MVI)
*niacin—vitamin B_3 (Niacor, Nicobid)
*phytonadione—vitamin K_1 (AquaMEPHYTON)
vitamin E (Aquasol E)

Topical Preparations

Topical preparations are frequently ordered for the eye or the ear, or to be applied to the skin.

Examples of Ophthalmic Preparations (for the eye):
bacitracin c̄ polymyxin B (Polysporin Ophthalmic)
bacitracin c̄ polymyxin B and neomycin (Neosporin Ophthalmic)
dipivefrin (Propine)
timolol (Timoptic)
tobramycin (Tobrex)

Examples of Otic Preparations (for the ear):
hydrocortisone c̄ ciprofloxacin (Cipro HC Otic)
Vosol HC otic solution

Examples of Preparations for the Skin:

Betadine spray	Lotrisone
Cortisporin ointment	Mycolog cream and ointment
desoximetasone (Topicort)	Neosporin ointment
gentamycin cream	Triamcinolone (Aristocort)
hydrocortisone	
(Cort-Dome, Hytone)	

EXERCISE 8

Briefly describe the general purpose of each of the following drug groups.

1. antidiabetics

   _____

2. anticoagulants

   _____

Look- or Sound-Alike Medications
Many drug names look or sound alike. Name confusion is to blame for 12% to 25% of errors voluntarily registered in the United States by health care professionals and patients. Confusion exists about generic and brand names for medications. The risk is increased when doctors who are writing prescriptions have illegible handwriting. Below are some examples of similarly spelled medications.

Medication Order Written by Doctor	Medication That Could Cause Confusion
quinine 200 mg PO	quinidine 200 mg PO
lamotrigine 150 mg	lamivudine 150 mg PO
Zyrtec 20 mg q day	Zantac 200 mg q day
indapamide 2.5 mgPO	isradipine 2.5 mg PO
Lamictal 25 mg q day	Lamisil 250 mg q day
hydroxyzine 25 mg PO	hydralazine 25 mg PO
Losec TM 20 mg PO qd	Lasix TM 20 mg PO qd
Klonopin 0.5 mg PO	clonidine 0.5 mg PO
lovastatin 40 mg q day	lisinopril 40 mg q day
Platinol	Paraplatin

3. anti-infectives

   _____

4. antisecretory agents or antiulcers

   _____

5. antineoplastics

   _____

6. sedatives

   _____

7. hypnotics

   _____

8. hormones

   _____

9. potassium replacements

   _____

10. narcotics or opioids, analgesics with narcotics, and non-narcotic analgesics

✎ TAKE NOTE

A Summary of Drugs Needed to Identify to Meet Objective 13

Analgesics, Narcotic
acetaminophen with codeine
  (Tylenol 1, 2, 3, or 4)
codeine (Contin)
hydrocodone with acetaminophen
  (Lortab, Vicodin)
meperidine (Demerol)
morphine sulfate (Roxanol)
oxycodone (OxyFast, OxyContin)

Analgesics, Non-Narcotic
acetaminophen (Tylenol)
acetylsalicylic acid
  aspirin (Ascriptin)
ibuprofen (Advil, Motrin)

Sedatives/Hypnotics
flurazepam (Dalmane)
temazepam (Restoril)
zolpidem (Ambien)

Antianxiety Drugs
alprazolam (Xanax)
diazepam (Valium)
lorazepam (Ativan)

Anticonvulsants
gabapentin (Neurontin)
phenobarbital (Luminal)
phenytoin (Dilantin)

Antihistamines
desloratadine (Clarinex)
fexofenadine (Allegra)

**Drugs Used to Treat
Asthma/Related Conditions**
albuterol (Proventil, Ventolin)
aminophylline
fluticasone salmeterol (Advair)

Antibiotics
amoxicillin
  (Amoxil, Polymox)
azithromycin (Zithromax)
ciprofloxacin (Cipro, Ciloxan)
doxycycline (Vibramycin)

Antidiabetic Drugs
metformin (Glucophage)
pioglitazone (Actos)
clindamycin (Cleocin, HCL, Dalacin)
insulin glargine (Lantus)

theophylline
(Slo-bid, Theo-Dur)
erythromycin base
(E-Mycin, Erythrotab)
penicillin VK (Apo-Pen VK, Pen VeK)

Subcutaneous Insulin
insulin lispro (Humalog)
NPH (Pork NH Iletin II,
  Humulin N, Novolin N)
regular insulin

Cardiovascular Drugs
Antiarrhythmics
digoxin (Lanoxin)
diltiazem (Cardizem)
metoprolol (Lopressor)
nitroglycerine (Nitro-Bid, Nitro-Dur,
  Nitrostat, Transderm-Nitro)

Antianginals
atenolol (Tenormin)
diltiazem (Cardizem)
hydrochlorothiazide
(Esidrix, HydroDIURIL)
propranolol (Inderal)

Diuretics
bumetanide (Bumex)
furosemide (Lasix)

Antihypertensives
atenolol (Tenormin)
carvedilol (Coreg)
fosinopril (Monopril)
irbesartan (Avalide)
lisinopril (Prinivil, Zestril)
nitroprusside (Nipride, Nitropress)
(hypertensive emergency agent)

Potassium Replacements
potassium chloride (Kaochlor,
  K-Lor, K-Lyte, Micro K, Slow-K)

Antihyperlipidemics
atorvastatin (Lipitor)
ezetimibe (Zetia)
gemfibrozil (Lopid)
lovastatin (Mevacor)
simvastatin (Zocor)

Vasopressors
Dopamine (Intropin)
norepinephrine (Levophed)

Anticoagulants
clopidogrel (Plavix)
enoxaparin (Lovenox)
heparin (Hepalean)
warfarin (Coumadin)

✏ TAKE NOTE—cont'd

Antacids
esomeprasole (Nexium)
lansoprazole (Prevacid)
omeprazole (Prilosec)

Laxatives
bisacodyl (Dulcolax)
magnesium citrate
(Citrate of Magnesia)
phosphates (Fleet enema Phosphosoda)
polyethylene glycol (GoLYTELY, Colyte)

Anti-inflammatories
Nonsteroidal (NSAIDs)
flurbiprofen
(Ansaid)
ibuprofen (Motrin)
naproxen (Anaprox, Naprosyn)

Antineoplastics
cyclophosphamide (Cytoxan)
interferon alfa (Intron A)
methotrexate (Folex, Mexate)

Antisecretory Drugs
cimetidine (Tagamet)
famotidine (Maalox H_2,
Mylanta AR, Pepcid)
ranitidine (Zantac)

Antiemetics/ Antinauseants
chlorpromazine
(Thorazine)
dimenhydrinate
(Dramamine)
hydroxyzine (Vistaril)
prochlorperazine (Compazine)

Muscle Relaxants
carisoprodol (Soma)
cyclobenzaprine (Flexeril)
orphenadrine (Norflex)

Vitamins
cyanocobalamin–vitamin B_{12}
(Hydro-Cobex)
multivitamin (MVI)
niacin–vitamin B_3 (Niacor, Nicobid)
phytonadione–vitamin K_1
(AquaMEPHYTON)

Antidiarrheals
diphenoxylate (Lomotil)

Anti-inflammatories Steroids
hydrocortisone
(Cort-Dome, Hytone)
prednisone (Deltasone)
prednisolone (Pred Mild)

11. antihistamines

_____

12. antihyperlipidemics

_____

13. antiarrhythmics

_____

14. antianginals

_____

15. antihypertensives

_____

16. diuretics

_____

17. laxatives

_____

18. antiemetics

_____

19. vasopressors

_____

REAGENTS USED FOR DIAGNOSTIC TESTS

The following diagnostic procedures are performed by the nursing staff. Supplies used to perform the tests are requisitioned from the pharmacy during the transcription procedure.

Skin Tests

Skin tests are administered intradermally or topically to detect allergens, to determine immunity, and to diagnose disease (Fig. 13-11). Types and explanations of common skin tests follow.

DOCTORS' ORDERS FOR SKIN TESTS

Allergy Skin Testing by Dr. Dermat Before Discharge
The most common method of skin testing involves the process of injecting small quantities of suspected allergens intradermally. Positive reactions (erythroderma) usually occur within

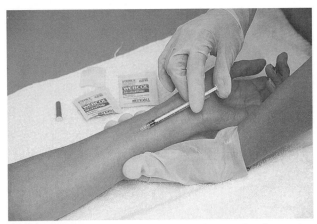

Figure 13-11 Intradermal injection in forearm for skin testing. (From Wilson SF, Thompson JM: *Respiratory disorders*, St. Louis, 1990, Mosby.)

20 minutes in varying degrees. Other methods include the scratch, patch, conjunctival, Prausnitz-Kustner (PK), radioallergosorbent (RAST), and **use** tests.

PPD Today

This is a screening test for tuberculosis. The test agent that is administered to the patient is purified protein derivative (PPD). Inter (intermediate) is the dosage strength.

Cocci 1:100 Now

This diagnostic test is used for coccidioidomycosis (valley fever). The ratio 1:100 refers to the dilution of the test material. It may also be administered in a 1:10 dilution.

Histoplasmin 0.1 mL Today

This skin test is employed as an aid in diagnosing histoplasmosis, a fungal disease. ■

MEDICATION STOCK SUPPLY

Hospitals store a supply of medications on nursing units, often in the (computerized medication) cart. This supply is often called the *medication stock supply*, and it includes such drugs as aspirin, acetaminophen, mineral oil, and milk of magnesia. When floor stock medicines are ordered from the pharmacy, they are charged to the unit budget.

RENEWAL MEDICATION ORDERS

Drugs such as narcotics and hypnotics, as well as other drugs controlled by federal or state laws, have an automatic stop date. Hospital medical committees may set automatic stop dates on anticoagulants and antibiotics. These drugs must be reordered before or when the stop date is reached. The HUC instructor or hospital pharmacist may provide a list of medications that have an automatic stop date in each specific hospital and the number of hours the drugs may be in effect before reordering is necessary.

A renewal stamp may be used by some hospitals as a reminder of the automatic stop date (Fig. 13-12). This stamp is placed on the doctor's order sheet by nursing personnel shortly before the order is due to expire; when completed, this is regarded as a new order and is transcribed as such. Where

DOCTOR, THE ___*Narcotic*___
HAS EXPIRED.   **DO YOU**

WISH THE ___*Demerol*___
RENEWED?   **THANK YOU.**

DR's. SIGNATURE ___*Dr. Starr*___

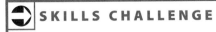

Figure 13-12 Drug renewal stamp.

permitted, this order may require changing the dates only on the MAR.

If the doctor wishes to discontinue the medication that is to be renewed, "No" may be written or chosen with a check mark on the renewal stamp. This automatically discontinues the medication. If the doctor does not choose an option to renew or discontinue an order or does not sign the renewal stamp, the patient's nurse usually calls to clarify if the doctor wishes to renew or discontinue the medication.

DISCONTINUING MEDICATION ORDERS

When a doctor discontinues a standing or standing prn order, a discontinue order is written on the doctor's order sheet: DC Achromycin 500 mg PO tid.

> ### SKILLS CHALLENGE
>
> To practice renewing and discontinuing medication orders, complete Activities 13-8 and 13-9 in the *Skills Practice Manual*.

MEDICATION ORDER CHANGES

A patient's medication order may have to be changed for any number of reasons. The change may involve the dosage, route of administration, or frequency of a drug already ordered. Whenever this is done, it is considered a new order and should be written as such on the MAR. It is illegal to erase or cross out parts of an order, or to write over an order on the MAR, because this is a record of what medication has been administered to the patient. This may result in a serious medication error. The old order must be discontinued according to the policy and the new order written. (See Fig. 13-3, *A* for discontinuing medication on the MAR.)

✓ DOCTORS' ORDERS FOR MEDICATION ORDER CHANGES

- Change meperidine 50 mg IM q4h prn to Demerol 50 mg PO q4h prn (change in route of administration)
- Decrease ciprofloxacin 250 mg IV q12h to 200 mg IV q12h (change in dosage)
- Change lorazepam 1 mg PO tid to 5 mg PO bid (change in frequency of administration) ■

SKILLS CHALLENGE

To practice transcribing medication order changes, complete Activity 13-10 in the *Skills Practice Manual*.

To test your skill in transcribing a review set of medication orders, complete Activity 13-11.

To test your skill in transcribing a review set of doctor's orders, complete Activity 13-12.

To practice locating medications in the *Physicians' Desk Reference*, complete Activity 13-13.

To practice recording telephoned doctor's orders and to practice recording telephoned messages, complete Activities 13-14 and 13-15.

KEY CONCEPTS

EMR and CPOE have changed the responsibilities of the HUC regarding the doctor's orders for medication. The HUC does not transcribe the medication orders but may have the responsibility of printing the home instructions for the discharged patient, including their medication orders. A basic knowledge of medications is very beneficial.

When the EMR and CPOE have not been implemented, transcribing medication orders requires extreme accuracy. Errors may result in serious consequences to the patient and liability to the hospital and all involved personnel. The HUC must be careful not to omit any orders during the transcription procedure. Each order must be transcribed exactly as written by the doctor. Each order should be written legibly, so it can be read easily by the nurse who is administering the medication.

An understanding of the type, form, and proper transcription procedure of medication orders should be acquired by all who work with drug orders. With experience comes familiarity with the more commonly administered medications and the groups to which they belong, such as laxatives, sedatives, and cardiac medications.

Whenever any doubt is expressed regarding a medication order or any order, always check with the nurse and/or pharmacist. If requested by the patient's nurse, place a call to the ordering doctor, so the nurse can clarify the order. Never hesitate to ask the nurse or pharmacist, or to call the doctor, whenever misinterpretation of the medication order is a possibility, or when the order cannot be read.

REVIEW QUESTIONS

1. Identify the underlined abbreviations in the following doctors' orders:

(1) (2) (3)

a. Coreg 25 <u>mg</u> <u>PO</u> <u>q</u> day   1. _____ 2. _____ 3. _____
(1)

b. <u>ASA</u> 81 mg PO q day   1. _____

(1)(2)(3)

c. bumetanide 0.1 mg/<u>kg</u>/dose <u>IV</u> q6<u>°</u>   1. _____ 2. _____ 3. _____

(1)(2)

d. budesonide 1 spray <u>ea</u> nostril <u>bid</u> A.M. & P.M.   1. _____ 2. _____

(1)(2)

e. albuterol 5mg/<u>mL</u> 1 puff q4-6h <u>prn</u>   1. _____ 2. _____

(1)(2)(3)

f. <u>NTG</u> 0.4 mg sub-<u>ling</u> prn, keep @ <u>BS</u>   1. _____ 2. _____ 3. _____

(1)(2)

g. meperidine 50 mg <u>IM</u> q4-6<u>h</u> for pain   1. _____ 2. _____

(1)

h. <u>TPN</u> orders to be written by Dr. Johnson   1. _____

(1)

i. <u>PCA</u> orders to be written by Dr. Doright   1. _____

   (1)

j. diazepam 5 mg/kg <u>IVP</u> now   1. _____

   (1)

k. cephalothin 0.5 g <u>IVPB</u> q8h   1. _____

   (1)(2)

l. add 1 <u>amp</u> <u>MVI</u> to TPN   1. _____ 2. _____

   (1)(2)

m. check blood sugar <u>ac</u> and <u>hs</u>   1. _____ 2. _____

   (1)(2)

n. add 40 <u>mEq</u> <u>KCL</u> to present IV   1. _____ 2. _____

   (1)

o. patient may have <u>LOC</u> prn   1. _____

   (1)

p. Compazine 5 mg IM q3-4h prn <u>N/V</u>   1. _____

   (1)(2)

q. Maalox 15 mL <u>tid</u> <u>pc</u>   1. _____ 2. _____

   (1)

r. ipecac <u>syr</u> 5 mL now   1. _____

2. List four abbreviations that are included in The Joint Commission's "do not use" list:

   a. _____   c. _____

   b. _____   d. _____

3. Explain how computer physician order entry (CPOE) with a clinical decision support system (CDSS) reduces errors in the medication ordering process.

_____

_____

_____

_____

4. List five components of a medication order (in order).

   a. _____   d. _____

   b. _____   e. _____

   c. _____

5. Identify the following orders as standing, standing prn, short-series order series, one-time, or stat.

a. meperidine 100mg IM now _____

b. hydrocodone 5 mg po q4-6h for pain _____

c. carvedilol 25 mg PO q day _____

d. Ambien 10 mg this hs _____

e. Fleets 1 bottle PO this hs and repeat in A.M. _____

6. List the five rights of medication administration:

a. _____

b. _____

c. _____

d. _____

e. _____

7. Match the definition from column 2 with the drug group listed in column 1. (Place the appropriate letter from column 2 on the line provided in column 1.)

1. diuretic _____

2. antihistamine _____

3. cardiovascular drug _____

4. antinauseants _____

5. antihyperlipidemic _____

6. potassium replacement _____

7. laxative _____

8. antibiotic _____

9. hormone _____

10. hypnotic _____

11. anticoagulant _____

12. analgesic, narcotic _____

13. analgesic, non-narcotic _____

14. antidiabetic _____

15. antianxiety _____

16. anticonvulsants _____

a. given to relieve moderate to severe pain

b. given to slow the clotting process

c. given to treat constipation

d. given to replace glandular secretion

e. given to induce sleep

f. given to lower blood sugar

g. given to lower cholesterol

h. given to treat infections

i. given to affect heart and vascular system

j. to replace potassium that has been lost

k. given to relieve mild aches and pain

l. to relive nausea and vomiting

m. given to induce urination

n. given to assist drying secretions, nasal stuffiness

o. given to prevent or relieve convulsions

p. given to treat anxiety

8. List four groups of medications that would have stop dates.

a._____

b._____

c._____

d._____

9. List two medication reference books that may be found on the nursing unit.

a._____

b._____

10. Match the medication from column 2 with the drug group listed in column 1. (Place the appropriate letter from column 2 on the line provided in column 1.)

1. diuretic _____

2. respiratory drug _____

3. cardiovascular drug _____

4. antinauseants _____

5. antihyperlipidemic _____

6. potassium replacement _____

7. laxative _____

8. antibiotic _____

9. hormone replacement _____

10. hypnotic _____

11. anticoagulant _____

12. analgesic, narcotic _____

13. analgesic, non-narcotic _____

14. anticonvulsant _____

15. antianxiety _____

16. antidiabetic _____

a. K-Lyte

b. acetaminophen (Tylenol)

c. atorvastatin (Lipitor)

d. fexofenadine (Allegra)

e. doxycycline (Vibramycin)

f. diltiazem (Cardizem)

g. zolpidem (Ambien)

h. trimethobenzamide (Tigan)

i. furosemide (Lasix)

j. oxycodone (OxyFast, OxyContin)

k. magnesium citrate (Citrate of Magnesia)

l. levothyroxine (Synthroid)

m. pioglitazone (Actos)

n. clonazepam (Klonopin)

o. warfarin (Coumadin)

p. lorazepam

11. List three skin tests and give the purpose of each:

a. _____ _____

b. _____ _____

c. _____ _____

THINK ABOUT...

1. Discuss the many benefits of the EMR and CPOE in regard to medications ordered by the physician.
2. Discuss the need for having a base knowledge of common medications prescribed by physicians (when the EMR and CPOE have been implemented).
3. Upon answering the telephone on the nursing unit, a physician on the other end begins giving you medication orders. The physician states that she does not have time to wait for the nurse, and you should just write them down. It is hospital policy that telephone orders may be given only to a licensed nurse. (In some hospitals that have implemented CPOE, telephone orders are not accepted at all, unless it is an emergency.) Discuss what you would say to the doctor.
4. Identify abbreviations used (other than those on the Joint Commission's "do not use" list) that could cause confusion or could be misinterpreted.

CHAPTER 14

Laboratory Orders and Recording Telephoned Laboratory Results

CHAPTER OBJECTIVES

Upon completion of this chapter, you will be able to:

1. Define the terms in the vocabulary list.
2. Write the meaning of each abbreviation in the Abbreviations list.
3. List the two general purposes of laboratory studies.
4. Name the three major laboratory divisions, and briefly state the purpose of each.
5. Name six studies performed in each of the three major laboratory divisions.
6. List five specimens that may be studied in the laboratory.
7. Describe the health unit coordinator's responsibilities in sending specimens to the laboratory.
8. Name three methods of obtaining urine specimens.
9. List the four tests generally performed as part of electrolyte studies.
10. List five laboratory specimens that may require a written consent form.
11. Describe the procedure for requisitioning stat blood tests from the laboratory.
12. Name the procedure that must be performed to order blood (packed cells) for transfusion.
13. Describe the health unit coordinator's responsibilities in an order for a 2-hr PP.
14. Explain the difference between fasting and NPO.
15. Identify the laboratory department that would perform each of the tests that are marked with an asterisk.

16. Explain the procedure for ordering peak and trough drug levels.
17. Name three common urine chemistry tests (marked with an asterisk).
18. Describe how errors may be avoided in recording telephoned laboratory results.

VOCABULARY

Amniocentesis A needle puncture into the uterine cavity to remove amniotic fluid, the liquid that surrounds the unborn baby

Antibody An immunoglobulin (protein) produced by the body that reacts with and neutralizes an antigen (usually a foreign substance)

Antigen Any substance that induces an immune response

Biopsy Tissue removed from a living body for examination

Clean Catch A method of obtaining a urine specimen using a special cleansing technique; also called a midstream urine

Culture and Sensitivity The growth of microorganisms in a special media (culture), followed by a test to determine the antibiotic to which they best respond (sensitivity)

Cytology The study of cells

Daily Laboratory Tests Tests that are ordered once by the doctor but are requisitioned by the health unit coordinator every day until the doctor discontinues the order

Differential Identification of the types of white cells found in the blood

Dipstick Urine The visual examination of urine using a special chemically treated stick

Electrolytes A group of tests done in chemistry, which usually includes sodium, potassium, chloride, and CO_2

Erythrocyte A red blood cell

Fasting No solid foods by mouth and no fluids containing nourishment (e.g., sugar, milk)

Guaiac A method of testing stool for hidden (occult) blood using guaiac as a reagent (may also be called a Hemoccult Slide Test)

Lumbar Puncture A procedure used to remove cerebrospinal fluid from the spinal canal

Occult Blood Blood that is undetectable to the eye

Pap Smear A test performed to detect cancerous cells in the female genital tract; the Pap staining method also can study body secretions, excretions, and tissue scrapings

Paracentesis A surgical puncture and drainage of a body cavity

Pathology The study of body changes caused by disease

Plasma The fluid portion of the blood in which the cells are suspended; it contains a clotting factor called fibrinogen

Postprandial After eating

Random Specimen A specimen that can be collected at any time

Reference Range Range of normal values for a laboratory test result

Serology The study of blood serum or other body fluids for immune bodies, which are the body's defense when disease occurs

Serum Plasma from which fibrinogen, a clotting factor, has been removed

Sputum The mucous secretion from lungs, bronchi, or trachea

Sternal Puncture The procedure to remove bone marrow from the breastbone cavity for diagnostic purposes; also called a bone marrow biopsy

Thoracentesis A needle puncture into the pleural space in the chest cavity to remove pleural fluid for diagnostic or therapeutic reasons

Timed Specimen A specimen that must be collected at a specific time

Tissue Typing Identification of tissue types to predict acceptance or rejection of tissue and organ transplants

Titer The quantity of substance needed to react with a given amount of another substance—used to detect and quantify antibody levels

Type and Crossmatch The patient's blood is typed, then is tested for compatibility with blood from a donor of the same blood type and Rh factor

Type and Screen The patient's blood type and Rh factor are determined, and a general antibody screen is performed

Urinalysis The physical, chemical, and microscopic examination of the urine

Urine Reflex Urine is tested; if certain parameters are met, a culture is performed

ABBREVIATIONS

Note: Many doctors' orders for laboratory tests are written on the doctors' order sheet as the abbreviation appears here; for example, CBC is the doctor's written order for complete blood (cell) count. Examples of doctors' orders are given only for those orders that require more than the abbreviation.

Abbreviation	Meaning	Example of Usage on a Doctor's Order Sheet
Ab	antibody	HIV Ab
ADH	antidiuretic hormone (chemistry)	
AFB	acid-fast bacillus (microbiology)	sputum for AFB Cx
Ag	antigen	CMV Ag
ALP *or* alk phos	alkaline phosphatase (chemistry)	
ANA	antinuclear antibody (serology)	
BC	blood culture (microbiology)	Blood cultures × 2-15 min apart
Bili	bilirubin	
BMP	basic metabolic panel (chemistry)	
BNP	brain natriuretic protein (chemistry)	
BUN	blood urea nitrogen (chemistry)	
Bx	biopsy (cytology)	Liver needle Bx
Ca or Ca^+	calcium (chemistry)	
CBC	complete blood (cell) count (hematology)	
CC, creat cl, or cr cl	creatinine clearance (chemistry)	24 hr urine Cr Cl
CEA	carcinoembryonic antigen (chemistry)	
Cl	chloride (chemistry)	
CMP	comprehensive metabolic panel (chemistry)	
CMV	cytomegalovirus (microbiology, serology)	CMV IgG and IgM
CO_2	carbon dioxide (chemistry)	
CPK *or* CK	creatine phosphokinase *or* creatine kinase (chemistry)	

Abbreviation	Meaning	Example of Usage on a Doctor's Order Sheet	Abbreviation	Meaning	Example of Usage on a Doctor's Order Sheet
C&S	culture and sensitivity (micro)	Sputum for C&S	Lytes	electrolytes (chemistry)	
CSF	cerebrospinal fluid (chemistry, hematology, microbiology)	CSF for serology	Mg or Mg+	magnesium (chemistry)	
			Na	sodium (chemistry)	
Cx	culture (microbiology)	Sputum Cx	NP	nasopharynx	NP smear for C&S
Diff	differential (hematology)	WBC $\bar{c}$ diff	O&P	ova and parasites (parasitology)	Stool for O&P × 3
EBV	Epstein-Barr virus (serology)		PAP	prostatic acid phosphatase (serology)	
ESR or sedrate	erythrocyte sedimentation rate (hematology)		PC	packed cells (blood bank)	Give 2 U PC now
FBS	fasting blood sugar (chemistry)		PCV	packed-cell volume (hematology; same as hematocrit)	
FPG	fasting plasma glucose (chemistry)		PKU	phenylketonuria (chemistry)	
Fe	iron (chemistry)	Fe $\bar{c}$ TIBC	PO_4 or phos	phosphate or phosphorus (chemistry)	
FS	frozen section (cytology)	Liver wedge Bx FS	POCT or PCT	point-of-care testing (performed on the nursing unit)	
GTT or OGTT	glucose tolerance test or oral glucose tolerance test (chemistry)		PP	postprandial (chemistry)	2 hr PP BS
HB_sAg	hepatitis B surface antigen (serology)		PSA	prostatic specific antigen (serology)	
hCG	human chorionic gonadotropin (test for pregnancy [chemistry])		PT	prothrombin time (coagulation–hematology)	
Hct	hematocrit (hematology)		PTT or APTT	partial thromboplastin time or activated partial thromboplastin time (coagulation–hematology)	
HDL	high-density lipoprotein (chemistry)				
Hgb	hemoglobin (hematology)		RBC	red blood cell count (hematology)	
H&H	hemoglobin and hematocrit (hematology)		RBS or BS	random blood sugar or blood sugar (chemistry)	
$HIVB_{24}Ag$	human immunodeficiency virus antigen screen (serology)		RDW	red cell distribution width (hematology)	
HSV	herpes simplex virus (serology)		Retics	reticulocytes (hematology)	
K	potassium (chemistry)		RPR	rapid plasma reagin (serology)	
LDL	low-density lipoprotein (chemistry)		RSV	respiratory syncytial virus (microbiology)	
LP	lumbar puncture (also called spinal tap)	LP in AM	S&A	sugar and acetone (urinalysis)	

Abbreviation	Meaning	Example of Usage on a Doctor's Order Sheet
T₃, T₄, T₇	thyroid tests (chemistry)	
T&X-match or T&C	type and crossmatch (blood bank)	T&C for 2 U of packed red cells
TIBC	total iron-binding capacity (chemistry)	
Trig or TG	triglycerides (chemistry)	
T&S	type and screen (blood bank)	
TSH	thyroid-stimulating hormone (chemistry)	
UA or U/A	(urinalysis)	
UC	urine culture cath urine for UC	
WBC	white blood cell count (hematology)	
WNL	within normal limits	

✎ **TAKE NOTE**

Most of the abbreviations listed previously apply to some commonly ordered laboratory tests. Many more abbreviations for laboratory tests are covered throughout this chapter. The words in parentheses indicate in which division of the laboratory the test is performed.

EXERCISE 1

Write the abbreviation for each term listed below.

1. fasting blood sugar _____

2. ova and parasites _____

3. hemoglobin _____

4. erythrocyte sedimentation rate *or* sedimentation rate _____

5. potassium _____

6. acid-fast bacilli _____

7. red blood cell count _____

8. postprandial _____

9. cerebrospinal fluid _____

10. iron _____

11. culture and sensitivity _____

12. type and crossmatch _____

13. complete blood (cell) count _____

14. prostatic acid phosphatase _____

15. glucose tolerance test _____

16. packed cells _____

17. prothrombin time _____

18. urinalysis _____

19. alkaline phosphatase _____

20. hepatitis B surface antigen _____

21. frozen section _____

22. human immunodeficiency virus _____

23. magnesium _____

24. human chorionic gonadotropin _____

25. within normal limits _____

26. partial thromboplastin time *or* activated partial thromboplastin time _____

27. thyroid tests _____

28. thyroid-stimulating hormone _____

29. sugar and acetone _____

30. antigen _____

31. basic metabolic chemistry panel _____

32. cytomegalovirus _____

33. herpes simplex virus _____

34. type and screen _____

35. antibody _____

36. culture _____

37. respiratory syncytial virus _____

38. comprehensive metabolic panel _____

39. electrolytes _____

40. biopsy _____

41. point-of-care testing _____

42. packed-cell volume _____

43. random blood sugar *or* blood sugar _____

44. rapid plasma reagin _____

45. reticulocytes _____

46. prostatic specific antigen _____

47. differential _____

48. white blood cell count _____

49. phosphorus _____

50. total iron-binding capacity _____

51. hematocrit _____

52. lumbar puncture _____

53. sodium _____

54. nasopharynx _____

55. hemoglobin and hematocrit _____

56. carbon dioxide _____

57. antinuclear antibody _____

58. high-density lipoprotein _____

59. blood urea nitrogen _____

60. calcium _____

61. creatinine clearance _____

62. chloride _____

63. carcinoembryonic antigen _____

64. brain natriuretic protein _____

65. low-density lipoprotein _____

66. antidiuretic hormone _____

67. creatine phosphokinase or creatine kinase _____

68. Epstein-Barr virus _____

69. antibody _____

70. red cell distribution width _____

71. triglyceride _____

72. bilirubin _____

EXERCISE 2

Write the meaning of each abbreviation listed below.

1. FBS

   _____

2. O&P

   _____

3. Hgb

   _____

4. ESR or sedrate

   _____

5. K

   _____

6. AFB

   _____

7. RBC

   _____

8. PP

   _____

9. CSF

   _____

10. Fe

    _____

11. C&S

    _____

12. T&X-match or T&C

    _____

13. CBC

    _____

14. PAP

    _____

15. GTT

    _____

16. PC

_____

17. PT

_____

18. UA or U/A

_____

19. ALP or alk phos

_____

20. HB_sAg

_____

21. FS

_____

22. HIV $B_{24}Ag$

_____

23. Mg or Mg+

_____

24. hCG

_____

25. WNL

_____

26. PTT or APTT

_____

27. $T_3T_4T_7$

_____

28. TSH

_____

29. S&A

_____

30. Ag

_____

31. BMP

_____

32. CMV

_____

33. HSV

_____

34. T&S

_____

35. Ab

_____

36. Cx

_____

37. RSV

_____

38. CMP

_____

39. lytes

_____

40. Bx

_____

41. POCT or PCT

_____

42. PCV

_____

43. RBS or BS

_____

44. RPR

_____

45. retics

_____

46. PSA

_____

47. Diff

_____

48. WBC

_____

49. PO$_4$ or phos

_____

50. TIBC

_____

51. Hct

_____

52. LP

_____

53. Na

_____

54. NP

_____

55. H&H

_____

56. CO$_2$

_____

57. ANA

_____

58. HDL

_____

59. BUN

_____

60. Ca or Ca$^+$

_____

61. CC, creat cl, or cr cl

_____

62. Cl

_____

63. CEA

_____

64. BNP

_____

65. LDL

_____

66. ADH

_____

67. CPK or CK

_____

68. EBV

_____

69. Ab

_____

70. RDW

_____

71. trig or TG

_____

72. bili

_____

✎ TAKE NOTE

When the electronic medical record (EMR) with computer physician order entry (CPOE) is implemented, the physicians' orders are entered directly into the patient's EMR and are automatically sent to the appropriate departments. The health unit coordinator (HUC) is responsible for sending labeled and bagged specimens to the laboratory department after they have been collected by nursing staff, residents, or doctors. Other HUC tasks may be indicated by an icon (usually a telephone) next to the appropriate patient's name on the computer census screen. An example of an additional task would be to hold a patient's tray for a glucose tolerance test.

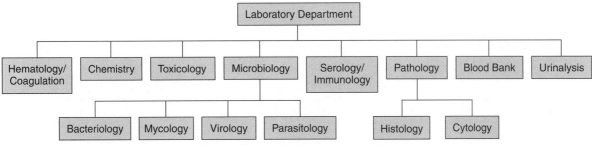

Figure 14-1 A laboratory divisional chart.

INTRODUCTION TO LABORATORY PROCEDURE

Tests performed by the laboratory are ordered for diagnostic purposes and for evaluation of a prescribed treatment. See the Evolve website for a comprehensive list of the studies that are performed in a laboratory.

Hospital size determines the number of divisions within the laboratory and the types of tests performed in each division. For example, a large hospital may have a microbiology division with subdivisions such as bacteriology, **serology**, parasitology, virology, and mycology. In smaller hospitals, all the tests performed in the divisions mentioned previously may be done in the microbiology division or sent to outside laboratories. (Figure 14–1 is a laboratory divisional chart.) Also, in some hospitals the division and some test names vary from those used in this book.

In this chapter, we will discuss three major laboratory divisions—hematology, chemistry, and microbiology—and five other divisions—toxicology, serology, pathology (including histology and cytology), blood bank, and urinalysis. The clinical laboratory also may perform tests related to nuclear medicine and gastroenterology when a hospital is not of sufficient size to maintain a separate nuclear medicine or gastroenterology department.

It is necessary for the HUC to interpret terms the doctor may use to write laboratory orders. The word *routine*, in a written laboratory order, usually would indicate that the test will be performed within a 4-hour period, because there is no urgency for the test results. For example, the doctor may write the order *Routine CBC*, meaning that the blood specimen for the complete blood count may be drawn according to the hospital (laboratory) policy. Nursing personnel or laboratory personnel may draw blood specimens.

The doctor also may use the word *daily*, as in the order *daily Hgb*; this means that the test is ordered once by the doctor but is requisitioned every day or entered into the computer for multiple days in advance by the HUC until the order is discontinued. Some hospitals have a policy that requires the doctor to renew daily laboratory orders every 3 days or discontinue the orders.

The word *stat*, as you recall, means "to be done immediately." Because of the urgency of a stat order, a different communication procedure is used. The procedure is to notify the laboratory by phone or verbally notify the appropriate nursing personnel on the unit. When calling the laboratory, supply the name of the patient, nursing unit, room number, and the test ordered. The order is entered into the computer immediately if a laboratory technician is to draw the blood. The order would be entered when the specimen is collected if collected by nursing personnel. When placing an order for a test that is to be drawn at a specified time, such as drug levels or a 2-hr PP blood sugar, the term "*Timed*" is used.

Specimens

All laboratory tests require a specimen. Blood, the most commonly used specimen, is most often obtained by nursing or laboratory personnel through venipuncture (puncture into the vein), finger stick (puncture into a capillary), or peripheral arterial or venous lines (Fig. 14-2). An additional source of blood is the umbilical cord. A "cord blood" specimen may be ordered on patients in the Labor and Delivery unit and is collected by nursing personnel.

Blood specimens may have to be collected in different containers depending on the test ordered. For example, coagulation studies and chemistry studies must be taken in different tubes. Cultures performed on blood for different types of organisms (aerobic versus anaerobic bacteria) also may require different tubes. Clear and complete information on all tests to be collected reduces the need for the patient to be redrawn for additional blood specimens. When asked by a nurse to call the laboratory to inquire about amount or means of collecting a specimen; document the information and the name of the person providing the information.

Other specimens for testing include urine, stool, sputum, sweat, wound drainage, discharge from body openings, and gastric washings (lavage). Nursing staff members usually collect these specimens (Fig. 14-3).

The doctor usually obtains specimens by entering parts of the body or a body cavity. Types of specimens and the names of the procedures used to obtain them are listed below. Most hospitals have a policy that requires written consent from the patient before these procedures are performed, except for pelvic examination. (Review "Preparing a Consent Form," Chapter 8.) It may be the HUC's responsibility to order trays, such as a lumbar puncture tray, or other equipment from the central supply department (CSD) for the doctor to use to perform these procedures.

Specimen	Procedure Performed to Obtain Specimen
Spinal fluid	Lumbar puncture; also called spinal tap
Bone marrow	Sternal puncture; also called bone marrow biopsy
Abdominal cavity fluid	Abdominal paracentesis
Pleural fluid	Thoracentesis or thoracocentesis
Amniotic fluid	Amniocentesis
Biopsy specimen	Biopsy of a part of the body
Cervical smear	Pelvic examination

All specimens obtained by the nursing staff or doctor usually will be bagged and labeled (not always possible during

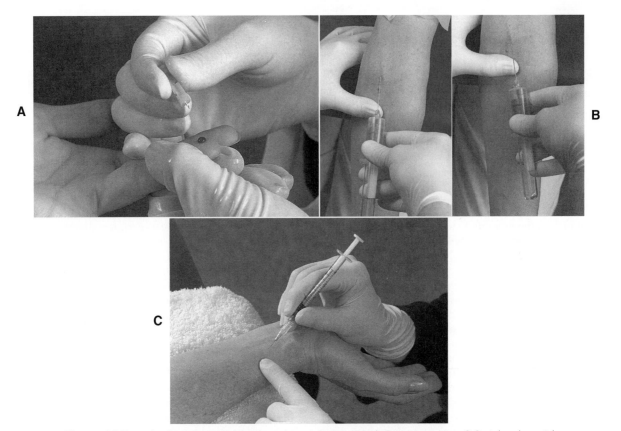

Figure 14-2 Methods of obtaining blood specimens: **A,** Finger stick. **B,** Venipuncture. **C,** Peripheral arterial draw. (From Sommer S, Warekois R: *Phlebotomy: worktext and procedures manual*, St. Louis, Saunders, 2001.)

an emergency) before they are handed to the HUC. It is recommended that the health unit coordinator keep plastic gloves in a drawer to use when specimens are not bagged and wash hands after handling specimens (even when placed in plastic bags). The label should include the date and time collected, along with the initials of the person who collected the specimen.

Requisitions for laboratory tests of specimens obtained by the nursing staff or doctor are kept on the nursing unit until the specimen is collected or the order is entered into the computer when the specimen is sent. The requisition or computer printout of the order is attached to the specimen bag, and then it is sent to the laboratory. It is essential that the HUC check the patient name on the specimen and on the computer order screen to compare with the doctor's order. Mislabeled specimens usually are discarded and the patient redrawn, causing a delay in diagnosis and treatment and causing the patient additional discomfort.

It is often the HUC's responsibility to take the specimen to the laboratory. This should be done as soon as possible. Some specimens (well wrapped) may be sent by the pneumatic tube system, especially when results are needed quickly (e.g., emergency department, surgery). Specimens that should *not* be sent by the pneumatic tube system are those that have been collected by an invasive procedure, such as cerebrospinal and amniotic fluids. When blood or urine is sent by the pneumatic tube system, specimens must be well wrapped and cushioned. Some facilities may have a policy that *any* specimens are not to be transported via the pneumatic tube system because of possible loss or spilling of the specimen.

> ### ✐ TAKE NOTE
>
> It is essential that the HUC check the patient's name on the specimen and computer order screen to compare with the doctor's order. Mislabeled specimens usually are discarded and the patient redrawn, causing a delay in diagnosis and treatment, and causing the patient additional discomfort.

Point-of-Care Testing

Many laboratory tests that were once only drawn and analyzed in the laboratory department may now be performed on the nursing unit. A laboratory test that is collected and analyzed on the hospital unit by nursing personnel is called a *point-of-care lab test*. Because of point-of-care testing (POCT), the procedure for ordering a test may change.

Results are obtained via several methods. These include analysis by portable automated analyzers, the use of reagents (chemicals), and microscopic visualization.

Portable automated analyzers may be used in departments that require immediate results; these decrease the need for stat specimens to be sent to the laboratory. Some tests that may be done on the unit by this method include **electrolytes**, blood glucose, BUN, hemoglobin, and hematocrit. A test to evaluate pulmonary function (see Chapter 16, pages 309 and 322), called arterial blood gases (ABGs), may be run on an automated analyzer on the unit.

Reagent-based tests may include a test for pregnancy or human chorionic gonadotropin (hCG) or activated clotting time

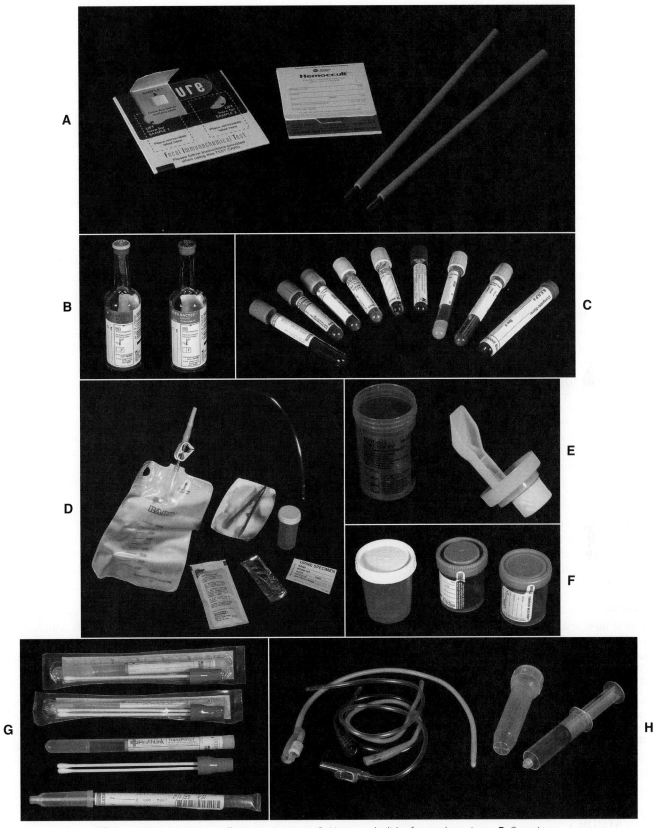

Figure 14-3   Specimen collection containers. **A,** Hemoccult slides for stool specimen. **B,** Containers for blood culture specimen. **C,** Various containers for blood specimen. **D,** Cath urine specimen container kit. **E,** Stool specimen container. **F,** Urine specimen containers: *Left,* voided specimen; *Right,* midstream specimen. **G,** Culturette and container for throat culture. **H,** Types of sputum collection containers.

(ACT), and a test for *Helicobacter pylori* (CLO test), a bacterium that has been indicated in ulcers of the gastrointestinal system. The CLO test actually uses a **biopsy** specimen obtained in the endoscopy department (see Chapter 16, pp. 318-319) and may yield positive results within 2 hours.

Some of the reagent-based tests that are considered point-of-care lab tests are those that are traditionally carried out by nursing personnel; these include blood and urine monitoring for the presence of ketones and for levels of glucose. Blood glucose monitoring is discussed in Chapter 10, p.172. **Guaiacs**, gastroccults, or hemoccults, which use reagents to detect hidden blood in gastric and stool specimens, also are considered point-of-care tests in some health care facilities.

A test that uses both a reagent and microscopic visualization is the fern test, which is used to indicate the presence of amniotic fluid (due to rupture of the amnion). The reagent portion uses a strip of paper that indicates acidity (pH paper), and the microscopic portion detects the characteristic fern pattern of crystallized amniotic sodium chloride (salt).

Communication With the Laboratory Department

All laboratory tests are communicated to the laboratory department through the ordering step of transcription.

DIVISIONS WITHIN THE LABORATORY

It may be necessary to identify the division in which a test is performed in order to complete the correct requisition or enter it into the computer. This information is also helpful in telephone communication when one is clarifying orders or requesting results.

Hematology

The hematology division performs tests related to physical properties of the blood (including blood cells and their appearance), tests related to clotting and bleeding disorders, and coagulation (clotting) studies done to monitor patients on anticoagulant therapy.

Specimen

Most of these tests are done on a blood specimen. However, bone marrow and spinal fluid also may be studied in the hematology division.

Fasting

Fasting generally is not required for tests performed in the hematology division of the laboratory.

Communication With the Laboratory

Hematology studies are ordered by computer or by completing a downtime requisition form (Fig. 14-4).

✓ DOCTORS' ORDERS FOR HEMATOLOGY STUDIES

It is impossible to list all doctors' orders related to this division of the laboratory. However, we have listed the more common ones in their abbreviated forms, along with an interpretation for reference. Refer to the abbreviations list at the beginning of the chapter if necessary.

Note: Unless stated otherwise, all of the following tests are performed on blood specimens; therefore, as mentioned previously, nursing or laboratory personnel obtain the specimen or POCT is performed.

CBC (Complete Blood Cell Count) or Hemogram

A CBC or hemogram is composed of a number of tests, including RBC; Hgb; Hct; RBC indices; WBC; and Diff, blood smear, and platelet count. These tests also may be ordered separately. The number of tests included in a CBC may vary among hospitals.

RBC (Red Blood Cell Count)

RBC is the measurement of red blood cells (**erythrocytes**) per cubic millimeter of blood.

HGB (Hemoglobin)

Hgb is the oxygen-carrying pigment of blood that gives it its red color. This test may determine the need for additional blood, or it may aid in diagnosing types of anemia.

HCT (Hematocrit)

Hematocrit, also called PCV (packed-cell volume), is a measurement of the volume percentage of red blood cells in whole blood.

RBC (Red Blood Cell) Indices

Measurement of RBC indices is a method for determining the characteristics of red blood cells. The measurements are reported as MCH (content of hemoglobin in average individual red cell), MCHC (average hemoglobin concentration per 100 mL of packed red cells), MCV (average volume of individual red cells), and RDW (red cell distribution width—a distribution of red cell volume).

WBC (White Blood Cell Count)

A WBC (leukocyte count) is the count of the number of white blood cells that are present in the blood to fight disease-causing organisms. This test often is used in the diagnosis of infection.

DIFF (Differential)

A **diff** reports the various types of WBCs (or leukocytes) found in the blood specimen. Some of these types are lymphocytes (lymphs), monocytes (monos), neutrophils (neutros), eosinophils (eos), and basophils (basos). A diff often is included in a CBC.

Blood Smear

A blood smear is an examination performed with special stains of the peripheral blood; it can provide a significant amount of information regarding drugs and disease that affect RBCs, WBCs, and platelets.

Platelet Count (Platelets)

Platelet count is the counting of clotting cells (platelets) that is essential for the coagulation process to take place.

ESR (Erythrocyte Sedimentation Rate)

An erythrocyte sedimentation rate, also called *sedrate*, determines the rate at which RBCs settle out of the liquid portion of the blood. This test is used to evaluate the progress of inflammatory diseases.

Doctor ordering _____   Stat

Today's date _____

Draw @ date _____ Time _____   Routine

Collection date _____ Time _____

Collected by _____

Requested by _____

Hematology	**Serology**	**Urinalysis/Urine Chemistry**
☐ Bleeding time, Ivy	☐ ANA	☐ Routine UA
☐ CBC c̄ diff	☐ ASO titer	☐ Reflex UA
☐ CBC c̄ manual diff	☐ CEA	☐ Amylase (2hr)
☐ Factor VIII	☐ CMV	☐ Bilirubin
☐ Fibrinogen	☐ IgG	☐ Calcium
☐ HCT	☐ IgM	☐ Chloride
☐ HGB	☐ Cocci screen	☐ Creatinine clearance
☐ H & H	☐ EBV panel	☐ Glucose tolerance
☐ Eosinophil Ct absolute	☐ Enterovirus Ab panel 1	☐ Nitrogen
☐ Eosinophil smear	☐ Enterovirus Ab panel 2	☐ Occult blood
☐ ESR	☐ FTA	☐ Osmolality
☐ LE cell prep	☐ Hepatitis screen	☐ Phosphorus
☐ Platelet Ct	☐ HbsAb	☐ Potassium
☐ PT	☐ HbsAg	☐ Pregnancy
☐ PTT (APTT)	☐ HIV	☐ Protein
☐ RBC	☐ Monospot	☐ Sodium
☐ RBC Indices	☐ PSA screen	☐ Sp gravity
☐ Reticulocyte Ct	☐ RA factor	☐ Uric Acid
☐ Sickle cell prep	☐ RPR	
☐ WBC	☐ RSV	
☐ WBC c̄ diff	☐ Rubella screen	
☐ WBC c̄ manual diff	☐ Strptozyme	
☐ Other		

Write in orders: _____

_____

Revised 9/10/07

Figure 14-4 Downtime requisition for hematology, serology, and urinalysis/urine chemistry.

Retics

The count of reticulocytes (immature red blood cells) determines bone marrow activity. It is used often in the diagnosis of anemia.

LE Cell Prep

LE cell prep is a diagnostic study for lupus erythematosus, an inflammatory disease.

PT (Prothrombin Time)

A PT measures the clotting ability of blood. This test assists the doctor in determining the dosages of the drugs—usually Coumadin—prescribed in anticoagulant therapy. The HUC may be required to telephone the test results to the doctor. (Telephoned results require a "read back" of the information and appropriate documentation.) How the results are reported depends on the testing method used, such as patient/control in seconds (e.g., 17 sec/13 sec); or patient/% of prothrombin activity (e.g., 14 sec/70% activity).

In addition to the PT result, a result called the international normalized ratio (INR) may be included. This is a calculation that uses the patient's PT result, the normal control result, and a coefficient factor that depends on the reagent used. The INR calculation is an attempt to standardize PT results.

APTT and PTT

An APTT (activated partial thromboplastin time) and a PTT (partial thromboplastin time) are coagulation studies. These are performed individually and are commonly used to monitor heparin dosage.

Bleeding Time

Bleeding time is the measurement of the time it takes for a standardized incision to cease bleeding. It differs from clotting time in that this test involves constriction of the smaller blood vessels. A standardized incision is an incision of specific length and depth. Several methods may be used, but template bleeding time (TBT) is preferred, in that the incision is standardized by the use of a cutting device called a *template.*

Clotting Time

Clotting time is the determination of the time it takes for blood to clot.

Refer to the Evolve website for other tests performed in the hematology division. ■

SKILLS CHALLENGE

To practice transcribing hematology and coagulation orders, complete Activity 14-1 in the *Skills Practice Manual.* To practice transcribing daily laboratory orders, complete Activity 14-2 in the *Skills Practice Manual.*

Chemistry

The chemistry division performs tests related to the study of chemical reactions that occur in living organisms. When a disease process occurs, the levels of chemicals within the body fluids vary from normal. Any variance permits a diagnosis or evaluation of the patient's health status.

Specimens

Blood and urine are the specimens that are collected most commonly for study in this division of the laboratory. Whole blood, **plasma**, or **serum** may be used for chemistry tests. Many tests of the same name can be done on either blood or urine; therefore, often the doctor uses the word *serum* to indicate that the test is to be performed on blood and uses the term *urine* if the test is to be done on a urine specimen.

Specimens for urine chemistries may require that the urine be collected over a specified period, such as 24 hours. This is often referred to as a 24-hour urine specimen (Fig. 14-5). It may be the HUC's responsibility to obtain the receptacle from the laboratory to be used for collection of the specimen. For some specimens that are to be kept for a period, a preservative is added to the collection bottle before it is sent to the unit. Other 24-hour specimens may have to be iced in the patient's bathroom until the collection is completed (see the Box *Chemistry Tests That May Require a 24-Hour Urine Specimen*).

Fasting

Many blood chemistry tests require that the patient fast or be assigned NPO status. Fasting means that the patient is given nothing to eat for 8 to 10 hours before the specimen to be tested is

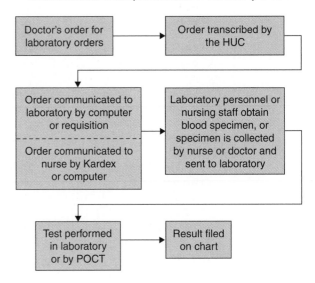

Communication and Implementation of Laboratory Orders

CHEMISTRY TESTS THAT MAY REQUIRE A 24-HOUR URINE SPECIMEN*

Albumin, quantitative and qualitative	Human chorionic gonadotropin (hCG)
Aldosterone	17-Hydroxycorticosteroids
Amino acids, quantitative-fractionated	5-Hydroxyindoleacetic acid, quantitative (5-HIAA)
Arsenic, quantitative	17-Ketogenic steroids
Calcium, quantitative	17-Ketosteroids
Catecholamines	Lactose[†]
Chlorides	Lead
Coproporphyrin, qualitative and quantitative	Metanephrines
Cortisol	Phosphorus
Creatine[†]	Porphobilinogen, quantitative
Creatinine clearance	Potassium
Epinephrine	Pregnanetriol
Epinephrine-norepinephrine	Protein, total
Estrogens, total	Sodium clearance
FIGLU (*N*-formiminoglutamic acid)	Uric acid[†]
Fluoride	Uroporphyrins, qualitative and quantitative
Follicle-stimulating hormone (FSH)	Vanillylmandelic acid (VMA)[†]
Glucose, quantitative[†]	Zinc
Homovanillic acid (HVA)	

Note: Check with your laboratory concerning these tests. Methods used may vary from hospital to hospital.
[†]Common test.

collected; the patient may have water. NPO means nothing by mouth—food or fluid—after midnight. It may be the HUC's responsibility to notify the nutritional care department and to obtain bedside signs to be posted to remind personnel that the patient is being prepared for a test. Table 14-1 lists chemistry and other laboratory tests that require the patient to fast or be NPO. (Because some of these tests are not considered fasting by all laboratories, students should check their instructor for their correct classification in specific hospitals.) Many fasting tests are ordered to be drawn during the routine morning draw time, because the patient is fasting naturally before breakfast.

Communication With the Laboratory

Chemistry tests are requisitioned by means of computer or by completing a downtime requisition form (Fig. 14-6).

Automated equipment permits many tests to be performed on a small sample of blood and in a short time. One requisition (or computer-entered laboratory request) is used to request a number of tests. Some of the automated instruments used are the Bayer Centaur, Dade RxL, Vitros, Paramax, Coulter (hematology), Stagos (coagulation), and Iris (urinalysis). In chemistry, these automated multicomponent studies are called *profiles*, *panels*, or *surveys*.

✓ **DOCTORS' ORDES FOR BLOOD CHEMISTRY STUDIES**

Many chemistry tests are ordered as a group; these are called *panels* or *profiles* (see the Box *Common Laboratory Panels*). These profiles are standardized nationally according to CPT (Current Procedures Terminology) or Healthcare Common Procedures Coding System (HCPCS) guidelines so a facility may receive Medicare reimbursement. Custom panels may be designed by a facility and must be approved on an annual basis.

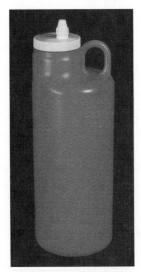

Figure 14-5   A 24-hour urine specimen container.

Table 14-1   **Fasting and/or NPO List for Laboratory Studies**

Procedure	Fasting	NPO	Laboratory Division
Bromsulphalein (BSP)	Yes	No	Chemistry
Cholesterol	Yes	No	Chemistry
Chromosomes	Yes	No	Blood bank
Deoxycorticosterone	Yes	No	Chemistry or nuclear medicine
D-Xylose (blood or urine)	Yes	Yes	Chemistry
Electrophoresis, lipids	Yes	No	Chemistry
Electrophoresis, lipoprotein	Yes	No	Chemistry
Factor VIII assay	Yes	Yes	Coagulation
Fasting blood sugar (FBS)	Yes	No	Chemistry
Gastrin (serum)	Yes	Yes	Chemistry or nuclear medicine
Glucose, fasting (FBS)	Yes	No	Chemistry
Glucose tolerance test (GTT)	Yes	Yes	Chemistry
Insulin tolerance test (ITT)	Yes	Yes	Chemistry
Iron (Fe)	Yes	Yes	Chemistry
Iron-binding capacity (IBC)	Yes	Yes	Chemistry
Lipids	Yes	Yes	Chemistry or GI lab
Neutral fat (lipid profile fractionization)	Yes	Yes	Chemistry or GI lab
Orinase tolerance test	Yes	Yes	Chemistry
Parathyroid hormone (PTH)	Yes	Yes	Chemistry or nuclear medicine
Phenolsulfonphthalein (PSP) urine	Yes	Yes	Chemistry
Phospholipids	Yes	Yes	Chemistry or GI lab
Plasma cortisol	Yes	Yes	Chemistry or nuclear medicine
Renin	Yes	Yes	Chemistry or nuclear medicine
Schilling test	No	Yes	Chemistry or nuclear medicine
Serum lipids	Yes	Yes	Chemistry or GI lab
Testosterone	Yes	Yes	Chemistry or nuclear medicine
Total iron-binding capacity (TIBC)	Yes	Yes	Chemistry
Triglycerides	Yes	Yes	Chemistry

Doctor ordering _____   □ Stat
Today's date _____   □ Timed
Draw @ date _____ Time _____   □ Routine

Chemistry	**Chemistry cont-**	**Toxicology**
Panels	**Tests cont-**	□ Acetaminophen
□ Electrolytes	□ Cortisol	□ Peak
□ BMP	□ Folic acid	□ Trough
□ CMP	□ Folate	□ Aminophylline
□ Renal	□ FSH	□ Peak
□ Hepatic	□ Glucose	□ Trough
□ Lipid	□ Glucose _____ Hr PP	□ Digitoxin
Tests	□ Glucose tolerance	□ Peak
□ Acetone	□ Iron	□ Trough
□ Ace level	□ Lactic Acid	□ Digoxin
□ ACTH	□ LDH	□ Peak
□ A/G Ratio	□ LH	□ Trough
□ Albumin	□ Lipase	□ Drug Screen
□ Aldolase	□ Magnesium	□ Gentamycin
□ Alk Phos	□ Phosphorous	□ Peak
□ Amylase	□ Potassium	□ Trough
□ ALT (SGPT)	□ Protein	□ Kanamycin
□ AST (SGOT)	□ Protein electrophoresis	□ Peak
□ Bilirubin, total	□ Sodium	□ Trough
□ Direct	□ TBG	□ Lidocaine
□ Indirect	□ Triglycerides	□ Peak
□ BNP	□ Troponin	□ Trough
□ BUN	□ TSH	□ Phenobarbital
□ Calcium	□ T_3	□ Peak
□ Carbon dioxide	□ T_4	□ Trough
□ Chloride	□ Uric Acid	□ Tobramycin
□ Chloesterol	□ VMA	□ Peak
□ Citrate		□ Trough
□ CK (CPK)		□ Vancomycin
□ CKMB		□ Peak
□ C-reactive protein		□ Trough
□ Creatinine		

Write in Orders: _____

Figure 14-6 Downtime requisition for chemistry and toxicology.

Note: Unless otherwise indicated, the specimen used for the following tests is serum, which is collected by nursing or laboratory personnel.

Standard Chemistry Panels:

Lytes (Electrolytes)
Na, K, Cl, CO_2

BMP (Basic Metabolic Panel)
Na, K, Cl, CO_2, glucose, BUN, creatinine, and Ca

Renal Panel
Na, K, Cl, CO2, glucose, BUN, creatinine, Ca, albumin, and phosphate

CMP (Comprehensive Metabolic Panel)
Na, K, Cl, CO_2, glucose, BUN, Creatinine, Ca, albumin, total bilirubin, Alk Phos, total protein, AST, ALT

Lipid Panel
Chol, trig, HDL, LDL

Hepatic (Liver) Function Panel

Alb, T. bili, D. bili, alk phos, T. protein, ALT (SGPT), and AST (SGOT)

An example of a custom panel is as follows:

Cardiac Enzymes or Cardiac Profile

CK (CPK) and CK-MB. A Troponin I also may be ordered. Additional tests may include CK-MB Isoenzymes or subforms a myoglobin or homocysteine level, and an LDH.

Each test in a panel may be ordered individually. Listed below are frequently ordered blood chemistry tests, written in abbreviated form as the doctor would write them on the doctors' order sheet. The full name of each test is given in parentheses. Normal values for common blood chemistry studies are given on p. 270.

Chemistry Tests

Alk phos (Alkaline Phosphatase)

The alkaline phosphatase level is used to evaluate bone and liver disease, among other uses.

ALT (Alanine Aminotransaminase)

Another name for ALT is serum glutamic-pyruvic transaminase (SGPT). This enzyme is released into the circulation by destroyed liver cells.

AST (Aspartate Aminotransferase)

Another name for AST is serum glutamic-oxaloacetic transaminase (SGOT). This enzyme is released into the circulation from destroyed skeletal or cardiac muscle, or the liver. The AST level is elevated in myocardial infarction, liver disease, acute pancreatitis, acute renal disease, and severe burns.

Amylase (Serum)

The level of amylase is elevated in acute pancreatitis, as well as in some other illnesses.

CPK (CK), and CK-MB

CPK (CK) and CK-MB are known as cardiac enzymes. These tests are ordered when a myocardial infarction (heart attack) is suspected.

Bilirubin

This test measures liver function. Bilirubin is the result of red blood cells that have broken down and are excreted by the liver. In diseases in which a large number of red blood cells are destroyed (e.g., liver disease, obstruction of the common bile duct), a high concentration of bilirubin is found in the blood serum. The doctor may order this test as total bilirubin, using the direct or indirect method of testing.

BMP (Basic Metabolic Panel)

A BMP is a chemistry panel that consists of eight chemistry tests, including glucose, BUN, Ca, creatinine, Na, K, Cl, and CO_2.

BNP (Brain Natriuretic Peptide)

Increased levels of BNP are released when ventricular diastolic pressure rises; this may indicate congestive heart failure, or increased risk of congestive heart failure or mitral valvular disease.

BS (Blood Sugar) or Glucose

A BS or glucose test is used to determine the amount of sugar in the blood. It is usually ordered at a specific time, such as 4 PM BS, also called an RBS. The patient is not fasting when this test is performed.

BUN (Blood Urea Nitrogen)

This test is useful in diagnosing diseases that affect kidney function.

Cholesterol

Cholesterol levels may be used to measure liver function. The patient is usually in a fasting state for this test. It is believed that cholesterol may sometimes be responsible for causing high blood pressure and hardening of the arteries (atherosclerosis). It is also important that the good blood lipids, or high-density lipoproteins (HDLs), be measured in relation to total cholesterol and low-density lipoproteins.

CMP

A comprehensive metabolic panel consists of 14 chemistry tests, including glucose, BUN, creatinine, albumin, total bilirubin, Ca, Alk Phos, total protein, AST, Na, K, Cl, CO_2, and ALT.

CPK or CK (Creatine Phosphokinase or Creatine Kinase)

CPK or CK is an enzyme found in heart, brain, or skeletal muscle that is released when damage results from a disease process. Specific isoenzymes or types of CK may be ordered: CK-BB for brain, CK-MB for heart, and CK-MM for skeletal muscle damage.

Creatinine Clearance Test (12- or 24-hour Creatinine Clearance)

A creatinine clearance test is done to study kidney function. It requires testing the blood and a timed urine specimen collected for 12 or 24 hours.

Electrophoresis

Electrophoresis is a procedure performed to determine protein or fatty acid levels. The doctor may order any of three tests that result in a serum protein pattern. These tests are protein electrophoresis, lipoprotein electrophoresis, and immunoelectrophoresis.

FBS (Fasting Blood Sugar)

An FBS, also called fasting glucose, determines the amount of sugar in the bloodstream after the patient has not eaten for 8 to 10 hours. This test is used in the diagnosis of diabetes and monitoring of diabetes treatment.

GTT (Glucose Tolerance Test) or OGTT (Oral Glucose Tolerance Test)

A GTT (OGTT) is performed to detect abnormalities in glucose metabolism. The patient is in a fasting state. The patient has an FBS drawn to establish baseline data and then is given a large amount (75 grams) of glucose solution to drink. A timed blood is taken 2 hours later. (The order has been communicated to the laboratory by requisition or computer to alert laboratory personnel to perform a fasting blood sugar test before administering the sugar solution.) An additional glucose tolerance test may include Gestational Diabetes Screen.

HbA$_{1c}$, GHb, or GHB (Glycosylated Hemoglobin or Glycohemoglobin)

A HbA$_{1c}$, GHb, or GHB test is a reflection of the blood glucose on red blood cells during the past 3 months. This test is used in monitoring patients with diabetes.

HDL (High-density Lipoprotein)

An HDL "good" cholesterol level is thought to be important in the total cholesterol profile.

LDH (Lactate Dehydrogenase or Lactic Acid Dehydrogenase)

LDH is an enzyme that is released into the circulation after tissue damage to heart, liver, kidney, brain, or skeletal muscle.

Lytes (Electrolytes)

Electrolytes consist of four tests: sodium (Na), potassium (K), chloride (Cl), and carbon dioxide (CO$_2$). These four tests may be performed separately.

COMMON LABORATORY PANELS	
Electrolytes	**CMP**
Na	Na
K	K
Cl	Cl
CO$_2$	CO$_2$
	BUN
BMP	Creatinine
Na	Gluc
K	Ca
Cl	Alb
CO$_2$	T. prot
BUN	AST
Creat	ALT
Gluc	T. bili
Ca	Alk phos
Renal Panel	**Lipid Panel**
Na	Chol
K	Trig
Cl	LDL
CO$_2$	HDL
BUN	
Creat	**CBC**
Gluc	RBC
Ca	WBC c̄ diff
Alb	Hb
Phosphate	Hct
	RBC indices
Hepatic Function Panel	
Albumin	**Acute Hepatitis Panel**
T. bili	HA Ab IgM
D. bili	HB$_c$Ab IgM
Alk phos	HB$_s$Ag
T. prot	Hep C Ab
AST	
ALT	**Epstein-Barr Virus Panel**
	EBV IgM
	EBV IgG
	EBV EA
	EBNA

PSA (Prostatic Specific Antigen)

A PSA measures the body's level of prostatic specific **antigen**. Increased PSA levels may indicate the presence of prostate cancer.

Serum Creatinine

A serum creatinine test is performed to diagnose kidney disease. It studies the creatinine level in the blood serum.

TIBC (Total Iron-binding Capacity)

A total iron-binding capacity test is useful in diagnosing anemia, some infections, and cirrhosis of the liver.

Troponin

Troponin is a test performed to diagnose acute myocardial infarction (AMI) from a few hours after onset to as long as 120 hours. It is more sensitive than CK-MB in detecting unstable angina with minor myocardial cell damage. Two subtypes may be ordered: Troponin I and Troponin T.

2-hr PP BS (2-hours Postprandial Blood Sugar)

A 2-hours **postprandial** blood sugar test is performed to assess the patient's response to carbohydrate intake. It is the HUC's responsibility to notify the laboratory when the patient has finished eating. The blood for this test may be drawn 2 hours after any meal and, if ordered for the laboratory to draw, is ordered as a *"Timed"* draw at the specified time.

Triglycerides

Triglycerides are the principal lipids (greasy organic substances) in the blood. The patient is in a fasting state for this study, which is important in diagnosing heart disease, hypertension, and diabetes.

Uric Acid

Uric acid levels are used principally to diagnose gout. ■

Special Chemistry Studies

Many of the tests previously included in the nuclear chemistry division of the clinical laboratory or the nuclear medicine laboratory now may be performed through a non–radioisotope-based method, and may be included in the chemistry division

NORMAL VALUES FOR FREQUENTLY PERFORMED HEMATOLOGY–COAGULATION STUDIES AND BLOOD CHEMISTRY STUDIES
Hematocrit (Hct)
• *Male:* 45-50 vol/dL
• *Female:* 40-45 vol/dL
Hemoglobin (Hgb)
• *Male:* 14.5-16 g/dL
• *Female:* 13-15.5 g/dL
White blood cell count (WBC): 6000-9000/mm^3
Prothrombin time (PT): 12-15 sec
Sodium (Na): 132-142 mEq/L
Potassium (K): 3.5-5.0 mEq/L
Fasting blood sugar (FBS): 70-120 mg/dL

as a special chemistry study. These tests are usually listed under the general heading of "Chemistry" on the computer order screen or on requisitions. The following studies are examples of tests that may be performed by these divisions (see the Evolve website):

- CEA (carcinoembryonic antigen)
  - An elevated level of CEA indicates liver, colon, or pancreatic cancer. CEA level also is used to monitor treatment of these conditions.

Examples of hormones that may be tested in special chemistry include the following:

- ACTH (adrenocorticotropic hormone)
- Cortisol
- Folate
- FSH (follicle-stimulating hormone)–urine
- GH (growth hormone)
- hCG (human chorionic gonadotropin)—a test for pregnancy
- LH (luteinizing hormone)
- PTH (parathyroid hormone)
- TBG (thyroxine-binding globulin)
- TSH (thyroid-stimulating hormone)
- T_3 (triiodothyronine)
- T_4 (thyroxine)
- T_7 (free thyroxine index)

✓ DOCTORS' ORDERS FOR URINE CHEMISTRY STUDIES

Urine chemistry tests are listed below. Refer to the list presented earlier for tests that require a 24-hour urine collection.

Urine Glucose
Urine glucose is ordered in conjunction with blood glucose for a glucose tolerance test. Determines the amount of glucose in the urine.

Urine Creatinine
Urine creatinine usually is ordered in conjunction with the blood chemistry portion of the creatinine clearance test but may be ordered separately.

Urine Protein
An elevated urine protein is found in inflammatory diseases of the urinary system and the prostate gland.

Urine Osmolality
Urine osmolality determines the diluting and concentrating abilities of the kidneys. ■

Toxicology

Toxicology is the scientific study of poisons, their detection, their effects, and methods of treatment for conditions they produce. Tests for detecting drug abuse and for monitoring drug usage also are performed in toxicology. Special consents, handling, and labeling may be required.

Specimen
Specimens include blood and urine.

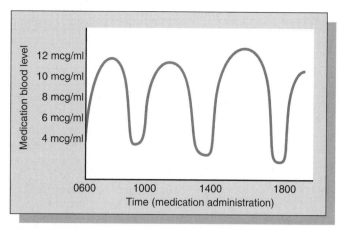

Figure 14-7 Graphic example of peak-and-trough levels of a medication.

 SKILLS CHALLENGE

For practice transcribing the following types of orders, please complete the following activities in the *Skills Practice Manual*:

- To practice transcribing blood chemistry orders, complete Activity 14-3.
- To practice transcribing stat laboratory orders, complete Activity 14-4.
- To practice transcribing fasting and NPO laboratory orders, complete Activity 14-5.
- To practice transcribing a review set of laboratory orders, including a toxicology order for peak and trough, complete Activity 14-6.

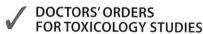 *TAKE NOTE*

Peak-and-trough, or random blood levels, are commonly drawn to check or monitor these medications:

- amikacin (Amikin)
- cyclosporine (Sandimmune)
- tacrolimus (Prograf)
- digoxin (Lanoxin)
- phenytoin (Dilantin)
- gentamicin
- kanamycin (Kantrex)
- tobramycin (Tobrex)
- vancomycin (Vancocin)

Communication With the Laboratory
Toxicology studies are ordered by computer or by completing a requisition form (see Fig. 14-6).

✓ DOCTORS' ORDERS FOR TOXICOLOGY STUDIES

When doctors want to check levels of certain medications the patient is receiving, they order peak-and-trough levels (Fig. 14-7). Sometimes, toxic blood levels accumulate instead of

✐ *TAKE NOTE*

Laboratory Divisions

- Hematology: Study of *physical properties* of blood, including blood cell studies and coagulation
- Chemistry: Study of *chemicals* of the blood and other body fluids
- Toxicology: Study of poisons, their detection, their effects, and methods of treatment for conditions they produce. Monitoring of drug use and detection of drug abuse
- Microbiology: Study of the *organisms* that cause disease; includes bacteriology, mycology, virology, and parasitology
- Serology/Immunology: Study of *immunologic* substances
- Pathology: Study of the nature and *cause of disease*, when changes in structure and function are noted
- Histology: Study of the microscopic structure of tissue
- Cytology: Study of *cells* obtained from body tissues and fluid
- Blood bank: *Blood typing* and crossmatching, storing blood and blood components for *transfusion*
- Urinalysis: Study of *urine*

being excreted. Antibiotics such as amikacin, gentamicin, kanamycin, and tobramycin are examples of medications ordered for peak-and-trough levels. Other medication levels may include Dilantin (random), digoxin (random), and tacrolimus (Prograf, trough level). For peak levels, the blood usually is collected 15 minutes after IV infusion and 30 to 60 minutes after IM injection. Trough levels usually require that blood be drawn 15 minutes before the next dose of medication is given to the patient. For peak-and-trough orders, the HUC must work closely with the laboratory and nursing staff to ensure proper scheduling of collections. When ordering peak-and-trough levels, the HUC would order them *"Timed,"* meaning that blood should be drawn stat at the specified time. In some cases, nursing staff will draw the peak level at the appropriate time.

- Gentamicin peak and trough around third dose

The HUC would have to check with the nurse to coordinate the times to order the gentamicin peak-and-trough and would order them *"Timed."*

Additional random toxicology tests may include screens for so-called "street drugs" (cocaine, opiates, and cannibanoids), as well as for ETOH (ethanol or alcohol) levels. ■

Microbiology

The terms *microbiology* and *bacteriology* sometimes are used interchangeably. However, large laboratories may use the broader term *microbiology* as a division name within the hospital, with areas in that division designated for bacteriology, parasitology, mycology, and virology, to name a few.

Microbiology is the study of microorganisms that cause disease. Specimens are cultured, are grown in a reproducing medium, and are identified with the use of biochemical tests. Identification of the causative organism of a specific disease

is important because isolation procedures are based on the methods by which organisms are spread.

Bacteriology is often the largest division of microbiology. Specimens are cultured, grown in a reproducing medium, identified with the use of biochemical tests, and then tested for antibiotic sensitivity.

Parasites, organisms that live off other living organisms, are dealt with in parasitology. Fecal specimens are studied here for ova and parasites.

In mycology, cultures are set up to isolate and identify fungi. Because a fungus must grow to produce spores, these cultures may take several weeks.

Virology is the study of viruses that cause disease.

Specimen

Almost any type of specimen, including blood, stool, urine, sputum, bronchial washes or other body fluids, catheter tips, eye/ear drainage, and wound drainage, may be studied in the microbiology division.

Fasting

Fasting is not required for tests performed in the microbiology division of the laboratory.

Communication With the Laboratory

Microbiology tests are requisitioned via computer or by completion of a downtime requisition form (Fig. 14-8). The requisition form for the test remains on the unit until the specimen is obtained.

✓ DOCTORS' ORDERS FOR MICROBIOLOGY STUDIES

Frequently ordered tests performed in the microbiology division, with an interpretation related to the HUC's role, are listed below. For assistance with abbreviations, check the Abbreviations list at the beginning of the chapter.

Bacteriology

Culture and sensitivity (C&S)

Can be ordered on almost any specimen, including blood, urine, stool, sputum, wound drainage, pleural fluid, bronchial wash fluid, cerebrospinal fluid, IV and urinary catheters, and nose and throat specimens. The specimen is placed on an appropriate medium for growth. If organisms grow, they are tested for antibiotic sensitivity, which determines those antibiotics that should be effective for treatment. Laboratory personnel, nursing staff, or the physician may be responsible for collection of the specimen.

Blood Cultures
Blood culture specimens may be collected as multiple specimens (at different times or different sites) to ensure accurate isolation and identification of the causative organism.

AFB Culture (Acid-fast Bacilli)
Performed to detect the presence of acid-fast bacilli such as *Mycobacterium tuberculosis*, which causes tuberculosis. The nursing staff is responsible for collection of the specimen (usually sputum). A special stain also may be performed.

Doctor ordering _____ ☐ Stat
Today's date _____ ☐ Routine
Collection date _____Time _____
Collected by_____
Requested by_____

Microbiology		**Fluids**	
Specimen Source	Test Requested	Specimen Source	Test Requested
☐ Abscess	☐ AFB culture	☐ Abdominal	☐ Cell count
_____	☐ AFB stain	☐ Amniotic	c̄ diff
☐ Blood	☐ C & S	☐ CSF	☐ Glucose
☐ Body cavity	☐ C & S	☐ Pericardial	☐ LDH
_____	Anaerobic	☐ Peritoneal	☐ Occult blood
☐ CSF	☐ C.diff	☐ Pleural	☐ Protein
☐ Ear drainage	☐ Fungal culture	☐ Synovial	☐ Sp gravity
☐ Right	☐ GC screen	☐ Other	☐ RPR (CSF)
☐ Left	☐ G-Stain		☐ Other
☐ Eye drainage	☐ Strep screen	# of Tubes _____	
☐ Right	☐ Viral culture		_____
☐ Left	☐ Other	**Cytology**	
☐ Nasal smear	_____		
☐ Sputum		Specimen Source	Test Requested
☐ Stool	☐ Stool	☐ Amniotic	☐ Pap
☐ Throat	☐ Fat	☐ Breast Bx	☐ Fungal
☐ Tissue	☐ Fiber	☐ Bronchial Asp	☐ Maturation
_____	☐ Occult blood	☐ Buccal	Index
☐ Urine	☐ Ova & parasites	☐ Cervical smear	☐ Other_____
☐ Voided	☐ #1 of 3	☐ Cervical Bx	
☐ Clean catch	☐ #2 of 3	☐ Colon Bx	
☐ St cath	☐ #3 of 3	☐ CSF	
☐ Foley cath		☐ Gastric fluid	
☐ Wound drainage _____		☐ Lung Asp	
☐ Other_____		☐ Pleural	
		☐ Pericardial	
		☐ Peritoneal	
		☐ Sputum	
		☐ Vaginal	
		☐ Other_____	Revised 9/10/07

Figure 14-8 Downtime requisition for microbiology, fluids, and cytology.

C diff or C difficile (Clostridium difficile) Toxin
Performed on stool specimens to identify an infection with *Clostridium difficile* bacteria. *C diff* is transmitted easily, and infection often occurs while in the hospital (nosocomially). A patient may be placed in isolation until three consecutive results for *C diff* toxin are negative. This test may be ordered through microbiology or serology, because it is a swab test for the antigen.

Urine for CC (Colony Count)
Done to determine the quantity of bacteria present in a urine specimen.

Gram Stain
Performed to classify bacteria into Gram-negative or Gram-positive groupings, thus allowing for differential diagnosis of the causative agent. Treatment can begin immediately, while awaiting the results of cultures.

Additional Culture Orders
Many cultures may be ordered to identify specific pathogens that cause infections. Some examples of opportunistic organisms that may be cultured and studied include *Nocardia* and *Acinetobacter*.

Parasitology

Stool for O&P (Ova and Parasites)
An order that is usually ordered times three, which requires three different stool specimens (three requisition forms must be prepared) to determine the presence of ova (eggs) or parasites in the stool. The nursing staff is responsible for the collection of stool specimens.

Mycology

Mycology Culture

A mycology culture is performed to detect the presence of fungi. It may be performed on blood or spinal fluid specimens. Results may take several weeks to determine. Studies may be performed to determine the presence of fungi such as *Histoplasma, Coccidioides, Candida,* and *Pneumocystis jiroveci.*

Virology

Virus Culture and Virus Serology

Virus cultures may be done on any specimen; virus serology is done on a blood specimen to detect the presence of viruses or antibodies to viruses.

CMV (Cytomegalovirus) Cultures

Performed to detect cytomegalovirus infection. The virus is widespread and common and may be an opportunistic pathogen in an immunocompromised patient. For culture specimens, a blood (buffy coat), urine, sputum, or mouth swab may be used as a specimen. Fresh specimens are essential. The results may take about 3 to 7 days to attain. ■

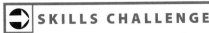

SKILLS CHALLENGE

To practice transcribing microbiology/bacteriology orders, complete Activity 14-7 in the *Skills Practice Manual.*

Serology/Immunology

Serology is the study of antibodies and antigens useful in detecting the presence and intensity of a current infection. It also may be useful in identifying a previous infection or exposure to an organism. Autoimmune diseases may be studied, and pretransplant and posttransplant conditions evaluated and treated. Tests for syphilis, rheumatoid arthritis, human immunodeficiency virus (HIV), some influenzae, and **tissue typing** are a few of the studies done in this area.

Immunology

The response of the body to a foreign substance may include mobilization of leukocytes (white blood cells) against the foreign substance, as well as the production of certain proteins that neutralize the substance. These proteins are immunoglobulins (or more commonly antibodies) that circulate in the blood. Five main types of immunoglobulins have been identified: IgG, IgM, IgA, IgD, and IgE.

An important characteristic of antibodies is that much of the time, they are produced specifically against a particular foreign substance, and they are ordered in reference to that substance. Any substance that elicits an immune response is called an *antigen.* Measurement of the **antibody** level may be ordered as a **titer.** Many serologic tests are done to detect antibody levels because antibodies are usually included in the serum portion of the blood. Serologic tests also can detect the presence of antigens.

Specimen

Most of these tests are done on the serum portion of a blood specimen. However, other body fluids such as spinal fluid and mucosal transudate (cheek swab) may be tested, along with biopsy specimens and secretions from wounds. Antigens also may be detected in stool specimens.

Fasting

Fasting is not required for tests performed in the serology division of the laboratory.

Communication With the Laboratory

Serology studies are ordered via computer or by completion of a laboratory requisition form (see Fig. 14-4).

✔ DOCTORS' ORDERS FOR SEROLOGY

ANA (Antinuclear Antibody)

An ANA test detects the presence of certain autoimmune diseases such as SLE (systemic lupus erythematosus).

ASO Titer (Antistreptolysin O Titer)

An elevated ASO titer usually indicates the presence of a streptococcal infection, such as acute rheumatic fever.

CMV IGG (Immunoglobulin G) and IGM (Immunoglobulin M) Antibodies

CMV IgG and IgM determine the levels of different types of antibodies (immunoglobulins) against cytomegalovirus. The presence of these antibodies may indicate exposure to or possible infection with cytomegalovirus.

EBV Panel (Epstein-Barr Virus)

An EBV panel determines various levels of antibodies (IgG and IgM) produced and directed against specific parts of the Epstein-Barr virus, such as viral capsid antigen (VCA) and Epstein-Barr virus nuclear antigen (EBNA). This can reveal whether the patient has had a recent or previous EBV infection. The specific tests in the panel are: EBV viral capsid antigen antibody IgM (EBV IgM), EBV viral capsid antigen antibody IgG (EBV IgG), EBV early antigen antibody (EBV EA), and EBV nuclear antigen antibody (EBNA).

FTA (Fluorescent Treponemal Antibody)

FTA is a serology test for syphilis.

HB$_s$AG (Hepatitis B Surface Antigen)

HB$_s$Ag is a serum study undertaken to identify the presence of hepatitis B in the blood.

Acute Hepatitis Panel

HAAb IgM, HB$_c$Ab IgM, HB$_s$Ag, HepC Ab

HIV-1 (Human Immunodeficiency Virus) Antibody Test

The HIV-1 antibody test uses oral mucosal transudate (OMT), a serum-derived fluid that enters saliva from the gingival crevice and across oral mucosal surfaces. This test is performed to screen for HIV. Additional tests (Western Blot or P24Ag) may be used for verification. A signed consent by the patient is required before HIV testing is conducted.

H pylori AB (Helicobacter pylori)

This is a test for the presence of antibodies against the bacterium *Helicobacter pylori,* which is implicated in the formation of gastric ulcers.

Heterophile Agglutination Test

A heterophile agglutination test is a diagnostic study for infectious mononucleosis.

RA (Rheumatoid Arthritis) Factor

An RA factor is a specific test for rheumatoid arthritis.

RPR (Rapid Plasma Reagin) Test

RPR tests are performed on blood and are screening tests for syphilis.

Method of Performing Immunologic Assays

Many physicians will specify which method they prefer the serology division to use in performing this test. The method by which the physician would like a test performed may be included in the physician's order.

ELISA (Enzyme-linked Immunosorbent Assay)

ELISA tests serum or plasma for antibodies and is widely used in the diagnosis of HIV and chlamydia. Also may be called EIA (enzyme immunoassay).

RIA (Radioimmunoassay)

RIA tests serum or plasma for antibodies with the use of radio-immune reagents.

FIA (Fluorescent Immunoassay)

FIA tests serum or plasma for antibodies with the use of fluorescent reagents.

COMP FIX (Complement Fixation) or Complement Fixation Titers

Complement fixation titers are done to detect various viral, fungal, and parasitic diseases.

PCR (Polymerase Chain Reaction) or RT-PCR (Real-time Polymerase Chain Reaction)

Polymerase chain reaction is a method by which relatively large quantities of DNA or RNA (nuclear material) may be produced from small amounts of original material. This test may be sensitive enough to detect very minute levels of antigen or antibody.

TITER

A titer is a measure of an antibody level. If positive, the level of antibody present is expressed as a ratio that indicates the dilution achieved before antibodies are undetectable. An example of a low titer is 1:8; an example of a high titer is 1:2048.

Refer to Appendix F for other tests performed in the microbiology and serology divisions. ∎

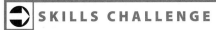

SKILLS CHALLENGE

To practice transcribing serology orders, complete Activity 14-8 in the *Skills Practice Manual*.

Blood Bank

The blood bank, which is usually a part of the clinical laboratory, has the responsibilities of typing and crossmatching patient blood, obtaining blood for transfusions, storing blood and blood components, and keeping records of transfusions and blood donors.

Before whole blood, packed cells, and some other blood components are administered, the patient must undergo a **type and crossmatch**. This is a test that determines the patient's blood type and compatibility. *The four major blood groups are A, B, AB, and O.*

- Patients with type A blood may receive transfusions of types A and O.
- Patients with type B may receive types B and O.
- Patients with type AB may receive types A, B, AB, and O.
- Patients with type O may receive only type O blood transfusions.

This laboratory division also performs several other blood studies, including Coombs' tests. DAT (the direct antiglobulin test) is a synonym for the Coombs' test. In a direct Coombs' test, a positive result is found in hemolytic disease of the newborn, hemolytic transfusion reactions, and acquired hemolytic anemia. The indirect Coombs' test detects the presence of antibodies to red blood cell antigens. This test is valuable in detecting the presence of anti-Rh antibodies in the serum of a pregnant woman before delivery.

✎ TAKE NOTE

An order for transfusion of whole blood, packed red blood cells, and some other blood components automatically indicates that blood will be typed and crossmatched.

Because the transfusion of blood and blood components is a treatment administered by nursing personnel, additional information on various types of blood transfusions (autologous, donor directed, and autotransfusion) is provided in Chapter 11.

Specimen

A specimen of blood is used for type and crossmatch.

Fasting

Fasting is not required for this procedure.

Communication with the Laboratory

Blood bank orders are requisitioned via computer or by completion of a downtime requisition form (Fig. 14-9). The number of units to be given and the names of the blood components are items that are included on this requisition. A blood transfusion consent must be signed before blood or blood products are administered. The patient also may sign a refusal of blood transfusion form.

✓ DOCTORS' ORDERS FOR BLOOD BANK

Listed below are examples of doctors' orders for blood component administration: (Refer to Chapter 11, p. 194, for examples of blood, blood components, and plasma substitutes.)

- T&C for 2 U packed cells
- Packed cells, 1 U (need type and crossmatching)

Doctor ordering _____	☐ Stat
Today's date _____	☐ Routine
Collection date _____ Time _____	
Collected by _____	
Requested by _____	

Blood Bank

☐ Routine   ☐ ASAP   ☐ Stat   ☐ For Hold

Date of surgery _____ Date of transfusion _____

Autologous blood? yes ____ no ____	☐ Whole blood	# of Units ____
Donor specific? yes ____ no ____	☐ Packed cells	# of Units ____
☐ Type and X-match	☐ Washed cells	# of Units ____
☐ Type and screen	☐ Frozen cells	# of Units ____
	☐ Fresh frozen plasma	# of Units ____
☐ Coombs' test	☐ Platelet concentrate	# of Units ____
☐ Other _____	☐ Cryoprecipitate	# of Units ____
	☐ Other _____	

Comments _____
_____
_____

Revised 3/11/03

Figure 14-9 Downtime requisition for blood bank.

- Plasma, 3 U stat
- Give washed cells 1 U (need type and crossmatching)
- Cryoprecipitate 1 U
- Give 2 U of platelets (no crossmatching needed, but donor plasma and recipient RBCs should be ABO compatible)
- Normal serum albumin 5% (no crossmatching)
- T&C 6 U pc—hold for surgery in AM ■

✎ TAKE NOTE

A blood transfusion consent must be signed before blood or blood products are administered. The patient also may sign a refusal of blood transfusion form.

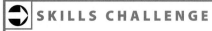 SKILLS CHALLENGE

To practice transcribing blood bank orders, complete Activity 14-9 in the *Skills Practice Manual*.

Urinalysis

The urinalysis division of the laboratory studies urine specimens for color, clarity, pH (degree of acidity or alkalinity), specific gravity (degree of concentration), protein (albumin), glucose (sugar), blood, bilirubin, and urobilinogen. Sediment is viewed microscopically for organisms, intact cells, and crystals.

Specimen

Urine is the specimen that is used for this test; however, the doctor may indicate that the nursing staff should follow a special procedure to obtain the specimen.

Procedures for Obtaining Urine Specimens:
- Voided urine specimen: The patient voids into a clean container.
- **Clean catch**, or midstream, urine specimen: The nursing staff uses a special cleansing technique to obtain this type of specimen.
- Catheterized urine specimen: This specimen is sterile and is obtained by catheterizing the patient. This procedure is usually done for culture and sensitivity testing, which is performed by microbiology.

Urine specimens that are collected at an unspecified time are called **random specimens**. However, the preferred collection time for a urine specimen is early morning upon rising.

Fasting

Fasting is not required for a urinalysis.

Communication With the Laboratory

Orders for urinalysis are entered into the computer or on a downtime requisition form (see Fig. 14-4) is used. Once again, the requisition is held on the nursing unit until the specimen has been collected, or the order is entered when the specimen has been obtained. The labeled specimen with the requisition or computer printout is sent to the laboratory.

DOCTORS' ORDERS FOR URINALYSIS

Listed below are examples of doctors' orders for urinalysis:

- Cath UA
- Clean catch UA
- **Dipstick urine** for ketones
- UA today
- **Urine reflex** (urine is tested in the laboratory; if certain parameters are met, the specimen is sent to microbiology to be cultured)

A urine specimen is sent to the laboratory. All regular urinalysis studies are performed, except the specimen is not examined microscopically.

 TAKE NOTE

Points to Remember When Ordering Laboratory Studies
- Determine whether the test ordered is a POCT, or whether the patient must be sent to the laboratory.
- All tests ordered require a specimen.
- Each specimen sent to the lab from the nursing unit requires a requisition and must be accurately labeled with patient ID label, and with the date, time, and initials of the person who collected the specimen written on the label.
- Include the date and time of collection on the requisition, as well as the name of the person who collected the specimens.
- Order tests as efficiently as possible to avoid the necessity for the patient to be redrawn (e.g., routines with stats).
- Communicate stat laboratory tests immediately to the lab and/or nursing personnel, and include all pertinent information.

SKILLS CHALLENGE

To practice transcribing urinalysis/urine chemistry orders, complete Activity 14-10 in the *Skills Practice Manual*.

The following tests may be sent to several of the laboratory departments for testing. ■

Studies Performed on Pleural Fluid

Studies are performed on pleural fluid to determine the cause and nature of pleural effusion, including hypertension, congestive heart failure (CHF), cirrhosis, infection, and neoplasms.

Specimen

Pleural fluid is obtained when the doctor performs a **thoracentesis**. The patient must sign a consent form for this procedure.

Fasting

Fasting is not required for tests performed on pleural fluid.

Communication With the Laboratory

The doctor orders tests to be done on the specimen, and the HUC enters the orders into the computer or completes a downtime requisition (see Fig. 14-8). As with any nonretrievable specimen obtained by invasive procedures, it should be transported to the laboratory immediately and should not be sent through a pneumatic tube system.

 DOCTORS' ORDERS FOR PLEURAL FLUID

Below are listed examples of doctors' orders for tests performed on pleural fluid:

- Thoracentesis, pleural fluid to lab for LDH, glucose, and amylase. CI: Cancer
- Pleural fluid for cell count, diff
- Pleural fluid for C&S ■

Studies Performed on Cerebrospinal Fluid

Studies are performed on cerebrospinal fluid to identify various brain diseases or injuries.

Specimen

Cerebrospinal fluid (CSF) is obtained when the doctor performs a lumbar puncture. The patient must sign a consent form before this procedure can be performed.

Fasting

Fasting is not required for tests performed on CSF.

Communication With the Laboratory

The doctor orders tests to be done on each specimen—possibly three or four. The HUC enters the respective tests into the computer or completes a requisition form. The doctor indicates in the orders the tube that should be used for each test (usually three or four tubes). The HUC enters this information into the computer or writes it on the requisition. It is sometimes the HUC's responsibility to transport these specimens to the laboratory. It is important to transport CSF specimens to the laboratory immediately. Because they are difficult to obtain and gathering them again would cause the patient further pain, never send the specimens via pneumatic tube.

 DOCTORS' ORDERS FOR CEREBROSPINAL FLUID

Below are listed examples of doctors' orders performed on CSF:

- Lumbar puncture, fluid to lab for cell count and diff
- CSF for serology
- CSF to lab for tube 1—cell count, protein, and glucose; tube 2—AFB and fungal culture; tube 3—Gram stain ■

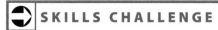

SKILLS CHALLENGE

To practice transcribing cerebrospinal fluid orders, complete Activity 14-11 in the *Skills Practice Manual*.

Pathology

Pathology is the study of the nature and cause of disease as seen in body changes. Histology and cytology are subdivisions of the pathology department. A pathologist is in charge of the pathology department.

Histology is the study of the microscopic structure of tissue. Cytology is the study of cells obtained from body tissues and fluids to determine cell type and to detect cancer or a precancerous condition.

Specimen

Organs, tissue, cells, and body fluids obtained from biopsies, centeses, **sternal punctures**, lumbar punctures, surgeries, and autopsies are studied in the pathology department. A **Pap**

smear is a staining method developed by Dr. George Nicolas Papanicolaou that can be performed on various types of specimens to identify the presence of cancer. However, cells from the cervix are the most frequently studied specimens (cervical smear). During a pelvic examination, the doctor may remove tissue or cells from the cervix for study.

RECORDING LABORATORY RESULTS

The results of laboratory tests are a valuable tool for the doctor in the diagnosis and treatment of patients; therefore, test result values are often communicated to the doctor before the computer report can be placed on the patient's chart. Stat and/or abnormal laboratory test results are communicated verbally or by telephone to the doctor by the HUC or nurse. Also, the doctor may request on the doctor's order sheet that laboratory test results be communicated to him by telephone immediately upon their completion.

To verbally communicate laboratory results, laboratory personnel call the HUC on the nursing unit, who records results on a telephone laboratory report sheet (Fig. 14-10). Laboratory

---

TELEPHONED LABORATORY RESULTS

Patient's name _____ Report called by _____

Room number _____ Report taken by _____

Date _____ Time _____

HEMATOLOGY	CHEMISTRY	URINE
RBC _____	GLUCOSE	COLOR _____
Hgb _____	Random _____	APPEARANCE _____
Hct _____	FBS _____	PH _____
WBC _____	E'LYTES	SP. GRAVITY _____
lymphs _____	Na _____	ACETONE _____
monos _____	K _____	GLUCOSE _____
neutros _____	Cl _____	BACTERIA _____
eos _____	CO_2 _____	WBC _____
basos _____	CARDIAC STUDIES	RBC _____
PLATELETS _____	SGOT _____	CASTS _____
RETICS _____	LDH _____	OCCULT BLOOD _____
SED RATE _____	CPK _____	OTHER
OTHER	BNP _____	
	Troponin _____	
	CALCIUM _____	
	PHOS _____	
	BUN _____	
	CREATININE _____	
	OTHER _____	

COAGULATION

BLEEDING TIME _____

COAGULATION TIME _____

PROTIME _____

  Patient _____

  Control _____

  % _____

PT

  Patient _____

  Control _____

  INR _____

PTT _____

TELEPHONED BLOOD GAS REPORT

Patient's name _____

Room number _____

Date _____ Time _____

Report called by _____

Report taken by _____

O_2 CONCENTRATION _____

O_2 TENSION _____

CO_2 TENSION _____

PH _____

ACT BICARB _____

BASE EXCESS _____

O_2 SAT _____

Figure 14-10 Telephoned laboratory test results form.

```
○                                                                                  ○
○              COLLEGE HOSPITAL                            PAGE 1                   ○
         A. MELZER MD & D. RUDOLPH MD PATHOLOGISTS
○                                                                                  ○
                      *** RESULT INQUIRY ***
○    PATIENT NAME: WADSWORTH, JENNIFER          PATIENT #: 437592                   ○
      LOC: 4W      AGE: 20    SEX: F    ADM PHY: PAYNE, IMA     ADM DATE: 10/9/04
○    --------------------------------------------------------------------------    ○
      CHEMISTRY PANEL          RESULT          UNITS       REFERENCE VALUES
○     ---------------          ----------      -------     ----------------        ○
         SODIUM             L     134          MMOL/L      (135-145       )
○        POTASSIUM          H     5.4          MMOL/L      (3.6-5.0       )         ○
         CHLORIDE                 96           MMOL/L      (96-110        )
○        CO2                      29           MMOL/L      (21-31         )         ○
         GLUCOSE                  103          MG/DL       (70-110        )
○        BUN                H     33           MG/DL       (6-20          )         ○
         CREATININE               1.2          MG/DL       (0.5-1.2       )
○        CALCIUM                  10.4         MG/DL       (8.5-10.5      )         ○
         URIC ACID               4.8          MG/DL       (3.9-7.8       )
○        CHOLESTEROL              166          MG/DL       (140-200       )         ○
         T. BILIRUBIN             1.0          MG/DL       (0.0-1.2       )
○        T. PROTEIN               6.9          G/DL        (6.1-8.0       )         ○
         ALBUMIN            L     2.4          G/DL        (3.5-4.8       )
○        ALK PHOS           H     132          U/L         (30-107        )         ○
         GGTP               H     195          U/L         (8-69          )
○        ALT (SGPT)               29           U/L         (0-55          )         ○
         LDH                H     398          U/L         (94-172        )
○        AST (SGOT)               29           U/L         (8-42          )         ○
         CPK                L     27           U/L         (38-224        )
○        TRIGLYCERIDES            154          MG/DL       (30-64         )         ○
         PHOSPHORUS               3.1          MG/DL       (2.4-4.3       )
○                                                                                  ○
      COMPLETE BLOOD COUNT
○     --------------------                                                         ○
         WHITE BLOOD CELL COUNT  H   14.9      X10^3       (4.8-10.8      )
○        RED BLOOD CELL COUNT    L   4.29      X10^6       (4.7-6.10      )         ○
         HEMOGLOBIN          L     12.6        G/DL        (14.0-18.0     )
○        HEMATOCRIT          L     37.3        %           (42.0-52.0     )         ○
         MCV                      87.0         U3          (80-94         )
○        MCH                      29.4         PG          (27-32         )         ○
         MCHC                     33.8         %           (33-37         )
○        RDW                 H     17.6        %           (11.5-14.5     )         ○
         POLYSEGMENTED NEUTROPHIL H  82        %           (50-70         )
○        BAND                     6            %           (0-10          )         ○
         LYMPHOCYTE          L     4           %           (20-40         )
○        MONOCYTE                 1            %           (0-10          )         ○
         METAMYELOCYTE       H     6           %           (0             )
○        ATYPICAL LYMPHOCYTE H     1           %           (0             )         ○
         PLATELET ESTIMATE        ADEQ
○        RBC MORPHOLOGY           SLT ANISO                                        ○
                                  SLT POLYC
○        PLATELET COUNT           220          X1000       (130-400       )        ○
○                                                                                  ○
```

Figure 14-11 Laboratory results printout.

results also may be accessed via computer and printed by the HUC. Results from an outside laboratory may be faxed to the nursing unit. Printed results also include the **reference range**, or range of normal values, for each laboratory test (Fig. 14-11). The HUC should report values to the patient's nurse, who may request that the results to be called in to the doctor's office. Although the task may appear simple to perform, it demands great responsibility, because the doctor may prescribe treatment according to the laboratory values conveyed. Consider for a moment what the consequences could be should the value be recorded inaccurately. To avoid errors, the HUC should always read the laboratory values they have recorded back to the person in the laboratory. Always have the person taking information in the doctor's office repeat recorded values back to you. The written report should be placed in the patient's chart in a timely manner. Accuracy in selection of the correct patient's chart and of the appropriate location in the chart is very important.

SKILLS CHALLENGE

For practice transcribing the following types of orders, complete the following activities in the *Skills Practice Manual*:

- To practice transcribing a review set of laboratory orders, complete Activity 14-12.
- To practice transcribing a review set of doctors' orders, complete Activity 14-13.
- To practice recording telephoned messages, complete Activity 14-15.

SKILLS CHALLENGE

To practice recording telephoned laboratory results, complete Activity 14-16 in the *Skills Practice Manual.*

KEY CONCEPTS

Laboratory studies are very useful in facilitating patient diagnosis and evaluation of treatment. Accuracy in ordering tests and sending specimens is of utmost importance because an error could result in a delay in diagnosis and/or treatment. It is imperative that all specimens are properly labeled according to hospital policy and sent or delivered to the laboratory in a timely manner.

One of the challenges for an HUC is to become familiar with the particular hospital's process of requisitioning laboratory orders. Become familiar with the various laboratory screens on the computer. It may be necessary to identify the division in which a test is performed before completing the correct requisition or entering the order into the computer. This information is also helpful in telephone communication when one is clarifying orders or requesting results. Most hospital units have a written laboratory procedure manual. If this is not the case, call the hospital laboratory Help Desk to have your questions answered.

REVIEW QUESTIONS

1. List two general purposes of laboratory studies.

a. _____

b. _____

2. State the purpose of the following divisions of the laboratory.

a. microbiology: _____

b. chemistry: _____

c. hematology: _____

3. Name three methods used by the nursing staff to collect urine specimens.

a. _____

b. _____

c. _____

4. List five common types of specimens collected for laboratory study.

a. _____

b. _____

c. _____

d. _____

e. _____

5. What is the procedure for ordering stat blood tests from the laboratory?

_____

6. What are the HUC's responsibilities for an order for a 2-hr PP BS?

_____

7. What is the difference between a stat order and a routine laboratory order?

_____

8. List five procedures that require consent forms and are performed by the doctor to obtain specimens for study.

a. _____

b. _____

c. _____

d. _____

e. _____

9. What procedure must be performed before some blood components, such as packed red cells, can be ordered for a patient for a transfusion?

_____

10. What is the HUC's responsibility regarding specimens collected on the unit to be sent to or delivered to the laboratory?

_____

11. What four laboratory studies make up the test called _electrolytes?_

a. _____

b. _____

c. _____

d. _____

12. Write the abbreviations for two cardiac chemistry studies.

a. _____

b. _____

13. Name six chemistry studies.

a. _____

b. _____

c. _____

d. _____

e. _____

f. _____

14. Name six hematology studies.

a. _____

b. _____

c. _____

d. _____

e. _____

f. _____

15. Name six microbiology studies.

a. _____

b. _____

c. _____

d. _____

e. _____

f. _____

16. Explain the difference between fasting and NPO.

_____

17. Define the following terms.

a. biopsy: _____

b. clean catch: _____

c. fasting: _____

d. lumbar puncture: _____

e. midstream: _____

f. occult blood: _____

g. postprandial: _____

h. sputum: _____

i. sternal puncture: _____

j. urinalysis: _____

k. voided specimen: _____

l. dipstick urine: _____

18. In the space provided, write in the laboratory division that performs each of the following tests:

a. FBS: _____

b. urine for C&S: _____

c. lytes: _____

d. CBC: _____

e. BMP: _____

f. APTT: _____

g. 1 unit of PC: _____

h. Hct & Hgb: _____

i. RPR: _____

j. triglycerides: _____

k. RA factor: _____

l. sputum for AFB: _____

m. RBC indices: _____

n. T3: _____

o. GTT: _____

p. Retics: _____

q. WBC & diff: _____

r. 2-hr PP BS: _____

s. PT: _____

t. protein electrophoresis: _____

u. T&C: _____

v. Coombs' test: _____

w. Na: _____

x. stool for O&P: _____

y. BNP: _____

z. CMP: _____

19. List three drugs for which a peak-and-trough is ordered to monitor levels.

a. _____

b. _____

c. _____

20. How may errors be avoided in recording of telephoned laboratory results?

_____

21. Rewrite the following doctors' orders using symbols and abbreviations. Or, to practice writing doctors' orders, have someone read the orders to you while you record them. Again, practice using symbols and abbreviations.

a. complete blood count and electrolytes every morning

_____

b. hemoglobin and hematocrit immediately

_____

c. type and crossmatch for six units of packed (red blood) cells—hold for surgery in the morning

_____

d. sputum specimen for culture and sensitivity and acid-fast bacillus

_____

e. lumbar puncture for cerebrospinal fluid: on tube number one, do protein and glucose levels; on tube number two, do cultures for cytomegalovirus and fungus; on tube number three, do an acid-fast bacillus stain

_____

f. comprehensive metabolic panel tomorrow morning

_____

THINK ABOUT...

1. Discuss possible consequences of labeling a laboratory specimen with the wrong patient's label.
2. Discuss the importance of washing your hands after handling laboratory specimens (even bagged specimens).
3. Discuss the importance of reading all of the doctors' orders before ordering laboratory tests.

CHAPTER 15

Diagnostic Imaging Orders

OUTLINE

CHAPTER OBJECTIVES

Upon completion of this chapter, you will be able to:

1. Define the terms in the vocabulary list.
2. Write the meaning of each abbreviation in the Abbreviations list.
3. Explain the benefits of picture archiving and communication systems for the patient and the doctor.
4. Name five patient positions that may be included in an X-ray order.
5. Identify X-ray orders that do not require preparation and X-ray orders that require preparation.
6. Name five X-ray orders that would require a signed patient consent form.
7. Prioritize provided diagnostic procedures ordered on the same patient.
8. Identify the appropriate division of diagnostic imaging that would perform provided procedures.
9. List ten special instructions about the patient that the health unit coordinator must include when ordering procedures from the diagnostic imaging department.
10. Explain why contrast media are used, and list types commonly used.
11. Explain how the health unit coordinator's responsibilities differ with the implementation of the electronic medical record and computer physician order entry versus use of the paper chart.
12. Explain the importance of following up on preparations required for diagnostic imaging procedures.

VOCABULARY

C-Arm A mobile fluoroscopy unit used in surgery or at the bedside

Cathartic An agent that causes evacuation of the bowel (laxative)

Clinical Indications Notations recorded when diagnostic imaging is ordered, to indicate the reason for doing the procedure

Computed Radiology Use of a digital imaging plate rather than film

Computed Tomography A radiographic process that uses ionizing radiation to create computerized images (scans) of body organs in sections or that can be coronal (referred to as a CT scan)

Contrast Media Substances (solids, liquids, or gases) used in diagnostic imaging procedures that permit the radiologist to distinguish between various body soft tissue structures; may be injected, swallowed, inhaled, or introduced by rectum

Fluoroscopy The direct observation of deep body structures made visible through the use of a viewing screen instead of film; contrast medium is required for this procedure

Magnetic Resonance Imaging A technique used to produce computer images (scans) of the interior of the body with the use of a powerful magnetic field and radiofrequency waves

Metastasis The process by which tumor cells spread to distant parts of the body

Modality A method of application or employment of any therapeutic agent, limited usually to physical agents and devices

Nuclear Medicine A technique that uses radioactive materials to examine anatomy and functional capacity of an organ

"On Call" Medication Medication prescribed by the doctor to be given before the diagnostic imaging procedure is performed; the department notifies the nursing unit of the time the medication is to be administered to the patient

Picture Archiving and Communication Systems Computers or networks dedicated to the storage, retrieval, distribution, and presentation of images. Full PACS handle images from various modalities, such as ultrasonography, magnetic resonance imaging, positron emission tomography, computed tomography, endoscopy, mammography, and digital radiography

Portable X-ray An X-ray taken by a mobile X-ray machine that is moved to the patient's bedside

Position Alignment of the body on the X-ray table that is favorable for taking the best view of the part of the body being imaged

Routine Preparation The standard preparation suggested by the radiologist to prepare the patient for a diagnostic imaging study

Scan An image produced with the use of a moving detector or a sweeping beam; image is produced by computed tomography, magnetic resonance imaging, nuclear medicine, and ultrasonography

Special Invasive X-ray Procedures Performed with the use of contrast media and under the direction of the radiologist or a surgeon with a radiologist present

Ultrasonography A technique that uses high-frequency sound waves to create an image (scan) of body organs (also may be referred to as sonography or echography)

ABBREVIATIONS

Abbreviation	Meaning	Example of Usage on a Doctor's Order Sheet
abd	abdomen	US of abd
AP	anteroposterior	chest AP & Lat
BE	barium enema	BE in AM
CI	clinical indications	BE-CI: tumor
CT	computed tomography	CT scan of abd
CXR	chest X-ray	CXR today
DSA	digital subtraction angiography	cerebral DSA
F/U	follow-up	F/U CXR in AM
Fx	fracture	X-ray CI: fx lt femur
GB	gallbladder	US of GB
GI	gastrointestinal	GI study in am
H/O	history of	CXR H/O chronic asthma
IVP	intravenous pyelogram	
IVU	intravenous urogram; synonymous with IVP	IVU CI: Kidney stones
KUB (also called a flat plate of abdomen)	kidneys, ureters, and bladder	KUB today

Abbreviation	Meaning	Example of Usage on a Doctor's Order Sheet
lat	lateral chest	PA & Lat today
LLQ	left lower quadrant	flat plate of abd att LLQ
LUQ	left upper quadrant	abd X-ray special attention to LUQ
L&S	liver and spleen	L&S scan tomorrow (nuclear medicine)
LS	lumbosacral	X-ray LS spine (X-ray)
Mets	metastasis	bone scan to determine mets
MRI	magnetic resonance imaging	MRI of brain
PA	posteroanterior	PA & lat chest X-ray
PACS	Picture Archiving and Communication System	The CXR may be viewed via PACS
PCXR	portable chest X-ray	PCXR stat
PET	positron emission tomography	PET scan tomorrow AM (nuclear medicine)
PTC or PTHC	percutaneous transhepatic cholangiography	PTC or PTHC tomorrow
RIS	radiology information system	X-ray report is available in RIS
RLQ	right lower quadrant	X-ray of abd: Compare c̄
RUQ	right upper quadrant	X-ray of 12/2/00: Check RUQ and RLQ
SBFT	small bowel follow-through	UGI c̄ SBFT
SNAT	suspected nonaccidental trauma	SNAT series CI: abuse
UGI	upper gastrointestinal	UGI p̄ IVU
US	ultrasound	US of GB

EXERCISE 1

Write the abbreviation for each term listed below.

1. intravenous pyelogram _____

2. right lower quadrant _____

3. kidneys, ureters, and bladder _____

4. barium enema _____

5. posteroanterior _____

6. upper gastrointestinal _____

7. lateral _____

8. lumbosacral _____

9. left upper quadrant   _____

10. anteroposterior   _____

11. gastrointestinal   _____

12. right upper quadrant   _____

13. computed tomography   _____

14. left lower quadrant   _____

15. gallbladder   _____

16. magnetic resonance imaging   _____

17. small bowel follow-through   _____

18. chest X-ray   _____

19. digital subtraction angiography   _____

20. portable chest X-ray   _____

21. percutaneous transhepatic cholangiography   _____

22. fracture   _____

23. history of   _____

24. follow-up   _____

25. clinical indications   _____

26. intravenous urogram   _____

27. ultrasound   _____

28. Picture Archiving and Communication System   _____

29. positron emission tomography   _____

30. liver and spleen   _____

31. radiology information system   _____

32. abdomen   _____

33. metastasis   _____

34. suspected nonaccidental trauma   _____

EXERCISE 2

The following is a list of orders for imaging procedures that may appear on patients' charts. Write the meaning of each underlined abbreviation.

1. BE tomorrow p̄ sigmoidoscopy

_____

2. Stat LS spine X-ray

_____

3. KUB this AM

_____

4. US for fetal age

_____

5. Abd X-ray c̄ attention to RLQ & LUQ

_____

6. IVU & UGI tomorrow. Check with radiologist for prep.

_____

7. CT of brain

_____

8. GI study c̄ barium swallow

_____

9. PA & lat chest now

_____

10. MRI of brain

_____

11. PCXR now

_____

12. UGI c̄ SBFT

_____

13. L & S scan in AM

_____

14. PET scan in AM

_____

15. CT c̄ DSA of head

_____

16. SNAT series CI: abuse

_____

COMMUNICATION WITH THE DIAGNOSTIC IMAGING DEPARTMENT

Many modalities, including radiography, nuclear medicine, ultrasound, **computed tomography (CT)**, and **magnetic resonance imaging (MRI)**, are included in the "diagnostic imaging department." Diagnostic imaging procedures are performed to diagnose conditions and/or diseases (or to rule them out) and to assist the doctor in determining treatment. Diagnostic imaging orders are communicated by the ordering step of transcription via computer or by completion of a downtime requisition form (Fig. 15-1). Because the patient usually is transported to the diagnostic imaging department for the procedure, it is important to indicate the mode of transportation—wheelchair or gurney (stretcher). The patient may be transported by the diagnostic imaging department staff, transport service, or nursing department staff.

✎ *TAKE NOTE*

When the electronic medical record (EMR) with the computer physician order entry (CPOE) is implemented, the physicians' orders are entered directly into the patient's electronic record, and the diagnostic imaging order is automatically sent to the diagnostic imaging department. The health unit coordinator (HUC) may have tasks to perform, such as coordinating scheduling, ordering special diets, and so forth. An icon may appear, indicating a HUC task, or it may signify a nurse request. The HUC will have to communicate with the nutritional care department (by e-mail or telephone) when ordering a diet for a patient who has completed a diagnostic procedure that required NPO status. *Some hospital nutritional care departments require that **all** diet orders be submitted in writing via computer.

A portable or mobile X-ray is an exception to the standard transportation procedure. A request for a portable X-ray requires the radiographer to take the portable equipment to the patient's room. A portable X-ray is ordered when movement might be detrimental to the patient's condition. A written order by the patient's physician is required for a portable X-ray.

When ordering the diagnostic procedure, indicate the following information about the patient:

a. reason for procedure (clinical indication)
b. transportation required
c. whether patient is receiving intravenous fluids
d. whether patient is receiving oxygen
e. whether patient needs isolation precautions
f. whether patient has a seizure disorder
g. if patient does not speak English
h. whether patient is diabetic
i. whether patient is sight or hearing impaired
j. whether patient is pregnant or pregnancy test results are pending

This information will assist personnel in the diagnostic imaging department to provide better care for the patient (see Fig. 15-1). The doctor may write the name of the radiologist who will perform an invasive procedure. The HUC should include this information when placing the order.

✎ *TAKE NOTE*

Clinical indications (the reason the doctor is ordering the procedure) must be recorded by the HUC when a diagnostic imaging procedure is ordered. Insurance companies require this information before they will provide reimbursement to health care facilities. Diagnostic imaging departments will not perform procedures until they have received the documented clinical indications.

✎ *TAKE NOTE*

Downtime requisitions are included in this chapter for learning purposes. The CD included in the *Skills Practice Manual* is a simulated hospital computer program that may be used as well.

✎ *TAKE NOTE*

A written order from the patient's physician is required to obtain a stat X-ray or a portable X-ray. The physician's original order for a routine X-ray cannot be changed to portable or stat for convenience, or because the original order was missed. If the nurse determines that the patient needs the X-ray stat or portable, the patient's physician would have to be called for a change to the original order.

BACKGROUND INFORMATION FOR RADIOLOGY

In 1895, Wilhelm Roentgen discovered a strange phenomenon that produced a photograph of the bones of his wife's hand. The exact mechanism for the production of these rays was unknown to Roentgen; therefore, he used the algebraic symbol for the unknown, *X*, to title his discovery.

X-ray studies performed in the radiology area of the diagnostic imaging department are carried out by a *radiographer*, a person with special education in the area of radiography. X-ray images are developed in the department and are interpreted by a *radiologist*, a doctor who is a specialist in this field. Some studies are done by observing the path of **contrast media** in the body by means of **fluoroscopy**. Physicians' orders do not always include the word "X-ray." For example, "Chest PA & Lat" indicates a chest X-ray that includes two views (posteroanterior and lateral). Some procedures scheduled in the radiology area must be carried out in specific sequence so that the contrast medium necessary for one procedure does not block the image of another.

PICTURE ARCHIVING AND COMMUNICATION SYSTEM

Picture archiving and communication systems (PACS) are computers or networks dedicated to the storage, retrieval, distribution, and presentation of images. Full PACS manage images from various modalities, such as ultrasonography, MRI, positron emission tomography, CT, endoscopy, mammography, and radiography (plain X-rays). PACS replace hard copy–based means of managing medical images, such

Doctor ordering _____

Date to be done _____ ☐ Stat ☐ Routine ☐ ASAP

Today's date _____ Requested by _____

| **Radiographic (X-ray) Procedures** |

Clinical indication _____

Transportation ☐ Portable ☐ Stretcher ☐ Wheelchair ☐ Ambulatory

O₂ ☐ Yes ☐ No   Diabetic ☐ Yes ☐ No   Hearing deficit ☐ Yes ☐ No

IV ☐ Yes ☐ No   Seizure disorder ☐ Yes ☐ No   Sight deficit ☐ Yes ☐ No

Isolation ☐ Yes ☐ No   Non-English speaking ☐ Yes ☐ No

Wirte out the entire doctor's order

Comments: _____

☐ Abdomen:_____

☐ Bone age study:_____

☐ Bone x-ray order:_____

☐ Chest order:_____

☐ IVP:_____

☐ KUB/flat plate of abdomen:_____

☐ KUB order:_____

☐ Mammogram:_____

☐ Sinus series order:_____

☐ SNAT series:_____

☐ Spine order:_____

☐ BE:_____

☐ SBFT:_____

☐ UGI:_____

☐ Write in order:_____

Figure 15-1   Downtime requisition for X-ray procedures.

as film archives. PACS provide off-site viewing and reporting (distance education, telediagnosis).

When a study has been reported by the radiologist, the PACS can mark it as read; this avoids needless double reading. Dictation of reports also can be integrated into a single system. The dictated recording is automatically sent to a transcriptionist workstation for typing; it also can be made available for access by physicians, avoiding typing delays for urgent results, or retained in cases of typing error. The report can be attached to the images and be viewable to the physician.

Physicians at various physical locations may access the same information simultaneously.

Global PACS networks enable images to be sent throughout the world. These systems provide growing cost and space advantages over film archives. PACS should interface with the existing hospital information systems (HIS) and radiology information system (RIS). An icon indicating a diagnostic medical image in a patient's medical record would allow the physician to view the image and the radiologist's report. Benefits for the doctor include faster results, ability to compare image versus a previous image (if applicable), ability to share with other physicians, and reduced risk of film loss. Benefits for the patient include reduction in treatment delays, reduced risk of film loss, and protection of confidentiality. An additional benefit is noted for the environment, in that X-ray photographic darkroom chemicals and toxins are eliminated from the process.

PATIENT POSITIONING

The doctor may wish an X-ray to be taken while the patient is placed in a specific **position** on the X-ray table or erect (e.g., chest studies) to allow the best view of the area to be exposed. The HUC must be careful to include all of the X-ray order without making any changes, and to be absolutely accurate when transcribing such orders. For example, the HUC should not write AP (anteroposterior) when the order calls for PA (posteroanterior) positioning. The wrong abbreviation can cause the radiographer to film a different view, which may obscure an abnormality.

Following is a list of the positions used most frequently in the writing of X-ray orders:

- *AP position:* This view may be taken while the patient is standing or lying on the back (supine); the machine is placed in front of the patient.
- *PA position:* This view may be taken while the patient is standing or lying on the stomach (prone) with the X-ray machine aimed at the patient's back.
- *Lateral position:* This view is taken with the patient standing or lying on the side.
- *Oblique position:* This picture is taken with the patient standing or lying halfway on the side in the AP or the PA position.
- *Decubitus position:* In this view, the patient is lying on the side with the X-ray beam positioned horizontally.

INFORMED CONSENT FORMS

Diagnostic imaging procedures that are invasive and those that require the injection of contrast medium are not performed until the patient has been informed of the procedure, risks, alternatives, outcomes, and so forth, and has signed a consent form. It is the responsibility of the HUC to prepare the consent form for the patient's signature. **Special invasive X-ray procedures** require signed consent because iodinated contrast media is used. Other diagnostic imaging procedures that require a consent form may vary among health care facilities. Maintaining a list of those requiring a signed consent form would assist the HUC in recalling which procedures require them.

✐ TAKE NOTE

Examples of procedures performed in each of the modalities of diagnostic imaging are included in this chapter. They are too numerous to list, but lists are a good representation of what procedures are performed in each **modality.**

RADIOGRAPHIC (X-RAY) PROCEDURES

X-rays That Do Not Require Preparation

X-rays can penetrate solid material, such as bone; this in turn produces a shadow that is recorded on film. Procedures that require the filming of bone structures or that are ordered to determine the position of other organs in relation to these structures can be performed by qualified radiology personnel without the need for preparation for the procedure (Fig. 15-2).

Listed below are X-ray studies as they commonly are written on a doctors' order sheet.

✓ DOCTORS' ORDERS FOR X-RAYS THAT DO NOT REQUIRE PREPARATION

Sinus Series Cl: Sinusitis

X-ray of the paranasal sinus structures.

Purpose: Used to identify infection, trauma, or disease in the paranasal sinuses.

PA and Lat Chest Cl: Pneumonia

Chest X-ray (Frequently, *X-ray* is not written on the order because some terms in the order are recognized as directions used only in radiography. The terms *PA* and *lat* indicate the angles from which the doctor wishes the film to be taken.)

Purpose: Used to diagnose or assess patients with pneumonia, pneumothorax, or atelectasis, or to check for infiltrates. A chest X-ray also is used to determine the size and position of the heart or for placement of invasive lines or tubes.

SNAT Series Cl: Evaluate for Child Abuse

Purpose: X-ray of long bones, skull, and spinal column to evaluate for hairline fractures and untreated fractures to identify child or adult abuse.

Bone Age Study Cl: FTT (Failure to Thrive)

Purpose: An X-ray of the wrist of an infant to evaluate the child's growth.

Communication and Implementation of Diagnostic Imaging

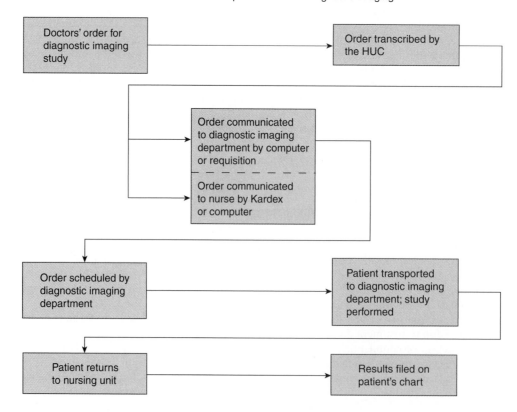

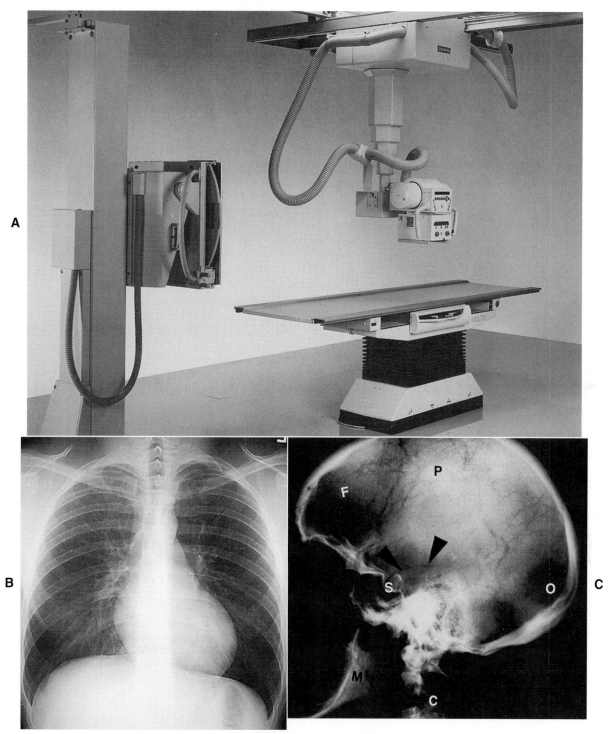

Figure 15-2 A, Radiographic table with chest unit (From Ballinger PW, Frank ED: *Merrill's atlas of radiographic positions and radiologic procedures,* ed 10, St. Louis, 2003, Mosby.). **B,** Chest X-ray. (From Bontrager KL, Lampignano JP: *Textbook of radiographic positioning and related anatomy,* ed 6, St. Louis, 2005, Mosby.). **C,** Skull X-ray, lateral view. Pointers indicate fracture line in temporal bone. (C, cervical vertebra; F, frontal bone; M, mandible; O, occipital bone; P, parietal bone; S, sella turcica.) (From Pagana KD, Pagana TJ: *Diagnostic testing and nursing implications: a case study approach,* ed 4, St. Louis, 1994, Mosby.).

LS Spine Series CI: Possible Fracture

X-ray of the lumbosacral area of the spine.

Purpose: Used to detect and evaluate abnormalities of the lumbosacral region.

Mammogram CI: Lump 10 Degrees Lt Breast

X-ray of the breast.

Purpose: Used to detect cancer or cysts in the soft tissue of the breast.

X-ray of the Tibia With Close Attention to the Distal Portion CI: Fracture

X-ray of the bone in the patient's lower leg. *Distal* indicates that the radiologist is to observe a particular portion of the bone. Remember to include the entire order on the requisition.

Purpose: Used to identify fractures.

KUB (also called a flat plate of abd) CI: General Survey of the Abd

X-ray of the abdomen.

Purpose: Used to detect and evaluate any abnormalities in the abdomen.

Portable Film of Rt Femur CI: Fx

A radiographer takes a portable X-ray machine to the patient's bedside to film the right upper leg of the patient. It is important for the HUC to write *portable* on the requisition form.

Purpose: Used to identify fractures.

Postreduction Study of the Lt Forearm

X-ray of the left forearm.

Purpose: Used to evaluate the alignment of a fracture after intervention.

AP and Lat Rt Hip CI: Postop Eval of Hip Replacement

X-ray of the right hip (*AP* and *lat* indicate the angles from which the doctor wishes the film to be taken).

Purpose: Used postoperatively to evaluate prosthetic replacement of the hip. Done at the bedside. ■

 SKILLS CHALLENGE

To practice transcribing radiology (X-ray) orders that require no preparation, complete Activity 15-1 in the *Skills Practice Manual.*

X-rays That Require Preparation and Contrast Media

When an X-ray is created, images of varying density appear on the exposed image. Differences in density are due to the degree of absorption offered by different tissues and air to the radiation. It is easy to differentiate bony structures because the bones offer resistance and therefore appear light on the image. The lungs, however, which contain air, do not offer much resistance to radiation and appear black on the image. Certain organs and blood vessels within the body are difficult for the radiologist to see because there is little difference in density between them and their surrounding parts. To increase the contrast, it is necessary for a *contrast medium* to be given to the patient.

Contrast media consist of organic iodine compounds, barium preparations, air, water, gas, and, with nuclear medicine procedures, radiopharmaceuticals. Contrast media may be injected or taken into the body by mouth, inhalation, or rectum. Contraindications to the use of iodine compounds include allergy to shellfish and previous reactions to iodinated studies. For contrast medium to prove most effective, the patient must be prepared for the procedure before it is scheduled. This process is known as a **routine preparation,** and the routine most often is established by the diagnostic imaging department.

The attending doctor may change the routine preparation if the patient's condition warrants. Specific changes to the routine preparation must be written on the doctors' order sheet by the patient's doctor. Sometimes, a contrast medium used for one procedure may interfere with results obtained in another scheduled procedure. Therefore, if multiple X-ray procedures are ordered, proper sequencing is necessary to obtain clear results. Sequencing is outlined by the diagnostic imaging department and may vary among hospitals.

Sequencing

Following are typical guidelines for scheduling X-ray studies:

1. X-ray studies of the lower spine and pelvis should be ordered first, before a barium enema or an upper gastrointestinal study is done. The presence of barium in specific parts of the body may obscure the portion of the body that is being studied.
2. Abdominal studies that use ultrasound or CT should precede studies that use barium.
3. Liver and bone scans and nuclear medicine studies may conflict with barium studies and should be done first.
4. Three X-ray studies that require contrast media frequently are ordered at the same time for diagnostic reasons. Only one or sometimes two can be done on the same day; thus, studies may have to be scheduled 3 or more days in advance. The order of scheduling is listed below:
   a. Intravenous urogram (IVU)
   b. Barium enema (BE)
   c. Upper gastrointestinal (UGI) or UGI and small bowel follow-through (SBFT)

✐ TAKE NOTE

When transcribing diagnostic imaging orders, the HUC should do the following:

1. Record the clinical indication when entering the order.
2. Record the necessary mode of transportation when entering the order.
3. Record necessary patient information when entering the order.
4. Check whether a consent form is necessary; if so, prepare one for signature.
5. Check whether patient preparation is required; if so, communicate this to the appropriate nursing personnel.
6. Check whether scheduling is required; if so, schedule the procedure for the proper day and/or time.

Accuracy in performing these steps is vital for reaching the expected outcome.

Preparation Procedure

To visualize internal organs with the use of contrast media, preparation usually is required. Most of the preparation is done by the nursing staff, and preparatory steps may begin the day before the X-ray study is scheduled.

Following are examples of doctors' orders for X-rays that require the patient to have some type of preparation. Each procedure and preparation is explained to help establish its relationship to the others and to clarify the role of a HUC.

Many hospitals have a computer system that automatically prints out the routine preparation when a procedure is entered. Some hospitals have preparation cards, that is, cards that list the tasks to be done to prepare the patient for the X-ray. When a patient is scheduled for one of the X-rays that require preparation, the computer printout or the preparation card usually is placed in the patient's Kardex form holder to remind the nursing staff of the tasks they need to perform.

Note: Preparation procedures may vary among hospitals.

✓ DOCTORS' ORDERS FOR X-RAYS THAT REQUIRE PREPARATION AND CONTRAST

Media

BE CI: Lesion of the Colon

Visualization of the large intestine (Fig. 15-3). The patient is given an enema with a barium contrast medium in the diagnostic imaging department.

Purpose: Used to identify diseases of the large intestine such as diverticula, cancer, or ulcerative colitis.

Patient Preparation:
• Cathartic PM & AM before the procedure
• Low-residue diet (jello, simple broths) 8 to 12 hours before the examination
• NPO 2400 hours

Transcribing the order: In addition to transcribing the order for a barium enema, the HUC would initiate diet changes and alert the nurse about any medications that are to be given in preparation. The doctor may wish to order an air contrast barium enema, which requires the same preparation as a barium enema but uses air as well as barium for the contrast medium.

IVU (synonymous with IVP; IVU is becoming the more common usage) CI: Ureterolithiasis

A procedure performed to outline the kidney, particularly the renal pelvis, ureters, and urinary bladder (Fig. 15-4). Contrast medium is established by injecting an iodinated contrast medium into the patient's vein. The injection takes place after the patient is transported to the diagnostic imaging department.

Purpose: Used to determine the size, location, and function of the kidneys, ureters, and bladder, and to identify the presence of abnormalities such as tumors or strictures.

AN EXAMPLE OF A PREPARATION FOR A BE

Barium Enema
Citrate of Magnesia 1 bottle 2 PM on day before examination
Fleets enema HS day before examination, & repeat @ 6 AM on day of examination
NPO 2400 hours

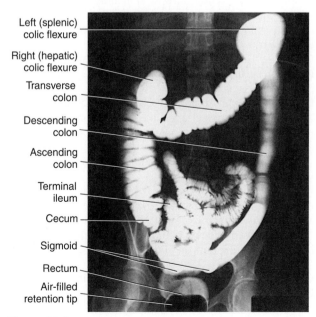

Figure 15-3 Barium enema showing contrast media (barium) filling the intestines. (From Ballinger PW, Frank ED: *Merrill's atlas of radiographic positions and radiologic procedures,* ed 10, St. Louis, 2003, Mosby.)

Labels on Figure 15-3:
- Left (splenic) colic flexure
- Right (hepatic) colic flexure
- Transverse colon
- Descending colon
- Ascending colon
- Terminal ileum
- Cecum
- Sigmoid
- Rectum
- Air-filled retention tip

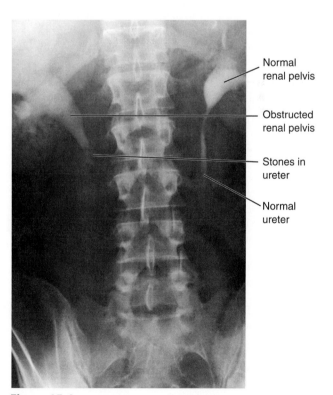

Figure 15-4 Intravenous urogram (IVU) showing a distended urinary collecting system obstructed by a stone in the right ureter *(left side of figure).* The left collecting system is normal in size and is unobstructed (intravenous pyelogram [IVP] and IVU are the same; IVU is used most commonly). (From Pagana KD, Pagana TJ: *Mosby's manual of diagnostic and laboratory tests,* ed 3, St. Louis, 2006, Mosby.)

Labels on Figure 15-4:
- Normal renal pelvis
- Obstructed renal pelvis
- Stones in ureter
- Normal ureter

OVERVIEW OF RADIOLOGY

X-rays are a form of electromagnetic radiation, similar to visible light. A computer or a special film is used to record the images that are created.

Examples of Radiology Procedures That Do Not Require Preparation or Contrast Media

Procedure	Purpose
Skeletal X-rays	To diagnose abnormalities, disease, and fractures of bones
Chest PA & LAT	To evaluate for surgery and diagnose obstructions, abnormalities, and disease
KUB	To diagnose abnormalities, obstructions, and disease within the abdomen
SNAT series	To idenfity abuse (child or adult)
Bone age study	To assess development/growth of child

Examples of Radiology Procedures That Do Require Preparation or Contrast Media

Procedure	Purpose
BE	To identify diseases of the large intestine (e.g., diverticula, cancer, ulcerative colitis)
IVU (IVP)	To diagnose abnormalities, strictures, disease of the urinary system
UGI	To detect hiatal hernia, strictures, ulcers, or tumors

 SKILLS CHALLENGE

To practice transcribing radiology (X-ray) orders that require preparation, complete Activity 15-2 in the *Skills Practice Manual*.

Patient Preparation:
- NPO 8 to 12 hours before the procedure is to be performed
- Some physicians write orders to hydrate the patient before the examination.

Transcribing the order: In addition to transcribing this order, the HUC would order the diet changes.

UGI c̄ SBFT CI: Peptic Ulcer

This procedure uses fluoroscopy, a viewing screen, and an X-ray machine to examine the distal portion of the esophagus, stomach, and small intestines.

Purpose: Used to detect hiatal hernia, strictures, ulcers, or tumors.

Patient Preparation:
- NPO 8 to 12 hours before the procedure

Transcribing the order: The HUC would transcribe the order and initiate the diet change.

SPECIAL INVASIVE X-RAY PROCEDURES

Special invasive X-ray procedures are performed under the direction of the radiologist or a surgeon with a radiologist present. A request for the use of a special X-ray room or operating room must be submitted in advance by the doctor, or the procedure may be scheduled by computer as part of the transcription procedure. A downtime requisition is shown in Fig 15-5. A contrast medium is used, and the patient is required to sign a patient consent form (see Chapter 8, p. 143, for use and preparation of a consent form).

Special invasive X-ray procedures may be performed with or without a general anesthetic. When a general anesthetic is used, the nursing staff follows specific preoperative and postoperative routines (see Chapter 19, p. 380). Preparations for these studies vary among hospitals.

The radiologist and/or surgeon may prescribe preprocedure medications to be given at a specific time or "on call." When medications are ordered *on call*, the doctor or department personnel, at the request of the radiologist and/or surgeon, notify the nursing unit to administer the medication.

DOCTORS' ORDERS FOR SPECIAL INVASIVE X-RAY PROCEDURES

PTC CI: Obstruction of the Bile Ducts

Visualization of the bile ducts through injection of iodine contrast directly into the biliary system.

Purpose: Usually done to determine the cause of obstruction, jaundice, or persistent upper abdominal pain after cholecystectomy.

Patient preparation: Special prep orders may or may not be ordered.

Transcribing the order: Routine transcription

Carotid Angiogram CI: Aneurysm

An angiogram is a visualization of vascular structures within the body after injection of contrast medium (Fig. 15-6). The specific name given to the study is determined by the vascular structure to be studied (e.g., renal angiogram, cerebral angiogram).

Purpose: Used to diagnose vascular aneurysms, malformations, and occluded or leaking blood vessels.

Lower Abdominal Angiogram CI: Angiodysplasia

X-ray of a blood vessel after injection of contrast medium (Fig. 15-7). An angiogram may be identified according to its anatomic location (e.g., femoral angiogram).

Purpose: Used to detect obstruction or narrowing of a blood vessel or aneurysm.

Arthrogram of the Left Knee CI: Torn Ligament

X-ray of a joint after injection of contrast medium.

Purpose: Used to detect trauma, such as bone chips or torn ligament, resulting from an injury.

Cholangiogram, Postoperative (T-Tube Cholangiogram) CI: Retained Stones

X-ray taken 1 to 3 days after a cholecystectomy to examine the bile ducts. Examination is done after contrast medium is injected through a T tube.

Doctor ordering _____

Date to be done _____ ☐ Stat ☐ Routine ☐ ASAP

Today's date _____ Requested by _____

| **Special Invasive X-ray Procedures** |

Clinical indication _____

Transportation ☐ Portable ☐ Stretcher ☐ Wheelchair ☐ Ambulatory

O₂ ☐ Yes ☐ No   Diabetic ☐ Yes ☐ No   Hearing deficit   ☐ Yes ☐ No

IV ☐ Yes ☐ No   Seizure disorder ☐ Yes ☐ No   Sight deficit   ☐ Yes ☐ No

Isolation ☐ Yes ☐ No   Non-English speaking ☐ Yes ☐ No

Write out the entire doctor's order

Comments: _____

☐ Angiogram _____

☐ Arteriogram_____

☐ Arthrogram_____

☐ Cervical myelogram_____

☐ Cholangiogram_____

☐ Hysterosalpingogram_____

☐ Lymphangiogram_____

☐ PTC _____

☐ Spinal myelogram_____

☐ Venogram_____

☐ Voiding cystourethrogram_____

☐ Write-in order_____

Figure 15-5 Downtime requisition for special invasive X-ray procedures.

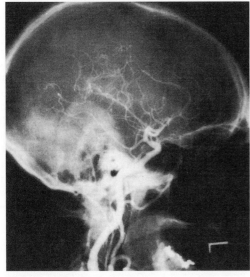

Figure 15-6 Carotid angiogram. (From Chipps E, Clanin N, Campbell V: *Neurologic disorders*, St. Louis, 1992, Mosby.)

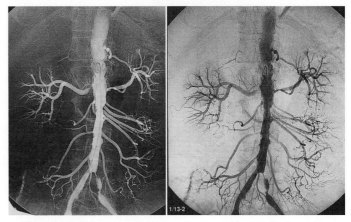

Figure 15-7 Lower abdomen angiogram, with digital subtraction angiogram (DSA) image on right. (From Bontrager KL, Lampignano JP: *Textbook of radiographic positioning and related anatomy*, ed 6, St. Louis, 2005, Mosby.)

Purpose: Used to rule out residual stones in the biliary tract after a cholecystectomy. It is called *T-tube cholangiogram* because the catheter placed in the biliary ducts during surgery is called a *T tube.*

Hysterosalpingogram CI: Obstruction of Fallopian Tubes

X-ray of the uterus and fallopian tubes taken after injection of contrast medium.

Purpose: Used in fertility studies and to confirm abnormalities such as adhesions, fistulas, and so forth.

Lymphangiogram Left Leg CI: Lymphatic Obstruction

X-ray of the lymph channels and lymph nodes taken after injection of contrast medium

Purpose: Used to identify metastatic cancer in the lymph nodes and to evaluate the effectiveness of chemotherapy.

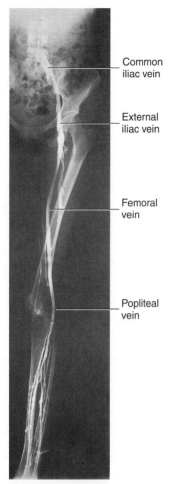

- Common iliac vein
- External iliac vein
- Femoral vein
- Popliteal vein

Figure 15-8 Normal venogram, lower left limb. (From Ballinger PW, Frank ED: *Merrill's atlas of radiographic positions and radiologic procedures,* ed 10, St. Louis, 2003, Mosby.)

Spinal Myelogram CI: Cord Compression Due to HNP (Herniated Nucleus Pulposus)

X-ray of the spinal cord after contrast medium has been injected between lumbar vertebrae into the spinal canal.

Purpose: Used to detect herniated disks, tumors, and spinal nerve root injuries.

Venogram of Left Leg CI: DVT (Deep Vein Thrombosis)

X-ray of a vein, usually in the lower extremities, taken after injection of contrast medium.

Purpose: Used to evaluate veins before and after bypass surgery and to investigate venous function when obstruction is suspected (Fig. 15-8).

Voiding Cystourethrogram (VCUG) CI: Bladder Dysfunction

X-ray films are taken to demonstrate the bladder filling then emptying as the patient voids.

Purpose: Used to demonstrate bladder dysfunction and urethral strictures.

Note: Endoscopies, including ERCP (endoscopic retrograde cholangiopancreatography), are covered in Chapter 16. ∎

OVERVIEW OF SPECIAL INVASIVE X-RAY PROCEDURES

Special invasive X-ray procedures are performed under the direction of the radiologist or a surgeon with a radiologist present. Contrast is given and a signed consent is required for special invasive X-ray procedures. "On call" medication may or may not be ordered by the patient's doctor.

Examples of Special Invasive X-ray Procedures

Procedure	Purpose
Arthrogram	To identify trauma, such as bone chips or torn ligaments, resulting from injury
Angiogram	To diagnose vascular aneurysms, malformations, occluded or leaking blood vessels
Voiding cystourethrogram	To demonstrate bladder and urethral strictures
Venogram	To evaluate veins before and after bypass surgery and for obstruction
Spinal myelogram	To detect herniated disks, tumors, and spinal nerve root injuries
Hysterosalpingogram	To confirm abnormalities, such as adhesions and fistulas, and to be used in fertility studies
Lymphangiogram	To identify metastatic cancer in lymph nodes and to evaluate chemotherapy treatment

---

COMPUTED TOMOGRAPHY

Computed tomography uses a type of ionizing radiation to provide a computerized image that can generate multiple two-dimensional cross sections (slices) of tissue and three-dimensional reconstructions (Fig. 15-9). Other contrast media may include gas or air introduced rectally for colon studies or water given orally for a CT of the stomach. Contrast medium may or may not be used. When writing the order, the doctor must indicate whether the procedure is to be performed with contrast. (Fig. 15-10 shows a downtime requisition for CT.)

 SKILLS CHALLENGE

To practice transcribing orders for special invasive X-ray procedures, complete Activity 15-3 in the *Skills Practice Manual.*

 DOCTORS' ORDERS FOR CT SCANS

CT of Head c̄ DSA CI: Aneurysm

Combines angiography, fluoroscopy, and computer technology to visualize the cardiovascular system without the interference of bone and soft tissue structures that may obscure the image.

Purpose: Used to evaluate postoperatively (e.g., endarterectomy) and to detect cerebrovascular abnormalities.

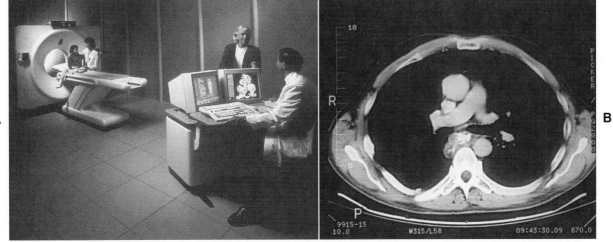

Figure 15-9 A, Computed tomography (CT) scanner. **B,** CT scan of the chest with intravenous (IV) contrast medium. (From Ballinger PW, Frank ED: *Merrill's atlas of radiographic positions and radiologic procedures*, ed 10, St. Louis, 2003, Mosby.)

Doctor ordering _____

Date to be done _____ ☐ Stat ☐ Routine ☐ ASAP

Today's date _____ Requested by _____

Computed Tomography

Clinical indication _____
☐ With contrast ☐ Without contrast

Transportation ☐ Portable ☐ Stretcher ☐ Wheelchair ☐ Ambulatory

O₂ ☐ Yes ☐ No   Diabetic ☐ Yes ☐ No   Hearing deficit ☐ Yes ☐ No
IV ☐ Yes ☐ No   Seizure disorder ☐ Yes ☐ No   Sight deficit ☐ Yes ☐ No
Isolation ☐ Yes ☐ No   Non-English speaking ☐ Yes ☐ No

Write out the entire doctor's order

Comments: _____

☐ CT scan of head _____
☐ CT scan of brain _____
☐ CT scan of abdomen _____
☐ CT scan of pelvis _____
☐ CT scan of spine _____
☐ CT of neck _____
☐ CT-guided liver biopsy _____
☐ DSA _____
☐ HIDA scan _____
☐ Write-in order _____

Figure 15-10 Downtime requisition for computed tomography.

CT Scan of Abd CI: Evaluate Carcinoma

A CT scan is often the preferred method for diagnosing many different cancers, because the image allows a physician to confirm the presence of a tumor and to measure its size, precise location, and extent of involvement with nearby tissue.

Purpose: Used to diagnose and determine stage of cancer and to follow its progress. CT also may be used to diagnose abdominal aortic aneurysm, bowel obstruction, and other conditions.

CT Scan of the Brain CI: Tumor

Computerized analysis of multiple images of brain tissue.

Purpose: Used to diagnose brain tumor, infarction, bleeding, and hematoma.

Patient Preparation: The patient is usually NPO for several hours before the procedure.

CT Scan of Abdomen and Pelvis CI: Retroperitoneal Lesion

CT images are obtained by passing X-rays through the abdominal organs from many angles.

Purpose: Used to diagnose tumors, abscesses, and bowel obstruction and to guide needles for biopsy.

Patient Preparation: Patient is usually NPO for 4 hours. These studies should be performed before barium studies are conducted.

CT of LS Spine CI: Spinal Stenosis

Scan of the lumbosacral area of the spine.

Purpose: Often ordered after myelogram. Used to confirm spinal stenosis, changes in the disks and vertebrae, and to confirm spinal infection.

CT of the Neck CI: Tumor

Scan of the neck.

Purpose: Used to identify soft tissue masses and/or to evaluate the larynx.

HIDA Scan (Cholescintigraphy) CI: Gallstones

Purpose: Used to diagnose obstruction of the bile ducts (by a gallstone or tumor), disease of the gallbladder, and bile leaks.

CT of Chest CI: Lung Cancer

A CT scan of the chest requires special equipment to obtain multiple sectional images of the organs and tissues of the chest. A CT scan produces images that are far more detailed than those produced by a conventional chest X-ray.

Purpose: Used to diagnose pulmonary embolism or aortic dissection, and to detect lung changes, pneumonia, and cancer.

CT-Guided Liver Biopsies

Used to identify the location of tissue for the biopsy, so needle placement is precise.

Purpose: Used to obtain tissue from the liver for diagnostic purposes. CT-guided lung and breast biopsies also are performed. ■

ULTRASONOGRAPHY (SONOGRAPHY)

Ultrasonography, also called *sonography*, uses high-frequency sound waves to create an image of body organs. Ultrasonography is a technique that is used to visualize muscles, tendons, and many internal organs, and to assess their size, structure, and the presence of pathologic lesions (Fig. 15-11). Ultrasonography is useful in the detection of pelvic abnormalities and can involve techniques known as abdominal (transabdominal) ultrasound, vaginal (transvaginal or endovaginal) ultrasound in women,

and rectal (transrectal) ultrasound in men. Ultrasound also is used (1) to guide procedures such as needle biopsy, in which needles are used to extract sample cells from an abnormal area for laboratory testing, imaging of the breasts, and biopsy sampling for breast cancer, (2) to diagnose a variety of heart and vascular conditions, and (3) to survey damage after a heart attack or other illness. Ultrasonography also is used to visualize a fetus during routine and emergency prenatal care, to date the pregnancy, and to check for the location of the placenta (afterbirth), the presence of multiple fetuses or physical abnormalities, the sex of the baby, and fetal movement, breathing and heartbeat.

OVERVIEW OF COMPUTED TOMOGRAPHY (CT)

Computed tomography (CT) uses a type of ionizing radiation to provide a computerized image that can generate multidimensional sections (slices) of tissue. Contrast medium may or may not be used.

Examples of Computed Tomography Procedures

Procedure	Purpose
CT of head c̄ DSA	To evaluate postoperatively (e.g., endarterectomy) and to detect cerebrovascular abnormalities
Chest CT	To detect lung changes, pneumonia, cancer, pulmonary embolism, aortic dissection, and other conditions
Abdominal CT	To detect cancer, aortic aneurysm, bowel obstruction, and other conditions
Head CT	To diagnose brain tumor, infarction, bleeding, and hematoma
LS spine CT	To confirm spinal stenosis and changes in disks and vertebrae, and to confirm spinal infection
HIDA scan	To diagnose obstruction of the bile ducts, diseases of the gallbladder, and bile leaks

---

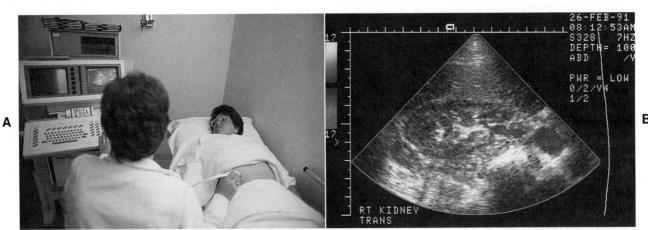

A   B

Figure 15-11 A, Ultrasound scanner. **B,** Ultrasound scan of the kidney. (From Brundage DJ: *Renal disorders*, St. Louis, 1992, Mosby.)

Ultrasonography also has therapeutic applications (e.g., treating benign and malignant tumors and other disorders) that can be highly beneficial when it is used with dosage precautions. High-intensity focused ultrasound (HIFU) (sometimes FUS or HIFUS) is a highly precise medical procedure by which high-intensity focused ultrasound is used to heat and destroy pathogenic tissue rapidly. This typically is performed under computerized MRI guidance, at which time it is referred to as magnetic resonance guided focused ultrasound, which often is shortened to MRgFUS. MRI is used to identify tumors or fibroids in the body, before they are destroyed by ultrasound. See Figure 15-12 for an ultrasound downtime requisition.

✓ DOCTORS' ORDERS FOR ULTRASONOGRAPHY STUDIES

US of Abd

Ultrasound of abdomen

Purpose: Used to detect liver cysts, abscesses, hematomas, and tumors.

Patient Preparation:
- NPO 8 to 12 hours before the procedure (for GB alone, may require only 4 to 6 hours NPO)
- If pelvis of female is included in abd study, full bladder, drink fluids—do not void
- No smoking AM of exam

US of Pelvis

Ultrasound of pelvis.

Purpose: Used during pregnancy to identify ectopic pregnancy, multiple births, and fetal abnormality. Used otherwise to identify ovarian cancer and other disorders.

Patient Preparation:
- Full bladder—drink fluids, do not void (usually only females)
- May require water enema

US of GB

Purpose: Used to diagnose cholelithiasis, cholecystitis, and to identify obstructive jaundice.

Patient Preparation:
- Fat-free evening meal
- Fast 4 to 6 hours

Note: Echocardiogram, echoencephalogram, and Doppler studies are covered in Chapter 16. ■

OVERVIEW OF ULTRASOUND (SONOGRAPHY)

Ultrasonography, also called *sonography* or *echography*, uses high-frequency sound waves to create an image of body organs. Female pelvic ultrasonography requires a full bladder.

Example of Ultrasound Procedures

Procedure	Purpose
Gallbladder	To diagnose cholelithiasis and cholecystitis, and to identify obstructive jaundice
Pelvis	To identify ovarian cancer and other disorders, and to identify ectopic pregnancy, multiple births, and fetal abnormalities
Abdomen	To detect liver cysts, abscesses, hematomas, and tumors

Ultrasonography is useful for examining other internal organs, including but not limited to the kidneys, heart and blood vessels, bladder, uterus, ovaries, unborn child (fetus) in pregnant patients, eyes, thyroid and parathyroid glands, and scrotum (testicles).

Doctor ordering _____

Date to be done _____ ☐ Stat ☐ Routine ☐ ASAP

Today's date _____ Requested by _____

Ultrasonography

Clinical indication _____

Transportation ☐ Portable ☐ Stretcher ☐ Wheelchair ☐ Ambulatory

O₂ ☐ Yes ☐ No	Diabetic ☐ Yes ☐ No	Hearing deficit ☐ Yes ☐ No
IV ☐ Yes ☐ No	Seizure disorder ☐ Yes ☐ No	Sight deficit ☐ Yes ☐ No
Isolation ☐ Yes ☐ No	Non-English speaking ☐ Yes ☐ No	

Comments: _____

Write out the entire doctor's order

☐ Cardiac US_____
☐ Fetal US_____
☐ HIFU_____
☐ MRI quided focused US_____
☐ US of abd _____
☐ US of pelvis _____
☐ US of GB _____
☐ Write-in order_____

Figure 15-12 Downtime requisition for ultrasonography.

MAGNETIC RESONANCE IMAGING

Magnetic resonance imaging (MRI) is a technique for viewing the interior of the body that uses powerful magnetic fields, radio waves, and a computer to produce images of body structures.

To perform an MRI scan, the patient is securely placed on an imaging table within a large tube surrounded by a giant magnet (Fig 15-13). The magnet creates a strong magnetic field that aligns the protons of hydrogen atoms, which then are exposed to a beam of radio waves. This excites the various protons of the body, which produces a faint signal that is detected by the receiver portion of the MRI scanner. Receiver information then is processed by a computer, and an image is produced.

MRI scanners can generate multidimensional sections (slices) of tissue. MRI gives doctors the ability to view all sorts of body structures, including soft tissues. Bones do not obscure the image as they do in X-rays. Studies are done on selected areas of the body, such as the brain, spinal cord, and bone. MRI frequently is used to detect cancers that otherwise would be difficult to diagnose and provides clinicians with the ability to detect cancers at early stages. Contrast medium may or may not be used and may be as simple as water (taken orally, for imaging the stomach and small bowel), although substances with specific magnetic properties may be used. When writing the order, the doctor must indicate whether the procedure is to be performed with contrast.

No adverse effects are associated because the procedure does not require radiation, but because of the strength of the magnet and the radiofrequency waves, MRI contraindications exist for patients with the following:

- Pacemaker
- Implanted port device
- Neurostimulator
- Intrauterine device (IUD)
- Insulin pump
- Older metal plates, pins, screws, or surgical staples
- Ear implant
- Older metal clips from aneurysm repair
- Metal clips in eyes
- Retained bullets
- Pregnancy

Any other large metal objects implanted in the body (e.g., tooth fillings, braces) usually are not a problem.

Note: Only ferrous (iron)-based devices are attracted by a magnet. In all, 99.9% of devices used today for MRI are safe. (The physician should be consulted.)

The HUC, when transcribing MRI orders, would prepare an interview form for the nurse to complete before sending the patient for an MRI. The form lists any contraindications that may prevent the patient from having the procedure.

Dental bridgework may have to be removed before the scan is performed, but permanent fillings and inlays are acceptable because they are not made of ferrous metals. Before the examination is conducted, the patient is asked to remove metallic jewelry, wristwatches, eyeglasses, hairpins, or wigs, if metal clips are present. Credit cards, bankcards, and similar devices with magnetically coded strips should be removed as well. This is especially important to remember in an outpatient diagnostic setting.

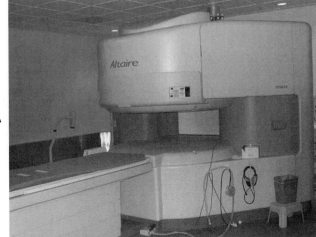

A

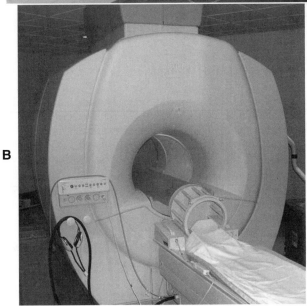

B

Figure 15-13 A, Open magnetic resonance imaging (MRI) machine. **B,** Closed MRI machine. Note that the tunnel is short and the edges are flared to minimize claustrophobia. (From Pagana KD, Pagana TJ: *Mosby's manual of diagnostic and laboratory tests*, ed 3, St. Louis, 2006, Mosby.)

OVERVIEW OF MAGNETIC RESONANCE IMAGINING

MRI is a technique that is used for viewing the interior of the body with the use of a powerful magnetic field, radio waves, and a computer to produce images of body structures. A contrast medium may or may not be used. A completed interview form is required.

Examples of Magnetic Resonance of Imaging Procedures

Procedure	Purpose
An MRI can be used to evaluate any part of the body	To diagnose internal injuries, conditions, or disease
	To monitor effects of medications and treatments inside the body

✓ DOCTORS' ORDERS FOR MAGNETIC RESONANCE IMAGING

- MRI of brain (Fig. 15-14) and cervical spine CI: malignancy
- MRI lumbar spine CI: HNP
- MRI rt shoulder CI: rotator cuff injury
- MRI lt knee CI: posterior cruciate ligament tear
   Fig 15-15 shows a downtime requisition for MRI. ■

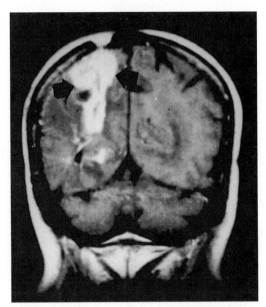

Figure 15-14 Magnetic resonance imaging (MRI) with arrows indicating a brain tumor accentuated by a Magnevist dye. (Courtesy Central Pennsylvania Magnetic Imaging, Williamsport, Pennsylvania; from Pagana KD, Pagana TJ: *Diagnostic testing and nursing implications: a case study approach*, ed 4, St. Louis, 1994, Mosby.)

NUCLEAR MEDICINE

Background Information

Nuclear medicine uses radioactive materials called *radiopharmaceuticals* to determine the functioning capacity of organs. Radioactive scanning materials are used to assist in diagnosing disease because of their ability to give off radiation in the form of gamma rays, which can be traced.

Depending on the study to be performed, the patient may take the radiopharmaceutical by mouth, or it may be injected within a vein. A gamma scintillation camera is the instrument used to form an image of the concentration of radioactive material within a specific organ of the body, thus producing a picture called a **scan** (Fig 15-16, *A*). It is possible to perform organ scans on the bone (Fig 15-16, *B*) with therapeutic doses of radiopharmaceuticals. Cancer of the thyroid and a blood condition called *polycythemia vera* respond to this treatment.

Radioactivity used in nuclear medicine differs from X-rays in that gamma radiation is transmitted from an outside source that passes the radiation through the body. In nuclear medicine, radioactive material is taken internally by mouth, inhalation, or intravenously, and it emits gamma radiation from the specific organ that is being studied.

To communicate the doctors' order to the nuclear medicine department, the HUC must enter the order on the computer or complete a nuclear medicine downtime requisition (Fig 15-17).

 SKILLS CHALLENGE

To practice transcribing orders for computerized tomography scans, ultrasound, and magnetic resonance imaging, complete Activity 15-4 in the *Skills Practice Manual*.

Doctor ordering _____

Date to be done _____ □ Stat □ Routine □ ASAP

Today's date _____ Requested by _____

Magnetic Resonance Imaging

Clinical indication _____

Transportation □ portable □ stretcher □ wheelchair □ ambulatory

O₂ □ Yes □ No   Diabetic □ Yes □ No   Hearing deficit □ Yes □ No

IV □ Yes □ No   Seizure disorder □ Yes □ No   Sight deficit □ Yes □ No

Isolation □ Yes □ No   Non-English speaking □ Yes □ No

Comments: _____

Write out the entire doctor's order

□ MRI of brain _____

□ MRI of spine _____

□ MRI shoulder _____

□ MRI knee _____

□ Write-in order _____

Figure 15-15 Downtime requisition for magnetic resonance imaging.

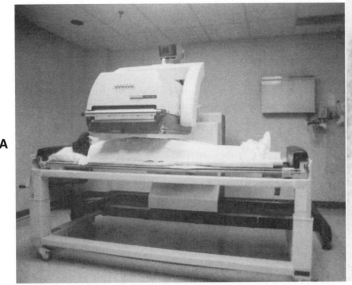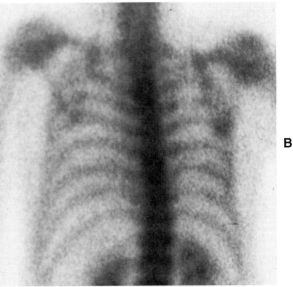

Figure 15-16 A, Patient prepared for bone scan. The patient's feet are tied to help maintain hips in position for maximal scanning uptake (From Mourad LA: *Orthopedic disorders*, St. Louis, 1991, Mosby.). **B,** Upper body bone scan (From Pagana KD, Pagana TJ: *Mosby's manual of diagnostic and laboratory tests*, ed 3, St. Louis, 2006, Mosby.).

Preparation may be required before the procedure is performed. Check health care facility's policy regarding preparation before scheduling the procedure.

Following are samples of nuclear medicine studies.

✓ DOCTORS' ORDERS FOR NUCLEAR MEDICINE STUDIES

Bone Scan—Total Body CI: Cancer, Prostate-Mets
Purpose: Performed to detect the presence of tumors, arthritis, or osteoporosis.

Bone Scan—Regional CI: Cervical Fx
Purpose: Performed to study a particular area of the body, such as vertebral compression fractures or unexplained bone pain.

Breast Scintigraphy (Breast Scan, Sestamibi Breast Scan) CI: Breast Cancer
Purpose: Used to identify breast cancer, especially in young women with dense breasts in whom the accuracy of mammography is diminished. Tracer doses of the isotope are used.

Contraindications: (1) Patients who are pregnant, unless the benefits outweigh the risk of fetal injury; (2) patients who are lactating, because of the risk of contamination of breast milk.

L&S (liver and spleen) Scan CI: Cirrhosis
Purpose: Performed to evaluate injury to the spleen, chronic hepatitis, and metastatic processes. It should be done before barium studies are performed. Other body scans may be performed on the brain, heart, lungs, kidneys, gallbladder, and pancreas.

Gallium Scan—Total Body CI: Lymphoma (also may be ordered regionally)
Purpose: Performed to stage gallium avid tumors (those that attract high concentrations of gallium, e.g., lymphoma, lung cancer). It is used to locate infection or inflammation in patients with fever of unknown origin. It also is used to monitor response to treatment for infection, inflammation, or tumor.

Preparation: Usually, administer a **cathartic** or enema to minimize increased gallium uptake within the bowel.

Thyroid Uptake and Scan CI: Check for Cold Nodules
Purpose: Performed to study thyroid gland performance. It demonstrates the ability of the thyroid gland to "take up" radioactive iodine.

Lung Perfusion/Ventilation Study CI: Embolism
Purpose: A diagnostic study for pulmonary embolism.

Scrotal Nuclear Imaging (Scrotal Scan, Testicular Imaging) CI: Rt Testicular Torsion
Scrotal imaging is helpful in the diagnosis of patients with sudden onset of unilateral testicular swelling and pain. Scrotal imaging can differentiate unilateral testicular torsion (twisting) from other causes of pain (e.g., torsion of the testicular appendage, orchitis, strangulated hernia, testicular hemorrhage). Tracer doses of isotopes are used.

Note: Testicular torsion is a surgical emergency that requires prompt surgical exploration to salvage the involved testicle. The surgeon must differentiate the condition from other causes of testicular pain that do not require surgery.

Gastrointestinal Bleeding Scan (Abdominal Scintigraphy, GI Scintigraphy) CI: GI Bleed
This study is used primarily to localize sites of GI bleeding.

PET (Positron Emission Tomography) Scan CI: Alzheimer's Disease
Purpose: Used to obtain information about blood flow to the myocardium, metabolism, glucose utilization, and schizophrenia. Isotopes are used.

Patient Preparation: Diet and medication adjustments are required before this procedure is performed.

Doctor ordering _____

Date to be done _____ ☐ Stat ☐ Routine ☐ ASAP

Today's date _____ Requested by _____

Nuclear Medicine

Clinical indication _____

Transportation ☐ Portable ☐ Stretcher ☐ Wheelchair ☐ Ambulatory

O₂ ☐ Yes ☐ No   Diabetic ☐ Yes ☐ No   Hearing deficit ☐ Yes ☐ No

IV ☐ Yes ☐ No   Seizure disorder ☐ Yes ☐ No   Sight deficit ☐ Yes ☐ No

Isolation ☐ Yes ☐ No   Non-English speaking ☐ Yes ☐ No

Comments: _____

Write out the entire doctor's order

☐ Adenosine/thallium scan _____

☐ Bone scan (total) _____

☐ Bone scan (regional) _____

☐ Breast scintigraphy _____

☐ Cardiac scan _____

☐ Liver and spleen _____

☐ Gallium scan _____

☐ GI bleeding scan _____

☐ Thyroid uptake and scan _____

☐ HIDA _____

☐ Neutrospec scan _____

☐ PET _____

☐ MUGA _____

☐ Scrotal nuclear imaging _____

☐ Thallium stress scan _____

☐ Sestamibi stress _____

☐ WBC scan _____

☐ Write-in order _____

Figure 15-17 Downtime requisition for nuclear medicine.

WBC Scan (White Blood Cell Scan) CI: Osteomyelitis

Purpose: Used to identify and localize occult inflammation or infection in patients who have fever of unknown origin, suspected osteomyelitis, or inflammatory bowel disease. Tracer doses of the isotope are used.

NeutroSpec Scan CI: Chest Infection

NeutroSpec scanning is performed to identify abdominal, chest, or deep space infections that otherwise are not clinically apparent.

Preparation: Encourage the patient to drink a lot of fluids, if possible, or administer increased intravenous fluids for patients who are NPO. ■

✓ DOCTORS' ORDERS FOR NUCLEAR CARDIOLOGY PROCEDURES

(Cardiac nuclear scanning includes myocardial scan, cardiac scan, nuclear cardiac scanning, heart scan, thallium scan, multigated acquisition [MUGA] scan, isonitrile scan, sestamibi cardiac scan, and cardiac flow studies)

MUGA Scan (also called *gated pool imaging*) CI: CAD

Scanning of the heart using computers and synchronized electrocardiogram. MUGA (multigated acquisition is the name of computer machinery).

Purpose: Used to calculate the cardiac ejection fraction.

Thallium Stress Scan CI: Infarction

A thallium stress test is a nuclear imaging method that provides a view of the blood flow into the heart muscle. A sestamibi stress test is the same test, but sestamibi is used as a radionuclide instead of thallium. Thallium and sestamibi tests also are called "MIBI stress test" and "myocardial perfusion scintigraphy"; these are used to evaluate how well the patient's heart is perfused (supplied with blood) at rest as compared with during activity.

Stress is induced by using the treadmill; if the patient cannot use the treadmill, medications are given to the patient to simulate the effects of exercise in the body. Drugs that simulate the effects of exercise are persantine, adenosine, or dobutamine.

Purpose: Used to monitor blood flow to the myocardium while at rest or after normal stress to diagnose coronary artery disease or to evaluate blood flow after a coronary bypass operation.

OVERVIEW OF NUCLEAR MEDICINE

Nuclear imaging examines organ function and structure, whereas diagnostic radiology is based on anatomy. Contrast agents are used.

Example of nuclear imaging procedures

Procedure	Purpose
Lung perfusion	Study to diagnose pulmonary embolism
Liver and spleen scan	Performed to evaluate injury to the spleen, chronic hepatitis, and metastatic processes
Renal scans	Used to examine the kidneys and to detect any abnormalities, such as tumor or obstruction of renal blood flow
Thyroid scans	Used to evaluate thyroid function
Bone scans	Used to evaluate degenerative and/or arthritic changes in the joints, to detect bone disease and tumor, and/or to identify the cause of bone pain or inflammation
Gallium scans	Used to diagnose active infectious and/or inflammatory diseases, tumors, and abscesses
Brain scans	Used to investigate problems within the brain and/or in the blood circulation to the brain
Breast scans	Often used with mammograms to locate cancerous tissue in the breast
OctreoScan	Used to find primary and metastatic neuroendocrine tumors
HIDA scan (cholescintigraphy)	Used to diagnose obstruction of the bile ducts, disease of the gallbladder, and bile leaks
NeutroSpec scanning	Performed to identify abdominal, chest, or deep space infections that are otherwise not apparent clinically
PET scan	Used to obtain information about blood flow to the myocardium, metabolism, glucose utilization, or schizophrenia
Scrotal nuclear imaging	Used to differentiate testicular torsion from other causes of pain
WBC scan	Used to identify and localize occult inflammation or infection
Heart Scans	
Myocardial perfusion	Identifies ischemic or infarcted heart muscle
Myocardial function (MUGA)	Most accurate method used to measure cardiac ejection fraction
Cardiac flow	Performed in children with suspected cardiac anomalies
Nuclear ventriculography	Evaluates muscle wall activity
Exercise stress test	Evaluates muscle wall activity during stress (physical or chemical)

Note: Exercise stress tests are discussed in Chapter 16.

 SKILLS CHALLENGE

For practice transcribing the following types of orders, complete the following activities in the *Skills Practice Manual:*

- For practice transcribing nuclear medicine orders, complete Activity 15-5.
- For practice transcribing a review set of doctors' orders, complete Activity 15-6.
- For practice recording telephone messages, complete Activity 15-7.

Adenosine/Thallium Scan or Persantine/Thallium Scan

Orders for a thallium scan using medications to simulate the effects of exercise.

Octreoscan

Purpose: Octreoscan is an imaging agent that can reveal primary and metastatic neuroendocrine tumors.

HIDA Scan (Cholescintigraphy) CI: Gallstones

Purpose: To diagnose obstruction of the bile ducts (e.g., by gallstone, by tumor), disease of the gallbladder, and bile leaks.

Cardiac Flow CI: Cardiac Anomalies

This is most commonly performed in children with suspected cardiac anomalies.

Purpose: Determines the direction of cardiac flow. ■

KEY CONCEPTS

The primary responsibility of the HUC in the transcription of diagnostic imaging orders, beyond ordering the requested study, involves communicating with the nursing staff about patient preparation and with the nutritional care department regarding diet changes. Accurate communication of the preparation procedure is vital to the expected outcome. An error may cause a procedure to be postponed or may result in an unclear or nonvisible diagnostic image; each of these outcomes is costly to the patient and hospital in terms of time and money. It is important to indicate, as part of the requisitioning process, the date on which the procedure is to be done. Health unit coordinators continue to have coordination responsibilities regarding scheduling of procedures when the electronic medical record is implemented.

REVIEW QUESTIONS

1. Write the name of the division of diagnostic imaging that would perform each of the following procedures:

a. chest PA & LAT _____

b. L & S scan _____

c. BE _____

d. CT of brain _____

e. head scan _____

f. pelvic US _____

g. KUB _____

h. UGI _____

i. LS spine X-ray _____

j. IVU _____

k. HIDA scan _____

l. SNAT series _____

m. sinus series _____

n. MRI of lt femur _____

o. angiogram _____

p. SBFT _____

q. US of GB _____

r. arthrogram _____

s. PCXR _____

t. X-ray rt femur _____

u. mammogram _____

v. tomogram _____

w. cerebral angiogram _____

x. PET scan _____

y. MRI LS spine _____

z. myelogram _____

2. Explain the benefits of picture archiving and communication systems for the patient and for the doctor.

_____

3. Name five positions that may be included in an X-ray order.

a. _____

b. _____

c. _____

d. _____

e. _____

4. Which of the following procedures would require a preparation (on nursing unit and other than NPO), and which would require a consent form? (Write yes or no on the lines provided.)

Procedure	Preparation	Consent
a. KUB	_____	_____
b. UGI	_____	_____
c. cerebral angiogram	_____	_____
d. CT of head	_____	_____
e. SNAT series	_____	_____
f. voiding cystourethrogram	_____	_____
g. US of GB	_____	_____
h. angiogram	_____	_____
i. mammogram	_____	_____
j. BE	_____	_____
k. myelogram	_____	_____
l. arthrogram	_____	_____

5. Medications predetermined by the diagnostic imaging department that should be given for certain procedures and routinely given to a patient by nursing personnel are called a _____.

6. Medications ordered by the patient's physician and given when the diagnostic imaging department calls with instructions that it be given are _____.

7. In the event the doctor ordered the following diagnostic procedures for the same patient, in what sequence would they be scheduled? IVU, UGI, pelvic ultrasound, BE

a. _____

b. _____

c. _____

d. _____

8. Rewrite the following doctors' orders using abbreviations.

a. magnetic resonance imaging of lumbosacral spine, CI: fracture

_____

b. posteroanterior and lateral chest X-ray, CI: pneumonia

_____

c. upper gastrointestinal X-ray, intravenous urogram, and barium enema, CI: abdominal mass

_____

   d. computed tomography of the right shoulder, CI: rotator cuff injury

   _____

   e. pelvic ultrasound, CI: age of fetus

   _____

   f. computed tomography of head $\bar{c}$ digital subtraction angiography

   _____

9. List ten items that the HUC would be required to include when ordering a diagnostic procedure.

   a. _____

   b. _____

   c. _____

   d. _____

   e. _____

   f. _____

   g. _____

   h. _____

   i. _____

   j. _____

10. Explain the reason why contrast media should be used when diagnostic imaging procedures are performed.

   _____

   _____

11. List five examples of contrast media used by the various divisions of diagnostic imaging.

   a. _____

   b. _____

   c. _____

   d. _____

   e. _____

12. Which division of the diagnostic imaging department would require that the patient be interviewed and a form completed by the nursing department?

   _____

13. Explain how the HUC's responsibilities would differ with the implementation of the electronic medical record from those required when paper charts are used.

_____

_____

14. Explain the importance of following up on the preparation required for diagnostic imaging procedures.

_____

_____

_____

THINK ABOUT...

1. Discuss why it is important to provide the correct transportation information when ordering a diagnostic procedure for a patient.
2. Discuss other information that may be written in the doctor's orders that would need to be included when the order is entered into the computer.

Other Diagnostic Studies

CHAPTER OBJECTIVES

Upon completion of this chapter, you will be able to:

1. Define the terms in the vocabulary list.
2. State the meaning of each abbreviation in the Abbreviations list.
3. Explain the purpose of provided diagnostic procedures.
4. Identify the hospital department that would perform provided procedures.
5. State two purposes of an electroencephalogram.
6. State what category of medication should be noted on the requisition when an electroencephalogram is ordered.
7. State the difference between an invasive procedure and a noninvasive procedure.
8. Name two noninvasive diagnostic studies related to the heart.
9. Name two invasive diagnostic studies related to the heart.
10. State what category of medication should be noted on the request when an electrocardiogram is ordered.
11. Name six endoscopies and the parts of the body visualized by each.
12. Discuss the importance of patient preparation before a sigmoidoscopy or any visual examination of the colon.

13. List two studies related to the gastrointestinal (GI) system that are performed in the endoscopy department.
14. List four diagnostic tests that are performed by the cardiopulmonary (respiratory care) department.
15. State what category of medication should be noted on the requisition when arterial blood gases are ordered.
16. Name two studies performed by the cardiovascular department to diagnose vascular diseases.

VOCABULARY

2-D (2-dimensional) Echocardiogram A technique used to "see" actual heart structures and their motions

Apnea The cessation of breathing

Arterial Blood Gases A diagnostic study to measure arterial blood gases (oxygen and carbon dioxide) to attain information needed to assess and manage a patient's respiratory status

Arterial Line (art line) A catheter placed in an artery that continuously measures the patient's blood pressure

B-scan An image made up of a series of dots, each indicating a single ultrasonic echo. The position of a dot corresponds to the time elapsed, and the brightness of a dot corresponds to the strength of the echo.

Caloric Study A test performed to evaluate the function of cranial nerve VIII. It also can indicate disease in the temporal portion of the cerebrum

Capillary Blood Gases A diagnostic study performed primarily on infants. Blood is obtained from the infant's capillary arterial vessel, usually from the heel

Cardiac Monitor Monitor of heart function that provides a visual and audible record of heartbeat

Cardiac Monitor Technician (CMT) A person who observes the cardiac monitors

Cardiac Stress Test A noninvasive study that provides information about the patient's cardiac function

Color Doppler An enhanced form of Doppler echocardiography; different colors are used to designate the direction of blood flow

Doppler Ultrasound A procedure used to monitor moving substances or structures, such as flowing blood or a beating heart. Used to locate vessel obstructions, to observe fetal heart sounds, to localize the placenta (afterbirth), and to image heart functions

Echo The reflection of an ultrasound wave back to the transducer from a structure in the plane of the sound beam

Echocardiogram (2-D M-mode echo) A diagnostic, noninvasive procedure in which ultrasound is used to study the structure and motion of the heart

Electrocardiogram A graphic recording of the electrical impulses that the heart generates during the cardiac cycle

Electroencephalogram A graphic recording of the electrical activity of the brain

Electromyogram A record of muscle contraction produced by electrical stimulation

Electroneurography (nerve conduction study) Similar to an EMG, except that it evaluates the integrity of the peripheral nerves. This test often is performed with EMG

Electronystagmography A test used to evaluate nystagmus (involuntary rapid eye movement) and the muscles that control eye movement

Electrophysiologic Study A method of studying evoked potentials within the heart

Endoscope A tubular instrument (rigid or flexible) with a light source and a viewing lens for observation that can be inserted through a body orifice or through a small incision.

Endoscopy The visualization of the interior of organs and cavities of the body with an endoscope. Biopsies may be obtained during an endoscopy. Endoscopic surgeries are discussed in Chapter 17

Evoked Potential Studies Tests used to evaluate specific areas of the cortex that receive incoming stimuli from the eyes, ears, and lower or upper extremities or sensory nerves

Gastrointestinal (GI) Study A diagnostic study related to the gastrointestinal system. GI studies often are performed in the endoscopy department

Holter Monitor A portable device that records the heart's electrical activity and produces a continuous EKG tracing over a specified period

Impedance Cardiography A flexible and fast-acting noninvasive monitoring system that measures total impedance (resistance to the flow of electricity in the heart)

Invasive Procedure A diagnostic or therapeutic technique that requires entry of a body cavity or interruption of normal body functions

Manometric Studies A procedure undertaken to evaluate certain areas of the body by using a manometric device to measure and record pressures; usually performed in the endoscopy department

M-mode Echo Image obtained with M-mode echocardiography shows the motion (M) of the heart over time. 2-D M-mode would be a two-dimensional study

Narcolepsy A chronic ailment that consists of recurrent attacks of drowsiness and sleep during the daytime

Nerve Conduction Study This study measures how well individual nerves can transmit electrical signals (often performed with an electromyogram)

Noninvasive Procedure A diagnostic or therapeutic technique that does not require the skin to be broken or a cavity or organ of the body to be entered

Obstructive Sleep Apnea The cessation of breathing during sleep

Occlusion A blockage in a canal, vessel, or passage of the body

Plethysmography (arterial) Usually performed to rule out occlusive disease of the lower extremities, or may identify arteriosclerotic disease in the upper extremity

Plethysmography (venous) Measures changes in the volume of an extremity; usually performed on a leg to exclude DVT (deep vein thrombosis)

Radiopaque Catheter A catheter coated with a substance that does not allow the passage of x-rays, thus allowing the movement of the catheter to be followed on the viewing screen

Real-Time Imaging An ultrasound procedure that displays a rapid sequence of images (like a movie) instantaneously while an object is being examined

Rhythm Strip A cardiac study that demonstrates the waveform produced by electrical impulses from the electrocardiogram

Spirometry A study conducted to measure the body's lung capacity and function

Telemetry The transmission of data electronically to a distant location

Transesophageal Echocardiography A procedure used to assess the heart's function and structures. A probe with a transducer on the end is inserted down the throat.

ABBREVIATIONS

Abbreviation	Meaning	Example of Usage on a Doctor's Order Sheet
ABG	arterial blood gases	ABG on RA
BAER	brain stem auditory evoked response; also called auditory brainstem evoked potential (ABEP)	BAER to evaluate hearing loss
CBG	capillary blood gases	CBG @ 10 AM

Abbreviation	Meaning	Example of Usage on a Doctor's Order Sheet
DVT	deep vein thrombosis	Venous plethysmography rt leg, CI: DVT
ECG, EKG	electrocardiography	ECG before surgery; EKG today
EEG	electroencephalography	Schedule EEG
EGD	esophagogastroduodenoscopy	EGD
EMG	electromyography	EMG tomorrow
ENG	electronystagmography (electrooculography)	Schedule for an ENG
EPS	electrophysiologic study	EPS today
ERCP	endoscopic retrograde cholangiopancreatography	Schedule for ERCP in AM
ICG	impedance cardiography	Place on ICG today
IPG	impedance plethysmography	IPG today
LOC	leave on chart (when it follows ECG, LOC ECG or EKG)	
NCS	nerve conduction studies	EMG c̄ NCS
OSA	obstructive sleep apnea	Sleep study to assess pt for OSA
PFT	pulmonary function test	PFT to evaluate COPD
RA	room air	ABG on RA
SEP	somatosensory evoked potential	Schedule for SEP
TEE	transesophageal echocardiography	Schedule for TEE this afternoon
VEP	visual evoked potential	Schedule VEP in AM

EXERCISE 1

Write the abbreviation for each term listed below.

1. electroencephalography _____

2. electrocardiography (2) _____

3. electromyography _____

4. room air _____

5. leave on chart _____

6. arterial blood gases _____

7. capillary blood gases _____

8. endoscopic retrograde cholangiopancreatography _____

9. esophagogastroduodenoscopy _____

10. electrophysiologic study _____

11. nerve conduction studies _____

12. obstructive sleep apnea _____

13. brainstem auditory evoked response _____

14. electronystagmography _____

15. somatosensory evoked potential _____

16. visual evoked potential _____

17. deep vein thrombosis _____

18. transesophageal echocardiography _____

19. pulmonary function test _____

20. impedance plethysmography _____

21. impedance cardiography _____

EXERCISE 2

Write the meaning of each abbreviation listed below.

1. ABG _____

2. ECG or EKG _____

3. EEG _____

4. LOC _____

5. EMG _____

6. RA _____

7. EGD _____

8. ERCP _____

9. EPS _____

10. CBG _____

11. NCS _____

12. OSA _____

13. BAER _____

14. ENG   _____

15. SEP   _____

16. VEP   _____

17. DVT   _____

18. TEE   _____

19. PFT   _____

20. IPG   _____

21. ICG   _____

> ✎ **TAKE NOTE**
>
> When the electronic medical record (EMR) with the computer physician order entry (CPOE) is implemented, the physicians' orders are entered directly into the patient's electronic record, and the diagnostic procedure order is automatically sent to the appropriate department. The health unit coordinator (HUC) may have tasks to perform, such as coordinating scheduling, ordering special diets, and so forth. An icon may indicate a HUC task, or it may signal a nurse request. The HUC will have to communicate with the nutritional care department (by e-mail or telephone) when ordering a diet for a patient who has completed a diagnostic procedure that required him to be NPO. *Some hospital nutritional care departments require that **all** diet orders be submitted in writing via computer.

> ✎ **TAKE NOTE**
>
> Treatments and therapeutic procedures included in this chapter that may take place during diagnostic studies or that may be scheduled after these studies are completed are discussed in Chapter 17.

ELECTRODIAGNOSTICS

Background Information

Electrodiagnostics include procedures used to evaluate the cardiovascular, nervous, and muscular systems to diagnose conditions and diseases. Indications to perform these procedures include patients with symptoms of numbness, tingling, weakness, muscle cramping, or pain. Most electrodiagnostic studies are performed with the use of electrical activity and electronic devices to evaluate disease or injury to a specified area of the body. Some type of electrode is applied to the patient to record electrical activity in most tests. Electrical impulses can be generated spontaneously or can be stimulated. The heart generates electrical impulses spontaneously during the cardiac cycle; these may be recorded by performing an **EKG (electrocardiogram)**. Electrical impulses may be stimulated by an electrical shock applied to the body when an **EMG (electromyogram)** is performed. The most common electrodiagnostics are discussed in this chapter.

> ✎ **TAKE NOTE**
>
> Downtime requisitions are included in this chapter for learning purposes. The CD included in the *Health Unit Coordinator Skills Manual* is a simulated hospital computer program that may be used as well.

Neurologic and Neuromuscular System Electrodiagnostics

Electrodiagnostic tests involving the neurologic system include procedures involving the brain, cranial nerves, and sensory pathways of the eyes, ears, and peripheral nerves. Electromyography often performed with electroneurography is used to diagnose diseases or conditions of the neuromuscular system. Neurologic electrodiagnostic procedures that may be performed include those discussed in the following sections.

Electroencephalography

An **electroencephalogram (EEG)** is a recording of the electrical activity of the brain. The procedure is performed to identify and assess patients with seizures, and to study brain function. Results of the study may be used to diagnose brain tumors, epilepsy, other brain diseases, or injuries, and to confirm brain death or cerebral silence (Fig. 16-1). The role of the HUC is to communicate the order to the EEG department via computer or by completion of a downtime requisition. Anticonvulsant medications such as phenobarbital (Luminal) and phenytoin (Dilantin) should be noted when a procedure involving the neurologic system is ordered (Fig. 16-2).

Preparation of the patient by the nursing staff is usually required. The patient's hair is washed the night before the test is to be done. The use of cola drinks, cocoa, coffee, or tea is restricted because these liquids may act as stimulants; however, food and other fluids are permitted. Some hospitals have special preparation cards that contain information regarding preparation of the patient for an EEG. The HUC places the preparation card in the patient's Kardex holder during the transcription procedure.

An EEG may be ordered to be done portable (an EEG machine would be brought to the patient's bedside), or the patient may be transported to the neurology department for the test, which is performed by the EEG technician. To order an electroencephalogram, the doctor usually writes *EEG* on the doctors' order sheet.

Evoked Potentials

Evoked potentials (EPs) constitute a group of diagnostic tests that measure changes and responses in brain waves that are evoked from stimulation of a sensory (visual, auditory, or somatosensory) pathway. Evoked potentials are objective in that voluntary patient response is not needed. This makes EPs useful with nonverbal and uncooperative patients and permits the distinction of organic from psychogenic problems. The

Communication and Implementation of Cardiovascular Diagnostics

```
┌─────────────────────┐        ┌─────────────────────┐
│ Doctor's order for  │ ─────▶ │ Order transcribed by│
│ cardiovascular      │        │ the HUC             │
│ diagnostics         │        │                     │
└─────────────────────┘        └─────────────────────┘
```

```
┌─────────────────────┐        ┌─────────────────────┐        ┌──────────┐
│ Order communicated  │        │ EKG technician from │        │ Results  │
│ to cardiovascular   │ ─────▶ │ cardiovascular      │ ─────▶ │ filed    │
│ diagnostics by      │        │ diagnostics or the  │        │ on       │
│ computer or         │        │ patient care        │        │ chart    │
│ requisition         │        │ technician performs │        └──────────┘
│- - - - - - - - - - -│        │ EKG at bedside      │
│ Order communicated  │        │- - - - - - - - - - -│
│ to nurse by Kardex  │        │ Patient sent to     │
│ or computer         │        │ cardiovascular      │
└─────────────────────┘        │ diagnostics         │
                               │ department for other│
                               │ cardiovascular tests│
                               └─────────────────────┘
```

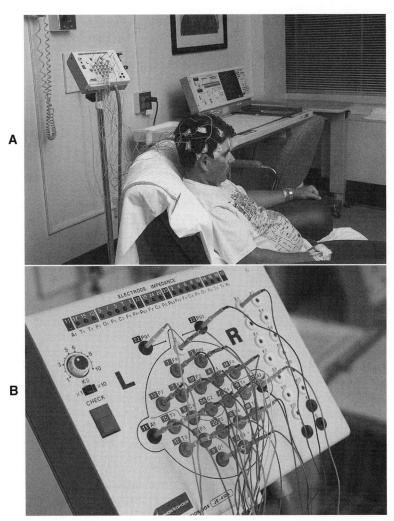

Figure 16-1 Electroencephalography (EEG). **A,** Electrodes are attached to the patient's head **(B)** with wires leading to corresponding areas on the equipment to record brain wave activity. (From Chipps E, Clanin N, Campbell V: *Neurologic disorders,* St. Louis, 1992, Mosby.)

```
Doctor ordering _____
Date to be done _____  □ Stat □ Routine □ ASAP
Today's date _____  Requested by _____

┌─────────────────────┐
│ Neurology Department │
└─────────────────────┘

Clinical indication _____
Transportation □ Portable □ Stretcher □ Wheelchair □ Ambulatory

O₂  □ Yes □ No      Diabetic  □ Yes □ No      Hearing deficit  □ Yes □ No
IV  □ Yes □ No      Seizure disorder  □ Yes □ No    Sight deficit  □ Yes □ No
Isolation □ Yes □ No   Non-English speaking  □ Yes □ No

Comments: _____

Write out the entire doctor's order

□ BAER _____
□ Caloric study _____
□ EEG _____
□ EMG _____
□ ENG _____
□ Nerve conduction studies _____
□ SEP _____
□ VER _____
Write in order _____
```

Figure 16-2 A neurology department downtime requisition.

projected future of evoked potentials is that they will aid in diagnosing and monitoring mental disorders and learning disabilities. Examples of EPs follow. These studies are performed by a physician in less than 30 minutes.

Visual Evoked Potential. The visual evoked potential (VEP) is a response to visual stimuli (e.g., a strobe light flash, reversible checkerboard pattern, retinal stimuli). It also can be called *visual evoked response (VER)*. Abnormal results may be seen in patients with neurologic disease (e.g., multiple sclerosis, Parkinson's disease). VEP may be used to detect lesions of the eye, disorders of neurologic development, and eyesight problems or blindness in infants. This test also may be used during eye surgery to provide a warning of possible damage to the optic nerve.

Brainstem Auditory-Evoked Response or Auditory Brainstem-Evoked Potential. The brainstem auditory-evoked response (BAER) or auditory brainstem-evoked potential (ABEP) usually uses clicking sounds to stimulate the central auditory pathways of the brainstem. Either ear can be evoked to detect lesions in the brainstem that involve the auditory pathway without affecting hearing. This test is commonly used in low-birthweight newborns to screen for hearing disorders. Recognition of deafness enables infants to be fitted with corrective devices as early as possible, often preventing speech abnormalities. This test also may be effective in the early detection of brain tumors of the posterior fossa.

Somatosensory Evoked Potential. Somatosensory evoked potentials (SEPs) usually are initiated by sensory stimulation of an area of the body. The time that it takes for the current of the stimulus to travel along the nerve to the cortex of the brain is measured. This test is used to assess patients with spinal cord injury and to monitor spinal cord functioning during spinal surgery. SEP also is used to monitor treatment of diseases (e.g., multiple sclerosis), to evaluate the location and extent of areas of brain dysfunction after head injury, and to pinpoint tumors at an early stage.

Caloric Study (Oculovestibular Reflex Study)

This test is used to evaluate the function of the vestibular portion of the eighth cranial nerve (CN VIII). The external auditory canal is irrigated with hot or cold water to induce nystagmus (rapid eye movement). A **caloric study** also can aid in the differential diagnosis of abnormalities that may occur in the vestibular system, brainstem, or cerebellum. When results are inconclusive, electronystagmography may be performed. A caloric study is performed by a physician or a technician and takes approximately 15 minutes to complete. Most patients experience nausea and dizziness during this test.

Electronystagmography (Electro-oculography)

Electronystagmography (ENG) is a test that is performed to evaluate nystagmus (rapid eye movement) and the muscles that control eye movement. Electrodes are taped to the skin around the eyes, and various procedures, such as pendulum tracking, changing of head position, and changing of gaze position, are used to stimulate rapid eye movement. This test is performed to evaluate patients with vertigo and to differentiate organic from psychogenic vertigo. An ENG can identify the site of a lesion if present and is used to evaluate unilateral deafness. The patient should avoid caffeine and alcohol for 24 to 48 hours before the test is performed. This procedure is performed by a physician or an audiologist and takes approximately 1 hour to complete.

Electromyography (EMG)

This test is used in the assessment of patients with diffuse or localized muscle weakness. An EMG often is combined with **electroneurography;** it can be used to identify primary muscle diseases and to differentiate them from primary neurologic pathologic conditions. A recording electrode is placed into a skeletal muscle to monitor its electrical activity. An EMG is performed by a physical therapist, a psychiatrist, or a neurologist and takes about 30 to 60 minutes. Slight pain may occur with insertion of the needle electrode.

Electroneurography (Nerve Conduction Studies—NCS)

This test is performed to identify peripheral nerve injury in patients with localized or diffuse weakness, to differentiate primary peripheral nerve disease from muscular injury, and to document the severity of injury in legal cases. It also is used to monitor nerve injury and response to treatment. This test is conducted by a physiatrist or a neurologist, takes about 15 minutes, and often is performed with an EMG. A mild shock that can be uncomfortable is required for nerve impulse stimulation.

 DOCTORS' ORDERS FOR NEUROLOGIC AND NEUROMUSCULAR ELECTRODIAGNOSTICS

- EEG tomorrow
- Schedule for ENG
- VER today
- EMG tomorrow AM
- Schedule BAER for tomorrow ■

OVERVIEW OF NEUROLOGIC AND NEUROMUSCULAR SYSTEM ELECTRODIAGNOSTICS

Electroencephalography (EEG)
Visual-evoked potential (VEP)
Brainstem auditory-evoked response (BAER) or auditory brainstem-evoked potential (ABEP)
Somatosensory-evoked potential (SEP)
Caloric study (oculovestibular reflex study)
Electronystagmography (ENG) (electro-oculography)
Electromyography (EMG)
Electroneurography (nerve conduction studies—NCS)

 SKILLS CHALLENGE

To practice transcribing neurologic and neuromuscular electrodiagnostics orders, complete Activity 16-1 in the *Skills Practice Manual.*

Cardiovascular Electrodiagnostics

Electrodiagnostic tests of the cardiovascular system include procedures involving the heart and the vascular system. The results of electrodiagnostic tests and other cardiovascular studies aid the physician in making a diagnosis and prescribing treatment.

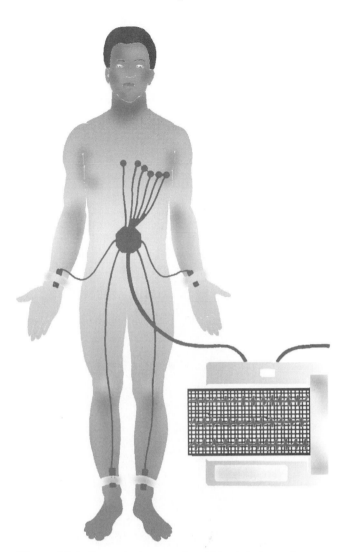

Figure 16-3 Electrode placement for a 12-lead electrocardiogram (ECG). (From Ignatavicius D, Workman L: *Medical-surgical nursing,* ed 5, Philadelphia, 2006, Saunders.)

Electrocardiogram

An **electrocardiogram (EKG or ECG)** is a **noninvasive procedure** that measures the electrical impulses that the heart generates during the cardiac cycle. The EKG lead system is composed of several electrodes that are placed on each of the four extremities and a varying site on the chest. Each combination of electrodes is called a *lead.* The doctor also may use the abbreviation *EKG* or *ECG* to order this study, which is performed at the bedside. *LOC* is a request to the EKG technician to leave a copy of the cardiac tracing on the patient's chart (Fig. 16-3). When ordering an EKG, the HUC should indicate whether the patient has a pacemaker or an automatic implanted cardiac defibrillator (AICD or ICD). Specific cardiac medications, such as digoxin (Lanoxin), diltiazem (Cardizem), and nitroglycerin (Nitro-Bid, Nitro-Dur, NitroStat, Transderm-Nitro), should be noted when an EKG is ordered. An EKG usually is performed at the bedside by a technician.

A rhythm strip shows the waveforms produced by electrical impulses from the heart. One lead of the EKG is used (usually lead II) (Fig. 16-4). A rhythm strip also may be printed from a continuous EKG when a patient is in a telemetry

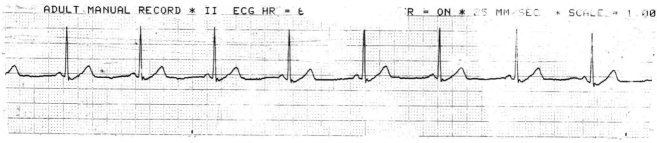

ADULT MANUAL RECORD * II ECG HR = 6   R = ON * 25 MM/SEC * SCALE = 1.00

Figure 16-4 A normal rhythm strip.

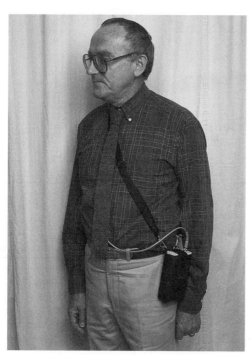

Figure 16-5 Patient wearing Holter monitor. (From Canobbio MM: *Cardiovascular disorders,* St. Louis, 1990, Mosby.)

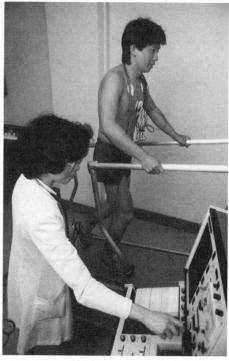

Figure 16-6 Patient taking exercise stress test while the nurse monitors the electrocardiogram (EKG) response. (From Canobbio MM: *Cardiovascular disorders,* St. Louis, 1990, Mosby.)

unit and is wearing a monitor. If the nurse or monitor technician detects an abnormality, or if the patient reports chest pain or discomfort, a rhythm strip may be printed for interpretation.

Impedance Cardiography

Impedance cardiography (ICG) is a noninvasive monitoring system that measures total impedance (resistance) to the flow of electricity in the heart. ICG is used to assess, plan, and individualize the treatment plan for patients with heart failure, severe trauma, or fluid management.

Holter Monitor

A **Holter monitor** is a portable continuous recording of the electrical activity of the heart for periods up to 72 hours. The patient's physician often orders this test when a patient is c/o (complaining of) syncope, palpitations, atypical chest pains, or unexplained dyspnea. The EKG tape recorder is worn in a sling or holder around the chest or waist (Fig. 16-5). The EKG is recorded on a magnetic tape during unrestricted activity, rest, and sleep. The Holter monitor includes a clock that permits accurate time monitoring on the EKG tape. While wearing

the monitor, the patient maintains a diary of activities and any symptoms experienced, including the time of occurrence.

Exercise Electrocardiography (also called treadmill stress test)

An exercise electrocardiogram or a treadmill stress test is a noninvasive study performed with the use of a treadmill or a stationary bicycle to evaluate cardiac response to physical stress. This study provides information on myocardial response to increased oxygen requirements and determines the adequacy of coronary blood flow. Occluded arteries are unable to meet the heart's increased demand for blood during testing (Fig. 16-6).

Electrophysiologic Study (EPS; Cardiac Mapping)

An electrophysiologic study (EPS) is an **invasive procedure** that is performed to study evoked potentials within the heart. A small plastic catheter (wire) is inserted through the groin (or arm, in some cases) and is threaded up into the heart with the use of a special type of X-ray, called *fluoroscopy,* which guides the catheter. Electrode catheters are used to pace the heart and potentially induce dysrhythmia. Mapping may be done to locate the point of origin of dysrhythmia.

Results of this study will help the physician select additional therapeutic measures, such as insertion of a pacemaker or defibrillator, or other treatments. The procedure is performed by a cardiologist in a cath lab.

Note: Treatments or therapeutic procedures that may be performed during or scheduled after this study are discussed in Chapter 17.

CARDIOVASCULAR/NUCLEAR MEDICINE STUDIES

Thallium and Sestamibi Stress Tests

These tests were discussed in Chapter 15 because they are two-step procedures involving both the nuclear medicine and cardiovascular departments. The HUC may have to coordinate procedures by communicating with both departments by phone, computer, or downtime requisition.

> ### ✐ *TAKE NOTE*
>
> When exercise testing is not advisable, or the patient is unable to exercise to a level that is adequate to stress the heart, **chemical stress testing** is recommended. Chemicals that may be used include Persantine, adenosine, or dobutamine. Pacing is another method of stress testing. In patients with pacemakers, the rate of capture can be increased to a rate that would be considered a cardiac stress.

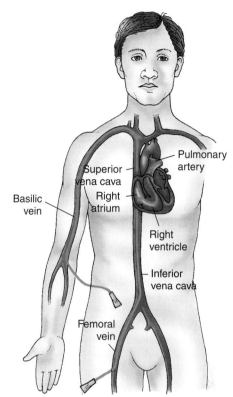

Figure 16-7 Right-sided cardiac catheterization. (From Ignatavicius D, Workman L: *Medical-surgical nursing,* ed 5, Philadelphia, 2006, Saunders.)

CARDIOVASCULAR/ULTRASOUND (SONOGRAPHY, ECHOGRAPHY) STUDIES

Echocardiography

The echocardiogram is a noninvasive ultrasound procedure that is used to create a graphic recording of the internal structure of the heart and the position and motion of the cardiac walls and valves. This study, which is completed by sending ultra–high-frequency sound waves through the chest wall, usually includes M-mode two-dimensional (2-D) recordings and a Doppler study. **M-mode** produces a one-dimensional recording of the amplitude and rate of motion (M) of heart structures in real time, allowing the various cardiac structures to be located and studied during a cardiac cycle. The 2-D mode moves the ultrasonic beam within one sector of the heart, producing a two-dimensional image of the spatial relationships within the heart. Color flow Doppler imaging demonstrates the direction and velocity of blood flow within the heart and great vessels. The procedure is performed by an ultrasound technician and may be performed at the bedside.

Transesophageal Echocardiography

Transesophageal echocardiogram (TEE) examines cardiac function and structure with the use of an ultrasound transducer placed in the esophagus. The transducer provides views of the heart structure and its major blood vessels.

CARDIAC CATHETERIZATION (CORONARY ANGIOGRAPHY, ANGIOCARDIOGRAPHY, VENTRICULOGRAPHY)

Cardiac catheterization is used to visualize the heart chambers, arteries, and great vessels. It is used most often to evaluate chest pain or abnormalities detected in a **cardiac stress test**. The procedure is used to locate the region of coronary **occlusion** (blockages) and to determine the effects of valvular heart disease. A catheter is passed into the heart through a peripheral vein (right-heart cath) (Fig. 16-7) or artery (left-heart cath). Pressures are recorded and radiographic dyes are injected through the catheter. With the assistance of computer calculations, cardiac output and other measures of cardiac function can be determined. The signed consent required for this procedure usually includes possible treatment or therapeutic procedure options.

Note: Treatments or therapeutic procedures that may be performed during or scheduled after this study are discussed in Chapter 17.

SWAN-GANZ CATHETER INSERTION

This is a special procedure that is performed by a doctor in a critical care unit. A balloon-tipped catheter is inserted through the subclavian vein into the right side of the heart. The catheter goes through the right ventricle past the pulmonic valve and into a branch of the pulmonary artery. Measurements revealed by this procedure are used to guide and evaluate therapy.

VASCULAR PLETHYSMOGRAPHY STUDIES

Venous plethysmography is a noninvasive method of determining venous thrombosis and deep vein thrombophlebitis (DVT). This test measures changes in the volume of an extremity and is usually performed on a leg to rule out DVT. Three blood pressure cuffs are applied to the proximal, middle, and distal portions of the extremity. A volume recorder (plethysmograph) attached to the cuffs then displays each pulse wave.

Note: Doppler studies also are used to identify DVT, but they are less accurate in evaluating the venous system below the knee.

Arterial plethysmography usually is performed to rule out occlusive disease of the lower extremities; it may also be used to identify arteriosclerotic disease in the upper extremity. Three blood pressure cuffs are applied to the proximal, middle, and distal portions of the extremity. A volume recorder (plethysmograph) attached to the cuffs then displays each pulse wave.

Impedance plethysmography (IPG) is a noninvasive study that is performed to estimate blood flow and quantify blood volumes. Electrodes are applied to the leg, and electric resistance changes are recorded. This technique is not accurate in detecting the presence or absence of partially obstructive thrombi in major vessels.

VASCULAR ULTRASOUND STUDIES (VENOUS/ARTERIAL DOPPLER ULTRASOUND)

Vascular ultrasound studies evaluate blood as it flows through a blood vessel, including the body's major arteries and veins in the abdomen, arms, legs, and neck. Nicotine can cause vasoconstriction, so cigarette smoking is prohibited before and during this test.

Vascular Duplex Scanning

Vascular duplex scanning is called "duplex" because it combines the benefits of Doppler with B-mode scanning. A computer provides a two-dimensional image of the vessel, along with an image of blood flow. **Color Doppler** ultrasound can be added to arterial duplex scanning, which assigns color for direction of blood flow within the vessel. This provides an accurate representation of vessel anatomy and blood flow within the vessel.

Vascular ultrasound studies and vascular duplex scans that may be ordered include the following:

Carotid Doppler flow analysis: A directional Doppler probe is used to detect the flow of blood in the major neck artery.
Carotid duplex Scan: A carotid duplex scan is a noninvasive ultrasound test that is used in the extracranial carotid artery to directly detect occlusive disease.
Vascular ultrasound studies (Doppler flow studies) on lower extremities: In these procedures, an ultrasound probe is placed over the major leg veins or arteries. A graphic tracing is produced, which shows flow changes caused by changes within the blood vessels.

See Figure 16-8 for a downtime requisition for noninvasive and invasive cardiovascular diagnostic procedures.

CARDIOVASCULAR DIAGNOSTIC TESTS

Noninvasive

- Electrocardiogram (EKG or ECG)
- Impedance Cardiography (IPG)
- Holter Monitor
- Cardiac Stress Test (exercise electrocardiogram or treadmill stress test)
- Thallium or Sestamibi Stress Test (discussed in Chapter 15)
- Echocardiogram
- Transesophageal Echocardiogram
- Plethysmography Vascular Studies
- Vascular Ultrasound Studies
- Vascular Duplex Scans

Invasive (usually requiring sedation of the patient)

- Electrophysiologic studies (EPSs)
- Cardiac Catheterization (Coronary Angiography, Angiocardiography, Ventriculography)
- Swan-Ganz catheter insertion

SKILLS CHALLENGE

To practice transcribing cardiovascular diagnostics orders, complete Activity 16-2 in the *Skills Practice Manual*.

DOCTORS' ORDERS FOR CARDIOVASCULAR ELECTRODIAGNOSTICS

- EKG stat LOC
- Schedule for heart cath 0800 in AM
- Arterial Doppler lower ext today
- 2-D M-mode echo this afternoon ■

ENDOSCOPY STUDIES

Endoscopy is an invasive procedure that is performed to visualize and examine a body cavity or hollow organ. The procedure is named for the organ or body area to be visualized and is performed by a doctor. Most hospitals have an endoscopy department. The **endoscopes** that are used to perform endoscopies are tubular instruments with a light source and a viewing lens for observation. Many endoscopic procedures now are performed with a video chip in the tip of a camera that is placed over the viewing lens. The color image then is transmitted to a nearby television monitor. Biopsies and surgical procedures often are performed during an endoscopy.

Note: Surgical procedures performed during endoscopy are discussed in Chapter 17.

In transcribing an endoscopy order, the HUC may call to schedule the procedure with the responsible department, or may order the procedure via computer or downtime requisition (Fig. 16-9). Endoscopies require a patient to sign a consent form. Preparation varies according to the type of endoscopy to be performed. When ordering the procedure, the doctor

Doctor ordering _____
Date to be done _____ □ Stat □ Routine □ ASAP
Today's date _____ Requested by _____

| **Cardiovascular Department** |

Clinical indication _____
Cardiac medications _____
Pacemaker? □ Yes □ No   Type _____   Ht _____Wt _____
Comments: _____
LOC? □ Yes □ No

Noninvasive Studies

□ Arterial plethysmography   □ EKG c̄ rhythm strip
□ Cardiac monitor   □ Holter monitor_____hours
□ Carotid Doppler flow analysis   □ IPG
□ Chemical stress test   □ Thallium stress test
□ Doppler flow studies_____   □ Sestamibi stress test
□ Echocardiogram 2D M-Mode   □ Transesophageal echocardiogram
□ EKG/ECG/2-lead   □ Treadmill stress test
□ Venous plethysmography   □ Vascular duplex scan
                                     □ Vascular us

Invasive Studies

□ Cardiac catheterization   □ EPS
□ Write in order_____

Transportation □ Portable □ Stretcher □ Wheelchair □ Ambulatory
O₂ □ Yes □ No   Diabetic □ Yes □ No   Hearing deficit □ Yes □ No
IV □ Yes □ No   Seizure disorder □ Yes □ No   Sight deficit □ Yes □ No
Isolation □ Yes □ No   Non-English speaking □ Yes □ No

Figure 16-8 Cardiovascular diagnostic downtime requisition.

usually will indicate if any preparation or "on call" medication is required.

The following is a list of endoscopic examinations that are commonly performed in a hospital setting on an inpatient or outpatient basis:

- **Arthroscopy:** A visual examination of a joint interior with a specially designed endoscope. **Usual prep:** NPO 8 to 12 hours before examination because a general anesthesia usually is used to diminish pain.
- **Bronchoscopy:** A visual inspection of the bronchi by means of a bronchoscope (Fig. 16-10). **Usual prep:** NPO for 4 to 8 hours before the procedure to reduce risk of aspiration.
- **Colonoscopy:** A visual examination of the large intestine from the anus to the cecum by means of a fiberoptic colonoscope. **Usual prep:** cathartic and/or enemas and NPO before examination.
- **Endoscopic retrograde cholangiopancreatography (ERCP):** This diagnostic procedure consists of inspection of the bile and pancreatic ducts and is performed with the use of a fiberoptic endoscope. **Usual prep:** NPO 8 to 12 hours before examination.
- **Esophagogastroduodenoscopy (EGD):** A visual examination of the esophagus, stomach, and duodenum. **Usual prep:** NPO for 8 to 12 hours before examination.
- **Sigmoidoscopy:** A visual examination of the sigmoid portion of the large intestine performed by means of a

sigmoidoscope. **Usual prep:** cathartic and/or enemas and NPO 8 to 12 hours before examination.

> ✎ *TAKE NOTE*
>
> The patient would have to be cleaned out (cathartics or enemas) before gastrointestinal endoscopy is performed because the presence of stool would obscure visualization of the intestinal walls. Barium studies would have to be performed after GI endoscopy because barium also would obscure visualization of the intestinal walls. Gastrointestinal endoscopic studies could not be done if the patient were not properly prepared.

✓ **DOCTORS' ORDERS FOR ENDOSCOPY**

Sigmoidoscopy tomorrow am.
- Fleet enema HS and repeat @ 0600
- NPO 2400 hours

Schedule for gastroscopy tomorrow am.
- NPO p̄ MN

Schedule ERCP for tomorrow.
- NPO p̄ MN

Doctor ordering _____

Date to be done _____ Time to be done _____

Today's date _____ Requested by _____

Endoscopy Department

Clinical indication _____

Transportation ☐ Portable ☐ Stretcher ☐ Wheelchair ☐ Ambulatory

O₂ ☐ Yes ☐ No   Diabetic ☐ Yes ☐ No   Hearing deficit ☐ Yes ☐ No

IV ☐ Yes ☐ No   Seizure disorder ☐ Yes ☐ No   Sight deficit ☐ Yes ☐ No

Isolation ☐ Yes ☐ No   Non-English speaking ☐ Yes ☐ No

Pre-op medication ☐ Yes ☐ No

Time given _____

Comments: _____

☐ Arthroscopy   ☐ Esophagoscopy

☐ Bronchoscopy   ☐ Fetoscopy

☐ Colonoscopy   ☐ Gastroscopy

☐ Colposcopy   ☐ Hysteroscopy

☐ Cystoscopy   ☐ Laparoscopy

☐ Enteroscopy ERCP   ☐ Mediastinoscopy

☐ EGD   ☐ Pelvioscopy

☐ Peritoneoscopy

☐ Proctoscopy

☐ Sigmoidoscopy

☐ Sinus endoscopy

☐ Thoracoscopy

☐ Write in order _____

Figure 16-9 Endoscopy downtime requisition.

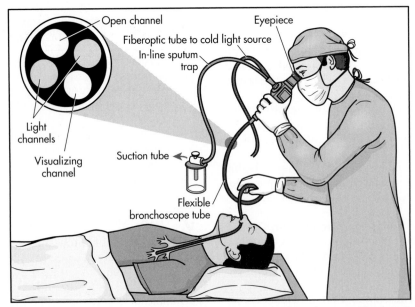

Figure 16-10 Bronchoscopy with the use of a flexible fiberoptic bronchoscope. The four channels consist of two that provide a light source, one vision channel, and one open channel that accommodates instruments or allows administration of an anesthetic or oxygen. (From Pagana KD, Pagana TJ: *Mosby's manual of diagnostic and laboratory tests*, ed 3, St. Louis, 2006, Mosby.)

TYPES OF ENDOSCOPIES

All endoscopies require a signed consent. Preparations vary according to the procedure and the doctor and whether a general anesthesia will be used.

Endoscopy	Area of Visualization	Prep
Arthroscopy	joints	NPO
Bronchoscopy	larynx, trachea, bronchi, alveoli	NPO
Colonoscopy	rectum, colon	yes
Colposcopy	vagina, cervix	no
Cystoscopy	urethra, bladder, ureters, (male) prostate	yes
Enteroscopy	upper colon, small intestines	yes
Endourology	bladder and urethra	no
Endoscopic retrograde cholangio-pancreatography	pancreatic and biliary ducts	NPO
Esophagogastro-duodenoscopy	esophagus, stomach, duodenum	yes
Fetoscopy	fetus	no
Gastroscopy	stomach	NPO
Hysteroscopy	uterus	NPO
Laparoscopy	abdominal cavity	yes
Mediastinoscopy	mediastinal lymph nodes	NPO
Sigmoidoscopy	sigmoid colon	yes
Sinus endoscopy	sinus cavities	NPO
Thoracoscopy	pleura, lung	NPO

Bronchoscopy tomorrow @ 9:30 am
• Have consent signed.
• Demerol 50 mg
• Atropine 0.8 mg IM @ 8:30 AM

Schedule colonoscopy for 8 am on Wednesday.
• Have consent signed.
• Clear liquids, NPO p̄ MN
• Fleet enema HS and repeat @ 0600

Note: The doctor may or may not write an order for a consent to be signed. A consent is required for endoscopy. ■

 SKILLS CHALLENGE

To practice transcribing endoscopy orders, complete Activity 16-3 in the *Skills Practice Manual.*

GASTROINTESTINAL STUDIES

Background Information

Some **gastrointestinal (GI) studies** are performed in the endoscopy department, usually on an outpatient basis, whereas others may be performed at the bedside by the nurse. The health unit coordinator may be asked to requisition the necessary equipment from the central service department for a bedside collection. Specimens collected by the nurse are sent to the hospital clinical laboratory for study, or they may be sent to a private laboratory.

GI studies are discussed in the following paragraphs.

Gastric Analysis

This study is performed to measure the stomach's secretion of hydrochloric acid and pepsin and to evaluate the stomach and check for duodenal ulcers. This test takes approximately 2½ hours to complete and may be performed in the endoscopy department.

Esophageal Manometry (Esophageal Function Study, Esophageal Motility Study)

An esophageal manometry is used to identify and document the severity of disease that affects the swallowing function of the esophagus. It also is used to document and quantify gastroesophageal reflux. The study includes measurement of the lower esophageal sphincter and a graphic recording of swallowing waves (motility). This study usually is performed in the endoscopy department. **Usual prep:** NPO 8 to 12 hours before examination.

Secretin Test

A secretin test evaluates pancreatic function after stimulation with the hormone secretin. The test measures the volume and bicarbonate concentration of pancreatic secretions. Lower than normal volume suggests an obstructing malignancy or cystic fibrosis. This test may be performed in the endoscopy department.

Note: Other GI studies are discussed in Chapters 14 and 15.

CARDIOPULMONARY (RESPIRATORY CARE) DEPARTMENT

Background Information

The cardiopulmonary (respiratory care) department evaluates, treats, and cares for patients with breathing or other cardiopulmonary (pertaining to the heart and lungs) disorders. The cardiopulmonary department also may perform presurgical evaluations. Patients who require respiratory care range from premature infants whose lungs are not fully developed to elderly people whose lungs are diseased. Cardiopulmonary diagnostic procedures are discussed in this chapter, and therapeutic options/treatments are discussed in Chapter 17.

The HUC communicates the doctors' order to the cardiopulmonary (respiratory care) department via computer or by completion of a requisition (Fig. 16-11).

No preparation is required for cardiopulmonary (respiratory care) tests unless the doctor has included special instructions with the order. For example, the doctor may discontinue respiratory medications before testing or may want the amount of oxygen adjusted or turned off before the patient's blood gas is obtained. *Example:* DC O_2 at 10 AM, ABG at 11 AM.

Diagnostic tests commonly performed by the cardiopulmonary (respiratory care) department include those discussed in the following paragraphs.

Doctor ordering _____

Date to be done _____ □ Stat □ Routine □ ASAP

Today's date _____ Requested by _____

┌───┐
│ **Cardiopulmonary (Respiratory Care) Department—Diagnostics** │
└───┘

Clinical indication _____

Anticoagulant medication? □ Yes Name of medication _____
                          □ No

Room air □ Yes □ No   Oxygen □ Yes □ No If yes _____ L/min

Comments: _____

□ ABG   □ Pre-op teaching
□ CBG   □ PFT
□ CPR teaching   □ Spirometry
□ Pulse oximetry
□ Write in order _____

Figure 16-11 A cardiopulmonary (respiratory care) diagnostics downtime requisition.

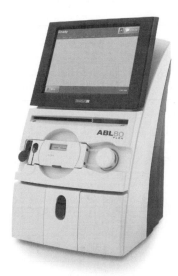

Figure 16-12 Radiometer's ABL80 FLEX point-of-care STAT analyzer measures blood gases as well as electrolyte and metabolite parameters. (Courtesy Radiometer Medical ApS, Westlake, OH.)

Oximetry (Pulse Oximetry, Ear Oximetry, Oxygen Saturation)

Oximetry is a noninvasive method that is used to monitor arterial O_2 saturation levels (SaO_2) in patients at risk for hypoxemia. Oximetry typically is used to monitor oxygenation status during the perioperative period (before, during, and after surgery) in patients who have a compromised respiratory status caused by illness or disease, and in those receiving heavy sedation or mechanical ventilation. A monitoring probe or sensor is clipped to the finger or ear (see Fig. 10-3). This study may be performed at the bedside by a respiratory therapist or nurse in a few minutes or may be left in place to serve as a continuous monitor.

Arterial Blood Gases

Arterial blood gases (ABGs) are used to monitor patients on ventilators or critically ill nonventilator patients, and to establish preoperative baseline parameters and regulate electrolyte therapy. The blood sample for this diagnostic study is obtained from the patient's artery by the respiratory care technician. ABG measurements provide valuable information for assessing and managing a patient's respiratory (ventilation) and metabolic (renal) acid/base and electrolyte homeostasis. They also are used to assess adequacy of oxygenation. Blood gases may be ordered for patients on room air (RA), or while they are receiving oxygen.

When ordering an ABG, the HUC must note whether the patient is on RA or, if on oxygen, the number of liters. If anticoagulants are being administered to the patient, the names of medications (e.g., enoxaparin [Lovenox], heparin [Hepalean], warfarin [Coumadin]) should be noted as well. The arterial blood specimen must be placed on ice immediately and taken to the pulmonary laboratory for analysis. A point-of-care (POC) ABG portable device may be used to perform ABG and pH measurements (Fig. 16-12).

Capillary Blood Gases

Capillary blood gases (CBGs) are performed primarily on infants. Blood is obtained from the infant's capillary arterial vessel, usually from the heel, by the respiratory care technician. The blood is then analyzed in the pulmonary function laboratory. Measurement of CBG also provides valuable information for assessing and managing an infant's respiratory (ventilation) and metabolic (renal) acid/base and electrolyte homeostasis. It also is used to assess adequacy of oxygenation.

Pulmonary Function Tests

Pulmonary function tests (PFTs) are performed to detect abnormalities in respiratory function and to determine the extent of pulmonary abnormality. Tests usually include spirometry, measurement of air flow rates, and calculation of lung volumes and capacities. Other tests may be requested by the ordering physician.

TAKE NOTE

Normal pH Values	Critical Values
Adult/Child: 7.35 to 7.45	pH: <7.25 to >7.55
Newborn: 7.32 to 7.49	PCO_2: <20, >60
2 months to 2 years: 7.34 to 7.46	HCO_3: <15, >40
PH (venous): 7.31 to 7.41	PO_2: <40
	O_2 saturation: 75% or lower
	Base/Excess: ±mEq/L

Spirometry

Spirometry is a procedure that uses a spirometer with a time element that can determine air volume and air flow rates. Air flow rates provide information about airway obstruction. The patient breathes through a sterile mouthpiece into a spirometer, inhaling as deeply as possible and then forcibly exhaling as much air as possible. This test may be repeated with the use of bronchodilators, if values are deficient. The doctor may order a prebronchodilator and postbronchodilator spirometry study.

✓ DOCTORS' ORDERS FOR RESPIRATORY TESTS

- ABG on O_2 @ 2 L/min
- Bedside spirometry study
- Prespirometry and postspirometry ■

➲ SKILLS CHALLENGE

- To practice transcribing cardiopulmonary (respiratory care) diagnostics orders, complete Activity 16-4 in the *Skills Practice Manual.*
- To practice transcribing a review set of doctors' orders, complete Activity16-5 in the *Skills Practice Manual.*
- To practice recording telephone messages, complete Activity 16-6 in the *Skills Practice Manual.*

SLEEP STUDIES (POLYSOMNOGRAPHY, MULTIPLE SLEEP LATENCY TESTS, MULTIPLE WAKE TEST)

The sleep study department performs studies to assess a patient's sleep patterns. Sleep studies are ordered for patients who snore excessively, experience **narcolepsy** (excessive daytime sleepiness), insomnia, or have motor spasms while sleeping, as well as in patients with documented cardiac rhythm disturbances limited to sleep time. Polysomnography is a comprehensive recording of the biophysiological changes that occur during sleep. The polysomnogram (PSG) monitors many body functions including brain (electroencephalogram–EEG), eye movements (electro-oculogram–EOG), muscle activity or skeletal muscle activation (electromyogram–EMG), heart rhythm (electrocardiogram–ECG), and breathing function or respiratory effort during sleep.

Inductive plethysmography is a noninvasive study that measures the patient's respiratory function and can differentiate central **apnea** from **obstructive sleep apnea** during a sleep study. Many hospitals have a sleep study department, and most sleep studies are performed on an outpatient basis. The doctor may order as follows: *Sleep study to assess patient for OSA.* During this procedure, electrodes for ECG, EEG, and EMG are applied to the patient. Excess hair may have to be shaved on male patients. Air flow, oximetry, and impedance monitors also are applied. The patient is allowed to sleep per normal routine and is monitored for respiratory disturbances such as apnea.

CARDIOPULMONARY (RESPIRATORY CARE) DIAGNOSTIC TESTS

- Oximetry (pulse oximetry, ear oximetry, oxygen saturation)
- Arterial blood gases (ABGs)
- Capillary blood gases (CBGs)
- Pulmonary function tests (PFTs)
- Spirometry
- Sleep studies

KEY CONCEPTS

Recognition of the need for and proper scheduling of all diagnostic studies are of utmost importance to the patient, the doctor(s), and the hospital. Both the patient whose condition is as yet undiagnosed and the patient who is awaiting test results are dependent on the knowledge and communication skills of the individual who is coordinating activities on the nursing unit. The HUC who can identify and order correctly all appropriate diagnostic studies is an asset to the unit.

REVIEW QUESTIONS

1. Explain the purpose of the following underlined diagnostic procedures.

  a. <u>Heart cath</u> @0800 tomorrow AM

  _____

  b. <u>EKG</u> stat

  _____

c. <u>ABG</u> on RA @ 4 PM today

_____

d. <u>Spirometry</u> prior to surg

_____

e. Schedule <u>BAER</u> for tomorrow

_____

f. Place on continuous pulse <u>oximetry</u>

_____

2. List two noninvasive cardiac studies that the doctor may request to diagnose cardiac abnormalities.

a. _____

b. _____

3. List two invasive cardiac studies that the doctor may request to diagnose cardiac abnormalities.

a. _____

b. _____

4. What category of medication should be noted on the request when one is ordering an electrocardiogram?

_____

5. Name six endoscopic procedures, and identify the portion of the body that is studied by each procedure.

Procedure	Area Visualized
a. _____	_____
b. _____	_____
c. _____	_____
d. _____	_____
e. _____	_____
f. _____	_____

6. Discuss the importance of properly preparing a patient for a sigmoidoscopy or any visual examination of the colon.

_____

7. What classification of medication would have to be noted on a blood gas requisition?

_____

8. List four diagnostic tests that are performed by the cardiopulmonary (respiratory care) department.

a. _____

b. _____

c. _____

d. _____

9. List two studies related to the gastrointestinal (GI) system that are performed (usually on an outpatient basis) in the endoscopy department.

   a. _____

   b. _____

10. Using the list in the left-hand column below for reference, identify the department that performs the studies indicated in the sets of doctors' orders in the right-hand column.

   Reference List
   a. Cardiovascular diagnostics
   b. Endoscopy department
   c. Neurology diagnostics (department)
   d. Cardiopulmonary (respiratory care) department
   e. Sleep study

   Doctors' Orders
   1. EMG and NCS
   2. Spirometry
   3. ABG on RA
   4. Sigmoidoscopy at 8 AM in clinic
   5. EEG tomorrow
   6. Colonoscopy
   7. EKG, LOC
   8. Echocardiogram
   9. Doppler flow studies
   10. Treadmill stress test
   11. Schedule for sleep study tomorrow
   12. Rhythm strip
   13. Schedule esophagoscopy for Monday
   14. Holter monitor for 24 hours
   15. IPG—left leg
   16. ERCP tomorrow
   17. Schedule BAER
   18. Place on oximetry

11. Name two studies that are performed by the cardiovascular department to diagnose vascular disease.

   a. _____

   b. _____

12. List two purposes of an electroencephalogram.

   a. _____

   b. _____

13. Identify the category of medication that should be noted on the request when one is ordering an electroencephalogram.

   _____

14. Define the following terms:

   a. invasive procedure _____

   b. noninvasive procedure _____

THINK ABOUT...

1. Discuss the importance of the HUC's noting anticoagulant medications on a requisition for an ABG.
2. Discuss the possible consequences of not transcribing doctors' orders for diagnostic tests in a timely manner.
3. Discuss the possible consequences of ordering a diagnostic test on the wrong patient and ways that this could be avoided.

Treatment Orders

CHAPTER OBJECTIVES

Upon completion of this chapter, you will be able to:

1. Define the terms in the vocabulary list.
2. Write the meaning of each abbreviation in the Abbreviations list.
3. Identify two procedures performed to repair obstructed coronary blood vessels.
4. State the purpose of the cardiopulmonary (respiratory care) department.
5. Explain the purpose of hyperbaric oxygen therapy.
6. Identify the two basic types of traction.
7. Name the traction setup used by patients to assist them to move in bed.
8. Given a list of treatments, identify which department would perform them.
9. State the purpose of the physical therapy department.
10. State the purpose of the occupational therapy department.
11. List the two main types of dialysis.

VOCABULARY

Active Exercise Exercise performed by the patient without assistance as instructed by physical therapist
Activities of Daily Living Tasks that enable individuals to meet basic needs (eating, bathing, and so forth)

Aerobic Living only in the presence of oxygen
Aerosol Liquid suspension of particles in a gas stream for inhalation purposes
Apnea Absence of spontaneous breathing
Auscultation The act of listening for sounds within the body to evaluate the condition of the heart, blood vessels, lungs, pleura, intestines, or other organs, or to detect fetal heart sounds
Cardiac Pacemaker An electronic device, temporary or permanent, that regulates the pace of the heart when the heart is incapable of doing it
Certified Respiratory Therapist (CRT) After completion of an approved respiratory therapy program, graduates may become credentialed by taking an entry level examination to become a CRT
Compressor Grip (C-GRIP) A tight, stretchy, tubular material used for temporary compression
Crackle A common, abnormal respiratory sound that consists of discontinuous bubbling noises heard on auscultation of the chest during inspiration (also called *rale*)
Débridement The process of removing dirt, foreign objects, damaged tissue, and cellular debris from a wound or a burn to prevent infection and to promote healing
Defibrillation Application of an electric shock to the myocardium through the chest wall to restore normal cardiac rhythm

Dialysis A mechanical process to remove toxic wastes from the blood, which would normally be filtered out by the kidneys

Dyspnea Difficult or labored breathing

Endotracheal Tube A tube inserted through the mouth that supplies air to the lungs and assists breathing. The ET tube is connected to a ventilator

Extubation Removal of a previously inserted tube (such as an endotracheal tube)

Hydrotherapy The use of water—including continuous tub baths, wet sheet packs, or shower sprays—to soothe pains and treat various conditions and diseases

Hyperbaric Oxygen Therapy A treatment that involves breathing 100% oxygen while in an enclosed system pressurized to greater than one atmosphere (sea level)

Hypertonic A concentrated salt solution (>0.9%)

Hypotonic A dilute salt solution (<0.9%)

Induced Sputum Specimen A sputum specimen obtained by performing a respiratory treatment to loosen lung secretions

Intervention Synonymous with treatment

Intubation Insertion and placement of a tube within the trachea (may be endotracheal or tracheostomy)

Isometric Of equal dimensions. Holding ends of contracting muscle fixed so that contraction produces increased tension at a constant overall length

Nebulizer A gas-driven device that produces an aerosol

Passive Exercise Exercise in which the patient is submissive and the physical therapist moves the patient's limbs

Positive Pressure Pressure greater than atmospheric pressure

Range of Motion The range in which a joint can move

Reduction The correction of a deformity in a bone fracture or dislocation

Resistive Exercise Exercise that uses opposition. A T band or water may be used to provide resistance for patient exercises

Splint An orthopedic device for immobilization, restraint, or support of any part of the body; may be rigid (metal, plaster, or wood) or flexible (felt or leather)

Stent A tiny metal or plastic tube that is placed into an artery, blood vessel, or other duct to hold the structure open

Tank Room A room where hydrotherapy is performed

Traction A mechanical pull to part of the body to maintain alignment and facilitate healing; traction may be static (continuous) or intermittent

Ultrasound Therapy A deep heating modality using high-energy sound waves that is most effective for heating tissues or deep joints and is performed by a physical therapist

Unit Dose Any premixed or prespecified dose; often administered with small volume nebulizer or intermittent positive-pressure breathing treatments

Ventilator A machine that is used to give the patient breaths through the ET or tracheostomy tube

ABBREVIATIONS

Abbreviation	Meaning	Example of Usage on a Doctors' Order Sheet
AA	active assisted	AA exercises B/L LE
ADL	activities of daily living	OT for ADL

Abbreviation	Meaning	Example of Usage on a Doctors' Order Sheet
ADS	adult distress syndrome	The patient's dx is ADS
AKA	above-the-knee amputation	AKA protocol
BiW	twice a week	PT 2 × a wk
BKA	below-the-knee amputation	consent for BKA
BLE	both or bilateral lower extremities	HBOT BLE
BUE	both or bilateral upper extremities	strengthening exercises BUE
CABG	coronary artery bypass graft	consent for CABG
CP	cold pack	CP L arm
CPAP	continuous positive airway pressure	CPAP 5 cm H$_2$O
CPM	continuous passive motion	CPM
CPR	cardiopulmonary resuscitation	CPR training for parents before child's discharge
CPT	Chest percussion therapy	DC CPT
DPI	dry powder inhaler	instruct patient on use of DPI
EPC	electronic pain control	EPC
ES	electrical stimulation	ES
ET	endotracheal tube	CXR for ET tube placement
FWW	front-wheel walker	provide c̄ FWW
HA	heated aerosol	HA T-piece @ 60%
HBOT	hyperbaric O$_2$ therapy	HBOT qd 3 × wk for 8 wk
HD	hemodialysis	HD BiW × 3 h
HP	hot packs	HP to neck
ICD	implantable cardioverter-defibrillator	Have consent signed for ICD
IPPB	intermittent positive-pressure breathing	IPPB q4h c̄ 0.5 mL Ventolin in 2 mL NS
IS	incentive spirometry	IS tid
ISOM	isometric	ISOM UE bid
lbs, #	pounds	bucks traction c̄ 5# weight
LE	lower extremities	ROM LE qd
LLE	left lower extremity	passive exercises LLE
LLL	left lower lobe	CPT—LLL only
L/min	liters per minute	↑O$_2$ to 4 L/min
LUE	left upper extremities	ROM LUE
LUL	left upper lobe	CPT to LUL

Abbreviation	Meaning	Example of Usage on a Doctors' Order Sheet
MDI	metered-dose inhaler	MDI c̄ ii puffs qid
NWB	non–weight-bearing	Crutch-walking NWB
O₂	oxygen	O₂ 6 L/min by mask
ORIF	open reduction, internal fixation	ORIF lt femur
OT	occupational therapy or occupational therapist	OT for ADL
PD	peritoneal dialysis	Tenckhoff cath for PD
PDPV	postural drainage, percussion, and vibration	PDPV to LUL
PEP	positive expiratory pressure	IS c̄ PEP
PROM	passive range of motion	PROM LUE bid
PT	physical therapy or physical therapist	To PT for crutch walking
PTA	physical therapy assistant	PTA to assist patient in amb
RLE	right lower extremities	ISOM to RLE
RLL	right lower lobe	CPT RLL
RML	right middle lobe	CPT RML
ROM	range of motion	ROM to upper extremities tid
RT	respiratory therapist	RT to obtain induced sputum specimen
RUE	right upper extremity	Hot pk to RUE
RUL	right upper lobe	CPT to RUL
SaO or O₂	oxygen saturation (on pulse	Titrate O₂ flow to SaO >95%
Sats	oximetry, not ABGs)	
SIDS	sudden infant death syndrome	The baby died of SIDS
STM	soft tissue massage	STM lt shoulder 20 min bid
SVN	small volume nebulizer	Δ SVN to bid
TENS	transcutaneous electrical nerve stimulation	Postop TENS
THR, THA	total hip replacement/ arthroplasty	follow THR protocol
TKR, TKA	total knee replacement/ arthroplasty	TKA protocol
TT	tilt table	TT for PT
TTOT	Transtracheal oxygen therapy	Start TTOT today
Tx	traction	Buck's Tx

Abbreviation	Meaning	Example of Usage on a Doctors' Order Sheet
UD	unit dose	UD Ventolin now
USN	ultrasonic nebulizer	USN 15 min tid
WBAT	weight bearing as tolerated	amb, WBAT rt leg
WP	whirlpool	WP to L leg bid
>	greater than	Call hospitalist if pH >7.4
<	less than	Call Dr. Jones if O₂ Sats <70%

EXERCISE 1

Write the abbreviation for each term listed below.

1. left upper lobe _____
2. occupational therapy or occupational therapist _____
3. physical therapy or physical therapist _____
4. liters per minute _____
5. oxygen _____
6. intermittent positive-pressure breathing _____
7. right upper lobe _____
8. range of motion _____
9. right lower lobe _____
10. activities of daily living _____
11. coronary artery bypass graft _____
12. right middle lobe _____
13. ultrasonic nebulizer _____
14. small-volume nebulizer _____
15. left lower lobe _____
16. pounds _____
17. non–weight-bearing _____
18. whirlpool _____
19. hot packs _____
20. transcutaneous electrical nerve stimulation _____
21. electronic pain control _____
22. electrical stimulation _____

23. continuous passive motion   _____

24. incentive spirometry   _____

25. metered-dose inhaler   _____

26. chest percussion therapy   _____

27. active assisted   _____

28. twice weekly   _____

29. above-the-knee amputation   _____

30. soft tissue massage   _____

31. lower extremities   _____

32. hemodialysis   _____

33. total hip replacement/arthroplasty   _____

34. open reduction, internal fixation   _____

35. traction   _____

36. tilt table   _____

37. isometric   _____

38. below-the-knee amputation   _____

39. endotracheal tube   _____

40. heated aerosol   _____

41. positive expiratory pressure   _____

42. postural drainage, percussion,
    and vibration   _____

43. oxygen saturation   _____

44. unit dose   _____

45. greater than   _____

46. total knee replacement/arthroplasty   _____

47. less than   _____

48. cold packs   _____

49. cardiopulmonary resuscitation   _____

50. hyperbaric oxygen therapy   _____

51. transtracheal oxygen therapy   _____

52. continuous positive airway pressure   _____

53. both upper extremities   _____

54. both lower extremities   _____

55. right upper extremity   _____

56. left upper extremity   _____

57. right lower extremity   _____

58. left lower extremity   _____

59. physical therapist assistant   _____

60. respiratory therapist   _____

61. passive range of motion   _____

62. weight bearing as tolerated   _____

63. front-wheel walker   _____

64. peritoneal dialysis   _____

65. implantable cardioverter-defibrillator   _____

66. adult distress syndrome   _____

67. dry powder inhaler   _____

68. sudden infant death syndrome   _____

EXERCISE 2

Write the meaning of each abbreviation listed below.

1. O_2

   _____

2. LUL

   _____

3. RLL

   _____

4. OT

   _____

5. PT

   _____

6. SIDS

   _____

7. ADL

   _____

8. lb or #

_____

9. RUL

_____

10. RML

_____

11. NWB

_____

12. ROM

_____

13. L/min

_____

14. SVN

_____

15. LLL

_____

16. IPPB

_____

17. USN

_____

18. HP

_____

19. WP

_____

20. CPM

_____

21. ES

_____

22. EPC

_____

23. TENS

_____

24. IS

_____

25. CPT

_____

26. MDI

_____

27. ORIF

_____

28. TT

_____

29. SaO or O_2 Sats

_____

30. AKA

_____

31. UD

_____

32. HA

_____

33. ISOM

_____

34. LE

_____

35. STM

_____

36. HD

_____

37. Tx

_____

38. PD

_____

39. >

_____

40. TKR, TKA

_____

41. THR, THA

_____

42. ET

_____

43. PD

_____

44. <

_____

45. BiW

_____

46. PEP

_____

47. CP

_____

48. AA

_____

49. CPR

_____

50. HBOT

_____

51. TTOT

_____

52. CPAP

_____

53. BUE

_____

54. BLE

_____

55. RUE

_____

56. LUE

_____

57. RLE

_____

58. LLE

_____

59. PTA

_____

60. RT

_____

61. PROM

_____

62. WBAT

_____

63. FWW

_____

64. CABG

_____

65. DPI

_____

66. ADS

_____

67. ICD

_____

68. PD

_____

When the electronic medical record (EMR) with computer physician order entry (CPOE) is implemented, the physicians' orders are entered directly into the patient's electronic record, and the treatment order is automatically sent to the appropriate department. The health unit coordinator (HUC) may have tasks to perform, such as coordinating and scheduling procedures, ordering special diets and cathartics for preparation, and so forth. An icon may indicate an HUC task, or it may signify a nurse request. The HUC will have to communicate with the nutritional care department (by e-mail or telephone) when ordering special diets or NPO for the patient.

Downtime requisitions are included in this chapter for learning purposes. The CD included in the *Health Unit Coordinator Skills Manual* is a simulated hospital computer program that may be used as well.

CARDIOVASCULAR

Cardiovascular conditions may be treated with medication and/or surgery, and/or placement of a pacemaker. Some of the surgical procedures required and the placement of pacemakers are discussed in this chapter.

Insertion of a Cardiac Pacemaker

A **cardiac pacemaker** is an electric apparatus that is used in most cases to increase the heart rate in severe bradycardia by electrically stimulating the heart muscle. A pacemaker may be permanent or temporary, may emit the stimulus at a constant and fixed rate, or may fire only on demand. Permanent pacemakers are implanted under a chest muscle during surgery. With temporary pacemakers, wires from outside the body lead into the heart (Fig. 17-1).

Insertion of an Implantable Cardioverter-Defibrillator

An implantable cardioverter-defibrillator (ICD) may be referred to as an automatic implantable cardioverter-defibrillator (AICD); it is implanted in the chest. An ICD is an electric device that monitors and restores proper rhythm by sending low-energy shocks to the heart when the heart begins to beat rapidly or erratically (Fig. 17-2).

Pacemakers usually are used to correct a heart rhythm that is bradycardia (slow heart rhythm), whereas implantable cardioverter-defibrillators (ICDs) are used to correct a heart rhythm that is tachycardia (fast heart rhythm).

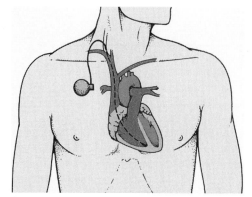

Figure 17-1 Pacemaker. (From Thibodeau GA, Patton KT: *Anatomy and physiology,* ed 6, St. Louis, 2007, Mosby.)

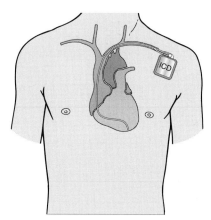

Figure 17-2 Implantable cardioverter-defibrillator. (From Lewis SM, Heitkemper MM, Dirksen SR: *Medical-surgical nursing,* ed 6, St. Louis, 2004, Mosby.)

Angioplasty (Balloon Angioplasty, Coronary Angioplasty, Coronary Artery Angioplasty, Cardiac Angioplasty, Percutaneous Transluminal Coronary Angioplasty, Heart Artery Dilatation)

Angioplasty is a medical procedure in which a balloon is used to open narrowed or blocked blood vessels of the heart (coronary arteries). Although it is an invasive procedure and a consent form is required, it is not regarded as a type of surgery. An angioplasty usually is performed during a heart catheterization, when it is deemed necessary. Traditional angioplasty involves the use of a balloon catheter—a small, hollow, flexible tube that has a balloon near the end of it. The balloon catheter is moved into or near the blockage, and the balloon on the end is blown up (inflated). This opens the blocked vessel and restores proper blood flow to the heart.

Stent

In most cases, a device called a **stent** is placed at the site of a narrowing or blockage in order to keep the artery open. Stenting (the implantation of a stent) is a common procedure. An intraluminal coronary artery stent is a small, self-expanding, metal mesh tube that is placed inside a coronary artery after balloon angioplasty to prevent the artery from reclosing

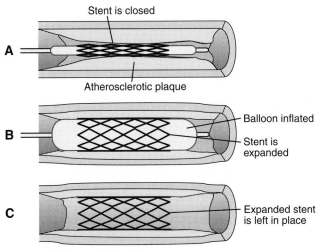

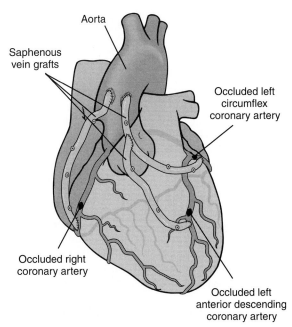

Figure 17-3 Coronary stent. (From LaFleur Brooks M: *Exploring medical language: a student-directed approach,* ed 6, St. Louis, 2005, Mosby.)

Figure 17-4 Coronary bypass (CBAG). (From Lewis SM, Heitkemper MM, Dirksen SR: *Medical-surgical nursing: assessment and management of clinical problems,* ed 5, St. Louis, 2000, Mosby.)

(Fig. 17-3). A drug-eluting stent is coated with medicine (sirolimus or paclitaxel) that helps to further prevent the arteries from reclosing. Similar to other coronary stents, it is left permanently in the artery.

Atherectomy

In a small number of cases, a special catheter with a small, diamond tip is used to drill through hard plaque and calcium that is causing the blockage. This is called *rotational atherectomy.*

Coronary Artery Bypass Graft

Coronary artery bypass graft surgery, or CABG (pronounced "cabbage"), has become a common treatment for blocked arteries when they are too severely blocked to be treated with angioplasty. Heart bypass surgery creates a detour or "bypass" around the blocked part of a coronary artery to restore the blood supply to the heart muscle (Fig. 17-4). After the patient has been anesthetized, the heart surgeon makes an incision in the middle of the chest and separates the breastbone. Through this incision, the surgeon can see the heart and the aorta (the main blood vessel leading from the heart to the rest of the body). After surgery, the breastbone is rejoined with wire, and the incision is sewn closed.

Artery and Vein Grafts

A vein from the leg, called the *saphenous vein,* may be used for the bypass; an incision is made in the leg and the vein removed. The vein is located on the inside of the leg, running from the ankle to the groin. The saphenous vein normally does only about 10% of the work of circulating blood from the leg back to the heart. Therefore, it can be taken out without harm to the patient or harm to the leg. The internal mammary artery (IMA) also can be used as the graft.

The IMA provides the advantage of staying open for many more years than vein grafts, but in some situations, it cannot be used. Other arteries also are being used now in bypass surgery. The most common of these is the radial artery. This is one of the two arteries that supply the hand with blood. It usually can be removed from the arm without resultant impairment of blood supply to the hand. Traditionally, the patient is connected to the heart-lung machine, or the bypass pump, which adds oxygen to the blood and circulates blood to other parts of the body during surgery.

Other surgical techniques for this procedure are being used more frequently. One popular method is called *off-pump coronary artery bypass,* or OPCAB. This operation allows the bypass to be created while the heart is still beating. Another alternative is the use of smaller incisions that avoid splitting the breastbone. This is referred to as minimally invasive direct coronary artery bypass, or MIDCAB. Coronary bypass surgery now can be performed with the aid of a robot, which allows the surgeon to perform the operation without even being in the same room as the patient. A surgical consent form is required, and the patient is admitted to the coronary intensive care unit after surgery.

> ✎ *TAKE NOTE*
>
> Usually, the consent form for heart catheterization includes all possible correction options, so the surgeon can proceed with the procedure or surgery as required.

> ➡ **SKILLS CHALLENGE**
>
> To practice transcribing cardiovascular treatment orders, complete Activity 17-1 in the *Skills Practice Manual.*

CARDIOPULMONARY (RESPIRATORY CARE) DEPARTMENT

Background Information

Diagnostic tests performed in the respiratory care department were discussed in Chapter 16. The cardiopulmonary (respiratory care) department also performs treatments to maintain or improve the function of the respiratory system. Treatments usually are performed by a respiratory therapist at the patient's bedside. It is important that the HUC enter all information regarding the order into the computer or onto the requisition form. The respiratory therapist then brings the needed equipment and medication to the unit, so the patient's treatment is not be delayed by having to obtain necessary items. The therapist reads the doctor's order before administering the treatment. Upon completion of treatment, the therapist documents the type of medication and treatment provided and other pertinent data on a respiratory therapy record sheet in the patient's chart.

To communicate the doctors' order to the cardiopulmonary (respiratory care) department, use the computer or complete a cardiopulmonary (respiratory care) treatment requisition (Fig. 17- 5). Listed below are examples of respiratory treatments provided by the cardiopulmonary (respiratory care) department.

Oxygen Therapy

Oxygen therapy is ordered to (1) treat hypoxemia (abnormal deficiency in the concentration of oxygen in arterial blood); (2) decrease the work of breathing; and (3) reduce myocardial (heart muscle) work. Oxygen is piped into the patient's room via a wall outlet and is administered under pressure (Fig. 17-6). A portable oxygen tank may be used when a patient is transported. Oxygen therapy may have a drying effect on the respiratory tract; therefore, oxygen is commonly humidified during administration. Oxygen supports combustion; therefore, no smoking is allowed in the room while oxygen is being administered. Most hospitals and other health care facilities have a general "no smoking" policy.

An oxygen order contains the amount of oxygen (flow rate or concentration) the patient is to receive and the type of delivery device to be used (mode of delivery). The flow rate is ordered in liters per minute.

Flow Rate or Concentration of Oxygen and Administration Devices

Oxygen may be administered with the use of a *low-flow system*, which provides only a portion of the total amount of gas the patient is breathing—the rest must be added from room air. Or *high-flow oxygen systems* may be used that provide enough gas flow to meet all of the patient's ventilatory demands.

Low-flow oxygen administration devices include the following:

(1) *Nasal cannula*, frequently referred to as *nasal prongs*, is the most commonly used method. Nasal cannulas should not be run over 6 L per minute because this may cause excessive drying of the nasal mucosa.
(2) *Simple mask* is a device generally used for emergencies and short-term therapies that fits over the patient's nose and mouth and acts as a reservoir for the next breath. The simple mask should be run at a minimum of 5 L per minute to ensure that the carbon dioxide the patient exhales is washed away and is not rebreathed.

Doctor ordering _____

Date to be done _____ □ Stat □ Routine □ ASAP

Today's date _____ Requested by _____

| Cardiopulmonary (Respiratory Care) Department Treatments |

Clinical indication _____

Comments: _____

□ O₂ _____ L/M   □ NP   □ Mask   □ Type   □ Other_____
□ Aerosol delivery type_____
□ Bi-level press.vent. _____
□ CPAP_____
□ CPT_____
□ IPPB_____
□ IS _____
□ SVN _____
□ USN _____
Write-in order_____

Ventilator orders
IMV mode _____ TV_____ FIO₂_____ PO₂_____ PS_____ Peep_____

Write in order _____

Figure 17-5 Downtime requisition for cardiopulmonary (respiratory care) treatment.

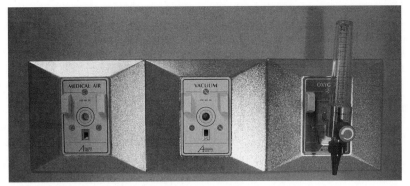

Figure 17-6 Wall outlet for oxygen.

(3) *Partial rebreathing mask* uses a simple mask connected to a bag reservoir with no valve between the bag and the mask. It is called a *partial rebreathing mask* because the first one third of exhalation enters the bag, mixes with source oxygen, and is consumed during the next inhalation.

(4) *Nonrebreathing mask* is designed to fit over the patient's nose and mouth as the simple oxygen mask does; however, a 500- to 1000-mL plastic bag is added to the mask, which has a series of one-way valves that permit the reservoir bag to fill only with pure oxygen (Fig. 17-7).

High-flow oxygen systems include the following:

(1) *Jet mixing mask*, also referred to as a **Venti mask**, delivers a total high flow by mixing oxygen with room air. The mask takes pure oxygen from the flow meter and mixes it with a certain proportion of room air to deliver a higher concentration of oxygen.

(2) *Large-volume nebulizer* is another example of a high-flow system. This device works much like the jet mixing mask, but it also provides bland (nonmedicated) **aerosol** therapy and can be connected to a variety of devices, including an aerosol mask, a face tent for patients with facial burns or who cannot tolerate a mask, a T piece or Briggs adapter for intubated patients, or a tracheostomy mask (collar) for those with a tracheostomy (Fig. 17-8).

Plastic tubing is used to carry oxygen from the wall outlet to the patient. Although cardiopulmonary (respiratory care) department personnel usually set up, take down, and handle the equipment for oxygen administration, nursing staff members also monitor this treatment.

✐ TAKE NOTE

Orders for oxygen therapy include the amount of oxygen (flow rate or concentration) and the type of delivery device.

It is important to recognize a new order for oxygen or a change in a previous order. An ABG on O_2 @ 4 L/min is *NOT* a new order for oxygen but is an arterial blood gas drawn while the patient's oxygen flow rate is at 4 L per minute. It may be necessary to notify nursing staff or the cardiopulmonary (respiratory care) department of the oxygen flow rate.

Aerosol Treatments
Aerosol Delivery Devices

Metered-Dose Inhaler (MDI). Metered-dose inhalers (MDIs), small portable aerosol canisters filled with medication, are the most common type of aerosol treatment. One or two puffs of the medication is inhaled with a deep breath and an inspiratory hold for a few seconds. Usually, MDIs are self-administered and require patient education and cooperation (Fig. 17-9).

Small-Volume Nebulizer (SVN) (Handheld Nebulizer [HHN]). Small-volume nebulizer treatments last between 8 and 12 minutes and allow for numerous breaths to administer the medication. The ideal breathing pattern is for the patient to inhale deeply with an inspiratory hold for a few seconds. Small-volume nebulizers also may be called *spontaneous nebulizer treatments* or *jet nebulizer treatments* or may be referred to by the brand name of the nebulizer device (Fig. 17-10).

Dry Powder Inhaler (DPI). Dry powder inhalers (DPIs) are devices that provide the drug in powder form to be delivered into the lungs for absorption. A total of 1 or 2 puffs of the medication is inhaled with a deep breath and an inspiratory hold for a few seconds. An example of a DPI is Advair. Usually, DPIs are self-administered and require patient education and cooperation (Fig. 7-11).

Hypertonic Ultrasonic Nebulizer (USN). An ultrasonic nebulizer with hypertonic solution often is used to induce a sputum specimen. It produces an aerosol that carries deep into the airways of the lung to loosen secretions so the patient may produce a sputum specimen. The solution used is a **hypertonic** (concentrated) salt solution of 5% sodium chloride (NaCl). This is called an *induced sputum specimen.*

A Lukens sputum trap often is used by a respiratory therapist to collect a sterile induced sputum specimen (Fig. 17-12).

Intermittent Positive-Pressure Breathing (IPPB). Intermittent **positive-pressure** breathing (IPPB) is a technique

---

✐ TAKE NOTE

Ultrasound diagnostic procedures are performed in the ultrasound division of diagnostic imaging (see Chapter 15).

An ultrasonic nebulizer is used as treatment by the cardiopulmonary (respiratory care) department. Ultrasound therapy is provided by the physical therapist. It is important to read the doctors' orders carefully so the order is sent to the appropriate department.

that is used to provide short-term or intermittent mechanical ventilation for the purpose of augmenting lung expansion, delivering aerosol medication, clearing retained secretions, or assisting ventilation. IPPB treatment usually is administered through the use of a pneumatically driven, pressure-triggered, pressure-cycled ventilator (Fig. 17-13).

Types of Aerosolized Drugs

Nasal Decongestants. Nasal decongestants are found primarily as over-the-counter (OTC) squeeze bottles that are sprayed into nostrils. These drugs are classified as vasoconstrictors. An example of a nasal decongestant is Neo-Synephrine.

Bronchodilators. Bronchodilators enlarge the diameter of the airway, usually by relaxing the smooth muscle that surrounds the airways. Examples of bronchodilators include Ventolin, Atrovent, Maxair, and Serevent.

Antiasthmatics. This is a relatively new category of drugs that desensitize the allergic response to prevent or decrease the incidence of asthma. Examples of antiasthmatics include cromolyn sodium and nedocromil sodium.

Corticosteroids. Corticosteroids are used in moderate and severe asthma attacks to reduce the inflammatory response within the lung. They also are used on a standing basis to prevent inflammation. Examples of corticosteroids include Pulmicort, Vanceril, Flovent, and Azmacort.

Mucolytics. Mucolytics break down secretions within the lungs to make it easier to expectorate and clear the lungs. Examples of Mucolytics include Pulmozyme and Mucomyst.

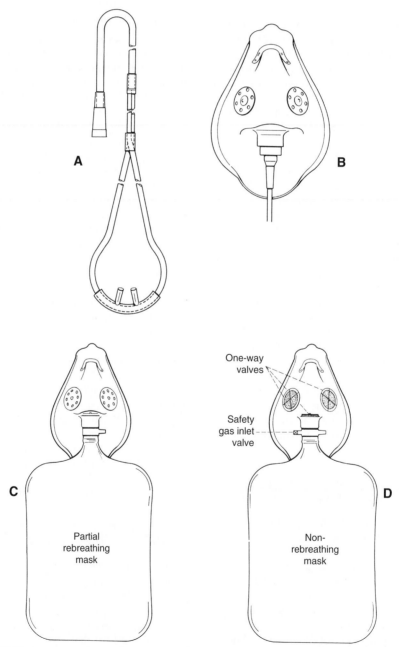

Figure 17-7 Devices used to administer low-flow system oxygen. (From Kacmarek RM: In-hospital administration of oxygen. In: Kacmarek RM, Stoller JK, editors: *Current respiratory care,* Toronto, 1988, BC Decker.)

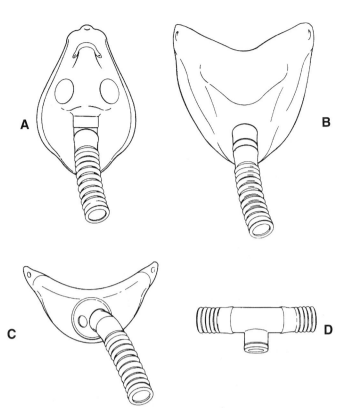

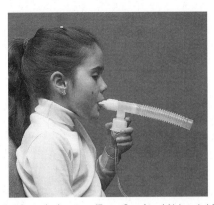

Figure 17-10 Nebulization. (From Sanders MJ, Lewis LM, Quick G, et al: *Mosby's paramedic textbook,* ed 2, St. Louis, 2000, Mosby.)

Figure 17-8 Various devices used to apply high-flow system oxygen. **A,** Aerosol mask. **B,** Face hood. **C,** Tracheostomy collar. **D,** Briggs T piece (From Kacmarek RM: In-hospital administration of oxygen. In: Kacmarek RM, Stoller JK, editors: *Current respiratory care,* Toronto, 1988, BC Decker.)

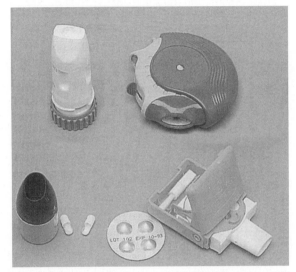

Figure 17-11 Dry powder inhalers. (Modified from Spiro S, Mac-Cochran G: Delivery of medication to the lungs. In: Albert R, Spiro S, Jett J, editors: *Comprehensive respiratory medicine,* St. Louis, 1999, Mosby.)

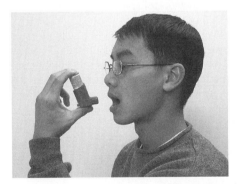

Figure 17-9 A metered-dose inhaler. (From Elkin MK, Perry AG, Potter PA: *Nursing interventions and clinical skills,* ed 3, St. Louis, 2004, Mosby.)

Antimicrobials. Antimicrobials are aerosolized antibiotics and antiviral agents that fight both bacterial and viral infections involving the respiratory system. Examples of antimicrobials include gentamicin, tobramycin, amphotericin B, ribavirin, and pentamidine.

Other Respiratory Treatments
Incentive Spirometry

Incentive spirometry (IS), also known as sustained maximal inspiration (SMI), often is used postoperatively to encourage and reinforce the patient to take protracted, slow, deep breaths. The benefits of IS include improving inspiratory muscle performance, thereby reestablishing or simulating the normal

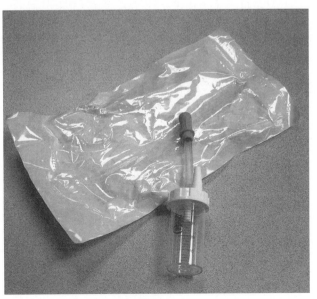

Figure 17-12 Lukens sputum trap, used to collect uncontaminated sputum specimens.

pattern of pulmonary hyperinflation. The devices used provide patients with visual positive feedback when they inhale at a predetermined flow rate or volume and sustain the inflation for a predetermined length of time (Fig. 17-14).

Chest Percussion Therapy

Chest percussion therapy (CPT), a technique of rhythmically tapping the chest wall with cupped hands (Fig. 17-15) or a mechanical device, is used to loosen secretions in the area underlying the percussion via the air pressure that is generated by the cupped hand on the chest wall. This treatment usually is performed in conjunction with postural drainage, a treatment of patient positioning that is designed to remove secretions from the lung.

Mechanical Ventilator

A mechanical ventilator is a device designed to provide mechanical ventilation to a patient. Ventilators are used chiefly in intensive care medicine, home care, and emergency medicine (as stand-alone units), and in anesthesia as a component of an anesthesia machine. Mechanical ventilation is indicated when the patient's spontaneous ventilation is inadequate to maintain life. It also is indicated to prevent imminent collapse of other physiologic functions or ineffective gas exchange in the lungs. Because mechanical ventilation serves only to provide assistance for breathing and does not cure a disease, the patient's underlying condition should be correctable and should resolve over time, although some conditions may warrant the use of mechanical ventilation for the duration of the patient's life. *Weaning* is a term that is used to describe the gradual removal of mechanical ventilation from a patient. Arterial blood gas tests will be ordered at intervals to monitor ventilator settings. Extubation orders will be written when the patient is to be removed from the ventilator. Postextubation orders will be written to monitor respiratory status after the patient has been removed from the ventilator.

Noninvasive Positive-Pressure Ventilation

Noninvasive positive-pressure ventilation (NIPPV) is the application of positive pressure by noninvasive means to a patient with acute or chronic respiratory failure, or while weaning a patient from ventilatory support.

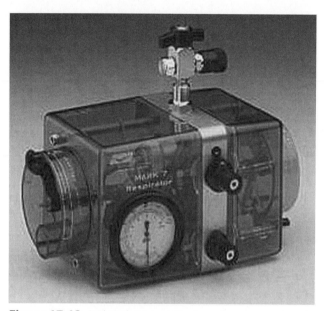

Figure 17-13 Bird Mark 7 intermittent positive-pressure breathing machine. (From Kacmarek RM, Dimas S, Mack CW: *The essentials of respiratory care*, ed 4, St. Louis, 2005, Mosby.)

AN EXAMPLE OF SETTINGS FOR A MECHANICAL VENTILATOR

COPD: Initial Ventilator Settings
Noninvasive
  Mode: Assist/control (pressure) or pressure support
  Tidal volume (TV): 6 to 8 mL/kg ideal body weight (IBW)
  Positive end-expiratory pressure (PEEP): 3 to 8 cm H_2O
  Ventilating pressure: 8 to 12 cm H_2O
  Inspiratory time: <1.0 second
  F_1O_2: to maintain $PaO_2 > 60$ mm Hg
  Backup rate: 8 to 10, actual patient rate determines baseline $PaCO_2$

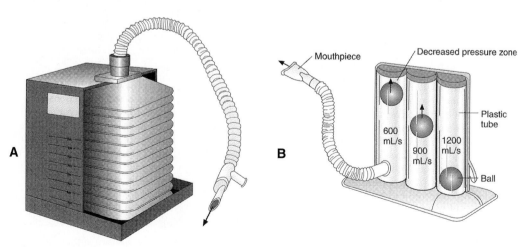

Figure 17-14 A, Volume-oriented incentive spirometer. **B,** Flow-oriented incentive spirometer. (From Eubanks DH, Bone RC: *Comprehensive respiratory care*, St. Louis, 1985, Mosby.)

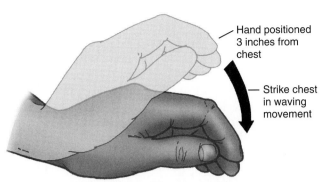

Hand positioned
3 inches from
chest

Strike chest
in waving
movement

Figure 17-15 Movement of cupped hand at wrist to percuss chest. (From Wilkins RL, Stoller JK, Scanlan CL: *Egan's fundamentals of respiratory care*, ed 8, St. Louis, 2003, Mosby.)

DOCTORS' ORDERS FOR RESPIRATORY TREATMENTS

The following orders include many instructions for the respiratory therapist. It is very important to be accurate in copying the order onto the cardiopulmonary (respiratory care) requisition or entering it into the computer, so the therapist will bring the correct equipment and/or supplies to carry out the order. The respiratory therapist also is required to read the physicians' orders before administering treatment.

O$_2$ 4 L/min NC cont
4 L per minute of oxygen is delivered continuously via nasal cannula.

SVN with UD albuterol tid c̄ CPT
This small-volume nebulizer (SVN) order includes a **unit dose** of albuterol and an order for chest percussion therapy.

SVN 0.5 mL terbutaline c̄ 2.5 mL NS qid
This treatment uses a simple device that produces an aerosol from liquid medication to be inhaled into the lungs.

✓ HYPERTONIC USN FOR SPUTUM INDUCEMENT

An ultrasonic nebulizer with hypertonic solution produces an aerosol that carries deep into the airways of the lung to loosen secretions so the patient may produce a sputum specimen.

> 🖋 *TAKE NOTE*
>
> The HUC must notify the cardiopulmonary (respiratory care) department when the doctor writes an order for an induced sputum specimen. Small-volume nebulizer or hypertonic ultrasonic nebulizer treatment is given by a respiratory therapist to loosen lung secretions. A Lukens trap often is used by a respiratory therapist to collect a sterile sputum specimen.

IPPB 0.5 mL Ventolin & 3 mL NS tid
This IPPB order includes medication (Ventolin) and dosage (0.5 mL). IPPB orders must include frequency and medication; duration and pressure used are optional.

MDI c̄ Ventolin qid i̇i̇i̇ puffs
MDI is a metered dose inhaler in which the medication is premeasured in the pharmacy.

HA @ 60% via T piece
A heated mist (heated aerosol) is produced for the patient to breathe in. It may be ordered for patients who are breathing through a tracheostomy or an **endotracheal tube**.

✓ INCENTIVE SPIROMETRY (IS) TID

IS c̄ PEP @ 5 cm H$_2$O
This incentive spirometry treatment includes positive expiratory pressure (PEP), which supplies resistance against exhalation (keeps air from coming out) in order to reinflate the alveoli in patients with atelectasis. PEP also may be ordered with SVN treatments.

Bilevel pressure I:10 E:5
Bilevel pressure ventilation is a treatment that uses a machine to push air into the lungs during inspiration (such as IPPB) and expiration (such as CPAP) in order to treat severe atelectasis or sleep **apnea**.

CPAP 5 cm H$_2$O
This continuous positive airway pressure treatment provides continuous positive pressure in the airway throughout the entire respiratory cycle. This approach prevents the lungs from completely returning to resting level and may be used to treat patients with sleep apnea and other respiratory syndromes. CPAP usually is provided noninvasively through a facial apparatus. It also can be used in weaning patients from a mechanical ventilator, or in treating those with inadequate oxygen intake.

✓ CARDIOPULMONARY (RESPIRATORY CARE) TO DO PREOPERATIVE TEACHING

The respiratory therapist will instruct the patient before surgery about incentive spirometry and other respiratory treatments that the doctor will order to be done after surgery. The patient will know then what to expect and will know what is expected in the performance of respiratory treatments.

✓ CARDIOPULMONARY (RESPIRATORY CARE) TO DO CPR TRAINING WITH PARENTS BEFORE A CHILD'S DISCHARGE

The respiratory therapist sometimes is asked to teach parents cardiopulmonary resuscitation (CPR) before a pediatric patient is discharged. ■

> **SKILLS CHALLENGE**
>
> To practice transcribing cardiopulmonary (respiratory care) orders, complete Activity 17-2 in the *Skills Practice Manual*.

WOUND CARE DEPARTMENT/CLINIC

Hyperbaric Oxygen Therapy

Hyperbaric oxygen therapy is a treatment in which the patient breathes 100% oxygen while in an enclosed system pressurized to greater than normal atmospheric pressure (3 times normal);

this is called a *hyperbaric chamber*. Hyperbaric oxygen therapy delivers oxygen systemically to injured areas quickly and in high concentrations. The increased pressure changes the normal cellular respiration process and causes oxygen to dissolve in the plasma. This stimulates the growth of new blood vessels, resulting in a substantial increase in tissue oxygenation that can arrest certain types of infections and enhance wound healing. Hyperbaric oxygen therapy generally is administered on an outpatient basis.

An Order for Hyperbaric Oxygen Therapy (HBOT)

• Hyperbaric oxygen therapy bid 3 × wk for 8 weeks

The patient will be enclosed in a hyperbaric chamber to breathe 100% oxygen twice a week for a period of 8 weeks.

TRACTION

Traction is the process of putting a limb, bone, or group of muscles under tension with the use of weights and pulleys, to align or immobilize, to reduce muscle spasm, or to relieve pressure. It is used to treat patients with fractures, dislocations, and long-duration muscle spasms, and to prevent or correct deformities. Traction can be used in short-term or long-term therapy. Two basic types include skin traction and skeletal traction.

Apparatus Setup
Bed

The apparatus that is attached to the patient's bed may include pulleys, rope, weights, and metal bars. The weights (metal disks or sandbags) provide the "pull" to a part of the body. The pulleys, rope, and metal bars are assembled to suspend the weights. Each type of traction requires a different assemblage of these parts; thus, a skilled person must perform this task. It is usually the responsibility of the nurse or an orthopedic technician to attach the traction apparatus to the bed. Physical therapy department personnel may assist with setting up traction equipment in smaller hospitals. The HUC

communicates a traction order verbally by telephone or via computer or requisition to the person or department (such as orthopedic equipment department) that is responsible for assembling the bed apparatus (Fig. 17-16).

Patient

The apparatus that is attached to the patient may consist of an external attachment, such as a halter, belt, or boot, or an internal attachment, such as a pin, tongs, or wires placed directly into the bone by the surgeon. The external apparatus is applied to the patient by the nursing staff, and sometimes the HUC must order necessary supplies from the central service department.

Although the types of supplies the HUC orders vary among hospitals. Moleskin tape, slings, and sandbags commonly are requisitioned from the central service department. Some hospitals have designated floors for the treatment of patients with orthopedic conditions and for those who have traction orders.

✓ DOCTORS' ORDERS FOR TRACTION

Traction Orders for Treatment of Bone Fractures

Two basic types of traction are used in orthopedics for the treatment of patients with fractured bones and for correction of orthopedic abnormalities. *Skin traction* applies pull to an affected body structure through straps attached to the skin surrounding the structure. Types include adhesive and nonadhesive skin traction. **Skeletal traction** is applied to the affected structure by a metal pin or wire inserted into the structure and attached to traction ropes. Skeletal traction often is used when continuous traction is desired to immobilize, position, and align a fractured bone properly during the healing process.

Skin Traction Orders

Skin traction 5 lb to left arm
Skin traction uses 5- to 7-lb weights attached to the skin to indirectly apply the necessary pulling force to the bone. The doctor may give additional directions regarding positioning.

Doctor ordering _____
☐ Stat ☐ Routine ☐ ASAP
Today's date _____ Requested by _____

| **Orthopedic Equipment** |

Diagnosis_____

Comments: _____
Write out the entire doctor's order
☐ Write in order_____
☐ Bryants_____
☐ Bucks _____
☐ Cervical _____
☐ Overhead frame and trapeze
☐ Russell's_____
☐ Skeletal tx_____
☐ Skin tx_____
☐ Split Russell's_____

Figure 17-16 Downtime requisition for orthopedic equipment.

Communication and Implementation of Traction Orders

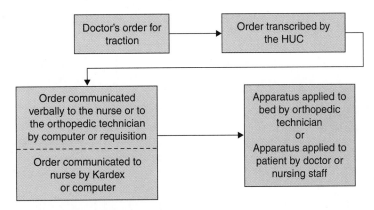

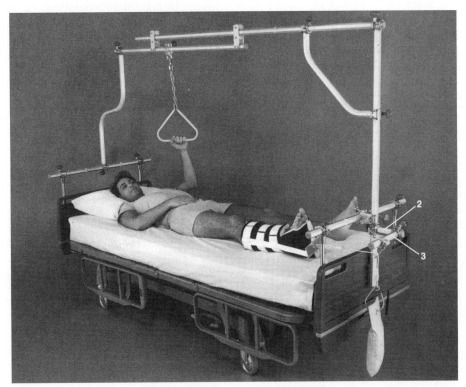

Figure 17-17 Unilateral Buck's traction.

Skin traction 7 lb to pelvis

Pelvic traction is applied to the lower spine, with a belt around the waist. This procedure is noninvasive and is the preferred treatment if traction is temporary, or if only a light or discontinuous force is needed. Weights usually are attached through moleskin tape, or with straps, boots, or cuffs.

Left unilateral Buck's skin traction 5 lb

A traction setup is used as temporary treatment of a patient with fractured hip, sciatica, or other knee and hip disorders (also may be called *Buck's extension*). *Unilateral* indicates that the traction is to be applied to one leg only (Fig. 17-17). Bilateral leg traction indicates that traction is to be applied to both legs. Traction is produced by applying regular or flannel-backed adhesive tape to the skin and keeping it in smooth close contact through circular bandaging of the part to

which it is applied. The adhesive strips are aligned with the long axis of the arm or leg, and the superior ends are about 1 inch from the fracture site. Weights sufficient to produce the required extension are fastened to the inferior end of the adhesive strips by a rope that is run over a pulley to permit free motion.

Russell's Traction rt leg c̄ 10# weight

Russell's traction is a combination of suspension and traction that is provided to immobilize, position, and align the lower extremity or extremities in the treatment of a fractured femur, hip and knee contractures, and disease processes of the hip and knee. Adhesive or nonadhesive skin traction may be used. **Split Russell's traction** suspends the traction weights from pulley-and-rope systems at the foot and head of the patient's bed. A jacket restraint often is incorporated to help immobilize the patient.

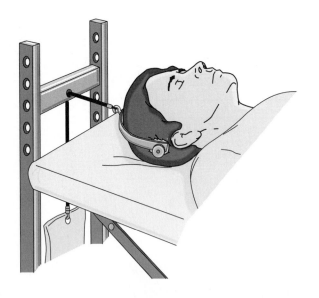

Figure 17-18 Crutchfield tongs. (From Phipps WJ, Monahan FD, Sands JK, et al: *Medical-surgical nursing,* ed 7, St. Louis, 2003, Mosby.)

Skeletal Traction Orders

Cervical traction c̄ Crutchfield tongs

Cervical traction is used in the treatment of fractures of the cervical vertebrae. Crutchfield tongs are attached to the skull to hyperextend the head and neck of patients with fractured cervical vertebrae for the purpose of immobilizing and aligning the vertebrae. The tips of the tongs are inserted into small burr holes drilled in each parietal region of the skull; the surrounding skin is sutured and covered with a dressing. A rope tied to the center of the tongs passes over a pulley at the head of the bed and is attached to a weight of 10 to 20 pounds, which hangs freely (Fig. 17-18). Other devices used for cervical traction include Gardner-Wells tongs and Vinke tongs. A special bed or Stryker frame may have to be obtained for the patient.

Thomas' leg splint c̄, Steinmann pin 20 lb of traction

A Thomas splint may be used to treat chronic joint disease through the use of a rigid **splint** constructed of steel bars curved to fit the involved limb that are held in place by a cast or a rigid bandage. A rigid metal splint that extends from a ring at the hip to beyond the foot may be used to treat a fractured

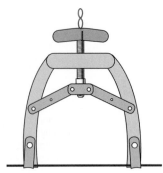

Figure 17-19 Steinmann pin. (From Elkin MK, Perry AG, Potter PA: *Nursing interventions and clinical skills,* ed 3, St. Louis, 2004, Mosby.)

leg and, in conjunction with various traction and suspension devices, to immobilize and position a fractured femur in a preoperative or postoperative patient. A Steinmann pin is a wide-diameter pin that is used for heavy skeletal traction; it is driven into the femur or tibia during surgery (Fig. 17-19).

Other Traction-Related Orders

Overhead Frame and Trapeze (Trapeze Bar)
An overhead frame and trapeze is used to help the patent move and support weight during transfer or position change. It also may aid in strengthening upper extremities (see Fig. 17-17). ■

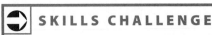
SKILLS CHALLENGE

To practice transcribing traction orders, complete Activity 17-3 in the *Skills Practice Manual.*

PHYSICAL MEDICINE AND REHABILITATION

Most hospitals have a physical medicine department that consists of physical therapy, occupational therapy, and speech therapy.

Physical Therapy

Background Information

Physical therapy is the division of the physical medicine department in the hospital that treats patients to improve and restore their functional mobility through methods such

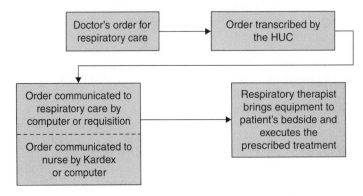

Communication and Implementation of
Respiratory Care Treatment/Therapy Orders

Doctor's order for respiratory care → Order transcribed by the HUC

Order communicated to respiratory care by computer or requisition
- - - - - - - - - - - -
Order communicated to nurse by Kardex or computer

Respiratory therapist brings equipment to patient's bedside and executes the prescribed treatment

as gait training, exercise, water therapy, and heat and ice treatments. Patients include those injured in accidents, sports, or work-related activities. Children affected by cerebral palsy and muscular dystrophy are assisted toward normal physical development through physical therapy. Individuals who experience strokes, spinal cord injuries, and amputations are assisted back to their highest level of physical function through therapy.

The physical therapist (PT), a person licensed to practice in this field, assesses the patient and initiates a plan of care. Physical therapy treatments may be carried out in the patient's room or in the physical therapy department by the PT or by the physical therapy assistant (PTA). The PT reads the order before administering treatment. The PTA may perform certain treatment tasks as directed by the PT. After treatment, the PT records treatment details and other pertinent data for inclusion in the patient's chart.

To communicate the order to the physical therapy division, use the computer, or complete a physical therapy requisition form (Fig. 17-20).

✔ DOCTORS' ORDERS FOR PHYSICAL THERAPY

Below are examples of doctors' orders for physical therapy. Brief descriptions and illustrations are included to assist you in interpreting the orders.

✐ TAKE NOTE

Two errors that commonly occur when doctors' orders are read involve interpretation of the abbreviation "PT." This may be an order for physical therapy or for a prothrombin time, which is a coagulation study (see Chapter 14). "PT" also can be confused with "patient," as in the order "PT to ambulate daily," which could be interpreted as patient (pt) to ambulate daily rather than physical therapy (PT) to ambulate the patient daily. It is important to fully understand doctors' orders during transcription.

Hydrotherapy Orders

Hubbard tank 30 min qd T 100°F, active underwater exercises to elbows and knees c̄ débridement
This treatment is used for underwater exercises and for cleansing wounds and burns (Fig. 17-21). **Hydrotherapy** treatments may be ordered to be done with a sterile solution. The physical therapy department will select an appropriate substance to use.

Whirlpool bath LLE bid
The whirlpool is smaller than the Hubbard tank. It is used for the same purposes.

Doctor ordering _____

Date to be done _____ Time to be done _____

Today's date _____ Requested by _____

Physical Therapy

Clinical indication _____

Transportation ☐ Portable ☐ Stretcher ☐ Wheelchair ☐ Ambulatory

O₂ ☐ Yes ☐ No   Diabetic ☐ Yes ☐ No   Hearing deficit ☐ Yes ☐ No

IV ☐ Yes ☐ No   Seizure disorder ☐ Yes ☐ No   Sight deficit ☐ Yes ☐ No

Isolation ☐ Yes ☐ No   Non-English speaking ☐ Yes ☐ No

Comments: _____

Write out the entire doctor's order

☐ CMP _____

☐ Crutch training _____

☐ ES _____

☐ Exercise orders: _____

☐ Evaluation _____

☐ Hot packs _____

☐ Hubbard tank _____

☐ Hyperburic oxygen tx _____

☐ Shortwave diathermy _____

☐ TENs _____

☐ Ultrasound c̄ massage _____

☐ Walker training _____

☐ Whirlpool _____

☐ Write in order _____

Figure 17-20 Downtime requisition for physical therapy.

Communication and Implementation of Physical Medicine Orders

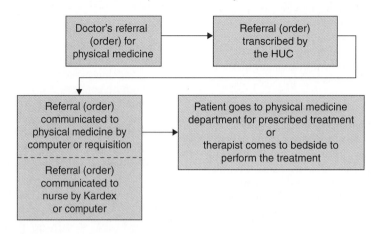

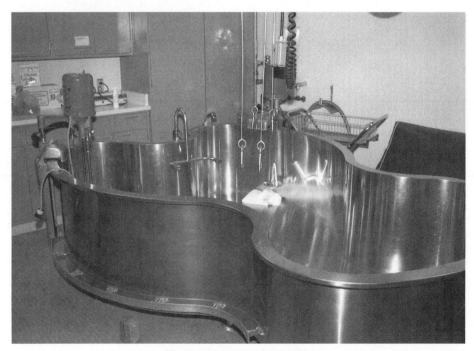

Figure 17-21 Hubbard tank.

Exercise Orders

Passive, active assistive, progressive, resistive, muscle reeducation, coordination, and relaxation are other types of exercises that may be ordered by the doctor.

AA exercise lt shoulder and elbow daily

Active assisted exercises would involve the patient's moving an extremity with assistance from the PT, as required.

ROM bid to UE

Range-of-motion exercises frequently are ordered for bedridden patients; therefore, they usually are performed in the patient's room. These exercises involve moving each joint of the upper extremities to the maximum extent in each direction.

PROM BLE bid

This passive range-of-motion exercise of both lower extremities would require the PT to move each joint of both lower extremities the maximum distance in each direction.

Joint mobilization to lt shoulder bid

The PT will mobilize (move) the patient's left shoulder.

Strengthening of all four extremities

The PT will evaluate the patient's condition and will recommend a series of exercises designed to strengthen the patient's extremities. The PTA may help the patient with these exercises.

PT to amb pt with walker as tol

The PT department often decides which equipment is best suited for the patient. For this order, the PT would assist the patient in using a walker for walking as tolerated.

PT to eval and treat

PT to evaluate and treat is the order most commonly written by the doctor. The PT will evaluate the patient and will initiate a plan of care.

ACL protocol per Dr. Melzer

Many physicians have preprinted courses of treatment (protocols) on file with the physical therapy department; these may be implemented throughout the patient's stay (precluding any complications). Programs of treatment include clinical pathways and goals that often are named after orthopedic surgery has been performed on the patient. Familiarity with orthopedic surgical procedures and abbreviations is helpful. An anterior cruciate ligament (ACL) protocol would follow an ACL repair.

Dr. Jen's BKA protocol

This preprinted protocol is used for rehabilitation after a below-the-knee amputation. Another physician's protocol may be different.

THA and TKA protocols

Many physicians have preprinted orders to be used when patients undergo total hip arthroplasty or total knee arthroplasty. The protocol is followed by physical therapy personnel.

Transfer training, wheelchair mobility

The PT teaches the patient how to transfer from the bed to the wheelchair and how to use the wheelchair; this training is ordered for patients who have had an amputation, stroke, or other physical disability.

Gait training with a walker, WBAT LLE

To carry out this order, the PT would train the patient to walk using a walker, with weight bearing on the left lower extremity as tolerated. Additional devices such as crutches and different types of canes may be used in patient ambulation.

Crutch walking, NWB daily

The PT instructs the patient to walk with crutches. Variations to this order may be noted regarding the amount of weight bearing permitted (such as full weight), any precautions that should be taken, or the type of crutch walking that should be taught to the patient (such as 4-point gait). Additional variations in the amount of weight bearing may be addressed in the doctor's order.

CPM 0 to 45 degrees, progress to 0 to 90 degrees by day 5

A continuous passive motion machine is used after joint replacement or total knee arthroplasty. It may be monitored by the PT or by nursing staff (Fig. 17-22). Additional motion orders may include active assistive **range of motion** (AAROM), active range of motion (AROM), and passive range of motion (PROM).

T-band exercises

With these exercises, a band of rubber or a Theraband is used for resistance.

Codman's exercises rt shoulder

These exercises for the shoulder are also called *pendulum exercises*.

Isometrics BUE (bilateral upper extremities)

Isometric exercises flex muscles without allowing actual movement of the limb. This order is performed on both upper extremities.

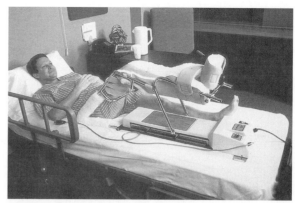

Figure 17-22 Continuous passive motion. (From Elkin MK, Perry AG, Potter PA: *Nursing interventions and clinical skills,* ed 2, St. Louis, 2000, Mosby.)

Heat and Cold Orders

- Ultrasound and massage to lower back
- Hydrocollator packs or hot packs to back bid
- Ice or cold packs to left leg bid

Pain Relief Orders

Postop TENS

Transcutaneous electrical nerve stimulation (TENS) is used to control pain by blocking transmission of pain impulses to the brain. Electrodes are applied to the skin surrounding the incision during surgery. Thin wires lead from the electrodes to a powered stimulator with a control. Usually, the patient is taught before surgery how to use the device. For nonsurgical use, the PT attaches external electrodes to the skin (Fig. 17-23).

FES or ES

Functional electrical stimulation or electrical stimulation may be used to reduce pain or swelling, promote healing, or assist in exercising muscles. Different types of machines are used to deliver this treatment.

Other Physical Therapy Orders

Apply foam cervical collar

A foam cervical collar is applied to the patient's neck.

Use abduction pillow between legs during treatment

An abduction pillow is placed between the patient's legs. The pillow is designed to help patients recuperate from hip surgery with minimal discomfort while providing protection from hip dislocation.

Apply knee immobilizer to lt knee

A knee immobilizer is used to stabilize the knee after injury or surgery (Fig. 17-24).

Note: These orders are often included in physical therapy orders or may be addressed by nursing personnel. ■

Occupational Therapy
Background Information

Occupational therapy (OT) is the division of the physical medicine department in the hospital that works toward rehabilitation of patients, in conjunction with other health

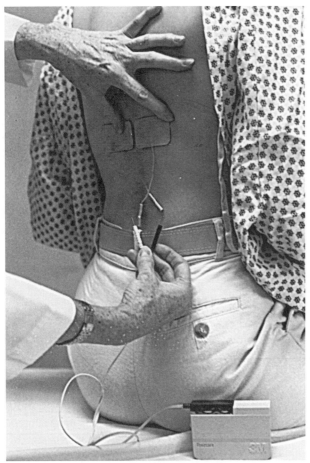

Figure 17-23 Transcutaneous electric nerve stimulation (TENS). (From Ignatavicius DD, Workman ML, Mishler MA: *Medical-surgical nursing*, ed 2, Philadelphia, 1995, Saunders.)

team members, to return the patient to the greatest possible functional independence. Creative, manual, recreational, and prevocational assessments are examples of activities used in rehabilitation of the patient. Occupational therapy activities are ordered by the doctor and are administered by a qualified occupational therapist, an occupational therapy technician, or an occupational therapy assistant. To communicate the order to the occupational therapy division, use the computer or complete an occupational therapy requisition form (Fig. 17-25).

✎ TAKE NOTE

Examples of basic skills to be achieved as a result of occupational therapy include toileting, bathing and dressing, cooking, and feeding oneself.

✓ DOCTORS' ORDERS FOR OCCUPATIONAL THERAPY

- OT for evaluation and treatment if needed daily
- Training in activities of daily living (ADLs)
- Supply and train in adaptive equipment such as button hooks and feeding utensils for ADLs

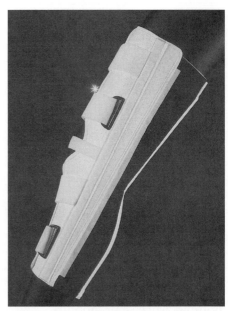

Figure 17-24 Knee immobilizer. (Courtesy Zimmer, Inc., Warsaw, Indiana; from Ignatavicius D, Workman L: *Medical-surgical nursing*, ed 5, Philadelphia, 2006, Saunders.)

- OT to increase mobility
- Fabricate cock-up splint for left upper extremity ■

⊜ SKILLS CHALLENGE

To practice transcribing physical medicine and rehabilitation orders, complete Activity 17-4 in the *Skills Practice Manual*.

✎ TAKE NOTE

Physical therapy, occupational therapy, and speech therapy are used to improve and restore function and/or enhance patient independence. Restorative programs may be run out of nursing homes and physical medicine and rehabilitation centers.

DIALYSIS

The kidneys are essential organs in the removal of toxic wastes from the blood. When the kidneys fail to remove those wastes, medical **intervention** is necessary to sustain life. The kidneys may fail temporarily (acute renal failure), or they may be permanently damaged and may become nonfunctional (chronic renal failure and end-stage renal disease [ESRD]). Two main types of **dialysis** have been identified: hemodialysis and peritoneal dialysis.

- *Hemodialysis* (also called *extracorporeal dialysis*) is the removal of waste products from the blood as attained by the utilization of a machine through which the blood flows. This procedure is performed regularly in a special outpatient

```
┌─────────────────────────────────────────────────────────────────────┐
│   Doctor ordering _____                  │
│   Date to be done _____ Time to be done _____                │
│   Today's date _____ Requested by _____                  │
│                                                                       │
│   ┌──────────────────────┐                                          │
│   │  Occupational Therapy │                                          │
│   └──────────────────────┘                                          │
│                                                                       │
│   Clinical Indication _____      │
│   Transportation □ Portable □ Stretcher □ Wheelchair □ Ambulatory   │
│                                                                       │
│   O₂ □ Yes □ No        Diabetic  □ Yes □ No                          │
│   IV □ Yes □ No        Seizure disorder □ Yes□ No    Hearing deficit □ Yes□ No │
│   Isolation □ Yes □ No  Non-English speaking □ Yes□ No  Sight deficit □ Yes□ No │
│                                                                       │
│   Comments: _____        │
│   Write out entire doctor's order                                    │
│                                                                       │
│   □ ADL                                                               │
│   □ Evaluation and treatment as needed                               │
│   □ Increase mobility                                                 │
│   □ Supply and train in adaptive equipment (e.g., Use ADL button hooks and feeding utensils) │
│   □ Write in order_____        │
└─────────────────────────────────────────────────────────────────────┘
```

Figure 17-25 Downtime requisition for occupational therapy.

dialysis facility and is completed commonly for 3- to 4-hour periods over 3 days a week. For the hospitalized patient, hemodialysis usually is performed in a special unit in the hospital. If the patient is too ill to be moved, a portable hemodialysis machine may be used.

- *Peritoneal dialysis* is the introduction of a fluid (dialyzing fluid) into the abdominal cavity that then absorbs the wastes from the blood through the lining of the abdominal cavity, or peritoneum. The dialysate is emptied from the abdominal cavity. This type of dialysis allows a greater level of freedom for the patient, as this fluid transfer may be performed outside of a health care facility. Some variations of peritoneal dialysis include continuous ambulatory peritoneal dialysis (CAPD), continuous cycling peritoneal dialysis (CCPD), and intermittent peritoneal dialysis (IPD).

 ## DOCTORS' ORDERS FOR DIALYSIS

Hemodialysis 3 × wk for 2 hours
The patient will undergo hemodialysis for 2 hours per session three times a week.

 ## CONSENT FOR TENCKHOFF CATHETER PLACEMENT FOR PERITONEAL DIALYSIS

This procedure involves surgical placement of a long-term catheter or tube into the patient's abdomen so that peritoneal dialysis can be performed.

 ## CONSENT FOR A-V SHUNT

Hemodialysis requires vascular access. With this surgical procedure, a cannula is inserted into an artery, and another into a vein. Both of these are then connected to tubing that allows easier needle insertion for hemodialysis. ■

RADIATION TREATMENTS

The area in the hospital where radiation therapy is performed may be a division of the diagnostic imaging department, or it may be a totally separate department.

Many of those who undergo radiation therapy are outpatients. However, the HUC may be called upon to schedule an appointment for an inpatient who requires treatment for a malignant neoplasm (cancer). Many hospitals require that units use a requisition form; others may schedule an appointment by telephone. After the initial visit, the radiation therapy department usually notifies the nursing unit of the patient's treatment schedule.

 ### SKILLS CHALLENGE

For practice transcribing the following types of orders, complete the following activities in the *Skills Practice Manual:*

- To practice recording a review set of doctors' orders, complete Activity 17-5.
- To practice recording telephone messages, complete Activity 17-6.

KEY CONCEPTS

Transcription of treatment orders involves communication of the order to the necessary department by computer or by requisition form, as well as communication of the order to the nursing staff verbally or through the kardexing step of the transcription procedure. Professionals in their respective departments then execute the orders.

1. Identify two procedures performed to repair obstructed coronary blood vessels.

a. _____

b. _____

2. State the purpose of each of the following hospital departments:

a. cardiopulmonary (respiratory care) department

_____

b. physical therapy department

_____

c. occupational therapy department

_____

3. Identify the information that is required when oxygen is ordered from the cardiopulmonary (respiratory care) department.

a. _____

b. _____

4. List the two basic types of traction.

a. _____

b. _____

5. State two purposes of an overhead frame and trapeze.

_____

6. Various types of treatments are listed in column 1, including treatments performed by the nursing staff. Write the health care personnel from column 2 who usually would perform each of these treatments.

Column 1	Column 2
a. IPPB	Physical Therapy
b. SSE	Cardiopulmonary (Respiratory Care)
c. USN	Occupational Therapy
d. ACL protocol	Nursing
e. O_2	
f. SVN	
g. CPT	
h. ADL	
i. IV therapy	
j. urinary catheterization	
k. ROM	
l. K-pad	
m. whirlpool	
n. TENS	
o. MDI	
p. gait training	

7. Define *dialysis*.

_____

8. Two types of dialysis are as follows:

a. _____

b. _____

9. Explain the purpose of hyperbaric oxygen therapy.

_____

_____

THINK ABOUT...

1. Discuss why it is important to list all of the information regarding a respiratory order when communicating the order to the cardiopulmonary (respiratory care) department.
2. Discuss why the respiratory therapist should read the doctors' order before administering treatment.
3. Discuss the reason why the patient's chart should accompany the patient when he is going to the physical therapy department for treatment.
4. Discuss solutions for keeping charts from being scattered and/or taken without your knowledge by personnel from ancillary departments (e.g., physical therapy, occupational therapy, respiratory therapy).

Miscellaneous Orders

CHAPTER OBJECTIVES

Upon completion of this chapter, you will be able to:

1. Define the terms in the vocabulary list.
2. Write the meaning of each abbreviation in the Abbreviations list.
3. List seven points of information that should be communicated to the consulting physician's office when a consultation order is transcribed.
4. Explain the health unit coordinator's responsibilities regarding requests for patient medical records to be obtained from or sent to another facility.
5. Explain the health unit coordinator's responsibilities regarding patient medical records received and orders for documents to be scanned into a patient's electronic medical record.
6. Describe the role of the case manager.
7. Name eight services rendered by the Social Services department.
8. List six tasks the health unit coordinator may have to perform when arranging for a patient to leave the hospital on a temporary pass.
9. List three reasons why a doctor may wish to transfer a patient to another hospital room and/or nursing unit.
10. Discuss the importance of reading the entire discharge order before the patient has been discharged.
11. Explain the purpose of a "parent teaching room" or "transition room" on a pediatric unit.

VOCABULARY

Consultation Order A request by the patient's attending physician for the opinion of a second physician with respect to diagnosis and treatment of the patient

Discharge Order A doctors' order that states that the patient may leave the hospital. A doctors' order is necessary for a patient to be discharged from the hospital (See Chapter 19 regarding "leaving hospital against advice")

Microfilm A film that contains a greatly reduced photo image of printed or graphic matter

Parent Teaching or Transition Room Many pediatric hospitals and/or units have a patient room with a bed so a parent can stay with the child 24 hours a day. Parents, after training, will assume full care of the child while they still have the support of the nursing staff. The child may then be discharged home to the parents' care

Transfer Order A doctors' order that requests that a patient be transferred to another hospital room and/or nursing unit, or to another facility

ABBREVIATIONS

Abbreviation	Meaning	Example of Usage on a Doctor's Order Sheet
appt	appointment	Schedule an appt with dental clinic

Abbreviation	Meaning	Example of Usage on a Doctor's Order Sheet
Disch	discharge	Disch today p̄ chest X-ray
DME	durable medical equipment	Contact DME supplier for hospital bed for home
DNR	do not resuscitate	DNR
NINP	no information, no publication	Pt requests NINP
Rx	take (treatment, medication, etc.) prescription	Disch c̄ Rx
wk	week	Disch, F/U appt in my office in 1 wk

EXERCISE 1

Write the abbreviation for each term listed below.

1. week   _____

2. no information, no publication   _____

3. durable medical equipment   _____

4. do not resuscitate   _____

5. discharge   _____

6. take (treatment, medication, etc.)   _____
   prescription

7. appointment   _____

EXERCISE 2

Write the meaning of each abbreviation listed below.

1. appt

   _____

2. DME

   _____

3. DNR

   _____

4. NINP

   _____

5. wk

   _____

6. Rx

   _____

7. disch

   _____

✎ TAKE NOTE

When the electronic medical record (EMR) with computer physician order entry (CPOE) is implemented, the physicians' orders are entered directly into the patient's electronic record. Many of the miscellaneous orders discussed in this chapter involve action taken by the health unit coordinator (HUC). When the doctor enters orders into the computer, an icon (usually a telephone) is displayed on the nursing unit census screen (next to the appropriate patient's name) to alert the HUC that there is a task to be performed.

CONSULTATION ORDERS

Background Information

The attending physician of a patient may wish to obtain the opinion of another doctor regarding diagnosis and treatment. The request for another doctor's opinion is written on the doctors' order sheet by the patient's doctor; this is called a **consultation order**.

The transcription process for consultation orders usually requires that the HUC must notify the office of the consulting doctor regarding the order. Prepare for the call to the doctor's office or answering service by writing the doctor's telephone number on a note pad; have the patient's chart close by so any additional requested information may be accessed easily. When the doctor's office is called, the patient's insurance information may be requested. If the doctor's office is closed and the consult is called to the answering service, the doctor's office secretary may call back for the patient's insurance information. It is important to document the time of notification and the name of the person or operator number (answering service) spoken to. Write this information next to the doctors' order on the doctors' order sheet, and initial it.

Note: Some hospitals may have a policy that requires the requesting doctor to notify the specialist personally, so patient history and additional information may be provided.

The following information should be communicated to the office of the consulting doctor:

- Hospital name
- Patient's name and age
- Patient's location (unit and room number)
- Name of the doctor requesting the consultation
- Patient's diagnosis
- Urgency of consultation and any additional information provided on the order
- Patient's insurance information, located on the patient's face sheet

After interviewing and evaluating the patient, the consulting doctor usually will dictate findings and recommendations. A hospital medical transcriptionist then will type the consultation report and send it to the nursing unit, and the HUC will file the report in the patient's chart (Fig. 18–1). When the EMR c̄ CPOE is implemented, the physician will enter findings and recommendations directly into the patient's EMR via computer. The consulting doctor usually will take a copy of the patient's face sheet back to the office for billing purposes.

 ## DOCTORS' ORDERS FOR CONSULTATION

Doctors' orders for consultation may be expressed in writing on the doctors' order sheet as follows:

Have Dr. Avery from Valley Anesthesia eval for CABG surg
Call Dr. Reidy for consultation
Call Dr. Casey to see patient re radiation therapy
Have Dr. Williams see patient today please ■

✐ TAKE NOTE

Document the time called and the name or operator number of the person spoken to when calling a specialist for consultation. Write this information next to the doctors' order on the doctors' order sheet, and initial it.

 SKILLS CHALLENGE

To practice transcribing a consultation order, complete Activity 18-1 in the *Skills Practice Manual*.

HEALTH INFORMATION MANAGEMENT SYSTEM ORDERS

Background Information

The health information management system department (HIMS), also called health information management, medical records or health records, stores the charts of patients who have been treated at the health care facility in the past.

Ordering and Obtaining Patient Medical Records

Records from recent hospital admissions are sent to the unit upon readmission of a patient automatically or when requested by the patient's doctor. The request is written on the doctors' order sheet, and the order is communicated to health information management by telephone or via computer by the HUC. Health information management system personnel then sends the old records or a printed hard copy if the record has been **microfilmed.** While old records are on the nursing unit, they are labeled with the patient's identification and stored

---

Date of consultation: 5/17/XX

Name of cosultant: John P. Rhine, MD

History: This 17-year-old woman was seen in consultation with her mother regarding problems referable to her nose. The patient has had progressive problems of congestion and sniffing, with difficulty moving air through her nose and sensation of pressure. She is a "mouth breather," and has history of allergy to pollens and dust. Patient feels these problems are becoming more severe. Her complaints are fairly consistent.

Examination: She presents with edema of her nasal mucosa, increase in the size of the turbinates, deviation of the nasal septum, and a rather narrow nasal airway.

Diagnosis:
  1. Probable allergic rhinitis with hypertrophy of the turbinates.
  2. Deviated nasal septum.
  3. Narrow, inadequate nasal airway.

Comments:
  1. I have discussed with this patient and with her mother the surgical approach to improving her nasal airway with septoplasty, and possible submucous resection of deviated portions of the septum, and possible reduction of the inferior turbinates. At the same time I would be performing a rhinoplasty procedure to smooth out the dorsal nose as well.
  2. Because of the history of allergies to pollens, dust, and environmental pollutants, it is quite possible the patient will continue to have some sniffing, and consequently, the degree of improvement of her nasal airway with surgery cannot be precisely determined.

_____
J. P. Rhine, MD

DD:
DT:
jpr/ct

Figure 18–1 Dictated and typed consultation report.

✎ TAKE NOTE

When the EMR is implemented, the patient's current and previous medical records become accessible to the patient's doctor and appropriate health care personnel.

in a designated area, rather than in the current patient's chart holder.

The doctor also may request medical records from the patient's previous stay in another hospital. Because this information is confidential, the patient must give written permission for release of the information from one hospital to another. To transcribe a doctors' order to obtain medical

records from another hospital, the HUC places a call to the health information management department of the other hospital to request records and prepares a consent form (Fig. 18–2) for the patient to sign. When signed, this form may be faxed to the health information management department in the other hospital, and the requested records then may be faxed to the nursing unit. The faxed records are usually placed in the patient's current chart if paper charts are used, or they are scanned into the patient's EMR if the EMR is used. After the records have been scanned into the patient's EMR the original documents are stamped as "scanned" with date and time and are placed in a bin or a box to be picked up by HIMS.

The doctor or nurse also may ask the HUC to scan into the patient's EMR electrocardiograms (EKGs), rhythm strips, handwritten histories and physicals, progress notes, and other

AUTHORIZATION TO OBTAIN MEDICAL INFORMATION

DATE __5/17/XX__

TO: _Memorial Hospital_   RE. _Marilee Owens_
                                              (NAME OF PATIENT)
_____   _1100 Ash St._
                                              (ADDRESS)
_____   _Phoenix_
_____   _7/7/XX_
                                              (BIRTHDATE)

THE ABOVE NAMED PERSON IS NOW A PATIENT IN THIS HOSPITAL UNDER THE CARE OF
DR. _Roosevelt Conklin_

WE WERE INFORMED THAT THIS PATIENT WAS IN YOUR INSTITUTION ON OR ABOUT
March 10–15   XX

WOULD YOU PLEASE SEND US A TRANSCRIPT OF ~~HIS~~ HER MEDICAL RECORD AS SOON AS POSSIBLE? WE ARE PARTICULARLY INTERESTED IN THE FOLLOWING REPORTS.

_____ HISTORY AND PHYSICAL EXAMINATION   _____ LABORATORY REPORTS

_____ OPERATION REPORTS   _____ PATHOLOGY REPORTS

_____ CONSULTATIONS   __X__ DISCHARGE SUMMARY

_____ X-RAY REPORTS   __X__ OTHER REPORTS
                                                                                 CT Brain

THANK YOU FOR YOUR COOPERATION

                                                                          SINCERELY YOURS,

KINDLY ADDRESS YOUR REPLY
ATTENTION OF
MEDICOLEGAL SECRETARY
MEDICAL RECORD DEPARTMENT   DIRECTOR
                                                                          HEALTH RECORDS SERVICES

I HEREBY AUTHORIZE _Memorial Hospital_ _____ TO GIVE TO THIS HOSPITAL A COPY OF MY HOSPITAL RECORDS OR ANY INFORMATION WHICH MAY HAVE BEEN ACQUIRED IN THE COURSE OF MY EXAMINATION OR TREATMENT.

                                              Marilee Owens
                                              (SIGNATURE OF PATIENT)
                                              __5/17/XX__
                                              (DATE)

Figure 18–2 Consent form to obtain records from another hospital.

documents. The HUC, after scanning these documents, stamps the originals with a "scanned" stamp with the date and time, and places them in a bin or a box to be picked up by HIMS.

✎ TAKE NOTE

When paper charts are used, the faxed patient records are placed in their current chart.

When the EMR is implemented, the faxed patient records are scanned into the patient's EMR by the HUC.

Photocopying, Sending, or Faxing Medical Records

When a patient is transferred to another facility or is sent to see another physician, the primary physician may write an order to have certain parts of the patient's record photocopied so they can be sent with the patient. The HUC may be responsible for photocopying the records, or it may be hospital policy that records must be sent to health information management to be photocopied. The policy for photocopying patient records is outlined in the hospital's policies and procedures. If EMRs have been implemented, the HUC prints the records from the computer. The HUC also may fax requested patient records to the facility or the doctor's office. The patient would need to sign a consent form for records to be photocopied, printed, or faxed to another facility or to a doctor's office.

✓ DOCTORS' ORDERS FOR HEALTH INFORMATION MANAGEMENT RECORDS

Doctors' orders for medical records may be expressed in writing on the doctors' order sheet as follows:

Send old records from admission 5 years ago to floor
Obtain records from all previous admissions
Obtain report on total body CT scan from St. Joseph's Hospital (done 2/28/XX)
Please copy all doctors' progress notes (last 3 days) and all diagnostic reports to be sent c̄ patient to Bryant's Rehab Center
Please scan attached progress notes into Mr. Robert's EMR ■

 SKILLS CHALLENGE

To practice transcribing a health information management order, complete Activity 18-2 in the *Skills Practice Manual*.

CASE MANAGEMENT ORDERS

Background Information

Case management is a nursing care delivery model in which the case manager (a registered nurse [RN] or a social worker) coordinates the patient's care to improve quality of care while reducing costs. The case manager interacts on a daily basis with the patient, the patient's family, health care team members, and payer representatives. Case management is not needed for every patient and usually is requested for chronically ill or seriously ill or injured patients, as well as for long-term high-cost cases. The case managers acts as the patient's advocate in getting home health services that best suit the patient's needs and in coordinating financial coverage through private insurers such as Medicare.

The doctor may write orders requesting that a case manager should access and prioritize the patient's needs, coordinate care conferences between the patient's family and physicians, identify and coordinate available resources, and arrange for home care, admission to a long-term care facility, or Hospice as needed. A patient with a life-limiting illness frequently can benefit from the services of Hospice. Hospice is a multidisciplinary organization that stresses a holistic approach to the care of patients during the final stage of life. The Hospice team comprises a physician, nurses, certified nursing assistants, social workers, a chaplain, and volunteers. Most hospice care can be rendered in the patient's home, although some hospice units are located in hospitals and freestanding Hospice facilities.

✓ DOCTORS' ORDERS FOR CASE MANAGERS

Case management for health assessment
Case management to arrange home care with patient's family for discharge in 2 days
Case management to arrange hospice care
Case management to arrange patient care conference ■

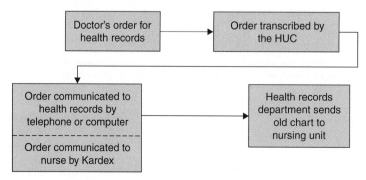

Communication and Implementation of Health Record Orders

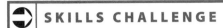

SKILLS CHALLENGE

To practice transcribing an order for case management, complete Activity 18-3 in the *Skills Practice Manual.*

SOCIAL SERVICE DEPARTMENT ORDERS

Background Information

Social service provides much-needed information regarding resources available to patients and their families as they transition from the health care facility back to their home. Social workers provide many of the same services as case managers and also may work as case managers. Social workers assist with the following:

- Solving patients' care-related financial matters
- Transportation home
- Meals for patients' families who are staying at the hospital
- In-home meals for patients after discharge
- Teachers for long-term pediatric patients
- Living arrangements for families who stay with patients
- Finding custodial care for patients
- Addressing psychosocial needs of patients
- Support for abuse victims, often by working with Protective Services

- Support for hospital staff after traumatic events (e.g., patient deaths, codes)

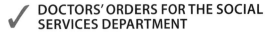 **DOCTORS' ORDERS FOR THE SOCIAL SERVICES DEPARTMENT**

Contact family re plans to place in custodial care facility
Arrange for home-bound teacher for 1 month
Social worker to call child protective services to evaluate home situation
Have social worker evaluate patient's home caregivers
Have social worker arrange for family to stay at Ronald McDonald House ■

SCHEDULING ORDERS

Background Information

Frequently, while the patient is in a health care facility, the doctor may write an order to schedule the patient for various types of tests or examinations to be performed in specialized departments or outside of the health care facility. It is usually the HUC's task to notify the department or facility that performs the test or examination, and schedule a time convenient for the involved department and the patient, as well as possibly arranging transportation to and from off-site testing. It is important to advise the patient's nurse to inform the patient and/or patient's family and to record the scheduled time on the patient's Kardex form.

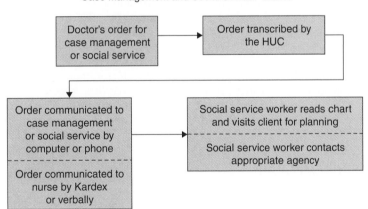

Communication and Implementation of
Case Management and Social Service Orders

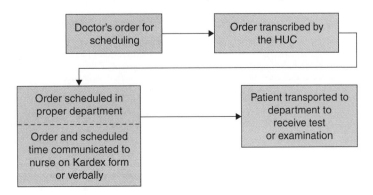

Communication and Implementation of
a Doctor's Order that Requires Scheduling

DOCTORS' ORDERS THAT REQUIRE SCHEDULING

Below are examples of doctors' orders that require scheduling. These vary greatly among health care facilities, according to the services available.

Schedule pt in outpatient department for radiation therapy
Schedule pt for psychological testing
Schedule pt for diabetic classes
Schedule pt for VER
Schedule appt for dental clinic for evaluation and care ■

> ### ⊜ SKILLS CHALLENGE
>
> To practice transcribing an order to schedule an examination, complete Activity 18-4 in the *Skills Practice Manual*.

TEMPORARY ABSENCES (PASSES TO LEAVE THE HEALTH CARE FACILITY)

Some long-term patients on rehabilitation units may be allowed to leave for 4 to 10 hours. Patients receive many benefits from visiting their homes or experiencing a recreational outing. A gradual return to society has therapeutic value for rehabilitating patients. A long-term patient also may be given a pass to attend a wedding, funeral, graduation, or similar event. A temporary pass requires the HUC to do the following:

- Arrange with the pharmacy for medications the patient is taking
- Note on the census worksheet when the patient leaves and returns
- Cancel meals for the length of the absence
- Cancel hospital treatments for the length of the absence
- Arrange for any special equipment that the patient may need
- Provide the nurse with a temporary absence release for the patient to sign (Fig. 18–3)

✓ DOCTORS' ORDERS FOR TEMPORARY ABSENCE

May have pass for tomorrow from 9 AM to 7 PM
Temporary hospital absence from 8 AM to 6 PM Friday; arrange for rental of wheelchair

May leave hospital from 10 AM to 1 PM today; have patient sign release

Note: Many insurance providers will not cover the patient's hospital stay if the patient is absent from the hospital for longer than 24 hours. ■

TRANSFER AND DISCHARGE ORDERS

If the doctor plans to transfer the patient to another room or another unit, or to discharge the patient to home or to another facility, the doctor writes an order for such on the doctors' order sheet.

To transcribe a **transfer** or **discharge order**, the HUC must notify the hospital admitting department by telephone or computer, or by completing a discharge or transfer slip. It is important to send or call a "pending discharge" or a transfer to the admitting department in a timely manner, especially when the hospital is full. Holding off on notifying admitting could cause a delay in another patient's admission and in the start of treatment.

Discharge orders may include orders to be carried out before the time of a patient's discharge or information such as instructions for the patient to follow after leaving the hospital, requests for appointments for the patient, and so forth. Often, a doctor will include other orders with a discharge order, such as the following: *discharge p̄ chest X-ray; disch p̄ mother has had CPR training; copy patients last 3 days of labs and diagnostic studies and send with patient to Bryant's Rehab Center;* or *discharge with Rx* (the prescription may be left in the patient's chart). Orders included in a discharge order often are missed and are discovered later, after the patient has left the hospital. The HUC must read the entire discharge or transfer order before the time of the patient's discharge, because often the patient's nurse will not see the order and will trust the HUC to review it.

The doctor may request the transfer of a patient for various reasons, such as for a different type of room accommodation (to private room) or for more intensive nursing care (regular unit to intensive care unit [ICU]) or less intensive nursing care (ICU to regular unit). Another reason for a transfer is that the patient's condition may require an isolation room.

Below are examples of how discharge or transfer orders may be expressed by the doctor on the doctors' order sheet.

Transfer
Transfer patient to 3E please

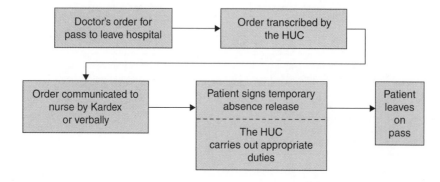

Communication and Implementation of Temporary Absence Orders

TEMPORARY ABSENCE RELEASE

The undersigned, being a patient of The Above Named Hospital, hereby confirms his (or her) agreement and understanding that neither the hospital, its employees, nor the attending physicians shall be responsible for his (or her) care or condition during any absences of the undersigned from the building or resulting from such absences.

Signed _____
PATIENT / PARENT / GUARDIAN

Date _____

Hour _____

Witness _____

09-0366   **TEMPORARY ABSENCE RELEASE**

Figure 18–3 Temporary absence release form.

Transfer patient to telemetry unit
Transfer patient to ICU after surgery
Transfer patient out of ICU to a medical unit

Transfer patient to isolation room
Transfer patient to Rehab Center
Discharge
Home today
Discharge p̄ chest x-ray
Home c̄ Rx
Home, make appt to see me in 2 wk
Home c̄ crutches
Disch c̄ mother p̄ car seat obtained
Arrange for CPR training for parents before the time of discharge

✎ *TAKE NOTE*

The procedures for transferring and discharging a patient and postmortem procedures are discussed in Chapter 20. This section deals only with transcription procedures for a transfer or discharge order.

OTHER MISCELLANEOUS ORDERS

Some orders do not relate to any department but are nevertheless deserving of mention. All should be Kardexed in their appropriate places. A few of the orders appear below:

Call patient's family to come to the hospital

When a patient is terminal, the doctor or nurse may request that the HUC call the family to come to the hospital. Usually, this will be a situation in which the family would already be expecting the call.

Diabetic nurse to do diabetic teaching with patient

Many hospitals employ nurses who specialize in diabetic teaching to work with newly diagnosed patients. The HUC notifies the diabetic nurse of the consult.

Have ostomy nurse work with and train patient in colostomy care

Many hospitals employ nurses who specialize in ostomy care and teaching. The HUC notifies the ostomy nurse of the consult.

Transfer patient to the parent teaching/transition room, and teach mother to change dressings; also, train in feeding tube care and feeding technique.

Many pediatric hospitals and/or units have a patient room with a bed for a parent to stay with the child. The parent, after training, will assume full care of the child. The child then may be discharged to the parent's care.

Cardiopulmonary (resp care) to do pre-op and post-op teaching

This order is a request for a respiratory technician to inform a patient before surgery (preoperatively) what to expect and to demonstrate the use of an incentive spirometer. The order also requests that the respiratory technician follow-up with the patient after surgery (postoperatively) to assist the patient with breathing techniques and in using the incentive spirometer.

Pre-op teaching

A pre-op teaching plan is designed for each patient's diagnosis and unique needs. This plan is reviewed and modified during the intraoperative and postoperative periods. Pre-op teaching may involve breathing exercises, as well as techniques for splinting an incision, moving in bed and transferring to a chair, and so forth.

No visitors, limited number of visitors, or have visitors speak c̄ nurse before seeing pt

A sign should be posted on the patient's door to see the nurse for further explanation. The switchboard and the information desk also should be notified.

DNR (do not resuscitate) or no code

This order means that no resuscitative measures are to be performed. A <u>Do</u> <u>Not</u> <u>Resuscitate</u> order may be requested by a patient upon admission. The order must be written on the patient's chart. A verbal request by a patient or a patient's family member is not legal. This order is not a complete refusal of care; it simply states that a resuscitation code should not be performed in the event of cardiac or respiratory arrest. If the physician writes an order for "do not resuscitate," the order should be visible on the Kardex and on the patient's chart. Some hospitals have DNR forms that specify extent of resuscitative measures to be taken. This information is placed in the front of the patient's chart. The DNR order also must be written on the patient's order sheet by the doctor, and, depending on the hospital's policy, it must be rewritten or renewed if the patient is transferred to another unit, or if there is a change in attending doctors.

NINP (no information, no publication)

Various hospitals may use different abbreviations, but whatever words or abbreviations are used, this order means that the hospital staff denies that the patient is admitted when asked by visitors, in person or by telephone. This order may be extended to include family members. Often, a code phrase or word is used for persons who are excluded from this restriction.

Notify Dr. Avery of pt's adm to ICU

This order is intended to inform the patient's primary physician of admission of the patient to the intensive care unit when another physician has admitted the patient.

Notify hospitalist (covered in Chapter 2) if systolic BP >190

This order is to notify the hospitalist if the patient's systolic blood pressure is above 190.

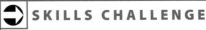 **SKILLS CHALLENGE**

To practice transcribing a review set of doctors' orders, complete Activity 18-5 in the *Skills Practice Manual*.

KEY CONCEPTS

This chapter has discussed a variety of doctors' orders. It concludes presentation of the transcription practice for all classifications of doctors' orders. Transcribing doctors' orders is a major HUC task. Repeated performance is necessary to gain expertise in this area.

When transcribing doctors' orders on the nursing unit of the hospital, it will be helpful to use the transcription procedures presented in this textbook as a reference.

Communication and Implementation of Transfer and Discharge Orders

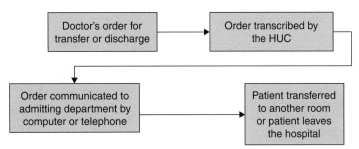

REVIEW QUESTIONS

1. Define the following terms:

a. transfer order

_____

b. discharge order

_____

c. consultation order

_____

2. The HUC is planning to call a doctor's office to notify the doctor of a consultation request. List the seven points of information to communicate to the consulting physician's office.

a. _____

b. _____

c. _____

d. _____

e. _____

f. _____

g. _____

3. Explain the responsibilities of the HUC in transcribing an order to obtain a patient's medical records from another facility.

_____

4. Explain the responsibilities of the HUC in sending a patient's medical record to another facility.

_____

_____

5. Describe the process of scanning a medical record into a patient's EMR.

_____

_____

6. The doctor may request to transfer a patient to another hospital room and/or unit because:

a. _____

b. _____

c. _____

7. List six tasks the HUC may need to perform for a patient who is given a 3-hour pass:

a. _____

b. _____

c. _____

d. _____

e. _____

f. _____

8. Two services that the case manager may perform for the hospitalized patient are:

a. _____

b. _____

9. List eight services rendered by the Social Services department:

a. _____

b. _____

c. _____

d. _____

e. _____

f. _____

g. _____

h. _____

10. Can a patient or a patient's family member verbally request that a DNR status be put into practice, if no, why?

_____

11. What is the purpose of a "parent teaching or transition room"?

_____

12. Explain the importance of reading the entire discharge order before the time of the patient's discharge.

_____

_____

THINK ABOUT...

1. Discuss why it is so important to document the time of call and the name or operator number of the person spoken to when calling a consultation to a doctor's office or to an answering service.
2. Discuss why documenting the name of the person from whom a report or a message is received or the name of the person who receives a report or a message is so important.
3. Discuss the consequences of not reading the entire discharge order before a patient leaves the nursing unit.

CHAPTER **19**

Admission, Preoperative, and Postoperative Procedures

CHAPTER OBJECTIVES

Upon completion of this chapter, you will be able to:

1. Define the terms in the vocabulary list.
2. Write the meaning of each abbreviation in the Abbreviations list.
3. List eight common components of a set of admission orders.
4. List 19 health unit coordinator tasks regarding the patient's admission that may apply when paper charts are used.
5. Name three items prepared by the registration department that are sent to the unit as part of the admission procedure.
6. List four types of admissions.
7. List at least eight registration tasks.
8. Describe the process for securing patient valuables.
9. Explain the health unit coordinator's responsibilities regarding the preoperative patient's orders and the patient's paper chart.
10. List seven components that may constitute part of a set of preoperative orders.
11. List five records or reports that may be on the patient's paper chart before the time of the patient's surgery.
12. List nine components that may constitute part of a set of postoperative orders.
13. List six tasks the health unit coordinator may perform regarding the postoperative patient's paper chart and Kardex.

14. Explain advance directives options.
15. Explain how the health unit coordinator's responsibilities regarding admission and preoperative and postoperative orders differ when the electronic medical record is implemented.

VOCABULARY

Admission Day Surgery Surgery scheduled on the day of the patient's arrival to the hospital; may be called *same-day surgery* or AM *admission*

Admission Orders Written (manually or electronically) instructions provided by the doctor for the care and treatment of the patient upon entry into the hospital

Admission Service Agreement or Conditions of Admission Agreement A form signed upon the patient's admission that sets forth the general services that the hospital will provide; also may be called conditions of admission, contract for services, or treatment consent

Advance Directives Documents that indicate a patient's wishes in the event that the patient becomes incapacitated and unable to make decisions regarding medical care

Allergy Identification Bracelet A plastic band with an insert on which allergy information is printed, or a red plastic band that has allergy information written directly on it, that the patient wears throughout the hospitalization

Allergy Information Information obtained from the patient regarding sensitivities to medications, food, and/or other substances (e.g., wool, tape)

Bariatrics The field of medicine that focuses on the treatment and control of obesity and diseases associated with obesity

Bariatric Surgery Surgery on part of the GI tract performed as a treatment for morbid obesity

Blood Transfusion Consent A patient's written permission to receive blood or blood products

Blood Transfusion Refusal A patient's written permission to refuse blood or blood products

Census A list of all occupied and unoccupied hospital beds

Color-coded "Alert" Wristbands Alert wristbands are used in many hospitals to quickly communicate a certain health care status or an "alert" that a patient may have. Red means "allergy alert," yellow means "fall risk," purple means "DNR (do not resuscitate)."

Comorbidity The presence of one or more disorders (or diseases) in addition to a primary disease or disorder, or the effect of such additional disorders or diseases

Direct Admission A patient who was not scheduled to be admitted and is admitted from the doctor's office, clinic, or emergency room

Elective Surgery Surgery that is not emergency or mandatory and can be planned at the patient's convenience

Emergency Admission An admission necessitated by accident or a medical emergency; such an admission is processed through the emergency department

Face Sheet A form initiated by the admitting department and included in the inpatient medical record that contains personal and demographic information, usually computer generated at the time of admission (also may be called the *information sheet* or *front sheet*)

HUGS Infant Protection System An example of an alarm system that includes monitoring software and an ankle bracelet that contains a tiny radio transmitter designed to prevent infants from being removed from a health care facility without authorization

Informed Consent The duty to inform a patient before a signature of permission is obtained

Intraoperative Pertaining to the period during a surgical procedure

Living Will A declaration made by the patient to family, medical staff, and all concerned with the patient's care, stating what is to be done in the event of a terminal illness; it directs the withholding or withdrawing of life-sustaining procedures

Medical Record Number The number assigned to the patient on or before admission; it is used for records identification and is used for all subsequent admissions to that hospital (also may be called health or medical records number)

Observation Patient A patient who is assigned to a bed on the nursing unit to receive care for a period of less than 24 hours; also may be referred to as a *medical short-stay* or *ambulatory patient*

Patient Account Number A number assigned to the patient to access insurance information; usually, a unique number is assigned each time the patient is admitted to the hospital

Patient Identification Bracelet A plastic band with a patient identification label affixed to it that is worn by the patient throughout hospitalization. In the obstetrics department, the mother and the baby would share the same identification label affixed to their ID bracelets

Perioperative Pertaining to the time of surgery

Postoperative Orders Orders written manually or electronically immediately after surgery. Postoperative orders cancel preoperative orders

Power of Attorney for Health Care The patient appoints a person (called a *proxy* or *agent*) to make health care decisions should the patient be unable to do so

Preadmit The process of obtaining information and partially preparing admitting forms before the time of the patient's arrival at the health care facility

Preoperative Care Unit A unit within the surgery area where a patient is prepared for surgery

Preoperative Health Unit Coordinator Checklist A checklist used by the health unit coordinator to ensure that the patient's paper chart is ready for surgery

Preoperative and Postoperative Patient Care Plan A plan that includes preoperative teaching, goals, and outcomes. This plan is reviewed and modified during the intraoperative and postoperative periods

Preoperative Nursing Checklist A checklist used to ensure that the paper or electronic chart and the patient are properly prepared for surgery

Preoperative Orders Orders that are written manually or electronically by the doctor before the time of surgery to prepare the patient for the surgical procedure

Registrar The admitting personnel who registers a patient to the hospital

Registration The process of entering personal information into the hospital information system to enroll a person as a hospital patient and create a patient record; patients may be registered as inpatients, outpatients, or observation patients

Scheduled Admission A patient admission planned in advance; it may be urgent or elective

Surgery Consent A patient's written permission for an operation or invasive procedure

Surgery Schedule A list of all the surgeries to be performed on a particular day; the schedule may be printed from the computer or sent to the nursing unit by the admitting department

Valuables Envelope A container for storing the patient's jewelry, money, and other valuables that is placed in the hospital safe for safekeeping

ABBREVIATIONS

Abbreviation	Meaning	Example of Usage on a Doctor's Order Sheet
BIBA	brought in by ambulance	Pt BIBA
DOA	dead on arrival	Pt was DOA
Dx	diagnosis	Dx: anemia
IVDU	intravenous drug user	Pt has hx of being an IVDU
MSSU	medical short-stay unit	Admit to: MSSU

Abbreviation	Meaning	Example of Usage on a Doctor's Order Sheet
OBS	observation	Pt to stay for 2 hr for OBS
OPS	outpatient surgery (ambulatory surgery)	Send pt to OPS
postop	after surgery	TCDB q2h postop
preop	before surgery	Call Valley Anesthesia for preop orders
SSU	short-stay unit	Pt to remain in SSU for 2°

EXERCISE 1

Write the abbreviation for each term listed below.

1. medical short-stay unit   _____

2. after surgery   _____

3. observation   _____

4. diagnosis   _____

5. before surgery   _____

6. outpatient surgery   _____

7. short-stay unit   _____

8. brought in by ambulance   _____

9. dead on arrival   _____

10. IVDU   _____

EXERCISE 2

Write the meaning of each abbreviation listed below.

1. OPS

_____

2. preop

_____

3. Dx

_____

4. OBS

_____

5. postop

_____

6. MSSU

_____

7. SSU

_____

8. BIBA

_____

9. DOA

_____

10. IVDU

_____

✏ TAKE NOTE

When the electronic medical record (EMR) is implemented, there willnot be a paper chart, and the health unit coordinator (HUC) will not have the responsibility of transcribing admission or preoperative or postoperative doctors' orders. The HUC may have the responsibility of escorting the newly admitted patient to the room, entering the patient's name into the computer, ordering a diet tray (if late admit), preparing the surgical consent form, and other tasks as indicated (with an icon) on the cmputer census screen. Scanning the signed consent and other documents as required or requested is also an important part of the HUC's role when the EMR c̄ computer physician order entry (CPOE) is used.

ADMISSION OF THE PATIENT

The HUC's role in the admission procedure is a very important one. Often, the HUC is the first person the new patient encounters on the nursing unit, which will serve as their "home" for several days or longer. This is an opportunity to demonstrate the caring nature of the hospital by greeting the patient warmly and making them feel welcome. In some instances, the HUC has the responsibility of admitting the patient. The ability to perform tasks in an efficient manner enables the health care team to provide the care and treatment ordered for the patient as soon as possible.

Types of Admissions

A person may become a hospital patient in a variety of ways. Types of admissions are discussed in the following sections.

Scheduled or planned admissions are admissions that are called into the admitting department before the patient arrives. Patients enter the hospital through the admitting department and usually are admitted to the service of their primary doctor. Scheduled admissions may be classified further as urgent, direct, or elective. Urgent or **direct admissions** occur when a doctor sees a patient in the office, decides that the person should be admitted to the hospital, and places a call to the hospital to arrange the admission. Another example of a direct admission is a pregnant woman who goes to the hospital and, after evaluation by a doctor, is immediately admitted to labor and delivery. Admission of a patient who has been transported by ambulance or helicopter from another health care facility such as an extended care facility also would be called a **direct admission**.

Elective scheduled admissions occur when the patient and the doctor decide when to schedule a nonemergency surgery or procedure. Patients may be admitted to the nursing unit on the day before their surgery/procedure or on the day their surgery/procedure is scheduled and will be admitted to a nursing unit after the surgery/procedure has been completed. A list of scheduled admissions may be available to print from the computer or may be sent to each nursing unit from the admitting department early in the day, allowing the nursing unit to plan for the admissions.

Emergency admissions are unplanned and are the result of an accident, sudden illness, or other medical crisis. Patients enter the hospital through the emergency department, are processed through the emergency department, and are referred to as *emergency admissions*. Emergency department personnel prepare an emergency department record (Fig. 19-1). Often, old records from the patient's prior admissions are requested from the health information management services department (HIMS) if the patient has had previous admissions. Should the patient's condition warrant admission to the hospital, the patient will be assigned to a nursing unit. The emergency department record is sent to the nursing unit with the patient and is placed in the patient's paper chart or is scanned into the EMR. The patient's old records also should be sent to the nursing unit with the patient and stored on the unit (if paper charts are used) until the patient is discharged or transferred. The HUC reviews the emergency department record to see whether all requested tests have been completed. For example, the emergency room doctor may have ordered a urinalysis, but the patient may not have voided yet. If tests have not been completed, the HUC processes those that remain to be done.

Some emergencies require that patients receive treatment before they are registered by the admitting department. Patients may be unconscious without identification and may be taken to an intensive care unit. An example is a near-drowning victim transported by ambulance from a public swimming pool or lake. The HUC would request that the patient be given an alias name and assigned a health record number by the admitting department, so tests may be ordered and lab specimens may be identified with a label and processed in the laboratory. When the patient's family arrives, family members may be sent to the admitting department so the patient can be admitted under the correct name. The patient's correct name then will be entered into the computer (the alias name will remain in the computerized record as well, for identification purposes). If an invasive procedure or surgery was immediately required to save the life of a patient who is unable to sign an informed consent, and no family is present, two medical doctors would sign the consent.

> ✐ **TAKE NOTE**
>
> Types of admissions include scheduled urgent, direct, elective, and emergency.

Types of Patients

Patients who receive medical care may be categorized as to type. Patient type may be assigned according to the purpose and length of hospitalization. The three patient types consist of inpatient, observation patient, and outpatient.

An inpatient is a patient who is admitted to the hospital for longer than 24 hours and is assigned to a bed on the nursing unit. The HUC will prepare a chart and process orders for the patient (see Chapter 8).

An observation patient is a patient who is assigned to a bed on a nursing unit to receive care for a period of less than 24 hours. An observation patient also may be referred to as a *medical short-stay* or an *ambulatory patient*. Some hospitals may have a specific unit such as a medical short-stay unit (MSSU) or ambulatory care unit that provides short-term care. If the patient requires further hospital care beyond 24 hours, the doctor must write an order for hospital admission. The criteria for observation patients may vary from facility to facility, and differences depend on the patient's insurance as well. The HUC may prepare a chart and process orders for the observation patient. It may be the HUC's task to monitor the time and notify the nurse that the patient needs to be discharged, or that an order was obtained for admission.

An outpatient is a patient who receives care in a hospital, clinic, or surgicenter but does not stay for longer than 24 hours. An outpatient usually is scheduled to receive treatments, therapies, or tests. The department that provides care for the outpatient processes the outpatient orders. Usually, the assembly of a chart is not required, although patients may receive outpatient services on a routine basis that do require a chart.

> ✐ **TAKE NOTE**
>
> Types of patients receiving medical care include inpatient, observation patient, and outpatient.

Types of Services

Service type refers to the type of nursing unit (see Chapter 3, "Hospital Nursing Units," pp 39-40), such as surgical, medical, and so forth. The patient may be classified as a teaching or a nonteaching patient, indicating whether residents and/or other health care students will be involved in the patient's care. Patients also may be classified according to the type of insurance coverage they have (e.g., Medicare, preferred provider organization [PPO], health maintenance organization [HMO]).

Admission Arrangement

In all types of admissions, a doctor with admitting privileges to the hospital must authorize the patient's admission. One of the following is responsible to arrange for the admission of a patient: the attending or primary doctor; the emergency

EMERGENCY ROOM

MEDICAL RECORD NO 1: 567-435	MED SERVICE: Orth	FINANCIAL CL 7	DATE 8: 5/23/XX	SOC SEC NO/MEDICARE NO: 527-48-XXXX
PATIENT NAME 2 LAST: Lowrey	FIRST: Holly	MIDDLE: Elinor		HOSPITALIZATION INSURANCE - 1: Sunstate; POLICY/GROUP NO: 100-0000
PATIENT'S PERMANENT ADDRESS: 10001 North	CITY: Mountain, Sky,	STATE: AZ	ZIP: 85000	TEL: 942-XXXX; ADDRESS: 2222 N.Tower Pl. Sky, AZ
PATIENT'S TEMPORARY ADDRESS	CITY	STATE	ZIP	TEL; HOSPITALIZATION INSURANCE 2; POLICY/GROUP NO
BIRTHDATE: 5/3/XX	AGE: 22	HAS PATIENT EVER BEEN TREATED IN THIS HOSPITAL: ☐ INPATIENT ☐ OUTPATIENT	WHEN; UNDER WHAT NAME	ADDRESS; EFFECTIVE DATE - 1: 1/06/XX; EFFECTIVE DATE - 2
SEX: ☐ MALE ☒ FEMALE	MARITAL STATUS: ☒ SINGLE ☒ MARRIED ☐ SEPARATED ☐ DIVORCED ☐ WIDOWED	RACE: ☐ WHITE ☒ BLACK ☐ INDIAN ☐ ORIENTAL ☐ OTHER	RELIGION: ☐ CATHOLIC ☐ JEWISH ☐ PROTESTANT ☒ OTHER	INDUSTRIAL - PATIENT'S EMPLOYER: ☐ YES ☒ NO
RESPONSIBLE PARTY NAME 3: SELF		RELATIONSHIP	TEL	ADDRESS; TEL
ADDRESS STREET P O BOX APT NO CITY 4 5		STATE	ZIP 6	RELATIVE NOTIFIED
SPOUSE OR NEAREST RELATIVE (NEXT OF KIN): Iris Lowrey		RELATIONSHIP: Mother	TEL: 943-XXXX	TIME: 1800 BY WHOM: M. Loor
ADDRESS STREET P O BOX APT NO CITY: 211 E. Sun Dr. Sky, AZ		STATE	ZIP: 85000	POLICE NOTIFIED
E R PHYSICIAN: Thomas V. Riggs	ATTENDING PHYSICIAN: B. Urself			TIME: 1730 BY WHOM: M. Loor

EVENTS AND CARE GIVEN PRIOR TO ARRIVAL / CHIEF COMPLAINT: Pt. states she was involved in an auto accident 10am to-day - no loss of consciousness - Complaint of pain Right shoulder - right knee - 3 inch lac. to left cheek area - abrasion (R) hand

VITAL SIGNS: TEMP 98⁴ ORAL/RECTAL P 88 R 24 BP 130/80

ALLERGIES: Codeine

LAST TETANUS: July 1971

	ADMIT	EXAM	CALLED	CALLED	CALLED	CONTACTED	ARRIVED
INITIAL							
TIME	5pm						
PHYSICIANS NAME	B. Urself		5:45p	5:55p		6:10p	7pm

	LAB	X-RAY	DISCHG
CALLED		5:30p	
SPEC TAKEN			
RESULTS OBY			

NURSE: HOME / DR OFF / OTHER / WORK; ADMIT TO ROOM

BROUGHT IN BY (NAME OF PERSON OR AMBULANCE): Associated ambulance

MEDICAL EXAMINER

DISPOSITION OF VALUABLES: to husband

NURSE'S SIGNATURE: Mable Jones RN

ORDERS	HISTORY: PHYSICAL FINDINGS & TREATMENT
	S. ↓ Rom (R) SHOULDER
1. CERVICAL - XTABLE 1ST	2° TO PAIN
2. SKULL	Obj 1. VS - STABLE
3 R SHOULDER	2. HEAD ① PERLA, EOM'S, disc NORMAL
R KNEE	② EAR'S - NO BLOOD
R HAND (done ML)	③ Ⅱ CRANIAL NERVE SENSATION L=R
4. 1% LIDOCAINE	4. 3" lac FACE
4-0 - NYLON WHITE	3. NECK - SUPPLE
6-0 NYLON - BLACK	4 CHEST - GOOD EXPANSION
(done ML) abrasions, laceration	LUNGS CLEAR
cleansed c̄ betadine soln	5. ABD - GOOD BS, NO HS MEGLY, NO
dressed c̄ neosporin, dry	TENDERNESS, REBOUND OR REFERRED
dressing.	PAIN.
	6 EXT - (R) SHOULDER - ECCHYMOSIS, ↓ ROM
	(R) KNEE - CONTUSION + ABRASION
	R-HAND - ABRASION
	7 XRAYS - SKULL, CERVICAL, R SHOULDER - NEG
	A&R, A/A, LACERATION, ABRASION + CONTUSION
FINAL DISPOSITION - DESCRIBE	FINAL DIAGNOSIS: PLAN instr/HEAD SHEET given to pt. MS / STITCHES OUT - 4 DAYS; ICE ↑
SIGNATURE OF E R PHYSICIAN: Thomas V. Riggs MD	SIGNATURE OF ATTENDING PHYSICIAN; CODE

00-2912 1-77

MEDICAL RECORDS

Figure 19-1 Emergency department record.

room doctor; the primary or attending doctor's office staff; or the HMO staff acting on instructions of the doctor. The doctor provides the admitting diagnosis or medical reason for admission. Many hospitals employ a hospitalist who may oversee the patient's care during the hospital stay. The hospitalist communicates with the patient's attending or primary doctor.

✎ TAKE NOTE

Whatever the patient's route to the hospital may be, a doctor with admitting privileges to the hospital must authorize the admission. In many hospitals, a hospitalist may oversee the patient's care during their stay in the hospital.

Bed Assignment

Most hospitals are open for admissions 24 hours a day. The admitting department or registration staff performs many tasks in relation to the admission of the patient to the hospital. Usually, the hospital **census** is computerized and provides an accurate, up-to-date list of occupied and unoccupied hospital beds. Nursing unit assignments for scheduled admissions usually are determined in advance. A list of scheduled patient admissions may be made available on the computer or may be printed and sent to each nursing unit that receives patients. Nursing assignments generally are determined for scheduled admissions in the morning. Direct admissions or emergency admissions are assigned beds when the patient arrives at the hospital and is ready for a room. The admitting diagnosis and/or patient age usually determine the type of nursing unit that is suitable, and the nursing staff usually decides on the specific bed. In many hospitals, staff members on the nursing unit decide bed assignment. Nursing personnel are familiar with staffing and roommate issues and can best decide which bed is appropriate for the new patient. After receiving patient information such as name, diagnosis, age, and sex, the HUC or nurse may assign the bed number.

✎ TAKE NOTE

It is important to notify the admitting department of pending discharges in a timely manner, especially when the hospital is low on open beds. Delaying notification could cause a delay in another patient's admission and treatment.

Patient Admission/Registration

Registration is the process of entering personal information into the hospital information system to register a person as a hospital patient and create a patient record. A **registrar** in the admitting department or the HUC may assume the patient admission/registration responsibilities.

Patient Admission/Registration Tasks

Patient admission/registration tasks include the following:

- Copy insurance cards.
- Verify insurance (may be done in advance when admission is scheduled).

- Ask patient or patient guardian to sign appropriate insurance forms.
- Interview patient or family to obtain personal information.
- Prepare admission forms (admission service agreement and face sheet) and obtain signatures.
- Ask patient whether he has an advanced directives document or would like to create one (required in most states).
- Prepare patient's identification bracelet.
- Prepare patient's identification labels.
- Secure patient valuables if necessary.
- Supply and explain required information, including a copy of the *Patient's Bill of Rights* and hospital privacy laws (required by the Joint Commission [TJC]).
- Include any test results, prewritten orders, or consents that were previously sent to the admitting department in the packet that accompanies the patient to the nursing unit.

Interview

When admissions are arranged in advance, such as for planned or **elective surgery**, preadmission information may be obtained by the registration staff by mail, by phone, or by computer. This information, including the patient's name, address, and telephone number; employer's name and address; insurance carrier; and doctor's name and diagnosis, is placed on a record called the *information sheet* or *face sheet* (see Chapter 8). If patient information was not obtained previously, this is done at the time of admission.

Interview Techniques. When interviewing a patient to obtain personal information, it is imperative to use the interpersonal skills discussed in Chapter 5. Being admitted to the health care facility is a stressful situation, and many patients also may be experiencing physical discomfort. The following guidelines should be observed when patients are interviewed:

- Protect confidentiality.
- Ensure privacy when asking for personal information.
- Be proficient and professional.
- Asking whether the patient was hospitalized previously can hasten the registration process and reduce the risk of error in assignment of health information management and patient account numbers (demographics would have to be verified in case of possible changes).
- Treat each patient as an individual.
- Listen carefully.
- Project a friendly, courteous attitude.
- Include family or significant other in the process.

✎ TAKE NOTE

Patient registration tasks should be completed before orders can be processed for the patient, unless a life-threatening emergency occurs.

Admission Forms

The admission service agreement or the conditions of admission agreement (COA or C of A) lists the general services that the hospital will provide. It is an agreement between the patient and the hospital and includes a legal consent for treatment (see Chapter 8). This consent may specify financial responsibility also. The patient is to sign the form upon admission. Patients who are unable to sign an admission service agreement may have a legal guardian sign for them. A copy of the admission service agreement is given to the patient after it is signed, and the original becomes part of the patient's paper medical record or is scanned into the patient's EMR by the HUC.

The **face sheet, front sheet, or information sheet** is the form that is generated after patient information, such as address, telephone number, nearest of kin, insurance carrier, and so forth, is entered into the hospital information system. It usually is filed as the first page of the patient's paper medical record or is scanned into the patient's electronic medical record by the health unit coordinator.

Advance Directives

Society now recognizes the individual's right to make decisions regarding care if he becomes incapacitated, and to die with dignity rather than be kept alive indefinitely by artificial life support. As a result, most states have enacted "right to die" laws and laws dealing with advanced directives. The term **advance directive** refers to an individual's desires regarding care if they should become incapacitated and require end-of-life care. An adult witness or witnesses or a notary must sign an advance directive. The notary or witness cannot be the person named to make the decisions or the provider of health care. If there is only one witness, it cannot be a relative or someone who will be the beneficiary of property from the patient's estate if the patient dies.

Most states require that patients be asked if they have or would like to have an advanced directive document. See Chapter 8 for an example of an advance directive checklist, which provides documentation that the patient was asked and what decision was made regarding health care. Advance directives include the following documents:

- A **living will** is a declaration made by the patient to family, medical staff, and all concerned with the patient's care stating what is to be done in the event of a terminal illness. It directs the withholding or withdrawing of life-sustaining procedures. The patient may define what is meant by *meaningful quality of life*, a phrase commonly used in living wills to describe the level of functioning the patient would be comfortable with.
- **Power of attorney for health care** allows the patient to appoint another person or persons (called a *proxy* or *agent*) to make health care decisions for him should the patient become incapable of making decisions. The proxy (agent) has a duty to act consistently with the patient's wishes. If the proxy does not know the patient's wishes, the proxy has the duty to act in the patient's best interests. Figure 19-2 is an example of a health care power of attorney and living will combined form. An advance directive becomes effective *only* when the patient can no longer make decisions for himself or herself. The patient may change or destroy any directive or living will at any time.

Routine admissions may have had tests performed before their admission. Test results are forwarded to the hospital admitting department and are sent to the nursing unit with the other chart forms. Doctors may manually or electronically write orders or obtain consents in advance; these also are forwarded

to the hospital admitting department and are sent to the nursing unit upon admission.

At the time of admission or before admission, each patient is assigned a health information management number that is unique for that patient. The health information management number identifies the patient and all chart forms and is used for all future admissions to that hospital. The patient account number is assigned at the time of admission and is used to reference insurance information; it is usually unique to each admission. The patient account number also serves to identify all charges for equipment, supplies, and procedures. The business office uses the patient account number for billing purposes.

Patient Identification Labels

Patient identification labels are self-adhesive labels used on the patient's identification bracelet to identify forms, requisitions, specimens, and so forth (see Chapter 8). Patient identification labels may be prepared by registration staff members who enter the information into the computer and may then print it through the computer on the nursing unit.

> ✎ *TAKE NOTE*
>
> If an imprinter and patient identification imprinter cards are used, forms, requisitions, and so forth, would be stamped (using an imprinter machine) with patient information instead of using labels. A cardboard insert with patient identification information printed on it may be inserted into the plastic identification bracelet.

Patient Identification Bracelet

A **patient identification bracelet** or band is prepared by registration staff upon admission of the patient to the hospital. The bracelet is usually a plastic band with the patient's identification label affixed to it, or a cardboard insert may be used (Fig. 19-3). Identifying information may consist of (1) the patient's name, sex, age, and date of birth, (2) the patient's attending doctor's name, (3) the health information management number, and (4) the patient account number. The patient's room and bed numbers are usually written in pencil so they may be changed easily if the patient is moved to a different room and/or bed number. The health information management number serves as the main identifier because it is a unique number assigned to that patient. Most hospitals have stopped using the patient's social security number as an identifying number to protect confidentiality. The bracelet is worn throughout the patient's hospitalization. All personnel

> ✎ *TAKE NOTE*
>
> Three color-coded wrist "alert" bands are now being used in many hospitals to quickly communicate a certain health care status or an "alert" that a patient may have. Each color has a certain meaning. A red wristband is used to indicate that the patient has an allergy, purple indicates "Do not resuscitate (DNR)," and yellow alerts that the patient is a "fall risk." The words for the alerts are also written on the wristband to reduce the chance of confusing the alert messages. The identification bracelet or wristband used is white.

HEALTH CARE POWER OF ATTORNEY & LIVING WILL
Combined Form

I, _____, as principal, designate _____ as my agent for all matters relating to my health care, including, without limitation, full power to give or to refuse consent to all medical, surgical, hospital, psychiatric and related health care. This power of attorney is effective whenever I am unable to make or to communicate health care decisions. All of my agent's actions under this power have the same effects on my heirs, devisees, and personal representatives as if I were alive, competent and acting for myself.

If my agent is unwilling or unable to serve or to continue to serve, I hereby appoint _____ as my agent.

In acting under this power, I want my agent to give great weight to the following statements: I am in favor of trial treatment. That means I want all necessary medical care to treat my condition until, and only until, my doctors and my agent reasonably decide that I am in an irreversible coma, or a persistent vegetative state, or a locked-in state, or that I cannot be expected to return to a fully conscious state. If, following the guidelines stated above, my doctors and my agent decide that further medical care is inappropriate:

1. I **want** only comfort care and I **do not want** to undergo artificial administration of food or fluids.

2. I **do not want** to be resuscitated in case I stop breathing or my heart stops beating.

If my doctors and my agent reasonably decide that I have a terminal illness, I want all decisions concerning my medical and surgical care to be made in light of the expected length and quality of life which would result from such care and the predictable effects on me of undergoing treatment. **If I cannot be expected to have a significant period of conscious life even after medical or surgical care, then I want comfort care only.** (Examples: I do not want any surgery or other care designed to prolong my life. I do not want artificially administered food or fluids and I do not want to be resuscitated.)

This combined health care directive is made under § 36-3221 and § 36-3261, Arizona Revised Statutes. It continues in effect for all who may rely on it, except those to whom I have given notice of its revocation.

_____   _____
Dated   Signature of Mark of Person Making Living Will or Granting Health Care Power of Attorney

Verification

I affirm that: (1) I was present when this living will was dated and signed or marked or (2) the person making this living will directly indicated to me that the living will expressed that person's wishes and that the person intended to adopt it at that time. The maker of this document appeared to be of sound mind and free from duress.

(If there is only one witness signing this document) I certify that: I have not been designated to make medical decisions for the person who signed this living will, I am not directly involved with providing health care to that person, I am not related to that person by blood, marriage, or adoption and I am not entitled to any part of that person's estate.

_____   _____   _____
Witness   Witness   Date

STATE OF ARIZONA   )
) ss.
County of   )

The maker of this document appears to be of sound mind and free from duress. It was subscribed and sworn to before me this _____ day of _____, 19_____.

_____   My Commission Expires _____
Notary Public

(A health care power of attorney and living will must be signed by a notary or by an adult witness or witnesses, who saw you sign or mark the document and who say that you appear to be of sound mind and free from duress. A notary or witness cannot be the person you name to make your decisions or your provider of health care. If you have only one witness, that witness cannot be related to you or someone who will get any of your property from your estate if you die.)

July 1995 • Arizona Hospital and Healthcare Association

Figure 19-2 Health care power of attorney and living will admission.

who perform services for the patient must read the identification bracelet before administering any service, to ensure correct patient identification.

Patients' Valuables

Patients who have a large quantity of money, expensive jewelry, or other items of value with them at the time of admission are requested to send them home with family or place them in the hospital safe. These items are placed in a numbered **valuables envelope** (Fig. 19-4), and the patient is given a duplicate numbered claim check. This number, which also may be written manually or electronically in the patient's chart, serves as a reminder that there are valuables in the hospital safe. A clothing and valuables form also is prepared, which lists clothing, eyeglasses, false teeth, prosthesis, and any other items of value (Fig. 19-5). The form is signed, the signature is witnessed, and the document is placed into the patient's paper chart or is scanned into the EMR.

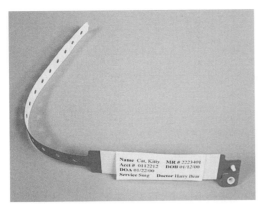

Figure 19-3 Patient identification bracelet.

> ✏ *TAKE NOTE*
>
> Most hospitals have discontinued use of the patient's Social Security number on patient identification labels and identification bracelets for confidentiality purposes. The medical record number serves as the main identifier because it is assigned to the patient and is unique to that patient. Information contained on patient ID labels may differ slightly among hospitals.

Provided Patient Information

The registration staff or the HUC will explain the registration process and hospital rules to the patient and/or the patient's family. Because of various state laws, the hospital may be required to inform the patient of specific information. Upon admission, the patient usually is supplied with a copy of patient rights and the hospital's privacy practices; other handouts may be provided regarding the hospital stay.

Escort to the Nursing Unit

Once the nursing unit and bed assignments have been made, a volunteer, a member of the hospital transportation department, or an admitting personnel staff member escorts the patient to the assigned unit. In some hospitals, the HUC may escort the patient to the room, advise him of visitation rules, and instruct him in use of the bed controls, the television control, and the Internet. If the patient has already been registered, the admitting papers are delivered to the receiving unit. The HUC greets the patient and tells the nurse who will be caring for the patient of the patient's arrival. The nurse completes the admitting nurse's notes (see Chapter 8), which the HUC may use to complete the patient profile with information such as allergies, height, and weight.

> ◑ **SKILLS CHALLENGE**
>
> To practice preparing the newly admitted patient's chart and Kardex forms, complete Activity 19-1 in the *Skills Practice Manual.*

ADMISSION ORDERS

Admission orders are written directions provided by the doctor regarding the care and treatment of the patient upon entry into the hospital. Most orders are written on the unit by the hospitalist, attending doctor, resident, or nurse practitioner, or they may be received by telephone immediately after the patient's arrival. However, at times, the admission orders arrive before the patient does. Doctors may have preprinted order sets or clinical pathways for certain types of admissions, such as a patient admitted for a CABG or total hip or knee replacement surgery. Some doctors may write admission orders before the time of arrival of the patient and leave them on the nursing unit. The HUC must ensure that these orders are identified with the patient's name, which should be written on the order sheet in ink. The orders are labeled with the patient's identification label later, when the patient arrives to the nursing unit. When the EMR with CPOE is implemented, the doctor enters the orders directly into the computer, or the preprinted order sets or clinical pathways may be computerized.

Admission Order Components

Common components of admission orders include the following:

- Admitting diagnosis
- Diet
- Activity
- Diagnostic tests/procedures
- Medications. Usually, medications are needed for the patient's disease condition, for sleeping, and/or for pain.
- Treatment orders
- Request for old records
- Patient care category or code status. The patient care category or code status may be indicated on the patient's admission orders. The patient care category or code status refers to the patient's wishes regarding resuscitation. Code status may be written as full code, modified support, or do not resuscitate. The doctor must follow any state-specific statute and the hospital's policies and procedures when writing a DNR status.

Figure 19-6 is an example of a set of admission orders. Health unit coordinator tasks performed during the admission procedure are listed in Procedure 19-1.

> **SKILLS CHALLENGE**
>
> To practice transcribing a set of admission orders for a medical patient, complete Activity 19-2 in the *Skills Practice Manual.*

THE SURGERY PATIENT

Information

The procedure for admission of a medical or surgical patient is the same, except that diagnostic tests ordered by the doctor are performed on surgery patients as soon as possible after their arrival to the hospital. This allows the time needed to

PATIENT'S VALUABLE ENVELOPE

01903
ENVELOPE NUMBER

IMPRINT AREA OR PATIENT'S NAME AND HOSPITAL NO

HOSPITAL TAKES ALL POSSIBLE PRECAUTIONS TO SAFEGUARD YOUR PROPERTY BUT DISCLAIMS RESPONSIBILITY FOR VALUABLES SURRENDERED TO WRONGFUL HOLDER OF IDENTIFICATION SLIP AND WILL NOT BE RESPONSIBLE FOR ANY CLAIM FOR LOSS

CONTENTS OF ENVELOPE
DEPOSITED WITH HOSPITAL

[X] CASH $100 ___ $20 _5_ $5 _1_   LOOSE CHANGE
          $ 50 ___ $10 ___ $1 _2_ .

[ ] CHECKS (LIST SEPARATELY) _____

[X] CREDIT CARDS (LIST SEPARATELY) _VISA_____

[ ] WATCH _____

[ ] RINGS _____

[X] WALLET _____

[ ] OTHER EXPLAIN _____

[ ] OTHER EXPLAIN _____

ARTICLES RETAINED BY
PATIENT OR RESPONSIBLE PARTY

[X] CASH   _$3.00_

[ ] WATCH _____

[ ] RINGS _____

[ ] WALLET _____

[ ] RAZOR _____

[X] DENTURES PARTIAL   _LOWER_

[X] GLASSES _____

[ ] OTHER EXPLAIN _____

00-1346 REV 5-77

I HAVE CHECKED THE ABOVE AND ACKNOWLEDGE THE LISTS TO BE CORRECT. I, THE PATIENT, OR RESPONSIBLE PARTY ASSUME FULL RESPONSIBILITY FOR THOSE ITEMS RETAINED IN MY POSSESSION DURING MY HOSPITALIZATION OR BROUGHT TO PATIENT AFTER SIGNATURES HAVE BEEN OBTAINED

| TIME _1400_ | DATE _11/2/xx_ | PATIENT'S SIGNATURE OR RESPONSIBLE PARTY X _Wendy Leigh_ | WITNESSED BY _Kay Iver, R.N._ |

VALUABLE ENVELOPE CHART COPY RECEIVED BY _Kay Iver, R.N._   HOSPITAL EMPLOYEE

CASHIER'S USE ▶ DATE _11/2, XX_   RECEIVED AND CERTIFIED _Mark Palmer_

EMERGENCY ROOM USE ▶ DATE ___   PROPERTY COLLECTED BY ___   WITNESSED BY ___

WITHDRAWALS

DATE	DESCRIPTION	CASHIER INITIALS	PATIENT SIGNATURE

NOT RESPONSIBLE FOR ARTICLES AFTER 30 DAYS FROM DISCHARGE
LOST RECEIPT DOCUMENTATION
CLAIMANT MUST PROVIDE SOME INDEPENDENT EVIDENCE OF HIS IDENTITY FOR RELEASE OF THE ENVELOPE CONTENTS PLEASE DESCRIBE THIS IDENTIFICATION

Figure 19-4 Valuables envelope.

perform diagnostic studies and have the test results added to the patient's chart before surgery is performed. An abnormal blood test result or a chest x-ray that is abnormal may require that surgery be postponed pending further evaluation.

Some surgeries, such as open-heart surgery or organ transplant surgery, may require additional diagnostic studies, patient preparation, preoperative teaching, and careful explanation of the procedure to the patient and the family. A tour of the intensive care unit may be arranged so that the patient will be aware of surroundings and activities that will take place after surgery.

Admission Day Surgery

Admission day surgery refers to patients who are scheduled for surgery on the day of their arrival to the hospital. The patient usually has been pre-admitted and has had all necessary pre-op labs, chest x-ray, and EKG completed before their admission. After completion of the patient's surgery and some time spent in the postanesthesia care unit (PACU), the patient is admitted

to a surgical nursing unit. Health insurance companies promote this type of admission because it eliminates a hospital day, which reduces the cost of the hospitalization. Other terms for this practice include **same-day surgery** and AM **admission**.

The doctor's office, the hospital admitting department, and the surgery-scheduling secretary usually coordinate the same-day surgery patient's admission. Laboratory tests, x-rays, and other diagnostic testing may be performed at the doctor's office, at an outside facility, or at the hospital on an outpatient basis before admission. The patient usually goes to the hospital admitting area to complete the registration process a few days before the actual admission day. Admitting personnel places the patient identification bracelet or band on the patient's wrist at that time.

On the day of surgery (several hours before the scheduled surgery), the patient reports to the registration desk and will be escorted to the preoperative care unit.

The patient's chart will contain the following:

- Doctors' orders
- All preadmission diagnostic reports that were performed

PATIENT VALUABLES

VALUABLES

QUANTITY	DESCRIPTION

☐ I have been informed that a safe is available in the Patient Accounts Department for the safekeeping of my valuables.

☐ I understand that the Hospital will assume responsibility for eyeglasses, bridgework, dentures and clothing (up to $50) lost or damaged due to negligence of Hospital personnel.

☐ I agree to assume full responsibility for any valuables not turned over to the Hospital for safekeeping in the Hospital safe by myself or my personal representative. I will hold the Hospital responsible for only those valuables listed above.

Signed: _____   Date _____ 20 ____
              (Patient or Representative)

Witnessed by: _____
                    (Admission Representative)

Received by: _____   Deposit Envelope No. _____
                 (Cashier or Nursing Office Representative)

Verified by: _____
                (Admissions Representative or Other Employee)

Safe Deposit Envelope No. _____ Date of Deposit _____ 20 ____

Comments: _____
_____

Patient Valuables

Figure 19-5 Clothing and valuables list. (Courtesy Rockford Memorial Hospital, Rockford, Illinois.)

PHYSICIANS' ORDER SHEET

DATE	TIME	SYMBOL	ORDERS
5/4/00	1300		Admit to med-surg unit
			DX: acute pulmonary edema
			BRP c̄ help
			VS q 2 for 8 then q4°
			1800 cal ADA NAS diet
			Daily wts
			I & O
			CBC, lytes & cardiac isoenzymes stat
			CMP in am
			ABG on RA now, then place on O_2 @ 2 L/M
			Repeat ABG in 2 hr—call me c̄ results
			Chest PA & lat today & in am CI infiltrates
			EKG today & in am
			Lung perfusion/ventilation scan in am CI embolism
			bepridil hydrochloride 300 mg qd
			bumetanide 2 mg PO now & qd
			Ambien 10 mg qhs prn for sleep
			Old records to floor
			Pt is a full code status
			Dr. John Stewart MD

Figure 19-6 Set of admission orders.

- Patient identification labels
- Admission forms

After spending time in surgery and the recovery room (PACU), the patient is assigned a bed and is transported to an inpatient surgical unit.

> ✐ *TAKE NOTE*
>
> Usually, preoperative care, operating rooms, and the PACU are contained in one complete area, separate from all inpatient activities.

Preoperative Care Unit

The preoperative care unit (located in the surgery area) is where a patient is prepared for surgery. This is also a waiting area for surgical patients. Preparation may include: shaving the surgical area if necessary, starting intravenous fluids, or inserting a catheter (may be done in the operating room). Preoperative breathing treatments may also be administered in this area. If the patient is a same day surgery admission, the surgical consent form will also be signed here.

Preoperative Orders

The doctor who will perform surgery on a patient manually or electronically writes orders relative to the surgery before the time the surgery is performed. For example, the surgeon who is performing an open-heart surgery may wish the patient to receive preoperative teaching as provided by the cardiopulmonary (respiratory care) department on the evening before surgery. The doctor also may order a heparin lock to be inserted or an intravenous (IV) line to be started before a patient leaves the nursing unit for surgery.

The surgeon may designate the anesthesiologist who will manually or electronically write preoperative preparation orders. The surgeon manually or electronically writes the surgical procedure on the physicians' order sheet for preparation of the surgery consent. If a discrepancy is found between the physicians' written order for the surgery consent, the **surgery schedule**, or information on the patient's chart, or if there is any confusion for the patient, the patient's nurse should be notified (if unaware) and the correct procedure must be verified by calling the doctor's office immediately. For example, the surgery consent as written by the physician may state that the patient is to have an "open reduction of the *left* femur," whereas the patient's diagnosis and physical examination indicate that the patient has a fracture of the *right* femur; obviously, such a discrepancy must be corrected

PROCEDURE 19–1

ADMISSION PROCEDURE

(Tasks may vary between facilities.) When CPOE has been implemented, all tasks related to preparing a paper chart or transcribing orders would not apply.

TASK	NOTES
1. Greet the patient upon his arrival to the nursing unit.	1. *Introduce yourself and give your status. Example: "I'm Ted Mart, the health unit coordinator for this unit."*
2. Inform the patient that the nurse will be notified of his arrival.	2. Notify the nurse caring for the patient of the patient's arrival.
3. Notify the attending doctor and/or hospital resident or the hospitalist of the patient's admission.	
4. Move the patient's name from the admission screen on the computer to the correct bed on the nursing unit.	
5. Record the patient's admission on the admission, discharge, and transfer sheet and the census board.	
6. Check the patient's signature on the admission service agreement form.	6. *Compare the spelling of the patient's name on the face sheet or front sheet and the patient identification labels with the signature on the admission service agreement form. Also check to see that the doctor's name is correct.*

7. Complete the procedure for preparation of the paper chart.
   a. Label all chart forms with the patient's identification labels (if paper charts used).
   b. Fill in all the needed headings (if paper charts used).
   c. Place all forms in the chart behind the proper dividers (if paper charts used).	

8. Label the outside of the chart (if paper charts used).	8. *Identify the chart with the patient's and doctor's names and the room number.*
9. Prepare any other labels or identification cards used by the facility.	
10. Place the patient identification labels in the correct place in the patient's paper chart, or place in the nursing unit patient label book if EMR is used.	
11. Fill in all the necessary information on the patient's Kardex form or enter it into the computer if Kardex is computerized (if paper charts used).	11. *The information is obtained from the front sheet or face sheet prepared by the admitting department and the admission nurse's notes.*
12. Place the Kardex form in the proper place in the Kardex file (if paper charts used).	
13. Enter appropriate required data into the computer or scan required forms into the patient's EMR if the EMR is used.	13. *A patient profile requires information found on the face sheet screen or face sheet and the nurse's admission notes, such as name, address, nearest of kin, height, weight, etc.*
14. Record the data from the admission nurse's notes on the graphic sheet (if paper charts used).	14. *The admission nurse's notes include data such as vital signs, height, and weight.*
15. Place the allergy information in all the designated areas, or write "NKA" (if paper charts used).	15. *Allergy information (the information obtained from the patient about any sensitivity to medication, food, or other substance) usually is placed on the front of the patient's chart, Kardex form, and medication record. The allergy information is obtained from the admission nurse's notes. Writing "NKA" indicates to the staff that the allergy information has been checked.*
16. Prepare an allergy bracelet with allergies written on it to be placed on the patient's wrist if necessary.	
17. Note code status on front of chart if necessary (if paper charts used).	
18. Place a label or a piece of red tape stating "name alert" on the spine of the chart if there is a patient on the unit with the same or a similar name (if paper charts used).	
19. Transcribe the admission orders according to hospital policy (if paper charts used).	

PHYSICIANS' ORDER SHEET

DATE	TIME	SYMBOL	ORDERS
5/13/XX	1400		Full liq diet tonight
			T & X match 2 u PC & hold for surgery
			CBC, Ua & chest x-ray PA & LAT Cl: pre-op
			ECG this pm
			Consent: partial gastrectomy, vagotomy
			& pyloroplasty
			Hibiclens shower this pm
			H & P by surgical resident
			Pre-ops per Dr. A. Sleep
			Start 1000mL% D/W 1 hr prior to surg.
			Dr. G. Astro MD.
5/13/XX	1600		NPO 2400
			Restoril 15 mg hs tonight MR x 1
			Demerol 100 mg
			Vistaril 25 mg } IM @ 0700
			Dr. A. Sleep MD

Figure 19-7 Set of preoperative orders.

before any orders are carried out. All charting rules must be followed when consent forms are prepared. The surgery consent must be written legibly in black ink and written exactly as the doctor wrote it, with the exception of abbreviations. Words cannot be added, deleted, or rearranged, and all abbreviations must be spelled out on the surgery consent. The first and last names of the patient and the doctor also are required.

The anesthesiologist manually or electronically writes orders on the physicians' order sheet before the surgery. These orders specify the time food and fluids are to be discontinued and the preoperative medication to be given to help relieve anxiety and aid in the induction of anesthesia.

Preoperative Order Components

Orders related directly to the surgery have certain common components.

Surgeons' Orders:

* *Name of surgery for surgery consent.* The consent must be signed before the patient receives any "mind-clouding" drugs. In the case of surgery that may result in sterility or in loss of a limb (amputation), two permits may be required.
* *Enemas.* The order for an enema depends on the type of surgery. For surgeries within the abdominal cavity, all wastes must be removed from the intestines. This

allows the surgeon more room for exploration and a clear field of vision, and it decreases the danger of contamination and infection.

* *Shaves, scrubs, or showers.* The site of the surgical incision must be prepared. This order requires the removal of body hair by shaving. The procedure is referred to as a *surgical prep.* The surgeon also may require a special scrub at the surgical site. In some facilities, the operating room staff members may do shaves and scrubs. Often, the doctor writes an order for the patient to take a shower before surgery using an antibacterial soap such as Hibiclens.
* *Name of anesthesiologist or anesthesiology group.* It is necessary to know the anesthesiologist's name or specific anesthesiology group in the event that preoperative medication orders are not received. The HUC then may call the anesthesiologist, group, or person responsible for writing the **preoperative orders.** (In hospitals where nurse anesthetists administer the anesthesia, the surgeon may write the preoperative anesthesia orders.)
* *Miscellaneous orders.* Other orders may include Ted hose, additional diagnostic studies, blood components to be given during surgery, or intravenous preparations to be started before surgery. Treatments and additional medications also may be ordered.

Anesthesiologists' Orders:

- *Diet.* When surgery is to be performed during the morning hours, the patient is usually NPO at midnight. For a patient who is having late-afternoon surgery, an order may be written for a clear liquid breakfast at 0600 and then NPO. Food and/or fluids by mouth are not allowed for 6 to 8 hours before surgery in which an anesthetic is used that renders the patient unconscious. The NPO rule is maintained to lessen the possibility that the patient may aspirate vomitus while under anesthesia.

- *Preoperative medications.* The anesthesiologist or the surgeon usually writes an order for preoperative medication for the patient who is scheduled for surgery. The preoperative medication order may include a hypnotic to ensure that the patient rests well the night before surgery and an intramuscular injection to be given approximately 1 hour before surgery to relax the patient. Figure 19-7 is an example of preoperative orders. Health unit coordinator tasks performed during the preoperative procedure are listed in Procedure 19-2.

SKILLS CHALLENGE

To practice transcribing a set of preoperative orders, complete Activity 19-3 in the *Skills Practice Manual.*

The Surgery Patient's Chart

The surgical patient's nurse usually designs a **pre-care and post-care plan** that integrates the nurse's knowledge, previous experience, and established standards of care. The plan usually includes preoperative teaching, goals, and outcomes. The plan is reviewed and modified during the **intraoperative** and postoperative periods. Outcomes established for each goal of care provide measurable evidence of the patient's progress. When the patient is involved in the development of the surgical care plan, surgical risks and postoperative complications are reduced.

It is the overall responsibility of the HUC to see that the surgery paper chart is properly prepared to send to surgery with the patient. The registered nurse (RN) completes a pre-op checklist; however, the HUC is involved in preparing the patient's paper chart. It is often hospital policy that surgery cannot begin if any of the required reports are missing. Therefore, the most important task is to have the following records on the chart:

- Current history and physical record (H&P): Essential in most health care facilities.

- Surgery consent: Before surgery is performed, an informed consent must be obtained that is accurate, includes patient's and surgeon's full names, is signed by the patient or legal guardian and dated, and includes a witness signature and date and time (see Chapter 8).

- Blood consent: A consent form must be signed to accept (see Chapter 8) or refuse (see Chapter 8) blood products.

- Admission service agreement (also called *conditions of admission*): Check to see whether this has been signed upon admission.

- Nursing preoperative checklist: Should be checked and signed by nursing personnel

- MAR: Current medication administration record should be placed in chart before transport to surgery.

- Diagnostic test results: Preoperative tests, including laboratory, diagnostic imaging, and so forth, that were ordered by the doctor

To ensure that each patient's paper chart is ready to be taken to surgery, an HUC may choose to create a preoperative checklist (Fig. 19-8). This checklist should not be confused with the nursing preoperative checklist (Fig. 19-9), which is checked and signed by the patient's nurse to ensure proper patient preparation for surgery. The nursing preoperative checklist is a legal chart form in most facilities.

✎ *TAKE NOTE*

After printing a surgery schedule from the computer or receiving a surgery schedule, the HUC highlights the patients going to surgery from that particular nursing unit.

Each nursing unit may print a surgery schedule from the computer or may receive a printed surgery schedule (Fig. 19-10) that lists all surgeries to be performed on the following day.

See Procedure 19-2 for HUC tasks required to prepare the patient's paper chart for surgery. Someone from surgery will call the nursing unit to determine whether the patient is ready to be picked up. After the HUC is given the okay from the patient's nurse and relays the message that the patient is ready, transportation is sent to pick up the patient. The patient's paper chart is sent to surgery with transport when the patient is taken to surgery. Examples of **perioperative** nurses' records may be found on the Evolve website.

Surgical Patients	3-C							
Rm#	Patient	Surg Time	Service Adm Agreement	H & P	5 Sheets Pt ID Labels	5 Face Sheets	Surgical Consent	Dx Reports
305	Pack, Fanny	0730	X	X	X	X	X	X
311	Juniper, Jack	0800	X	X	X	X	X	X
312	Harris, Susan	1100	X	X	X	X	X	X

Figure 19-8 A preoperative checklist for the health unit coordinator.

PREOPERATIVE CHECK LIST   DATE

NURSING UNIT CHECK LIST	YES	NO
1. Pre-op bath/Oral hygiene given	✓	
2. Make-up/Nail polish removed	✓	
3. Bobby Pins, Combs, Hair Pieces Removed Disposition:	✓	
4. Sanitary Belt removed	—	
5. Jewelry, Rings, Religious Medals, or other items removed (May be worn during cardiac catheterization) when removed disposition is:	✓	
6. Voided/Retention catheter	✓	
7. Preoperative medicine given as ordered	✓	
8. Addressograph with chart	✓	
9. Pre-anesthetic patient questionnaire completed	✓	

10. Where family can be located during and immediately after surgery   *Surgery Waiting room*

NURSING UNIT AND OPERATING ROOM NURSES CHECK LIST	UNIT NURSE		O.R. NURSE	
	YES	NO	YES	NO
11. Surgical consent for: Rt. (Lt.) *Inguinal hernieorrhaphy*	✓			
as obtained from Doctor's Order sheet	✓			
12. Special Consents Consultation				
13. History and Physical Dictated On Chart	✓			
14. Allergies Noted	✓			
15. Hematology	✓			
16. Urinalysis	✓			
17. Surgical/Cardiac cath prep done	✓			
18. Type and Cross Match / Units *P.C.*	✓			
19. Culture site: Results:				
20. Admission Chest X-Ray Report	✓			
21. EKG Report if over 40 years	✓			

22. Prosthetic Teeth May be worn during cardiac catheterization	REMOVED			
	YES	NO	YES	NO
Permanent cap or caps				
Permanent bridge				
Removable bridge				
Removable plate or plates				
Loose teeth				
23. Prosthesis and Disposition:				
Artificial eye in out				
Contact lens in out				
Pacemaker				
Other				

none

none

R.N. Signature

00-6015 Rev. 12-79

O.R. Nurse Signature

PATIENT IDENTIFICATION ON UNIT

A. Person from surgery calling for patient

1. Ask for patient by name

2. Check patient's chart

3. Check patient's chart with call slip (not necessary with cardiac catheterization)

B. Person from unit must accompany

1. Ask patient his/her name
   Ask patient his/her doctor's name

2. Check chart face sheet for patient's name and hospital number with patient identiband

3. Check call slip with identiband (not necessary for cardiac catheterization)

Winifred Marshall, R.N.
Signature Nursing Unit Personnel

Bill Standard, Ord.
Signature Surgery Personnel

SPECIAL COMMENTS TO OPERATING ROOM AND RECOVERY ROOM NURSES FROM NURSING UNIT: (PLEASE SIGN YOUR COMMENT)

B.P.:H.S. *130/76* a Pre-op *140/82* p Pre-op *136/80*

Pre-op TPR ____ NPO p *Mn.* WT. *136*

Pertinent Drug Therapy:

Demerol 75 mg } *I.M.*
Atropine 0.4 mg } *8:30 am*

PREOPERATIVE CHECK LIST

Figure 19-9 Nurse's preoperative checklist.

Postoperative Orders and Routine

Immediately after surgery, most patients spend 1 or more hours in the recovery room or the PACU. A record of patient progress is kept on the recovery room record. This record, along with other surgery records, is included in the patient's chart. **Postoperative orders** (written by the surgeon to be carried out immediately after surgery) often are initiated here. For example, the recovery room staff may carry out the doctors' order for antiembolism elastic hose (or stockings) to be placed on the patient's legs. Recovery room personnel will indicate on the physicians' order sheet those orders that have already been executed (note order No. 7 on Fig. 19-11).

Postoperative Order Components

Postoperative orders that relate to the patient's treatment after surgery usually contain the following components:

- **Diet:** The patient may remain NPO or may be given sips of water or ice chips ("sips and chips"). The diet then is increased as tolerated.

SURGERY SCHEDULE FRIDAY JUNE 10, 0000

Time	Surgeon	Procedure	Patient's Bed Number
Operating Room 1			
0730	Dr. Singsong	Anterior Colporrhaphy; left Bartholin's cystectomy	412A
0930	Dr. Prossert	Dilatation & curettage; FS, possible vag. hysterectomy, bil. salpingo-oophorectomy	321
1130	Dr. Broad	Laparoscopy	621B
1330	Dr. Street	Rt. breast biopsy, FS, Poss. rt. radical mastectomy	416
Operating Room 2			
0730	Dr. Patellar	Arthrotomy lt. knee, open reduction, internal fixation with plateau medial meniscectomy	502B
0930	Dr. Home	Arthroplasty rt. elbow, insertion of prosthesis; reconstruction rheumatoid rt. hand	511
1330	Dr. Bowl	Bone graft lt. radius	516A
Operating Room 3			
0730	Dr. Branch	Cystoscopy, TURP	212
0930	Dr. Signe	Cystoscopy, manipulation ureteral stone	222A
1130	Dr. Blake	Circumcision	316B
Operating Room 4			
0730	Dr. Throat	Tonsillectomy	304A
0930	Dr. Ober	Hemorrhoidectomy	601
Operating Room 5			
0730	Dr. Love	Cholecystectomy, biopsy rib cage	617B
0930	Dr. Solano	Repair of lt. inguinal hernia	600

Figure 19-10 Surgery schedule.

TAKE NOTE

Recovery room personnel (or an HUC working in surgery) will call the surgery waiting room (where patients' families are waiting) and the nursing unit to advise of the patient's arrival in the PACU, and they will call again when the patient is ready to return to their room.

It is important to notify the patient's nurse of the patient's arrival in the PACU and of the time when the patent is to return to the nursing unit.

- **Intake and output:** The patient's intake and output is closely watched for 24 to 48 hours (see Chapter 10).
- **Intravenous fluids:** For most surgery patients, at least one bag of intravenous fluids is ordered after surgery. A record of the intake of intravenous fluids is maintained on a parenteral fluid sheet (see Chapter 8).
- **Vital signs:** The patient's vital signs are monitored carefully after surgery—usually every 4 hours for 24 to 48 hours.
- **Catheters, tubes, and drains:** Postoperative patients may have a retention or indwelling urinary catheter. Other orders may pertain to intermittent catheterization of the patient, as necessary. Some patients may require suctioning when nasogastric or other tubes are in place.
- **Activity:** Activity after surgery may consist of only bedrest, and this may be increased as the patient continues to recuperate.

- **Positioning:** Some surgeons require that the patient's position be changed frequently. Elevation of the bed also may be very important.
- **Observation of the operative site:** It is imperative that the sites of the operation or the bandages be observed closely for bleeding, excessive drainage, redness, and swelling.
- **Medications:** Medications to relieve pain (narcotics) and nausea and vomiting (antiemetics) and to help the patient sleep or rest (hypnotics) may be prescribed for a period after surgery. Other medications are ordered as needed. (Figure 19-11 provides an example of postoperative orders.)

Postoperative orders cancel all previous orders. See Procedure 19-3, Postoperative Procedure, for HUC tasks that are involved in postoperative procedures.

SKILLS CHALLENGE

To practice transcribing a set of preoperative orders, complete Activity 19-4 in the *Skills Practice Manual*.

KEY CONCEPTS

For most patients, admission to the hospital can be a stressful experience. The HUC can do much in the field of public relations for the hospital at this time. The HUC is usually the first person on the nursing unit with whom the new patient has contact. A warm welcome and a pleasant smile may help to relieve anxiety. The expediency with which the patient's paper chart is prepared and the new

PHYSICIANS' ORDER SHEET

DATE	TIME	SYMBOL	ORDERS
6/7/03			Post op
			NPO
			NG tube to Low Suction
			Follow present IV c̄ 5% D/LR @ 125cc/h
			Demerol 75 mg IM q 4 h prn pain
			Compazine 10 mg IM q 4 h prn N/V
			Encourage to TCDB
			Knee length elastic hose ✓done / RR @1050
			May dangle this evening
			Dr. G. Astro

Figure 19-11 Set of postoperative orders.

orders transcribed determines the ability of the health care team to initiate care and treatment sooner. When the EMR is used, it is important to monitor the nursing unit census screen for HUC tasks and to scan documents in a timely manner.

The HUC must be familiar with the common components in an admission, as well as with preoperative and postoperative order sets. As with all orders, quick, accurate, and thorough transcription is a must toward ensuring quality care for the patient.

PROCEDURE 19-2

PREOPERATIVE PROCEDURE

(Tasks may vary between facilities.) When CPOE has been implemented, all tasks related to preparing a paper chart or transcribing orders would not apply.

TASK	NOTES
1. Label the surgery forms with the patient's identification labels and place them within the patient's paper chart (if paper charts used).	1. *The surgery forms include the nurse's preoperative checklist, the operating room record, the anesthesiologist's record, the recovery room record, etc. See the Evolve website for examples of operative records.*
2. Check the patient's chart for the history and physical report (if paper charts used).	2. *If the history and physical report is not found on the chart, call the HIMS to check whether it has been dictated. Notify the patient's nurse and doctor if the report is not located.*

3. Check the patient's paper or electronic chart for the following signed consent forms:
  a. Surgical consent
  b. Blood transfusion consent or refusal form
  c. Admission service agreement
	3. *Check the consent forms for patient and witness signatures and for the correct spelling of the surgical procedure.*

4. Check the patient's paper chart for any previously ordered diagnostic studies such as laboratory tests, X-rays, and so forth. If the EMR is used, check the computer screen for HUC tasks.	4. *If the diagnostic test results are not on the patient's chart, locate the results on the computer, print them, and place in patient's chart. If unable to locate results, notify patient's nurse.*
5. Chart the patient's latest vital signs (if paper charts used).	
6. File the current medication administration record in the patient's chart (if paper charts used).	
7. Print at least five face sheets to place in the paper chart. If the EMR is used, maintain five face sheets in a notebook to provide to consulting doctors and other health care providers as requested.	7. *Face sheets are removed and are used by doctors and other health care providers to bill patients.*
8. Place at least three sheets of patient identification labels in the patient's paper chart. If the EMR is used, maintain three sheets of labels in a notebook to label specimens as necessary.	8. *Patient identification labels are used to label specimens.*
9. Notify the appropriate nursing personnel when surgery calls for the patient.	9. *Usually, surgery personnel will call before transport is sent, to verify that the patient is prepared to be picked up.*

PROCEDURE 19-3

POSTOPERATIVE PROCEDURE

(Tasks may vary between facilities.) When CPOE has been implemented, all tasks related to preparing a paper chart or transcribing orders would not apply.

TASK	NOTES
1. Inform the patient's nurse of the patient's arrival to the PACU as soon as possible.	1. *PACU personnel usually notify the unit when the patient arrives from the operating room. The nurse then may plan and be prepared for the patient's return to the unit.*
2. Inform the patient's nurse of the expected arrival of the patient from the recovery room.	2. *PACU personnel will notify the nursing unit before returning the patient to the room and will give a report of the patient's condition to the appropriate nurse.*
3. Place all operating records behind the proper divider in the patient's chart.	
4. Write the date of surgery and the surgical procedure in the designated places on the patient's Kardex form or in the computer.	
5. Write in the date of the surgery on the patient's graphic sheet.	
6. Transcribe the doctors' postoperative orders. Notify the nurse who is caring for the patient of stat doctors' orders.	6. *All preoperative orders are automatically discontinued postoperatively. The HUC usually starts a new Kardex form for the patient.*

REVIEW QUESTIONS

1. Place the letter of the correct answer in the second column in the space provided in the first column.

1. admission orders	a. admission necessitated by an accident or a medical emergency
2. admission service agreement	b. entry into hospital planned in advance
3. emergency admission	c. directions for care and treatment written by the doctor on patient's entry into hospital
4. scheduled admission	d. contains general services the hospital will provide
5. direct admission	e. a patient who was not scheduled to be admitted and is admitted from the doctor's office, clinic, or emergency room

2. Define the following:

a. patient health information management number

_____

b. patient identification bracelet

_____

c. preoperative nursing checklist

_____

d. surgery schedule

_____

e. patient account number

_____

f. valuables envelope

_____

g. preoperative orders

_____

h. postoperative orders

_____

i. allergy information

_____

j. face sheet or front sheet

_____

k. preoperative HUC checklist

_____

l. elective surgery

_____

m. allergy identification bracelet

_____

n. pre-admit

_____

o. registration

_____

3. List at least six common components of a set of admission orders.

a. _____

b. _____

c. _____

d. _____

e. _____

f. _____

4. Three items prepared by the registration staff that are sent to the unit as part of the admission procedure are:

a. _____

b. _____

c. _____

5. List 19 HUC tasks that are related to the patient's admission when paper charts are used.

a. _____

b. _____

c. _____

d. _____

e. _____

f. _____

g. _____

h. _____

i. _____

j. _____

k. _____

l. _____

m. _____

n. _____

o. _____

p. _____

q. _____

r. _____

s. _____

6. List nine HUC responsibilities that are related to the preoperative patient's paper chart.

a. _____

b. _____

c. _____

d. _____

e. _____

f. _____

g. _____

h. _____

i. _____

7. Five records or reports that might be included in the patient's paper or electronic chart before surgery are:

a. _____

b. _____

c. _____

d. _____

e. _____

8. List seven components that may be included as part of preoperative orders.

a. _____

b. _____

c. _____

d. _____

e. _____

f. _____

g. _____

9. List nine components that may constitute part of a set of postoperative orders.

a. _____

b. _____

c. _____

d. _____

e. _____

f. _____

g. _____

h. _____

i. _____

10. List six tasks that the HUC may perform to assist with the postoperative patient's paper chart and Kardex.

a. _____

b. _____

c. _____

d. _____

e. _____

f. _____

11. Define *advance directives*.

_____

_____

12. List at least eight patient registration tasks.

a. _____

b. _____

c. _____

d. _____

e. _____

f. _____

g. _____

h. _____

13. What is the difference between a living will and power of attorney for health care?

_____

_____

14. When does an advance directive become effective?

_____

15. Explain why it is important for the HUC to monitor the patient's census screen consistently for HUC tasks when the EMR c̄ (with) CPOE is implemented.

_____

_____

16. Explain what the HUC's responsibility would be regarding the patient's signed consent forms, handwritten progress notes, and reports from other facilities faxed to the nursing station when the EMR c̄ (with) CPOE is implemented.

_____

_____

THINK ABOUT...

1. Discuss the consequences of a surgery that is canceled because it is discovered that the surgical consent form is not accurate, or that the condition of admission form was not signed before the patient was sedated.
2. Discuss how the first person encountered in a health care facility or doctor's office may influence a patient's overall opinion of that facility.
3. Discuss the importance of relating to the patient's nurse in a timely manner that a patient is ready to return to the room from the PACU.

CHAPTER 20

Discharge, Transfer, and Postmortem Procedures

CHAPTER OBJECTIVES

Upon completion of this chapter, you will be able to:

1. Define the terms in the vocabulary list.
2. Write the meaning of each abbreviation in the Abbreviations list.
3. List 14 tasks that may be required to complete a routine discharge. (Tasks involving paper chart forms, the temperature, pulse, and respirations [TPR] sheet, and the diet sheet would not be necessary when the electronic medical record [EMR] $\bar{c}$ computer physician order entry [CPOE] is used.)
4. Describe health unit coordinator (HUC) tasks that may be added to the routine discharge procedure when the EMR with CPOE is used.
5. List six additional tasks that may be required when a patient is discharged to a nursing home. (Tasks involving paper chart forms, the TPR sheet, and the diet sheet would not be necessary when the EMR $\bar{c}$ CPOE is used.)
6. Describe the tasks necessary to prepare the discharged patient's paper chart for the health information management department.
7. Explain what the HUC should do if a patient approaches the nursing station desk and states, "I am unhappy with the care I am receiving, and I am going home now."

8. List nine tasks performed by the health unit coordinator upon the death of a patient. (Tasks involving paper chart forms, the TPR sheet, and the diet sheet would not be necessary when the EMR $\bar{c}$ CPOE is used.)
9. List 14 tasks that are performed in the transfer of a patient from one unit to another. (Tasks involving paper chart forms, the TPR sheet, and the diet sheet would not be necessary when the EMR $\bar{c}$ CPOE is used.)
10. List eight tasks performed by the health unit coordinator in the transfer of a patient from one room to another room on the same unit. (Tasks involving paper chart forms, the TPR sheet, and the diet sheet would not be necessary when the EMR $\bar{c}$ CPOE is used.)
11. List nine tasks that are performed by the health unit coordinator when a transferred patient is received on the unit. (Tasks involving paper chart forms, the TPR sheet, and the diet sheet would not be necessary when the EMR $\bar{c}$ CPOE is used.)

VOCABULARY

Autopsy Examination of a body after death; it may be performed to determine the cause of death or for medical research purposes

Census Sheet A daily listing of all patient activity (admissions, discharges, transfers, and deaths) within the hospital; may also be referred to as the admissions, discharges, and transfers sheet (ADT)

Clinical Death Occurs when no brain function is present

Coroner's Case A death that occurs because of sudden, violent, or unexplained circumstances, or a patient who expires unexpectedly within the first 24 hours after admission to the hospital

Custodial Care Care and services of a nonmedical nature, which consist of feeding, bathing, watching, and protecting the patient

Discharge Planning Centralized, coordinated, multidisciplinary process that ensures that the patient has a plan for continuing care after leaving the hospital

Expiration A death

Extended Care Facility A medical facility for patients who require expert nursing care or custodial care; may also be referred to as a skilled nursing facility

Organ Donation Donating or giving one's organs and/ or tissues after death; one may designate specific organs (e.g., only cornea) or may donate any needed organs

Organ Procurement The process of removing donated organs; may also be referred to as harvesting

Patient Care Conference A meeting that includes the doctor or doctors caring for the patient, the primary nurses, the case manager or social worker, and other caregivers involved in the patient's care

Postmortem After death (a postmortem examination is the same as an autopsy)

Release of Remains A signed consent that authorizes a specific funeral home or agency to remove the deceased from a health care facility

Terminal Illness An illness ending in death

ABBREVIATIONS

Abbreviation	Meaning	Example of Usage on a Doctor's Order Sheet
AMA	against medical advice	Patient D/C AMA
ECF or SNF	extended care facility	Please have case mgt arrange for transfer to ECF
	skilled nursing facility	Arrange for ambulance transport to SNF (discussed in Chapter 2)

EXERCISE 1

Write the abbreviation for each term listed below.

1. against medical advice   _____

2. extended care facility   _____

EXERCISE 2

Write the meaning of each abbreviation listed below.

1. AMA

    _____

2. ECF

    _____

> ✎ *TAKE NOTE*
>
> Procedures for discharge, transfer, and postmortem processes when paper charts are used differ from the procedures used when the electronic medical record (EMR) with computer physician order entry (CPOE) is used only in that the health unit coordinator (HUC) does not have the responsibility of transcribing the doctor's orders or the paper forms. Health unit coordinator tasks may be added to the discharge procedure when the EMR c̄ CPOE is used; these are discussed in this chapter.

DISCHARGE PLANNING

Discharge planning is a centralized, coordinated, multidisciplinary process that ensures that the patient has a plan for continuing care after leaving the hospital. Discharge planning begins the moment a patient is admitted to the hospital and usually is handled by case managers or social workers who assist patients and their families with arrangements for post-hospitalization care. The case manager or social worker assists patients and their families and physicians in developing a discharge plan of care that is tailored to meet the specific needs of the patient. Once the plan has been developed, the case manager secures the necessary post-hospitalization services and can provide information about additional community resources when necessary.

A **patient care conference** is a meeting that includes the doctor or doctors caring for the patient, the primary nurses, the case manager or social worker, and other caregivers involved in the patient's care. The purpose of the conference is to review and evaluate the goals and outcomes of the patient's recovery progress and to modify the care plan as needed. Often a patient care conference is scheduled before the time of a patient's discharge so that a post-hospitalization care plan can be developed. The HUC should be made aware when the patient's chart is taken into the conference room.

DISCHARGE OF A PATIENT

Once a patient has received a written discharge order from the doctor, the prompt attention of the HUC is required. Most patients prefer to leave the hospital as soon as possible after the discharge order is written, and often, patients are waiting to be admitted. Environmental Services (or housekeeping) must prepare the vacated room and bed for the admission of a new patient. There are five types of discharges:

1. Discharge home
2. Discharge to another facility
3. Discharge home with assistance
4. Discharge against medical advice (AMA)
5. Expiration

All discharges require a doctor's order. When a patient insists on leaving AMA, the doctor usually writes a discharge order that documents that the patient is leaving AMA.

✐ TAKE NOTE

It is important to read a discharge order carefully before a patient leaves the unit. The doctor may write "discharge after chest x-ray" or other directions and/or may leave a prescription on the chart that must be given to the patient.

Routine Discharge Procedure

Most discharges from the hospital are routine in nature, that is, the patient is discharged alive to go home in the company of a family member, a friend, or alone. See Procedure 20-1 and Figures 20-1 through 20-4.

Discharge to Another Facility

Insurance reviewers are employed by insurance companies to review hospitalized patients' charts to advise doctors regarding what the insurance will cover and how many hospital days will be covered. When paper charts are used, the HUC should always ask the insurance reviewer to show identification (required) before allowing any access to look at a patient's chart. When the patient no longer needs expert nursing care but still requires custodial care, the doctor is requested to transfer the patient from the hospital to an assisted living facility or nursing care home. **Custodial care** is care of a nonmedical nature, such as feeding, bathing, watching, and protecting the patient. The insurance reviewer places a sticker on the cover of the patient's chart binder to indicate

---

PROCEDURE 20-1

ROUTINE DISCHARGE PROCEDURE

TASK	NOTES
1. Read the entire order when transcribing the discharge order.	1. *The order may be written on the doctor's order sheet the day before or the day of the expected discharge. Read the order carefully. Sometimes the doctor will write disch c̄ chest x-ray or other diagnostic test. Check for any Rx that may have been left on the chart by the doctor.*
2. Notify the discharged patient's nurse.	2. *The patient's nurse will provide the patient with discharge instructions. When the EMR c̄ CPOE is implemented, the HUC may print the discharge instructions from the computer for the patient. The HUC also may print out the medication information sheets for medications that the patient will be taking after discharge (Fig. 20-1 A, B).*
3. Enter a "pending discharge" with the expected departure time into the computer.	3. *Notification may be made by telephone or by computer. Entering a "pending discharge" with expected departure time notifies the business department to prepare the patient's bill. Some patients may be required to stop at the business office before leaving the hospital. The "pending discharge" notification also alerts the admitting department that a patient who is waiting to be admitted may be placed into a room slot. Holding notification of a discharge could delay another patient's admission and the start of treatment.*
4. Explain the procedure for discharge to the patient and/or the patient's relatives.	4. *Explanation of the discharge procedure may also be given by the nurse; however, many patients come to the nurse's station and ask the HUC for the explanation.*
5. Notify other departments that may be giving the patient daily treatments.	5. *Departments such as physical therapy and cardiopulmonary (respiratory care) may have to be notified. Communication may be made by telephone or by computer.*
6. Communicate the patient's discharge to the nutritional care department by computer.	6. *If the patient is not planning to leave the hospital during regular discharge hours (usually before lunch), type in the expected departure time.*
7. Arrange for any appointments requested by the doctor.	7. *Write out the appointment date and time on a piece of paper and give it to the patient's nurse. The appointment date and time may then be written on or typed into the discharge instruction sheet.*

PROCEDURE 20-1—Cont'd

ROUTINE DISCHARGE PROCEDURE

TASK	NOTES
8. Arrange transportation if needed.	8. *Patients who do not have family or friends available to provide transportation may have to have a call made for a taxi. Many hospitals provide taxi vouchers for patients.*
9. Prepare credit slips for medications returned to the pharmacy or equipment and supplies returned to the central services department (CSD).	9. *Supplies specifically ordered for the patient from CSD, but not used by the patient, must be returned to CSD with a credit slip (see Fig. 20-2).*
10. Notify nursing personnel or transportation service to transport that patient to the discharge area when the patient is ready to leave.	10. *Patients should never be allowed to go to the discharge area without an escort from the hospital staff. Also, the patient should be transported via wheelchair.*
11. Write the patient's name on the admission, discharge, and transfer sheet.	11. *An example of an admission, discharge, and transfer sheet is shown in Figure 20-3.*
12. Delete the patient's name from the unit census board and TPR sheet.	12. *Draw a line through the patient's name on the TPR sheet and erase the name from the census board. (Applicable when paper charts are used)*
13. Notify environmental services to clean the discharged patient's room.	13. *Notification may be made by telephone, by computer, or by informing environmental services personnel on the unit.*
14. Prepare the patient's paper chart for the health information management department (HIMS).	14. *Many hospitals issue a discharge checklist (see Fig. 20-4) to prepare the chart for HIMS. (Applicable when paper charts are used)*
a. Check the summary/DRG worksheet for the doctor's summation and the patient's final diagnosis. It is important to have this information upon patient discharge so that coding of diagnosis-related groups may be placed on the chart by HIMS personnel.	*(Applicable when paper charts are used)*
b. Check for the correct patient identification labels on chart forms.	*(Applicable when paper charts are used)*
c. Shred all chart forms that have been labeled and have no documentation on them.	*(Applicable when paper charts are used)*
d. Check for old records or split records and send with the chart to HIMS.	
e. Arrange chart forms in discharge sequence according to hospital policy.	
f. Send the chart of the discharged patient to HIMS, along with any old records of the patient. Paper charts of discharged patients must be sent to HIMS on the day of discharge.	*After the patient's paper chart has been sent to HIMS, nurses, doctors, residents, and other health care providers will have to go to there to complete charting or sign forms, if necessary.*

how many more days will be covered by the patient's insurance. If the doctor believes that the patient needs additional hospitalization, the reasons for the additional days will have to be documented.

Other patients may be discharged to an assisted living facility, a nursing care home, or an **extended care facility**/skilled nursing facility (ECF/SNF). Frequently, the hospital case manager or social service worker makes the arrangements for long-term care. The discharge of a patient to another facility is the same as a routine discharge but with additional steps Fig. 20-5 (Procedure 20-2).

Many patients require care or assistance provided at home as part of their recovery process. Additional steps are required when a patient needs home health care. The hospital case manager or social service worker arranges home health care and home health equipment. See Procedure 20-3.

✎ **TAKE NOTE**

A patient may be restrained from leaving the hospital if two doctors certify that the patient poses a threat to self or others.

DISCHARGE AGAINST MEDICAL ADVICE

A patient may feel that the care being provided is not acceptable, or perhaps the patient believes that the care provided has not resulted in an improvement in their condition. Whatever the reason, the patient may decide to leave the hospital without the doctor's approval.

The patient may appear at the nurse's station and may announce, "I am not happy with the care I am receiving, and I'm

DISCHARGE INSTRUCTIONS

DIAGNOSIS: _____

_____

SURGERY/PROCEDURE: _____

1. **ACTIVITY**	NO LIMIT	LIMIT
Bathing		
Driving		
Sexual		
Work		
Exercise		
Ambulation		

2. **MEDICATION:**

____ Patient/family knows what medications are for.

____ Prescriptions sent with patient or family.

NAME OF MEDICATION	**DOSAGE**	**FREQUENCY/TIMES**

3. **DIET:**

Your diet will be _____

Please call dietition at _____ if you have any questions.

4. **SPECIAL INFORMATION:** (include wound care, further treatments, referrals, equipment, etc.)

5. **RETURN VISIT TO PHYSICIAN:** Please call Dr. _____ Phone: _____

to make an appointment in _____ days. Please call the doctor if you cannot take your medicine

or to answer any questions.

6. **INSTRUCTION SHEETS GIVEN:** (Please list pamphlets, written instructions or other standardized information.)

The above was discussed with me and
I understand all of the information.

_____
Signature of R.N.

_____
Date

_____
Signature of Patient/Guardian

Patient (original)   Medical Records (yellow)   Other (pink)   DISCHARGE INSTRUCTIONS

Figure 20-1 A, Discharge instruction sheet. (From Rockford Memorial Hospital, Rockford, Illinois.)

Opportunity Medical Center - Pharmacy

DRUG: Zithromax 250 mg Tabs (Z- PAK)
INGREDIENT NAME: Azithromycin (az-ith-rie-MYE-sin)

COMMON USES: This medicine is a macrolide antibiotic used to treat bacterial infections.

BEFORE USING THIS MEDICINE: Some medicines or medical conditions may interact with this medicine. INFORM YOUR DOCTOR OR PHARMACIST of all prescriptions and over-the-counter medicine that you are taking. DO NOT TAKE THIS MEDICINE if you are also taking propafenone or pimozide. ADDITIONAL MONITORING OF YOUR DOSE OR CONDITION may be needed if you are taking anticoagulants (such as warfarin), digoxin, nelfinavir, cyclosporine, ergotamine, hexobarbital, phenytoin, rifampin, theophylline, triazolam, certain drugs for high cholesterol (such as lovastatin), medicines for irregular heartbeat (such as amiodarone, disopyramide, quinidine, or procainamide), or medicines that may affect your heartbeat. Ask your doctor if you are unsure if any of the medicines you are takingmay affect your heartbeat. Inform your doctor of any other kidney problems, liver problems, allergies, pregnancy, or breastfeeding. Contact your doctor or pharmacist if you have any questions or concerns about taking this medicine.

HOW TO USE THIS MEDICINE: Follow the directions for using this medicine provided by your doctor. This medicine may be taken on an empty stomach or with food. DO NOT TAKE THIS MEDICINE within 1 hour before or 2 hours after aluminium- or magnesium–containing antacids. STORE THIS MEDICINE at room temperature, away from heat and light. TO CLEAR UP YOUR INFECTION COMPLETELY, continiue taking this medicine for the full course of treatment even if you feel better in a few days. DO NOT MISS ANY DOSES. Taking this medicine at the same time each day will make it easier to remember. IF YOU MISS A DOSE OF THIS MEDICINE, take it as soon as possible. If it is almost time for your next dose, skip the missed dose and go back to your regular dosing schedule. If you miss a dose, do not take 2 doses at once.

CAUTIONS: DO NOT TAKE THIS MEDICATION if you have had an allergic reaction to it or are allergic to any ingredient in this product. DO NOT TAKE THIS MEDICINE IF YOU HAVE HAD A SEVERE ALLERGIC REACTION to erythromycin or any macrolide or ketolide antibiotic. A severe reaction includes a severe rash, hives, breathing difficulties, or dizziness. If you have a question about whether you are allergic to this medicine, contact your doctor or pharmacist.

IF YOU EXPERIENCE difficulty breathing; tightness of chest; swelling of eyelids, face or lips; or if you develop a rash or hives, tell your doctor immediately. Do not take any more of this medicine unless your doctor tells you to do so. IF MODERATE TO SEVERE DIARRHEA OCCURS during or after treatment with this medicine, check with your doctor or pharmacist. Do not treat it with non-prescription (over-the-counter) medicines. BEFORE YOU BEGIN TAKING ANY NEW MEDICINE, either prescription or over-the-counter, check with your doctor or pharmacist. FOR WOMEN: IF YOU PLAN ON BECOMING PREGNANT, discuss with your doctor the benefits and risks of using this medicine during pregnancy. IT IS UNKNOWN IF THE MEDICINE IS EXCRETED in breast milk. IF YOU ARE OR WILL BE BREAST-FEEDING while you are taking this medicine, check with your doctor or pharmacist to discuss the risks to your baby.

POSSIBLE SIDE EFFECTS: SIDE EFFECTS that may go away during treatment include mild diarrhea, nausea, or stomach pain. If they continue or are bothersome, check with your doctor. CHECK WITH YOUR DOCTOR AS SOON AS POSSIBLE if you experience vomiting, hearing loss, or ringing in the ears. CONTACT YOUR DOCTOR IMMEDIATELY if you experience swelling of your hands, legs, face, lips, eyes, throat, or toungue; difficultly swallowing or breathing; hoarseness; irregular heartbeat; reddened blistered, or swollen skin; or severe diarrhea. An allergic reaction to this medicine is unlikely, but seek immediate medical attention if it occurs. Symptoms of an allergic reaction include rash, itching, swelling, dizziness, or trouble breathing. If you notice other effects listed above, contact your doctor, nurse,or pharmacist.

OVERDOSE: If overdose is suspected, contact your local poison control center or emergency room immediately. Symptoms of overdose may include nausea, vomiting, and diarrahea.

ADDITIONAL INFORMATION: DO NOT SHARE THIS MEDICINE with others for whom it was not prescribed. DO NOT USE THIS MEDICINE for other health conditions. KEEP THIS MEDICINE out of reach of children.

Figure 20-1 Cont'd—B, Perscription information printout.

going home now." The health unit coordinator should ask the patient to be seated until the nurse is advised. The hospitalist, resident, or admitting doctor may be called to speak with the patient. The patient may be advised that insurance may not cover the hospital bill if the patient leaves against medical advice. Everything possible is done to encourage the patient to remain in the hospital until treatment has been completed. However, if the patient does not pose a threat to self or others, the patient cannot be restrained from leaving, and usually, the admitting doctor, resident, or hospitalist will write a discharge order to document that the patient is leaving against medical advice.

In the event that the patient is not convinced to stay, a release form (Fig. 20-6) is prepared. This form is signed by the patient or their representative, and the signing is witnessed by an appropriate member of the hospital staff. The patient is then permitted to leave the hospital, and the discharge procedure is the same as for a routine discharge.

DISCHARGE OF THE DECEASED PATIENT

Patient Deaths

Not all patients who enter the hospital for care and treatment are discharged alive. Some patients who enter the hospital are well advanced in age. Other patients, in any age group, may have a **terminal illness** that results in expected death.

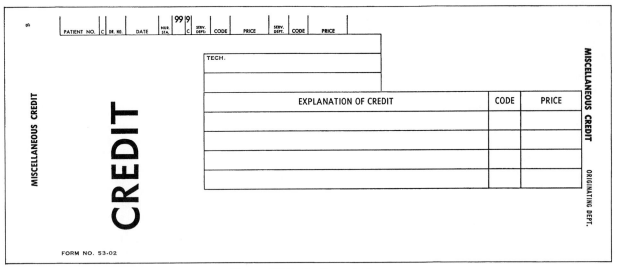

Figure 20-2 Credit requisition.

Admission/Discharge/Transfer Sheet

Nursing Unit _____   Date _____

Admissions   **Discharges**

103   Jackson, Henry   109   Pack, Fanny

110   Smith, Mary   102   Johnson, John

105   Packer, Penny

_____   _____

_____   _____

_____   _____

_____   _____

Transfers

101-1   Jones, Thomas to 303

_____   _____

_____   _____

Figure 20-3 Census sheet or admission, discharge, and transfer sheet.

Occasionally, death is unexpected, as in the case of complications from surgery, traumatic injuries, or sudden onset of a life-threatening condition, such as a heart attack. In other instances, the patient's death is slow, and health care staff members have the opportunity to offer support to family members as time permits.

The HUC may be asked to call a member of the clergy from a specific religion to speak with the patient or to perform final rites. Most facilities have a list of representatives from various denominations and nondenominational groups who can assist patients and families, and many hospitals employ a chaplain to address the religious needs of patients. A notation should be made on the patient's Kardex form of any final rites

that have been performed. It is important to remind clergy that a lighted candle may not be used when oxygen is in use in the patient's room.

Certification of Death

In cases in which a death is expected, the nurse or family members may be with the patient at the time of **expiration** (death). At other times, the patient may die unexpectedly. In either instance, the hospitalist, resident, or doctor must be notified to pronounce the patient dead. The patient is examined for any signs of life. If none can be detected, the patient is pronounced dead and the official time of death is recorded on the doctors'

DISCHARGE CHECKLIST

(To be completed and sent with chart to the Medical Records Department by end of shift on which the patient is discharged. Check Yes or No box.)

Date of Admission ___12/4/XX___

Check List

HISTORY & PHYSICAL

Yes No

☒ ☐ 1. History and Physical on chart within 48 hours. Due ___12/6/XX___
       (IF NO, ANSWER NUMBER TWO.)

☐ ☐ 2. History and Physical Notification Form # 00-0531 sent to Medical Records. Date sent___

Health Unit Coordinator Signature ___Ima Clerke___

Check List

FINAL DISPOSITION OF CHART

Yes No

☐ ☐ 1. All sheets embossed with correct patient master card and legible, and all reports are for this patient.

☐ ☐ 2. Portions of chart that have been removed are replaced in proper order, with chart dividers removed.

☐ ☐ 3. Reports are correctly inserted or attached.

       4. FRONT SHEET:

☐ ☐   a. Discharge diagnosis written on Front Sheet by Doctor. If No, answer 4b.

☐ ☐   b. Final diagnosis noted on Telephone Tentative or Final Discharge Diagnosis Form #00-0523 attached
          to chart and send to Medical Records with check list. If unable to complete, state reason on form.

☐ ☐ 5. Previous Medical Records returned to Medical Record Department.

☐ ☐ 6. Accordion folders used for sending records to Medical Record Department.

☐ ☐ 7. Discharge entered in Unit Transit Book.

Date of Discharge ___

Health Unit Coordinator Signature ___

☐ ☐ 8. Nurses notes are complete.

R.N. or L.P.N. Signature: ___

Figure 20-4 Discharge checklist.

progress notes. The patient's doctor must complete a death certificate, and a report of the death must be filed with the Bureau of Vital Statistics.

Release of Remains

The patient's family or guardian must indicate the funeral home to which the body will be released. Usually, the family must sign a form (see Evolve) before the patient can be released to the funeral home. The nursing staff or the HUC (when requested to do so) may notify the funeral home of the expiration. The HUC may be asked to call hospital morgue personnel to transport the deceased patient to the morgue. Most hospitals have a stretcher with a lower compartment that may be covered with a sheet to transport a deceased patient, making it unnecessary to close the doors to patient rooms on the unit when the patient is being transported to the morgue. Funeral home personnel may pick up the patient from the unit or the hospital morgue. A hospital security officer may have to accompany funeral home personnel.

Organ Donation

Many patients indicate their wishes for **organ donation** before the time of their death. A patient may designate specific organs (e.g., only cornea) or may indicate that any needed organs or

(Use Typewriter or Ballpoint Pen — Press Firmly)   *(See Instructions on back of Page 3)*

CONTINUING CARE TRANSFER INFORMATION

TO BE COMPLETED AND SIGNED BY NURSING SERVICE (Please attach a copy of the Nursing Care Plan)

PATIENT'S NAME   Last   First   MI   DATE OF BIRTH   SEX   RELIGION   HEALTH INSURANCE CLAIM NUMBER

PATIENT'S ADDRESS (Street number, City, State and Zip Code)   ATTENDING PHYSICIAN   Name   Address

RELATIVE OR GUARDIAN   Name   Address   Phone Number

Name and Address of Facility Transferring FROM   Dates of Stay at Facility Transferring FROM   Facility Name and Address Transferring TO
     Admission   Discharge

PAYMENT SOURCE FOR CHARGES TO PATIENT:

☐ Self or Family   ☐ Private Insurance ID Number _____   ☐ Blue Cross/Blue Shield ID Number _____   ☐ Employer or Union

☐ Public Agency _____   ☐ Other (specify) _____

PATIENT EVALUATION:

SPEECH: ☐ Normal ☐ Impaired ☐ Unable to speak   HEARING: ☐ Normal ☐ Impaired ☐ Deaf   SIGHT: ☐ Normal ☐ Impaired ☐ Blind   MENTAL STATUS: ☐ Always Alert ☐ Occasionally Confused ☐ Always Confused   FEEDING: ☐ Independent ☐ Help with Feeding ☐ Cannot Feed Self

DRESSING: ☐ Independent ☐ Help with Dressing ☐ Cannot Dress Self   ELIMINATION: ☐ Independent ☐ Help to Bathroom ☐ Bedpan or Urinal ☐ Incontinent   BATHING: ☐ Independent ☐ Bathing with Help ☐ Bed Bath with Help ☐ Bed Bath   AMBULATORY STATUS: ☐ Independent ☐ Walks with Help ☐ Help from Bed to Chair ☐ Bed Bound

NURSING ASSESSMENT AND RECOMMENDATIONS: TREATMENTS:

Last Medication: _____ /Dose: _____

Date: _____ Time: _____

APPLIANCES OR SUPPORTS: or check none ☐

_____ Signature   Title   Date

TO BE COMPLETED AND SIGNED BY THE ATTENDING PHYSICIAN

ECF Admitting Diagnosis: Please send a copy of the following records with patient:

☐ Summary Sheet (face sheet)
☐ Discharge Summary
☐ Physical Examination and History
☐ Consultation
☐ Other (specify) _____

Patient knows diagnosis: ☐ Yes ☐ No   Transfer by: ☐ Ambulance ☐ Car ☐ Other (specify) _____

Surgical Procedures: (current admission)   Allergies: ☐ No ☐ Yes (specify) _____

VDRL: ☐ Positive ☐ Negative

Anticoagulant: ☐ Taking now ☐ Previously

Orders: Diet, medication and special therapy *(To be renewed in 48 hours)*   Chest X-Ray Diagnosis: _____

I will care for this patient after admission to new facility: ☐ Yes ☐ No

Medication Regimen is stabilized: ☐ Yes ☐ No

Anticipated length of stay for extended care _____ days

_____ Physician's Signature   Date

If necessary, attach order sheet — The above constitutes valid temporary orders only if signed by a physician.   _____ Address   Telephone Number

Figure 20-5 Continuing care transfer form.

tissues may be donated. Because of state laws, the nursing staff may be required to ask the family about organ donation. It will be necessary to check the hospital's policies regarding organ donation. Additional consent forms (see Evolve) are necessary for the harvesting of an organ (**organ procurement**).

AUTOPSY OR POSTMORTEM EXAMINATION

An **autopsy**, or **postmortem** examination, of the body is performed to determine the cause of death or for medical research purposes (see Evolve). The family may ask that an autopsy be done, or the doctor may request it. Before an

PROCEDURE 20-2

ADDITIONAL STEPS REQUIRED TO DISCHARGE PATIENT TO ANOTHER FACILITY

TASK	NOTES
1. Notify case management or social service of the doctor's orders to discharge to another facility.	
2. Transportation usually will be arranged by the case manager or social worker.	2. *The patient who is confined to bed or who has other special medical needs may require an ambulance when requested.*
3. Complete the continuing care form or transfer form.	3. *The continuing care form requires some information that the HUC may obtain from the face sheet. The nurse and the doctor must complete their sections of the form (see Fig. 20-5).*
4. Photocopy or print from the computer patient chart forms as indicated in the doctor's orders.	4. *Requirements for forms vary from facility to facility. The patient's doctor will write an order that indicates the specific forms to be photocopied or printed from the computer. It is also necessary to check hospital policy to determine who is responsible for making photocopies or for printing them from the computer (i.e., the HUC or HIMS). Once the copies have been made, it is important to place the paper originals back into the chart in proper sequence.*
5. Distribute continuing care form and copies as required.	5. *The photocopies and a copy of the continuing care form are placed in a sealed envelope to be given to the ambulance driver or a family member. This person delivers the envelope to the nurse at the nursing care facility.*
6. Now, perform all routine steps as shown in Procedure 20-1.	

PROCEDURE 20-3

ADDITIONAL STEPS FOR DISCHARGE HOME WITH ASSISTANCE

TASK	NOTES
1. Notify case management or social service of the doctor's order.	1. *The responsible personnel will vary depending on patient type.*
2. Prepare the continuing care form.	2. *The HUC will complete the personal information section.*
3. Obtain a release of information signature from the patient.	
4. Photocopy or print forms as indicated in the doctor's order.	
5. Distribute the continuing care form and copies as required.	
6. Now, perform routine discharge steps.	

autopsy can be performed, however, the family must grant permission. A consent for autopsy form must be signed by the next of kin.

Coroner's Cases

A **coroner's case** is one in which the patient's death is due to sudden, violent, or unexplained circumstances, such as an accident, a poisoning, or a gunshot wound. Deaths that occur less than 24 hours after hospitalization is begun may also be called coroner's cases. State, county, and local governments have regulations that define a coroner's case in their particular localities. The law gives the coroner permission to study the body by dissection to determine whether evidence of foul play is present. Signed consent provided by the nearest of kin is not required when a death is ruled a coroner's case. See Procedure 20-4 for tasks related to the death of a patient that may be performed by the HUC.

> ✎ *TAKE NOTE*
>
> Five Types of Discharges
> Home
> To another facility
> Home with assistance
> Against medical advice
> Expiration

TRANSFER OF A PATIENT

A variety of circumstances may necessitate a patient transfer. A patient's condition may change, a patient may improve and may be transferred out of intensive care, a patient's condition may deteriorate and an intensive care unit stay may be required, or the patient may have to move to a specialty unit to receive a particular type of care (e.g., when an orthopedic

LEAVING HOSPITAL AGAINST ADVICE

Date_____

This is to certify that_____,
a patient in The Above Named Hospital, is leaving the hospital against the advice
of the attending physician and the hospital administration. I acknowledge that I
have been informed of the risk involved and hereby release the attending physician,
and the hospital, from all responsibility and any ill effects which may result from
this action.

_____
PATIENT

_____
OTHER PERSON RESPONSIBLE

_____
RELATIONSHIP

Witness_____

Witness_____

00-0434

LEAVING HOSPITAL AGAINST ADVICE

Figure 20-6 Form for discharge against medical advice.

patient develops cardiac problems). A patient may need a private room for infection control or isolation purposes. A patient may be transferred if the room they originally requested becomes available, for example, when the patient wanted a private room that is now available. A patient also may be transferred because of roommate incompatibilities.

The duties performed in a series of tasks allow for an orderly transfer of the patient from one area to another. Transfer may occur from one unit of the hospital to another, or it may occur from one room to another on the same nursing unit. Tasks that may be performed for the transfer of a patient from one hospital unit to another are listed in Procedure 20-5. Tasks to be performed when a patient is transferred from one room to another on the same unit are listed in Procedure 20-6. Tasks to be performed when a transferred patient is received on a nursing unit are listed in Procedure 20-7.

PROCEDURE 20-4

POSTMORTEM PROCEDURE

TASK	NOTES
1. Contact the attending doctor, hospitalist, or resident when asked by the nurse to do so, to verify the patient's death.	
2. Notify the hospital operator of the patient's death.	
3. Prepare any forms that may be needed.	3. *These forms may consist of a release of remains/request for autopsy (see Evolve) and/or consent for donation of body organs (see Evolve). Some hospitals use a postmortem checklist (Fig. 20-7) to ascertain whether all postmortem tasks have been completed.*
4. Notify the mortuary that has been requested by the family.	4. *If the family is not familiar with mortuaries in the area, a list of mortuaries is usually available from the hospital telephone switchboard operator. Nursing office personnel may notify the funeral home.*
5. Check the chart or ask the patient's nurse to determine whether the body is to be taken to the morgue or is to remain there until the mortuary arrives.	5. *Sometimes the family will request that the patient remain in the hospital room so that additional family members can see the deceased patient.*
6. The nurse will gather the clothes of the deceased and will place them in a patient belongings bag to be labeled with the patient's name, the room number, and the date.	6. *The clothing is given to the family or to the mortician. A postmortem checklist is completed by the patient's nurse.*
7. Obtain the mortuary book from the nursing office, or have a mortuary form prepared when the mortician arrives.	7. *The mortician who claims the body must also complete forms to show that he has claimed the body, the clothing, and/or any valuables (Fig. 20-7).*
8. Notify all doctors who were involved with the patient's care.	
9. Now, perform the routine discharge steps shown in Procedure 20-1.	

PROCEDURE 20-5

PROCEDURE FOR TRANSFER FROM ONE UNIT TO ANOTHER

TASK	NOTES
1. Transcribe the order for a transfer.	1. *The transfer order may be handwritten when paper charts are used or may be indicated by an icon on the computer census screen next to the appropriate patient's name when the EMR is used.*
2. Notify the nurse who is caring for the patient of the transfer order.	
3. Notify the admitting department of the transfer order to obtain a new room assignment.	
4. Communicate new unit and room assignment to the nurse who is caring for the patient.	
5. Notify the receiving unit of the transfer by telephone or by computer.	
6. Record the transfer on the unit admission, discharge, and transfer sheet.	
7. Send all thinned records, old records, (if paper charts are used), and x-rays with the patient to the receiving unit.	
8. Send the patient's chart, Kardex form, and current MAR with the patient to the receiving unit (if paper charts are used).	8. *An empty chart will be given by the receiving unit in exchange for the patient's chart (if paper charts are used).*
9. Usually, the nurse may put medications in a bag to send with the paper chart.	
10. Erase the patient's name from the census board.	
11. Notify all departments that perform regularly scheduled treatments on the patient.	
12. Indicate the transfer on the diet sheet or in the computer and on the TPR sheet (if paper charts are used).	
13. Notify environmental services to clean the room.	13. *Environmental services may be notified by telephone, by computer, or in person.*
14. Notify the attending doctor, all other doctors involved with the patient's care, and the information desk of the transfer.	

CHECK LIST
Post-Mortem Care

1) Telephone Notification
   ☐ Family
   ☐ ALL physicians involved in patient care
   ☐ Whether or not an autopsy is to be done
   ☐ Switch Board (name, room number, time, mortuary)
   ☐ Police in event of Coroner's Case (check to see if physician called)
   ☐ Mortuary if known - and if mortician is to come to the unit

2) Forms
   Mortuary Form
     When mortician comes to unit
     ☐ White copy to chart
     ☐ Yellow to mortician
     ☐ Pink to Business office with discharge requisition
     ☐ Patient Information Form remains on the unit
     When patient goes to morgue
     ☐ Entire completed form goes with patient
     ☐ Patient Information Form attached to mortuary form
   Autopsy
     ☐ Single copy remains on chart - send to Medical Records as soon as possible

3) Preparation of Body
   When patient goes to Morgue
     ☐ Shroud and tag properly
     ☐ Mark on the shroud tag if patient is in isolation and causative organism, if known
     ☐ Complete #1 and 2
   If a Coroner's Case
     ☐ Do not remove drains, IV's, etc., until police come. They may take the body with them.
     ☐ Notify mortuary of this
   When patient goes to mortuary from the unit
     ☐ Do not shroud unless isolated
     ☐ Mark on tag causative organism

4) Transport Patient
   ☐ Patient elevator on E Wing 7:00 a.m. to 3:30 p.m., Mon. thru Fri.
   ☐ A, B, and C to 5th floor and cross to elevator #8 to 1st floor of S Building, S-4
   ☐ If body goes to refrigerator, mark 3 x 5 card on door
   ☐ Two people go with patient and their names are charted

5) Chart
   ☐ Complete all of Check List for Medical Records
   ☐ All of items noted in "Telephone Notification"
   ☐ Who takes body to morgue
   ☐ Name of mortuary
   ☐ Follow Discharge Procedure

6) Please refer to Procedure Book for clarification of any and all of the above points, especially in reference to Coroner's Case, fetal death and autopsy.

_____ R.N.
                Signature

00-0585

Figure 20-7 Postmortem checklist.

PROCEDURE 20-6

PROCEDURE TO TRANSFER TO ANOTHER ROOM ON THE SAME UNIT

TASK	NOTES
1. Transcribe the order for the transfer.	1. *The transfer order may be handwritten when paper charts are used or may be indicated by an icon on the computer census screen next to the appropriate patient's name when the EMR is used.*
2. Notify the nurse who is caring for the patient of the request for transfer.	
3. Place the patient's chart in the correct slot in the chart rack after correcting the labels on the patient's chart and replacing patient ID labels with corrected labels (if paper charts are used).	
4. Place the Kardex form in its new place in the Kardex form file (if paper charts are used).	
5. Move the patient's name to the correct bed on the computer census screen. Send the change to the nutritional care department and change the room number on the TPR sheet (if paper charts are used).	
6. Record the transfer on the unit admission, discharge, and transfer sheet.	
7. Notify environmental services to clean the room.	7. *Environmental services may be notified by telephone, by computer, or in person.*
8. Notify the switchboard and the information center of the change.	

PROCEDURE 20-7

PROCEDURE FOR RECEIVING A TRANSFERRED PATIENT

TASK	NOTES
1. Notify the nurse who is caring for the patient of the expected arrival of a transferred patient.	
2. Introduce yourself to the transferred patient upon their arrival to the unit.	
3. Notify the nurse who is caring for the patient of the transferred patient's arrival.	
4. Place the patient's paper chart in the correct slot in the chart holder, print corrected patient ID labels, and label the patient's chart (if paper charts are used).	4. *Provide the empty chart to the unit from which the patient was transferred.*
5. Place the Kardex form in the proper place (if paper charts are used).	
6. Record the receiving of a transfer patient on the unit admission, discharge, and transfer sheet, and write the patient's name on the census board.	
7. Place the patient's name on the TPR sheet (if paper charts are used), and notify the nutritional care department of the patient's transfer.	
8. Move the patient's name from the unit the patient came from and place it in the correct bed on the computer census screen.	
9. Transcribe any new doctors' orders (if paper charts are used).	9. *When the patient is transferred from an intensive care unit to a regular unit, or from a regular unit to an intensive care unit, the doctor must write new orders. The intensive care unit orders are no longer valid.*

KEY CONCEPTS

The HUC's tasks for discharge and transfer procedures are many when the paper chart is used. Some tasks remain the same, and additional tasks may be required when the EMR is used. If the HUC learns these procedures in a particular order and does not deviate from the learned sequence, the tasks will always be performed thoroughly and completely.

REVIEW QUESTIONS

1. List 14 tasks that are performed during a routine discharge of a patient from the hospital. (Tasks involving paper chart forms, the TPR sheet, and the diet sheet would not be necessary when the EMR c̄ CPOE is used.)

   a. _____

   b. _____

   c. _____

   d. _____

   e. _____

   f. _____

   g. _____

   h. _____

   i. _____

   j. _____

   k. _____

   l. _____

   m. _____

   n. _____

2. Describe two HUC tasks that may be added to the routine discharge procedure when the EMR c̄ CPOE is used.

   a. _____

   b. _____

3. What action should the HUC take if a patient approches the nursing station desk and states, "I am very upset with the care I am receiving and I am leaving the hospital now!"

   _____

   _____

4. Describe the HUC tasks involved in the preparation of the discharged patient's paper chart for HIMS.

   _____

5. List six additional tasks that must be performed when a patient is discharged to another facility. (Tasks involving paper chart forms, the TPR sheet, and the diet sheet would not be necessary when the EMR c̄ CPOE is used.)

a. _____

b. _____

c. _____

d. _____

e. _____

f. _____

6. List six additional tasks that must be performed when a patient is discharged home with assistance. (Tasks involving paper chart forms, the TPR sheet, and the diet sheet would not be necessary when the EMR c̄ CPOE is used.)

a. _____

b. _____

c. _____

d. _____

e. _____

f. _____

7. Define the following terms.

a. terminal illness:

_____

b. expiration:

_____

c. postmortem:

_____

d. custodial care:

_____

e. autopsy:

_____

f. organ donation:

_____

g. release of remains:

_____

h. coroner's case:

_____

i. extended care facility:

_____

j. patient care conference:

_____

k. discharge planning:

_____

8. List nine tasks performed upon the death of a patient. (Tasks involving paper chart forms, the TPR sheet, and the diet sheet would not be necessary when the EMR c̄ CPOE is used.)

a. _____

b. _____

c. _____

d. _____

e. _____

f. _____

g. _____

h. _____

i. _____

9. Describe eight duties performed in the transfer of a patient from one room to another room on the same unit. (Tasks involving paper chart forms, the TPR sheet, and the diet sheet would not be necessary when the EMR c̄ CPOE is used.)

a. _____

b. _____

c. _____

d. _____

e. _____

f. _____

g. _____

h. _____

10. List 14 tasks that are performed in the transfer of a patient from one unit to another unit. (Tasks involving paper chart forms, the TPR sheet, and the diet sheet would not be necessary when the EMR c̄ CPOE is used.)

a. _____

b. _____

c. _____

d. _____

e. _____

f. _____

g. _____

h. _____

i. _____

j. _____

k. _____

l. _____

m. _____

n. _____

11. List nine tasks that are performed when a transferred patient is received on the unit. (Tasks involving paper chart forms, the TPR sheet, and the diet sheet would not be necessary when the EMR c̄ CPOE is used.)

a. _____

b. _____

c. _____

d. _____

e. _____

f. _____

g. _____

h. _____

i. _____

THINK ABOUT...

1. Discuss the consequences of not reading the entire doctor's order when one is discharging a patient.
2. Discuss the consequences of not notifying consulting doctors that a patient has expired.
3. Discuss the importance of communicating orders to the case manager or social worker regarding a patient's discharge or transfer.

CHAPTER 21

Recording Vital Signs, Ordering Supplies, Daily Diagnostic Tests, and Filing

CHAPTER OBJECTIVES

Upon completion of this chapter, you will be able to:

1. Define the terms in the vocabulary list.
2. Write the meaning of each abbreviation in the Abbreviations list.
3. Describe the health unit coordinator's responsibilities for recording vital signs and other information on the patient's graphic sheet when paper charts are used.
4. Demonstrate the correct procedure for correcting three types of errors on the graphic sheet when paper charts are used.
5. Convert Fahrenheit scale to Celsius scale, and Celsius scale to Fahrenheit scale.
6. List two reasons for efficient, accurate filing of records on the patient's paper chart or timely scanning of records into the patient's electronic medical record.
7. List five guidelines for filing records on the patient's paper chart.
8. List three guidelines for scanning records into the patient's electronic medical record.

9. Describe the health unit coordinator's responsibilities for ordering daily diagnostic tests when paper charts are used.
10. Explain the process of retrieving diagnostic test results with the computer.
11. Name five hospital departments that may provide supplies to the nursing unit, and list the types of supplies that may be obtained from each department.

VOCABULARY

Bowel Movement The passage of stool from the bowel
Celsius A scale used to measure temperature in which the freezing point of water is 0° and the boiling point is 100° (formerly called Centigrade)
Daily TPRs Taking each patient's temperature, pulse, and respiration at certain times each day
Fahrenheit A scale used to measure temperature in which 32° is the freezing point of water and 212° is the boiling point

Pulse Deficit The difference between the radial pulse and the apical heartbeat

Stool or Feces The body wastes from the digestive tract that are formed in the intestine and expelled through the rectum

ABBREVIATIONS

Abbreviation	Meaning
BM	bowel movement
C	Celsius
F	Fahrenheit
PO day	postoperative day
PP	postpartum
TPR(s)	temperature, pulse, and respiration

EXERCISE 1

Write the abbreviation for each term listed below.

1. temperature, pulse, and respiration   _____

2. postpartum   _____

3. postoperative day   _____

4. Fahrenheit   _____

5. Celsius   _____

6. bowel movement   _____

EXERCISE 2

Write the meaning of each abbreviation listed below.

1. PO day

   _____

2. PP

   _____

3. F

   _____

4. BM

   _____

5. C

   _____

6. TPR

   _____

RECORDING VITAL SIGNS AND OTHER DATA ON THE GRAPHIC RECORD WHEN PAPER CHARTS ARE USED

Chapter 10 includes a discussion of what vital signs are, different methods for obtaining them, and doctors' orders related to them.

Review the terms and abbreviations related to vital signs presented in the vocabulary and abbreviations lists, and the doctors' orders related to vital signs written in the Doctors' Orders for Nursing Observation section (see Chapter 10).

It is hospital routine to take each patient's temperature, pulse, and respiration (TPR) and blood pressure (BP) usually three times each day or according to specific hospital policy, to monitor the patient's condition. This process is often referred to as "routine vital signs." The doctor's written or printed order will indicate the frequency with which the doctor wishes vital signs to be observed, if more often than the routine set forth by the hospital.

"Normal vital signs" vary from one person to another; however, the following values are considered normal: temperature—98.6°F or 37°C; pulse—60 to 80; respiration—16 to 20; and blood pressure—<120/80.

It is hospital routine to record each patient's **bowel movements** along with the daily vital signs. If the doctor has ordered the patient to be weighed daily, this is also done routinely, usually when the morning vital signs are taken. The patient's intake and output is also recorded on the graphic record.

Vital signs are often included in the nursing record, and the nurse or the certified nursing assistant is responsible for recording the patient's vital signs when paper charts are used (Fig. 21-1). In some hospitals, the nursing personnel record patient vital signs on a TPR sheet. It then may be the health unit coordinator's (HUC'S) task to record data from the TPR sheet onto each patient's graphic record form. This process is often referred to as recording vital signs and would only occur when paper charts are used.

The HUC should record vital signs and other data as soon as they are recorded on the TPR sheet, so the information is readily available to doctors when they make rounds to see their patients. *Accuracy in the transfer of vital signs information is a must,* because the doctor may use this information to prescribe treatment for the patient.

Most often, the temperature is taken and recorded using the Fahrenheit scale, but it is sometimes taken and recorded on the Celsius scale, also known as the Centigrade scale. There may be times when the HUC will have to convert the temperature from one scale to another. The conversion formulas in Table 21-1 are used to convert Fahrenheit to Celsius and Celsius to Fahrenheit. With the use of this formula, a temperature of 98.6° Fahrenheit converts to 37.0° on the Celsius scale.

Table 21-1   Celsius–Fahrenheit Conversion

Conversion From Fahrenheit to Celsius	Conversion From Celsius to Fahrenheit
Subtract 32	Multiply by 9
Multiply by 5	Divide by 5
Divide by 9	Add 32

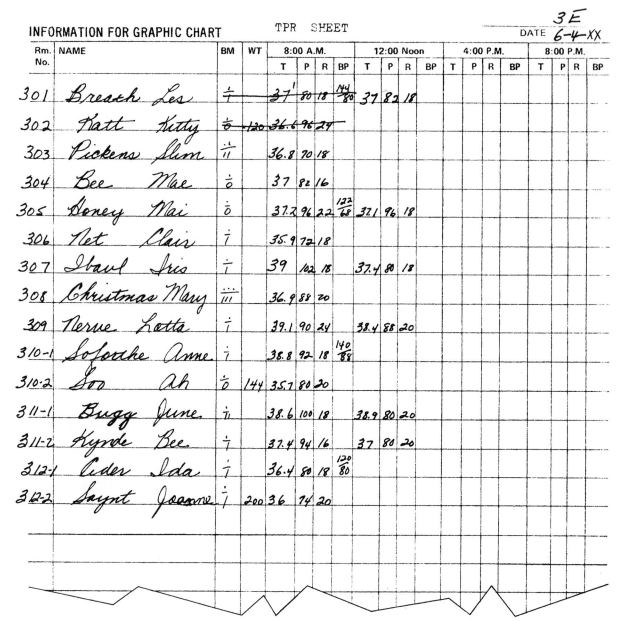

Figure 21-1 A temperature, pulse, and respiration (TPR) sheet with 8:00 A.M. and 12:00 P.M. data recorded on it. The straight line drawn through the values indicates that the information has been recorded (Celsius temperature scale).

✎ TAKE NOTE

Accuracy in the transfer of vital signs information is a must, because the doctor may use this information to prescribe treatment for the patient.

Method for Correcting Errors on the Graphic Record in Paper Charts

Minor graphic errors may be corrected on the original graphic record. However, correction of major errors may require that the original graphic record be recopied. The following procedure for correcting errors should be followed.

1. To correct a *minor error on the graphic portion* of the record, write "mistaken entry" or "error" in ink on the incorrect connecting line, and record your first initial, your last name, and status about the error; then graph the correct value (Fig. 21-2).

2. To correct a *numbered entry*, such as the respiration value, draw a line through the entry in ink, and write in ink "mistaken entry" or "error," your first initial, your last name, and status near it. As close as possible, insert the correct numbers (see Fig. 21-2).

3. To correct a *series of errors* on the graphic record, the entire record must be recopied to show the correct data (Fig. 21-3, *A*).
   a. Prepare a new graphic record and label with the patient's ID label (Fig. 21-3, *B*).
   b. Transfer in ink *all* the information onto the new graphic record, including the correction of errors (see Fig. 21-3, *B*).
   c. Draw a diagonal line through the old graphic record in ink, and record in ink on the line "mistaken entry" or "error" (see Fig. 21-3, *A*).

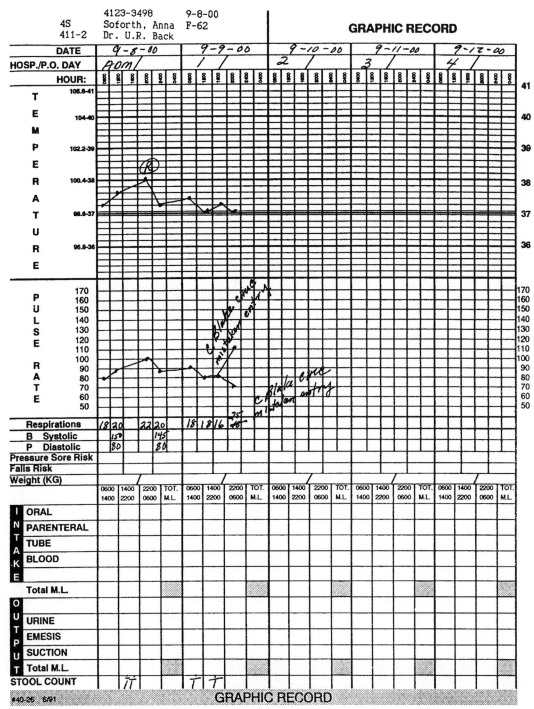

Figure 21-2 Correction of minor errors on the graphic record.

d. Place the old record behind the recopied record because it must remain as a permanent part of the chart.

e. In ink, write "recopied," followed by your name, status, and the date on the new graphic record

(see Fig. 21-3, *B*); place it behind the correct divider in the patient's chart.

RECORDING VITAL SIGNS AND OTHER DATA ON THE GRAPHIC RECORD WHEN THE ELECTRONIC RECORD IS USED

When the electronic medical record (EMR) is used, vital signs and other data may be entered directly into the patient's EMR by the nurse on a Pen Tab or Tablet Computer, or with the use of a computer on wheels (COW) at the patient's

---

SKILLS CHALLENGE

To practice recording the vital signs and other data on the graphic record, complete Activities 21-1 and 21-2 in the *Skills Practice Manual.*

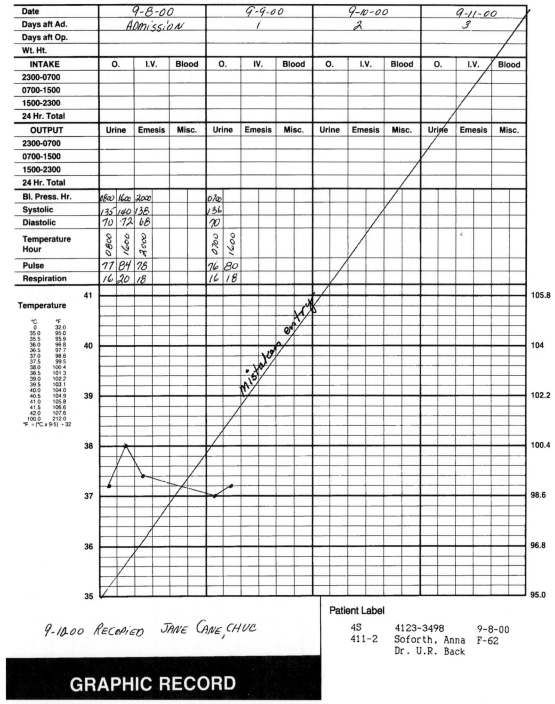

Date	9-8-00			9-9-00			9-10-00			9-11-00		
Days aft Ad.	ADmission			i			2			3		
Days aft Op.												
Wt. Ht.												
INTAKE	O.	I.V.	Blood	O.	IV.	Blood	O.	I.V.	Blood	O.	I.V.	Blood
2300-0700												
0700-1500												
1500-2300												
24 Hr. Total												
OUTPUT	Urine	Emesis	Misc.	Urine	Emesis	Misc.	Urine	Emesis	Misc.	Urine	Emesis	Misc.
2300-0700												
0700-1500												
1500-2300												
24 Hr. Total												
Bl. Press. Hr.	0800	1600	2000	0700								
Systolic	135	140	138	136								
Diastolic	70	72	68	70								
Temperature Hour	0800	1600	2000	0800	1600							
Pulse	77	84	78	76	80							
Respiration	16	20	18	16	18							

Mistaken entry

Temperature

°C.   °F
0.0   32.0
35.0   95.0
35.5   95.9
36.0   96.8
36.5   97.7
37.0   98.6
37.5   99.5
38.0   100.4
38.5   101.3
39.0   102.2
39.5   103.1
40.0   104.0
40.5   104.9
41.0   105.8
41.5   106.6
42.0   107.6
100.0 212.0
°F. = (°C. x 9/5) + 32

9-10-00 RECOPIED   JANE CANE, CHUC

Patient Label

4S   4123-3498   9-8-00
411-2   Soforth, Anna F-62
         Dr. U.R. Back

GRAPHIC RECORD

Figure 21-3   Recopied graphic record used to correct a series of errors. **A,** The original graphic record.

bedside. See Chapter 10 for descriptions and pictures of the various computers that may be used by nurses at the patient's bedside.

FILING RECORDS ON THE PATIENT'S PAPER CHART

Each day, the nursing unit receives many typed and computer-generated records, such as diagnostic results, history and physical reports, pathology reports, and others, to be filed on the patient's chart. Efficient, timely filing of these records on the patient's chart is necessary for two reasons. First, during the patient's

hospital stay, filed written records are readily available for use viewing by the attending doctor and other hospital personnel. Diagnosis and/or treatment/therapy are often dependent on these records. Second, upon the patient's discharge, the health information management department (HIMS) personnel have the legal responsibility of assembling and storing *all* records produced during the patient's hospital stay. Correct filing methods used during the patient's hospitalization assist HIMS personnel in completing this task.

Guidelines for filing records on the patient's chart on the nursing unit are listed on the following page.

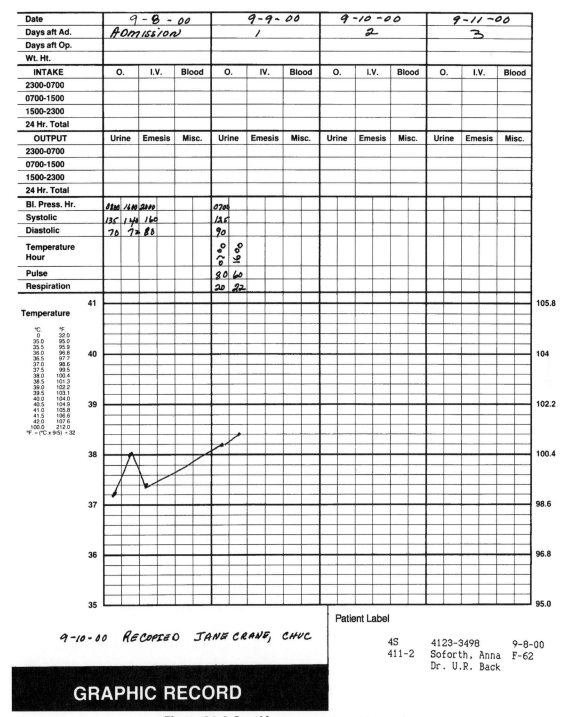

Date	9-8-00			9-9-00			9-10-00			9-11-00		
Days aft Ad.	Admission			1			2			3		
Days aft Op.												
Wt. Ht.												
INTAKE	O.	I.V.	Blood	O.	IV.	Blood	O.	I.V.	Blood	O.	I.V.	Blood
2300-0700												
0700-1500												
1500-2300												
24 Hr. Total												
OUTPUT	Urine	Emesis	Misc.	Urine	Emesis	Misc.	Urine	Emesis	Misc.	Urine	Emesis	Misc.
2300-0700												
0700-1500												
1500-2300												
24 Hr. Total												
Bl. Press. Hr.	0200 1600 2000			0700								
Systolic	135 140 160			135								
Diastolic	70 72 80			90								
Temperature Hour				0800 0900								
Pulse				80 60								
Respiration				20 22								

Temperature

°C.	°F.
0	32.0
35.0	95.0
35.5	95.9
36.0	96.8
36.5	97.7
37.0	98.6
37.5	99.5
38.0	100.4
38.5	101.3
39.0	102.2
39.5	103.1
40.0	104.0
40.5	104.9
41.0	105.8
41.5	106.6
42.0	107.6
100.0	212.0

°F. = (°C x 9/5) + 32

9-10-00 RECOPIED JANE CRANE, CHUC

Patient Label

4S 4123-3498 9-8-00
411-2 Soforth, Anna F-62
Dr. U.R. Back

GRAPHIC RECORD

Figure 21-3 Cont'd—B, A copied graphic record

Guidelines for Filing Records on the Patient's Paper Chart

When possible, file at the same time each day. Filing near the end of the shift allows all records received during the shift to be filed at one time. It is important for the patient's nurses to have ready access to all laboratory results as soon as they arrive on the nursing unit.

Separate the records according to the patient's name. In this way, all records for a given patient are prepared at one time, so the chart holder must be accessed only once.

Always check the patient's name within the chart with the name on the record before filing it. Never select the patient's chart just by the room number on the record, because the room number on the record will be incorrect if the patient has been transferred to another bed on the nursing unit after the records were initiated. Often a doctor prescribes treatment according to test results which may be delayed when records have been filed in the wrong patient's chart.

Be especially alert when two patients on the unit have the same name. When this happens, both patients' charts are flagged with a "name alert" sticker. File all medical records by their health records number. Many times, patients on the nursing unit will have the same or very similar names. The medical records number will never be duplicated.

Place the record behind the correct chart divider. Use consistent sequencing in filing the reports on the patient's chart to make it easier for the doctor and other health care personnel to locate them. Reports are usually filed with the latest report in front or on top of previously filed reports, right behind the divider.

Initial each record before filing. Follow the hospital's policy as to where to place initials if this practice is used.

Never discard any patient's records. Records that have not been filed for patients who have been discharged should be forwarded to the HIMS. Records that have not been filed for patients who have been transferred within the hospital should be forwarded to the receiving unit.

 SKILLS CHALLENGE

To practice filing records on the patient's paper charts, complete Activity 21-3 in the *Skills Practice Manual*.

SCANNING RECORDS INTO THE PATIENT'S ELECTRONIC MEDICAL RECORD

The HUC is responsible for scanning electrocardiogram reports, telemetry strips, medical records, and reports from outside facilities when requested, along with handwritten physician progress notes and any other relevant documents related to the patient's medical record.

Guidelines for Scanning Records Into the Patient's Electronic Medical Record

Label the document with the appropriate patient's ID label, and scan the records using the nursing unit scanner as required or requested in a timely manner. **After the documents have been scanned, they will be certified by an HIMS specialist and will be entered into the patient's EMR.**

Stamp the original documents as "scanned," and write the date, time, and your initials.

Place the original documents in a box or bin to be delivered to HIMS.

✎ *TAKE NOTE*

Some nursing units require that reports should be filed or scanned when received.

ORDERING DAILY DIAGNOSTIC TESTS WHEN PAPER CHARTS ARE USED

In Chapters 14 through 16, practice of transcription of many different types of diagnostic orders, including doctors' orders for daily laboratory tests, was provided. Chest X-rays and ECGs may be ordered to be performed daily.

The doctor may specify the number of days, such as chest X-ray or ECG × 3 days, or may write a standing order, such

as daily fasting blood sugar. Daily diagnostic tests may be ordered for several days in advance on most computer systems or may be ordered each day until the doctor cancels the order.

To order daily laboratory tests or diagnostic imaging procedures, look at each patient's Kardex form (Fig. 21-4) and enter the test or procedure into the computer every day. Note on the Kardex that the daily laboratory test or diagnostic imaging procedure has been ordered for the following day. Each unit has a method of indicating that daily orders have been entered and sent. "Order inquiry" is a computer screen that may be used to verify whether a patient's order has been entered and sent. This computer screen will display all of the patient's orders from the time of his admission. The HUC chooses "Order inquiry" from the master or home screen and then chooses a patient from the census screen to locate a list of all orders entered for the chosen patient.

Ordering of daily tests may be the task of the day shift or the evening shift HUC. Ordering should be done at a specified time each day to avoid omission or duplication of orders; if done on the day shift, it should be scheduled toward the end of the shift, to allow for possible cancellation of the order by the doctor. Daily diagnostic tests are ordered until the doctor writes an order to discontinue the tests.

✎ *TAKE NOTE*

Daily laboratory tests should be ordered for the first laboratory draw in the morning, so the patient will not have eaten breakfast and the results will be available when the doctors make their A.M. rounds.

✎ *TAKE NOTE*

Daily diagnostic tests may be ordered in advance on most hospital computer systems. When this is not possible or preferable, each nursing unit has a method of indicating that daily diagnostic tests have been ordered. When a test is ordered in advance, the date the order was written by the doctor is entered on the Kardex form, and a 3 × 5 card with patient label is affixed to it or to a separate book for daily diagnostic tests. A series of dates are written next to or below the test, and each day when the HUC orders tests for the following morning, he places a diagonal line across that date to indicate that tests have been ordered.

Example: 2/14 Daily H & H 2/15, 2/16, 2/17, 2/18.

This would indicate that the H & H was ordered for 2/15 and 2/16.

To verify that a test has been ordered, choose "Order inquiry" from the computer master screen (which will show the patient census on the nursing unit), and choose the patient's name. All of that patient's orders will be displayed on the computer screen.

DATE ORD.	TREATMENTS	DATE ORD.	DIAGNOSTIC STUDIES	TO BE DONE
6-1	K-pad to left shoulder	6-1	CBC UA Chest xray	
		6-2	T3 uptake	
		6-1	* Daily Hg + Hct	

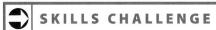

| | DATE | DIAGNOSTIC RESULTS |

860 - 25

Figure 21-4 Kardex form with a daily laboratory order recorded on it.

When the EMR c̄ CPOE is used, the doctor's order entered into the computer for daily diagnostic tests will automatically be sent to the appropriate departments. The doctor's order entered into the computer to discontinue daily diagnostic tests also will be automatically sent to the appropriate department. The HUC will not have the responsibility of transcribing these orders or discontinuing them but may be involved in sending laboratory specimens as they are collected by the nursing staff.

RETRIEVING DIAGNOSTIC TEST RESULTS

Most diagnostic test results may be retrieved from the computer by selecting "Laboratory results" or "Diagnostic imaging results," and then selecting the patient's name. The results will be displayed on the computer screen and may be printed. The HUC may print daily laboratory or diagnostic imaging results as requested. A summary of results may be printed daily for physicians to review on rounds or, if needed, to be sent to another facility if a patient is being transferred. Recorded diagnostic test results also may be obtained by telephone in some hospitals by calling a specified number.

✎ *TAKE NOTE*

When the EMR c̄ CPOE is used, the patient's doctors and nurses will have access to these records, and other health care staff, including the HUC, may have limited access to them.

⊙ **SKILLS CHALLENGE**

To practice ordering daily diagnostic tests, complete Activity 21-4 in the *Skills Practice Manual*.

ORDERING SUPPLIES FOR THE NURSING UNIT

A busy nursing unit stocks a variety of supplies to keep the unit functioning smoothly. Nursing unit supplies are obtained from the purchasing department, the central service department, the nutritional care department, the pharmacy, and the laundry department.

Two systems are used for restocking supplies. One system is used by the HUC or a unit aide to determine the supplies needed and to order them from the supplying department; the other is used by the supplying department to make daily rounds throughout the hospital and to restock supplies as needed (similar to restocking of shelves in a grocery store).

One aspect to be considered regarding supplies is who pays for them. The patient is charged for some items, such as catheter trays and medications, whereas other items, such as requisition forms, hand soap, paper clips, and so forth, are charged to the nursing unit budget. Downtime requisition forms often are used for items charged to the patient for billing and restocking purposes. Failure to complete the requisition form on items normally charged to the patient usually results in deduction of the cost from the nursing unit's budget. Carelessness in this area may play havoc with the overall management of money for nursing unit supplies.

Purchasing Department Supplies

Purchasing department supplies consist of non-nursing items, such as chart and requisition forms, pencils, staples, flashlights, and numerous other items. Figure 21-5 illustrates an example of a purchasing department order form. Items received

Form header fields: NAME OF REQUESTOR · TELEPHONE NO. · AUTHORIZED SIGNATURE · DATE ORDERED · DEPARTMENT NAME · BUILDING/LOCATION · FLOOR · COST CENTER **.460**

STANDARD REGISTER
STOCKLESS FORMS REQUISITION

NO. 01132

Column 1 — Standard Register Stockless Forms Requisition

QTY	UNIT OF MEASURE	FORM NUMBER	DESCRIPTION
	500/BX	2044	ENV BLUE #9 SPEC WINDOW
	500/BX	2045	ENV INTER OFFICE BLUE #10
	1/EA	2046	ENV INTER OFFICE MAN/10x13
	500/BX	2051	ENV MANILLA PAYROLL WIND
	500/BX	2061	ENV WHITE ST JOSEPH #10
	900/ROLL	2093	LABEL WHT 2-7/8 x 1-7/16
	500/PK	2177	ST JOSEPH LETTERHEAD
	500/BX	2881	ENV WHITE #9 OUTGOING
	1000/CTN	3224	PURCH 5 PT PAPER COLOR
	500/BX	3387	ENV WT WINDOW #10 PAT ACT
	2000/PK	3481	LABEL-ADDRESSOGRAPH-PACK
	25/PK	3623	HIV CONSENT FORM
	3000/CTN	61911G	WARD REPORT
	25/PD	ADM-1-4	CLASS ATTENDANCE SHEET
	25/PK	ADM-1-104	ST JOE OCCURRENCE RPT
	10/PK	ADM-1-196	ESP GRAM
	25/PK	ADM-1426	EMPL EXP REINBURSE
	50/PK	ADM-1775	PATIENT COMPLAINT SHEET
	100/PK	ADM-3-140	WHILE YOU WERE OUT PAD
	100/PK	ADM-503-127	REQ SPEC FOOD SERV
	100/PK	ADM-505	SPEED MEMO
	1930/CTN	ADMIT 1271	PATIENT INFO
	1000/CTN	ADMIT-1637	4 PT REQ INFO
	100/PK	BUS-1-222	OCCUPATIONAL THPY CHG
	100/PK	BUS-10	222 X-RAY CHGS
	100/PK	BUS-1000	GENERAL X-RAY
	200/PK	BUS-1001	RADIOLOGY CONSULT
	100/PK	BUS-1002	SP PROC X-RAY
	100/PK	BUS-1007	DEPT RAD CARDIO NUC MED
	100/PK	BUS-1008	GEN SERG DRUG CHGS
	50/PK	BUS-1016	CDV DIAG LAB
	10/PK	BUS-1040	CONTROLLED DRUGS ORAL A
	10/PK	BUS-1045	CONTROLLED DRUGS II
	10/PK	BUS-1055	CONTROLLED DRUGS-INJECT
	100/PD	BUS-1057	MEDICARE AS 2nd PAYOR
	100/PK	BUS-1057A	MEDICARE ADDENDUM A
	100/PK	BUS-1280	OP/PT CHRG-PROCEDURE
	200/PK	BUS-1476	BLOOD GAS LAB
	50/PK	BUS-15	EEG CHARGE SLIP
	100/PK	BUS-1597	PERINATAL AMNI BLOOD TEST
	100/PD	BUS-16-134	PHYS MED CHGE SLIP
	100/PK	BUS-178	CONDITIONS FOR TREATMENT
	100/PD	BUS-18	PHARMACY CHARGE SLIP
	100/PD	BUS-29-2	MISC CHARGE SLIP

Column 2

QTY	UNIT OF MEASURE	FORM NUMBER	DESCRIPTION
	5700/CTN	BUS-30-135	CREDIT SLIP
	1300/CTN	BUS-33	SPEECH OTOLOGY CHARGE
	3000/CTN	BUS-35-295	MEMO PADS
	100/PD	BUS-35-295A	FULL SIZE MEMO PAD
	2500/CTN	BUS-42	BLOOD BANK CONTINUOUS
	100/PD	BUS-42B	OUTPUT LAB REQUISITION
	100/PD	BUS-447	NEW INV CODING SHEET
	100/PD	BUS-448	PREPAID A/C CODE
	100/PD	BUS-50B	MICRO URINE FLDS LAB REQ
	100/PK	BUS-510-143	REQ FOR CK OR CASH
	100/PK	BUS-53B	CHEM, HEMA, SEROLO LAB REQ
	50/PK	BUS-60A	CYTOLOGY
	100/PK	BUS-61	TISSUES FORM
	25/PK	BUS-63	GENERAL SURGERY CHARGES
	250/PK	BUS-641	SPD CHARGE CARD
	100/PK	BUS-674	ER MEDICATION CHARGES
	100/PK	BUS-677	DELIVERY ROOM CHARGES
	1350/CTN	BUS-817	OCCUP THERAPY CHG SLIP
	100/PK	CRS-1421	GENERAL DIAGNOSTIC-CRS
	950/CTN	CRS-1483	CRS MTST PAPER
	100/PD	CS-3-291	NURSING CARE PLAN
	100/PK	DORM-508	DORM VISITATION SLIP
	100/PK	DORM-510	PRENATAL REC 2A MT ST
	250/PK	DP-2-163	BATCH HEADER/TRAILER
	250/PK	DP-2-163C	BATCH HEADER/TRAILER BLUE
	100/PD	DP-960	CREDIT/DEBIT RECORD
	100/PD	DP-962	BALANCE TRANSFER
	100/PD	DP-963	CREDIT/DEBIT SHEET
	250/PK	DP2-163B	BATCH HEADER/TRAILER PBS
	100/PD	EEG-609	PHYSICIAN TRANSCRIPTION
	25/PK	ENG-445	PLANT SERV SERVICE CALL
	100/PD	ER-508-172	PHONE REPORT OF LAB
	500/PK	ER-514	ER C/SERV ITEMS CHG SLIP
	5000/CTN	FS-1427	MENU LABEL
	100/PD	HB-17-96	WORK ORDERS
	200/PK	HB-1720	A/P BLUE
	250/PK	HB-54	RECEIPTS-PEGBOARD
	250/PK	HB-55	JOURNAL-PEGBOARD
	100/PK	HRS-2027	OPERATING ROOM PATH CONST
	100/PK	LAB-1684	1 PART LAB REPORT
	2500/CTN	LAB-1352	LAB LABEL-GREEN, MULTI-CUT
	5000/CTN	LAB-1353	LAB LABEL-WHT, SINGLE CUT
	5000/CTN	LAB-1354	LAB LABEL-RED
	1600/CTN	LAB-1428	12 PART CANARY-CONTINUOUS

Column 3

QTY	UNIT OF MEASURE	FORM NUMBER	DESCRIPTION
	50/PD	MR-41-282	CONSENT PHOTOG-PUBLS
	100/PK	MR-417	REQ FOR PRIOR ORDERS
	100/PK	MR-43-216	MEDICATION RECORD
	100/PD	MR-46-158	DIABETIC CHART
	2850/CTN	MR-47	DISCHARGE FINAL REPORT
	2850/CTN	MR-48	WEEKLY LAB SUMMARY
	100/PK	MR-480	PHYS PARENTERAL NUT ORDER
	200/PK	MR-5	LAB REPORT
	100/PK	MR-509-98	ADMISSION ASSESSMENT
	500/CTN	MR-522	6-PLY MTST PAPER/CBNLESS
	650/CTN	MR-522	MTST 5-PT PAPER CBN
	50/PD	MR-533	MEDICAL RECORD OUT CARD
	100/PK	MR-571	VENTILATOR RESP THERAPY
	100/PK	MR-581	PATIENT RECORD
	100/PD	MR-583	CDV ICU FLOW SHEET
	100/PD	MR-593	DEFICIENCY RECORD
	100/PD	MR-595-179	PROBLEM SHEET
	100/PD	MR-600-643	PREOP CHECK LIST
	1000/CTN	MR-616	PULMONARY LAB REPORT
	2500/CTN	MR-616A	PULMONARY LAB REPORT 1-PT
	100/PD	MR-650	VITAL SIGNS
	100/PK	MR-671-730	PRE-ANESTHESIA QUES
	100/PK	MR-675	NEONATAL RECORD I
	100/PK	MR-676	NEONATAL II
	100/PK	MR-677	OB SUMMARY
	100/PK	MR-684	CONDITIONS OF ADMISSION
	100/PK	MR-685-755	NURSING DISCHARGE ASSESS
	100/PD	MR-692-783	X-RAY CASSETTES
	100/PK	MR-717	PERIOPERATIVE RECORD
	100/PD	MR-803	DIET SERVICE PROG NOTE
	100/PK	MR-895	CRITICAL CARE FLOWSHEET
	100/PK	MRS-1157	BACKING SHEET
	100/PK	NS-12-240	NOURISHMENT ORDER FORM
	100/PD	NS-507-114W	REV TEAM ASSIGNMENT
	100/PD	NS-510-215	WEEKLY SCHEDULES
	100/PD	NS-518-14	RN CLINICAL REPORT
	50/PK	NS-529-478	TREAT AND TEST PLAN
	100/PD	NS-530-115	FLUID FORMS
	100/PD	NS-7-100	TPR RECORD
	100/PD	NS-9-21	INTAKE/OUTPUT SHEETS
	1/EA	NSY-325	INFO ABOUT YOUR BABY
	50/PK	NSY-761	NURSERY ICU KARDEX
	200/PK	OPD-19	CLINICAL PRESCRIPTIONS
	100/PK	OPD-60-253	PED-PROGRESS NOTES

Column 4

QTY	UNIT OF MEASURE	FORM NUMBER	DESCRIPTION
	100/PK	PER-1-196	EMPLOYMENT APPLICATION
	25/PD	PER-13-37	ACCIDENT EXPOSURE RC
	50/PK	PER-663-793	EMP/POS CHG REQUEST
	100/PD	PH1-299	PRESCRIPTION BLANKS
	100/PD	PH-2-637	PHONE ORDER FOR MEDS
	4900/CTN	PRD-1923	NOTICE OF DEPOSIT
	100/PD	PULF-526	PULF TELEPHONE REPORTS
	100/PK	PUR-1	PURCHASE ORDERS
	25/PK	PUR-1622	OFFICE SUPPLY REQ
	25/PK	PUR-203	REQUISITION TO PURCHASE
	100/PD	PUR-4-53	GEN REQUISITION SM
	100/PK	PUR-IV	PURCHASE ORDER TOP COPY
	25/PK	PUR-9	FORMS REQUISITION
	2500/CTN	QA-1247	RSOUM WORKSHEET
	10/PK	QA-842	MONITORING SYSTEMS
	1/EA	RO-11-214	RADIATION ONCOLOGY BROCH
	25/PD	RAD-18	CAT HISTORY FORM
	100/PK	RAD-511-667	RADIOLOGY PRELIM REPT
	250/PK	RAD-516	DAYLIGHT FLASHER CARD
	250/PK	RAD-516A	BLANK DAYLIGHT FLASHER
	200/PK	RTD-504	RESP THERAPY CHG
	400/CTN	RTD-507	RESP THERAPY SCHEDULE
	100/PD	SSD-104-283	MED RECORD
	100/PK	TRAN-363	TUBE ROOM ROUTE SLIP
	100/PK	TRAN-564	TRAN CALL SLIP

PROCEDURE FOR COMPLETING FORM

1. FILL IN QUANTITY OF FORMS DESIRED. COMPLETE ALL BLANKS AT TOP OF FORM.
2. FOR ITEMS NOT APPEARING ON THIS REQUISITION, CONSULT FORMS CATALOG AND WRITE IN BELOW. (FOR NON-CATALOG FORMS, SPECIAL ORDERS OR NEW FORMS, CONTACT PURCHASING).
3. KEEP "REQUESTOR'S COPY" FOR YOUR RECORDS.
4. SEND ALL REMAINING COPIES TO PURCHASING.
5. FOR ASSISTANCE, CALL EXT. 3443.

QTY	UNIT OF MEASURE	FORM NUMBER	DESCRIPTION

Figure 21-5 Purchasing department order form.

from the purchasing department are usually paid for from the nursing unit budget. A cost control center number for the nursing unit is placed on all requisitions issued by the unit. Restocking of purchasing department supplies is done weekly or bimonthly and is the most demanding of all supply tasks. It is important to order what is needed in a timely manner.

Central Service Department Supplies

Central service department (CSD) supplies consist of items used for nursing procedures that are charged to the patient or charged to the nursing unit's budget. Items charged to the patient, such as catheter trays and irrigation trays, usually have a requisition form with them. (See Fig. 11-2 for an example of a CSD computer screen.) Smaller items, such as Band-Aids, tongue blades, alcohol, and sponges, are covered by the nursing unit's budget.

In a recent trend, many frequently used disposable nursing items (such as catheter trays and enema bags), usually supplied by the CSD, may be obtained directly from the purchasing department. As you know, the purchasing department originally buys all hospital supplies; therefore, this method of bypassing the CSD is both efficient and economical.

Pharmacy Supplies

Pharmacy supplies include all medications administered to patients. Medications are kept on the nursing unit in three classifications: (1) controlled substances, which are locked in the narcotics cupboard or in a computerized dispensing cart; (2) other daily and prn medications that are currently being administered to patients according to doctors' orders; and (3) a unit stock supply of frequently used medications, such as aspirin. Restocking of daily medications usually is performed on a daily basis, and the stock supply is replenished as needed. Medications are charged to the patients who received them; therefore, pharmacy supplies are not covered by the nursing unit's budget. Charges cover the cost of administration supplies, such as needles and syringes, and usually are determined on the basis of information found on the patient's medication record sheet.

Nutritional Care Department Supplies

Nutritional care department supplies include food items such as milk, juices, soda pop, and crackers that are stored in the nursing unit kitchen and issued to patients as needed. These supplies are restocked daily and usually are charged to the nursing unit's budget. Figure 21-6 illustrates an example of a nutritional care department stock supply order form.

Laundry/Linen Department Supplies

Laundry/linen department supplies include linens and bedding such as pillows, sheets, blankets, towels, washcloths, and patient gowns. The cost of linen supplies usually is absorbed into the charge for the patient's room. Most hospitals employ a laundry service to supply linen that is then delivered to each nursing unit by hospital personnel. If supplies run low during the day, the HUC may have to call the linen department or page personnel from the laundry department for additional items.

NOURISHMENT ORDER FROM NUTRITIONAL CARE	
UNIT_____ ORDERED BY_____	
DATE_____ _____ ____	

DESCRIPTION	ORDER
Whole Milk	
Skim Milk	
Chocolate Milk	
Orange Juice (unsw) (qts)	
Apple Juice	
Cranberry Juice	
Prune Juice	
Tomato Juice	
Nectar	
Decaffeinated Coffee (pkg of 20)	
Tea Bags (pkg of 30)	
Graham Crackers (pkg of 12)	
Saltines (pkg of 20)	
Powdered non-dairy Creamers (50 per box)	
Sugar (per 100 ind.)	
Ice Cream	
Sherbet	
Jello	
Custard	
Margarine (ind.)	
Bouillon -Beef or Chicken (pkg/12)	
7-Up (6 pk)	
Cola (6 pk)	

NOTE: BETWEEN MEAL FEEDINGS, TUBE FEEDINGS OR LIQUID SUPPLEMENTS ARE TO BE ORDERED VIA COMPUTER CARD.

NS-12-240   Received by_____

Figure 21-6 Nutritional care department stock supply order form.

PREPARING DAILY FORMS

It may be the HUC's task to prepare forms for use by nursing team members, such as the patient assignment sheet (see Fig. 3-5, pp. 42-44) and work schedules. Because preparing these forms usually involves recording data pertinent to the individual nursing unit, this topic is not discussed further here. Daily tasks when paper charts are used may include preparing nurse's progress records by labeling with patient ID labels and filling in the headings, labeling CSD cards, and recopying MARs as needed. If preparing and filling out forms is an HUC responsibility, plan to do this at the same time each day when possible.

KEY CONCEPTS

The HUC's job is to coordinate activities at the nursing station by efficiently completing the tasks discussed in this and previous chapters. When paper charts are used, accuracy and efficiency are extremely important when one is charting vital signs, filing reports on patients' paper charts, and ordering daily tests and procedures. Performing these tasks at the same time each day (when possible) is necessary for efficient time management. When the EMR is used, it is equally important to scan patient records into the electronic file. Additional tasks may be added to the HUC's job description when the EMR $\bar{c}$ CPOE is implemented; these tasks may include tracking and monitoring of certifications and licensure of the nursing staff, documenting and monitoring of compliance with the Joint Commission (TJC) requirements by nursing staff, and completion of other record keeping tasks as requested by the nurse manager.

REVIEW QUESTIONS

1. Why is it important for the HUC to record vital signs in a timely manner when paper charts are used?

_____

_____

2. Why is accuracy important in the recording of vital signs?

_____

3. Describe how an incorrect entry of a patient's temperature would be corrected on a graphic record.

_____

4. Describe how an error made 2 days prior on a graphic sheet that resulted in a series of errors would be corrected (e.g., vital signs are recorded under incorrect dates).

_____

_____

5. When a graphic record is recopied, explain what is done with the original graphic record.

_____

_____

6. Convert the following Fahrenheit temperatures to Celsius.

a. 98.6° _____ b. 101.4° _____ c. 99.8° _____ d. 96.7° _____

7. Convert the following Celsius temperatures to Fahrenheit.

a. 38.2° _____ b. 39.5° _____ c. 36.4° _____ d. 37.8° _____

8. List two reasons for the need for efficient, accurate filing of records on the patient's paper chart.

a. _____

b. _____

9. List five guidelines for filing records on the patient's paper chart.

a. _____

b. _____

c. _____

d. _____

e. _____

10. List three guidelines for scanning records into the patient's electronic record.

a. _____

b. _____

c. _____

11. Name five hospital departments that may provide nursing unit supplies, and list the types of supplies that may be obtained from each department.

a. _____

b. _____

c. _____

d. _____

e. _____

12. Define the following terms:

a. pulse deficit

_____

b. Celsius

_____

c. stool or feces

_____

d. Fahrenheit

_____

THINK ABOUT...

1. Discuss the problems that carelessness in charting vital signs could cause.
2. Discuss the possible consequences of reports being filed in the wrong patient's chart or behind the incorrect divider.
3. Discuss the importance of restocking supplies on the nursing unit.

CHAPTER 22

Reports, Infection Control, Emergencies, and Special Services

CHAPTER OBJECTIVES

Upon completion of this chapter, you will be able to:

1. Define the terms in the vocabulary list.
2. Write the meaning of each abbreviation in the abbreviations list.
3. List three conditions that may cause a patient to become immunocompromised.
4. List four categories of events that require a written incident report.
5. Explain the importance of incident reports.
6. Name three methods by which bacteria may be spread.
7. Name three pathogenic microorganisms that are frequently responsible for hospital-acquired infection.
8. List four types of personal protective equipment used with standard precautions.
9. Explain how human immunodeficiency virus may be transmitted.
10. Name two opportunistic diseases related to acquired immune deficiency syndrome.
11. List nine tasks that the health unit coordinator may perform in a medical emergency.
12. Explain the duties carried out during a fire or fire drill.
13. List six guidelines that should be followed for electrical safety.
14. Describe how to handle mail and flowers delivered to the unit.

VOCABULARY

Airborne Precautions/Isolation The required use of a mask and a private room with monitored negative air pressure and high-efficiency filtration, in conjunction with standard precautions

Cardiac Arrest The patient's heart contractions are absent or insufficient to produce a pulse or blood pressure (may also be referred to as code arrest)

Centers for Disease Control and Prevention Division of the U. S. Public Health Service that investigates and controls diseases that have epidemic potential

Code Blue A term used in hospitals to summon additional help for a patient who has stopped breathing and/or whose heart has stopped beating (cardiac arrest)

Code or Crash Cart A cart stocked by the nursing and pharmacy staff with emergency medication, advanced breathing supplies, intravenous solutions and appropriate tubing, needles, a heart monitor and defibrillator, an oxygen tank, and a suction machine (used in emergency situations)

Communicable Disease A disease that may be transmitted from one person to another

Disaster Procedure A planned procedure that is carried out by hospital personnel when a large number of people may have been injured or exposed to hazardous materials

Epidemiology The study of the occurrence, distribution, and causes of health and disease in humans; the specialist is called an *epidemiologist*

Hepatitis B Virus An infectious blood-borne disease that is a major occupational hazard for health care workers

Human Immunodeficiency Virus The virus that causes acquired immunodeficiency syndrome

Incident An episode that does not normally occur within the regular hospital routine

Isolation The placement of a patient apart from other patients for the purpose of preventing the spread of infection, or protecting a patient whose immune system is compromised

Material Safety Data Sheet (MSDS) A basic hazard communication tool that gives details on chemical dangers and safety procedures

Medical Emergency An emergency that is life threatening

Nosocomial Infections Infections that are acquired from within the health care facility

Occupational Safety and Health Administration A U.S. governmental regulatory agency that is concerned with the health and safety of workers

Pathogenic Microorganisms Disease-carrying organisms that are too small to be seen with the naked eye

Protective Care Another term for isolation

Respiratory Arrest When the patient ceases to breathe, or when respirations are so depressed that the blood cannot receive sufficient oxygen, and therefore, the body cells die (also may be referred to as *code arrest*)

Reverse Isolation A precautionary measure taken to prevent a patient with low resistance to disease from becoming infected

Risk Management A department in the hospital that addresses the prevention and containment of liability regarding patient care incidents

Standard Precautions The creation of a barrier between the health care worker and the patient's blood and body fluids (also may be called universal precautions)

Tuberculosis A disease caused by *Mycobacterium tuberculosis*, an airborne pathogen

ABBREVIATIONS

Abbreviation	Meaning
AIDS	acquired immunodeficiency syndrome
ARC	AIDS-related complex
CDC	Centers for Disease Control and Prevention
HBV	hepatitis B virus
HIV	human immunodeficiency virus
MRSA	methicillin-resistant *Staphylococcus aureus*
OSHA	Occupational Safety and Health Administration
PPE	personal protective equipment
R *A *C *E	*Rescue* individuals in danger. *Alarm*: Sound the alarm. *Confine* the fire by closing all doors and windows. *Extinguish* the fire with the nearest suitable fire extinguisher.
TB	tuberculosis

INCIDENT REPORTS

An **incident** is an event that does not normally occur within the regular health care facility routine and may involve patients, visitors, physicians, hospital staff, or students. The incident may be the result of an accident, such as a patient's falling while on the way to the bathroom, or it may involve a situation such as spilled liquids in a hospital corridor that cause someone to slip and sustain an injury. Events other than accidents that occur within the hospital or on hospital property are also reportable.

Incidents that require written reports include the following:

* Accidents
* Thefts from persons on hospital property
* Errors of omission of patient treatment or errors in administration of patient treatment, including medication
* Exposure to blood and body fluids, as may be caused by a needle stick

When an incident or event occurs, the health unit coordinator (HUC) prepares an incident report form for the person who is reporting the incident or event. Many facilities may use computer programs by which incident/event reports are generated electronically.

An incident report form (Fig. 22-1) should be completed for all incidents that occur to anyone, no matter how insignificant they may seem. Documentation of all incidents is important for identifying hazards and preventing continuing problems, and in the case of a lawsuit that may arise from them. The names and home addresses of witnesses are required in case the incident should become a lawsuit and the witnesses are no longer employed at the hospital when the case is brought to court.

The attending doctor, hospitalist, or resident may be called to examine the patient involved in an incident. All incidents involving patients are reported to the attending doctor. Copies of the incident report are sent to the nurse manager, to risk management, and to quality assurance. If the incident involves another department, a copy is sent to the manager of that department. The incident report never becomes a part of the patient's permanent record.

Employee hospital incidents must be documented and the employee seen by the employee health nurse or evaluated by a doctor to be eligible for coverage by the State Workman's Compensation Commission. Hospital employees who fail to put into writing something that may appear trivial, such as a finger puncture with a needle, have no evidence to present should an infection develop after the injury is incurred. Exposure to blood and body fluids as may be caused by a needle stick may require the employee to be tested for human immunodeficiency virus (HIV) if the patient who is involved has not been tested.

Risk management personnel may interview witnesses to a patient incident in preparation for a lawsuit. Risk management staff also study patient incidents to look for trends and to prevent future similar incidents.

✒ TAKE NOTE

Patient incident reports are not a part of the patient's permanent record.

Confidential Information
INCIDENT REPORT
(Patient or Visitor)
Not a Part of Patient's Permanent Chart

1. Date of Admission

2. Diagnosis

3. Date of Incident   Time   M | Room No., Name, Age, Sex, Hospital Number, Attending Physician

4. Were Bed Rails up?   5. Hi Lo Bed Position
                  (YES OR NO)   (UP OR DOWN)

6. Were a Safety Belt or Restraints in use?
                                                    DESIGNATE SPECIFICALLY

7. Activity (Complete Bed Rest, Bathroom Privileges, Etc.)

8. Sedatives   Dose   Time   M ⎫ Given
                                                                                    ⎪ within
9. Narcotics   Dose   Time   M ⎬ 12 hours
                                                                                    ⎪ previous
10. Tranquilizers   Dose   Time   M ⎭ to incident

11. Nurse's Account of Incident (State incident, where discovered, condition of patient, etc.)

12. History of Incident as related by Patient

13. List Witnesses or Persons Familiar with Details of Incident (Include roommate's name and hospital number.)

Name   Address

Name   Address

Name   Address

14. Time Doctor was called   AM   PM   15. Time Doctor Responded   AM   PM

16. Time Supervisor called   AM   PM

17. Date of Report

18. _____
              SIGNATURE OF PERSON REPORTING

19. _____
           SIGNATURE OF DEPARTMENT SUPERVISOR

20. _____
           SIGNATURE OF DEPARTMENT HEAD

A   Complete **IMMEDIATELY** for **EVERY** incident and send to Administrator via Department Head.

Figure 22-1 An incident report **A,** General information.

The HUC is responsible for maintaining a supply of incident report forms for the nursing unit.

INFECTION CONTROL

For statistical purposes, records of infectious diseases must be maintained. A report should be submitted to the infectious disease department or to personnel in the hospital (Fig. 22-2). Most hospitals employ an epidemiologist or an infection control officer, who maintains all infection records and investigates all hospital-acquired infections. Infection control is essential for providing a safe environment for patients and health care workers. Patients are at risk for acquiring infection because of lowered resistance to infectious microorganisms and increased exposure to numbers and types of disease-causing microorganisms, and because

PHYSICIAN'S STATEMENT

21. State injuries or other result, if any, from this incident _____

_____

_____

22. How, if at all, did the results of this incident affect the patient's original condition? _____

_____

_____

23. What treatment was given? _____

_____

24. Were X-rays or other tests ordered (specify) _____

_____

_____

25. Results of X-ray or other tests _____

_____

_____

26. Patient Examined: Date _____ Hour _____ AM _____ PM

27. Signed _____ M.D. (House Physician)

B

28. Signed _____ M.D. (Attending Physician)

Figure 22-1 Cont'd—B, Doctor's statement.

they must undergo invasive procedures. The presence of a pathogen does not mean that an infection will begin. Development of an infection depends on six components called the *chain of infection,* as listed below (Fig. 22-3):

1. Infectious agent or pathogen (bacteria)
2. Reservoir or source in which pathogen can live and grow (human body, contaminated water or food, animals, insects, etc.)
3. Means of escape (blood, urine, feces, wound drainage, etc.)
4. Route of transmission (air, contact, and body excretions)
5. Point of entrance (mouth, nostrils, and breaks in the skin)
6. Susceptible host (individual who does not have adequate resistance to the invading pathogen)

If infection is to be prevented, the chain must be broken. By following infection prevention and control techniques, health care workers can prevent the spread of microorganisms to patients and can also protect themselves. Infections can be prevented or controlled through hand hygiene, disinfection/sterilization, and the use of barriers. Proper hand hygiene is the most important method of prevention because the hands of health care workers are the primary site through which disease is transmitted from patient to patient. The **Centers for**

✎ TAKE NOTE

Hand hygiene is the most important intervention in preventing infection because health care workers' hands are the primary means by which disease is transmitted from patient to patient. Most hospitals have a policy that bans artificial fingernails for all health care professionals.

Disease Control and Prevention (CDC) recommends a ban on artificial fingernails for health care professionals when they are caring for patients at high risk for infection.

Standard Precautions

In 1987, the CDC developed and presented a concept to protect health care workers from blood-borne pathogens such as HIV, hepatitis B virus, and hepatitis C virus. At that time, a quiet panic arose among health care workers. They were not sure of how HIV was spread or how they could protect themselves. The CDC called this new concept "universal precautions" (for blood and body fluids). Nationwide, hospitals and other health care facilities accepted and taught this new concept to their employees. "Universal precautions" are now usually referred to as "standard precautions."

Report # _____

REPORT OF INFECTION

COMPLETE ALL BLANKS IN TOP SECTION   UNIT

1. Diagnosis is: _____

_____

_____

2. Date of admission: _____

3. Evidence of Infection on admission?
   Yes ☐ No ☐

4. Date of last previous admission here: _____

5. Hospitalized at another hospital?
   Yes ☐ No ☐
   If yes, name hospital?

_____

   Date: _____

6. Date of surgery/delivery _____

7. Procedure done: _____

_____

8. Culture sent? Yes ☐ No ☐
   (If yes, what was cultured?)
   _____ Blood
   _____ Urine
   _____ Sputum
   _____ Drainage from _____
   _____ Other(specify) _____

9. *Fever?   Yes ☐   No ☐
   NOTE: *Fever = temp. greater than
   100.4°F (38°C) Oral
   101°F (38.4°C) Rectal

10. Pt. Isolated? Yes ☐   No ☐
    If yes, enter date next to type initiated
    _____ a. Limited
    _____ b. Respiratory
    _____ c. Wound & Skin
    _____ d. Enteric
    _____ e. Strict
    _____ f. Protective

11. Date of Discharge: _____

CHECK **ALL** THAT APPLY:

DIARRHEA:
_____ Over 3 stools/24 hrs. for more than 2 days s̄ laxatives, enemas, x-rays preps, cardiac drugs or antibiotics

PHLEBITIS: Location _____

Non-Suppurative:
_____ Mechanical Intracath
_____ Drug
_____ Possible focal site of infection
_____ Observed by Nurse
_____ Diagnosis by Physician

Suppurative:
_____ Purulent drainage

POST PARTUM:
_____ *Fever(exclude 1st PP day)
_____ Purulent vaginal discharge
_____ Diagnosis by Physician

POST-OP:
_____ Continuous *Fever for 2 consecutive days
_____ Abscess(usually documented at time of surgery)

RESPIRATORY TRACT:
Upper
_____ Coryza(profuse nasal drainage)
_____ Pharyngitis
_____ Diagnosis by Physician

Lower:
_____ Sudden on set of cough
_____ Purulent sputum
_____ Suppuration of trachea
_____ X-ray Dx - Pneumonia
_____ Diagnosis by Physician

SKIN:
_____ Abscess
_____ Boil
_____ Cellulitis
_____ Purulent decubiti
_____ Suppuration

BLOOD:
_____ HAA Pos.
_____ HAA Neg.
_____ Positive Culture

Report completed by: _____

URINARY TRACT:
Asymptomatic:
_____ No clinical symptoms
_____ Positive bacteriology X 100,000/ml
_____ Positive bacteriology X 10,000/ml c̄ previous urine culture negative
_____ Pyuria X 10 WBC

Symptomatic:
_____ Frequency
_____ Burning
_____ Urgency
_____ CVT(costo-vertebral tenderness)

WOUND:
_____ Abscess(usually documented at surgery time)
_____ Continuous *Fever for 2 consecutive days
_____ Stitch abscess
_____ Suppuration of wound
_____ Diagnosis by Physican
_____ Other _____

Date: _____

COMMENTS: _____

(DO NOT WRITE IN THIS SECTION. FOR USE BY INFECTION CONTROL OFFICER ONLY)

Figure 22-2 Infection report.

Standard precautions involve the creation of a barrier between the practitioner (health care worker) and the patient's body fluids. Standard precautions are used with all patients in health care settings, under the assumption that all body excretions and secretions are potentially infectious. Body fluids include blood, semen, vaginal secretions, peritoneal fluid, pleural fluid, pericardial fluid, synovial fluid, cerebrospinal fluid, amniotic fluid, urine, feces, sputum, saliva, wound drainage, and vomitus.

The *barrier* in standard precautions is created by the wearing of personal protective equipment (PPE), consisting of such items as gloves, gown, mask, goggles or glasses, pocket masks with one-way valves, and moisture-resistant gowns (Fig. 22-4 shows a nurse with PPE). *Every health care employee should practice standard precautions as required with every single patient.*

Airborne Precautions (Isolation)

Airborne precautions (isolation) are used for patients in whom infections such as tuberculosis are transmitted through the air. Airborne precautions reduce the risk that droplet nuclei or contaminated dust particles may travel over short distances (less than 3 feet) and land in the nose or mouth of a susceptible person. The patient is placed in a private room

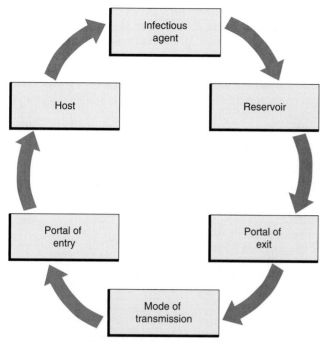

Figure 22-3 Chain of infection.

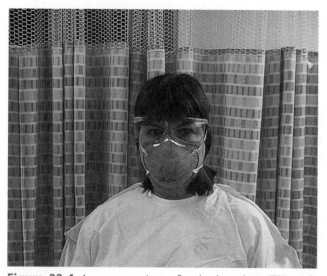

Figure 22-4 A nurse wearing a fitted tuberculosis (TB) mask, gown, and goggles. Gloves also would be worn (personal protective equipment [PPE]). (From Potter PA, Perry AG: *Fundamentals of nursing*, ed 6, St. Louis, 2005, Mosby.)

with monitored negative air pressure and high-efficiency filtration. The room usually has a door, an entryway or ante-room with a sink, and another door, with both doors remaining closed. Individuals who enter the room are required to wear masks, gloves, and gowns. Hand washing is also required. Linen and trash are bagged to prevent contamination.

Examples of patients who would be placed in airborne isolation are those with active tuberculosis (TB), measles, chicken pox, or meningitis. A culture is the most definitive way to confirm and identify microorganisms; sensitivity testing determines which antibiotics will destroy the identified microbes. See Chapter 14 for more information regarding cultures and sensitivities.

Reverse Isolation

Reverse isolation is used to protect patients with decreased immune system function by reducing their risks of exposure to potentially infectious organisms. Reverse isolation is also known as immunocompromised isolation. Patients who are immunocompromised include organ transplant recipients, burn victims, and those receiving chemotherapy.

DISEASES TRANSMITTABLE THROUGH CONTACT WITH BLOOD AND BODY FLUIDS

AIDS

AIDS stands for *acquired immunodeficiency syndrome*. AIDS is caused by a virus called **human immunodeficiency virus**, also called **HIV**. The AIDS virus attacks the immune system and thereby reduces the body's ability to defend itself against infection and disease. Persons who have AIDS become open to many opportunistic infections that are not usually a threat to persons with a normally functioning immune system. These infections are called *opportunistic* because the organisms take advantage of the patient's weakened immune system. As the immune system becomes weaker, these opportunistic illnesses may overwhelm the patient with AIDS and cause death.

AIDS is transmitted by blood, vaginal fluids, and semen and is not spread though casual contact. AIDS is spread in four primary ways. The first is by sexual contact. The second is by the use of needles that were previously injected into someone who carried the AIDS virus. The third is from an infected mother to her infant during pregnancy or birth. The fourth is by transmission of the virus through blood transfusions; this mode is especially common if the patient received the transfusion before blood was routinely tested for the virus (prior to the late 1980s). Surgical patients, hemophiliac patients, and mothers who received transfusions during or after birth have contracted the HIV virus in this way. AIDS also may be transmitted through the blood of an infected person that enters another person's bloodstream through a cut, an open sore, or blood that is splashed into the mouth or the eye. Appropriate PPE must be worn when one is coming into contact with body fluids from all patients.

An *AIDS virus carrier* is a person who carries the AIDS virus in the blood, but who may stay healthy for a long time. Some may never get sick. The only indication of AIDS infection in the carrier is usually a positive blood test for antibodies to the AIDS virus. Once infected with the AIDS virus, a person remains infected for life.

Months or years after initial infection, some people who carry the virus develop symptoms that may include tiredness, fevers, night sweats, swollen lymph glands, or mental deterioration resembling Alzheimer's disease. Often, the symptoms are recurrent and disable the person. This person is said to have ARC, or AIDS-related complex.

AIDS is the most severe form of the infection. A full-blown case may not appear until months or years after the initial infection. ARC symptoms may or may not have appeared. The two most frequent opportunistic illnesses that may overtake the AIDS patient are (1) *Pneumocystis carinii* pneumonia (PCP), a pneumonia caused by *Pneumocystis carinii*; and (2) Kaposi's sarcoma (KS), an otherwise rare skin cancer.

Hepatitis B Virus

Hepatitis B is an inflammation of the liver that is caused by the **hepatitis B virus (HBV).** It was formerly called serum hepatitis. Similar to AIDS, hepatitis B is spread by body fluids, but it is even more contagious than AIDS. Health care providers are at risk for exposure. Standard blood and body fluid precautions must be practiced.

OSHA (the Occupational and Safety Health Administration) mandates that employers provide hepatitis B vaccine for all employees who have an occupational exposure risk. The vaccines are given in three doses over a 6-month period. An employee has the right to refuse the hepatitis B vaccine but must sign a form that states this refusal.

Tuberculosis

Tuberculosis (TB) is caused by *Mycobacterium tuberculosis*, an airborne pathogen. Working with patients who have tuberculosis requires the use of special PPE, such as special masks fitted to the individual health care worker, so that one can avoid inhaling the tiny droplets that carry the virus through the air. TB has increased in the United States, and some viruses have become resistant to drug therapy.

Nosocomial Infections

Nosocomial infections are infections acquired from within the health care facility that often are transmitted to the patient by health care workers. Three **pathogenic microorganisms** that are frequently responsible for hospital-acquired infections are *Streptococcus*, *Staphylococcus*, and *Pseudomonas*. **Methicillin-resistant Staphylococcus aureus (MRSA)** is a variation of the common bacteria, *Staphylococcus aureus*. It has evolved the ability to survive treatment with beta-lactam antibiotics, including penicillin and methicllin. Patients with open wounds and weakened immune systems are at greater risk for infection than the general public. Excellent hand washing technique is the best way for health care workers to stop the spread of nosocomial infection.

HEALTH UNIT COORDINATOR TASKS PERFORMED TO CONTROL INFECTION

The HUC tasks for infection control and isolation vary from institution to institution. It is necessary in any health care facility for the HUC to have a basic understanding of infection control policies and standard precautions. *Accurate* information must

be given to inquiring visitors. If the HUC is unable to answer a question or is unsure of what to say, a nurse should be asked to speak with the visitor. All infectious or **communicable diseases** on the unit must be reported to infection control. Nurses will ask the HUC to order PPE and isolation packs as needed. The HUC should wear gloves when handling or transporting specimens and should practice good hand washing technique throughout the working day. Eating, drinking (open cups), and handling of contact lenses should not be done at the nursing station. Food should not be stored in refrigerators with specimens. The HUC transcribes laboratory orders that pertain to infection control. Below is a list of doctors' orders and the division of the laboratory to which they are sent:

Cerebrospinal fluid (CSF) for the following:
    Cell count—hematology
    Protein—chemistry
    Glucose—chemistry
    Lactate dehydrogenase (LDH)—chemistry
    Potassium hydroxide (KOH) and fungus culture—microbiology
    Acid-fast bacilli (AFB) and tuberculosis (TB)—microbiology
    Lyme titer—chemistry

Another area about which the HUC must be fully aware of institutional policy involves disclosure of information, such as in cases of AIDS. Laws regarding AIDS and confidentiality vary from state to state, as do laws regarding disclosure of HIV-positive persons. When in doubt, *do not disclose information*. In many health care facilities, guidelines have been established to assist the health care worker. Examples of some of these guidelines include the following:

Not putting "diagnosis of AIDS" or "rule out AIDS" on the computer; the primary diagnosis is the infection, symptoms, or cancer. AIDS becomes the secondary diagnosis and appears on the medical record but not in the computer.

Family, friends, and other persons may not know about the AIDS diagnosis and must not be told by any health care employee unless so advised by the doctor. Confidentiality and knowledge of the health care facility's policies and guidelines are essential if the HUC is to complete tasks and offer quality patient care in the area of infection control.

EMERGENCIES

Chemical Safety

All employees will receive chemical safety training during orientation regarding OSHA requirements for hazardous chemicals. Chemicals must be labeled with a statement of warning and a statement of what the hazard is, in order to eliminate risk and facilitate first aid measures undertaken in the event of a spill or exposure. A **material safety data sheet (MSDS)** is a communication tool that provides details on chemical dangers and safety procedures. Chemicals should not be stored above eye level or in unlabeled containers. Never add water to acid or mix chemicals indiscriminately. Never use chemicals in ways other than intended. Appropriate PPE should be worn when chemicals are used. Spill kits must be available and must comply with OSHA guidelines. It is unlikely that a HUC will be handling chemicals, but it is important to be informed so one will know what to do in case of a spill or an employee incident involving chemicals.

Fire and Electrical Safety

Fire and electrical safety is also a part of employee orientation. The term *fire* is not used because it may trigger responses that could be fatal to a patient or could create panic among patients. A code number such as Code 1000 or a name such as "Code Red" usually is announced by the hospital telephone operator to alert all hospital personnel when a fire or fire drill is taking place. It is essential that all employees be aware of the location of fire extinguishers. The HUC may be expected to assist with the evacuation of patients who are endangered by the fire. If the fire is not on the unit, the HUC may help nursing personnel to close the doors to patient rooms. All hospital units or sections of the hospital are separated by fire doors. These doors are constructed to help contain the fire in one area. They also must be closed during a fire. Most hospitals teach the RACE system because it is easy to remember:

R   Rescue individuals in danger.
A   Alarm: Sound the alarm.
C   Confine the fire by closing all doors and windows.
E   Extinguish the fire with the nearest suitable fire extinguisher.

Classes of Fire

Class A: wood, paper, clothing
Class B: flammable liquids and vapors
Class C: electrical equipment
Class D: combustible or reactive metals

The HUC often is asked to call maintenance when electrical equipment used for patient care needs repair. Electrical equipment used in the nursing station must be well maintained for safety purposes.

Guidelines for Electrical Safety

- Avoid the use of extension cords.
- Do not overload electrical circuits.
- Inspect cords and plugs for breaks and fraying.
- Unplug equipment when servicing.
- Unplug equipment that has liquid spilled in it.
- Unplug and do not use equipment that is malfunctioning.

Medical Emergencies

Two medical emergencies—that is, life-threatening situations—that require calm, swift action, and good communication on the part of the HUC are cardiac arrest and respiratory arrest. (It is common hospital terminology to refer to these as *code arrests*.) When either of these conditions occurs, the hospital telephone operator is notified immediately to announce the code so that personnel who need to respond will also be notified. Some hospitals have a call system installed in patients' rooms that allows hospital personnel to alert the hospital operator, as well as the nursing station, of a patient's code (Fig. 22-5). In **cardiac arrest,** the patient's heart contractions are absent or are grossly insufficient, and no pulse and no blood pressure are detected. In **respiratory arrest**, the patient may cease to breathe, or respirations may become so depressed that the patient does not receive enough oxygen to sustain life. Both

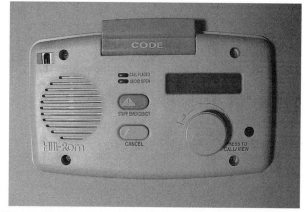

Figure 22-5 A call system installed in patients' rooms to alert the hospital operator and the nursing station of a patient's code.

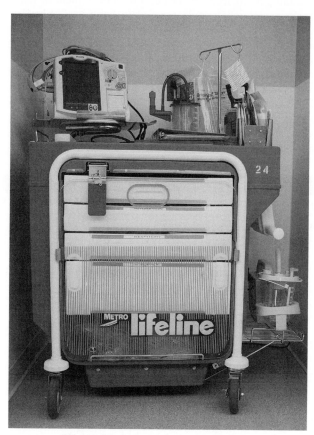

Figure 22-6 An example of a crash cart.

> ### ✎ *TAKE NOTE*
>
> It is helpful when the HUC who is working on a nearby nursing unit offers assistance to the HUC on the unit where the code is announced.

conditions require quick action by hospital personnel and the use of emergency equipment. Treatment must be instituted within 3 to 4 minutes because brain cells deteriorate rapidly from lack of oxygen.

Each hospital nursing unit and department maintains a **code** or **crash cart** (Fig. 22-6). This is taken to the code arrest patient's room immediately. It is important for HUCs to know the location of the code or crash cart and any other emergency equipment so it can be brought quickly to the nursing unit when needed.

Hospitals have designated hospital personnel who report to each code arrest. These individuals are members of the code arrest team. They may be employed in various hospital departments, such as intensive or coronary care, other nursing units, the cardiopulmonary (respiratory care) department, the pulmonary function department, surgery, and so forth.

As a member of the health care team, the HUC may be asked to perform the tasks outlined in Procedure 22-1.

Disaster Procedure

A **disaster procedure** is a planned procedure that is carried out by hospital personnel when a large number of persons have been injured. The disaster may occur during a flood, a fire, a bombing, or an accident such as a train derailment or plane crash. A group of people exposed to hazardous chemicals also would be considered a disaster situation. Every hospital maintains a disaster plan book. Disaster drills are held once or twice a year to keep hospital personnel informed and in practice. Announcing a code such as "Code 5000" on the hospital public address system activates the disaster procedure.

The HUC usually is designated to handle communication and to call off-duty health care personnel to assist in caring for hospital patients and disaster victims and in handling communications. The role of the HUC may vary among hospitals.

> ### ✎ TAKE NOTE
>
> Fire and disaster drills must be taken seriously so that all personnel will be prepared in case a fire or a disaster actually happens.

SPECIAL SERVICES

Flowers

When a health care facility is large enough to include a specific area where all flowers are delivered, the task of delivering flowers to patients may be assigned to a hospital volunteer. In this case, the HUC may need only to direct the volunteer to the correct room.

In hospitals in which the representative from the florist delivers the flowers directly to the unit, the HUC should ascertain that the patient is still on the unit or within the hospital before signing for and accepting the flowers. After signing the delivery slip, the HUC may deliver the flowers to the patient's room.

The HUC must be aware of any restrictions, for example, flowers are not allowed on some nursing units, such as intensive care or cardiopulmonary (respiratory care) units, and latex balloons are not allowed in most hospitals (especially not on

---

PROCEDURE 22-1

PROCEDURE FOR PERFORMING TASKS RELATED TO MEDICAL EMERGENCIES

Task	Notes
1. Notify the hospital telephone operator to announce the code.	1. *Notification is made by pressing a special button on the telephone, stating code arrest, and giving the location. Be very specific when stating unit, such as 4A-Apple, 4B-Boy, 4C-Charlie, or 4D-David. Some health care facilities use the expression "Code Blue" to designate a cardiac or respiratory arrest.*
2. Direct the code arrest team to the patient's room.	
3. Remove the patient information sheet from the patient's chart, and take or send the chart to the patient's room.	
4. Notify all doctors connected with the patient's case (attending doctor, consultants, and residents).	
5. Notify the patient's family of the situation if requested to do so.	5. *If the HUC does communicate with the family, the conversation should be carried on in as controlled a manner as possible, so as to not cause panic. The dialogue might be, "Mr. Whetstone, your brother's condition has changed, and the doctor thought you would like to know. The doctors are with him now. Will you be coming to the hospital?"*
6. Label laboratory specimens with the patient's ID label, enter the test ordered in the computer, and send the specimen to the laboratory stat.	
7. Call the appropriate departments for treatments and supplies as needed.	7. *Usually, cardiopulmonary (respiratory care), diagnostic imaging, and the central services department (CSD) are the departments involved.*
8. Alert the admissions department and the intensive care unit (ICU) about the possibility of a transfer to ICU.	8. *If the code procedure is successful, the patient is transferred to ICU or possibly to the critical care unit (CCU), where they can be monitored closely.*
9. For a successful code, follow Procedure 20-5 regarding transfer to another unit.	9. *See Chapter 20, p. 397.*
10. For an unsuccessful code procedure, follow Procedure 20-4 regarding postmortem care.	10. *See Chapter 20, p. 397.*

pediatric units). If family members are present, flowers and balloons may be sent home with them.

Mail

Mail is delivered to the nursing unit daily. The mail is checked and the patient's room and bed numbers are written on each envelope. In the event that the patient has been discharged, you would write "Discharged" in pencil on the envelope and return it to the mailroom. The mail may be distributed to patients as time allows, or the task may be designated to a hospital volunteer.

KEY CONCEPTS

Although the new HUC needs to learn many things upon starting employment, it is very important to know the routines and to be able to perform the tasks related to medical emergencies, fires, and disasters. When emergencies occur, there is no time to look in a book for directions about what should be done. The other tasks discussed in this chapter may not be part of the HUC's regular routine; therefore, the procedures for these can be reviewed in the hospital as time permits.

REVIEW QUESTIONS

1. Write the meaning of each abbreviation listed below in the space provided.

a. AIDS

_____

b. ARC

_____

c. CDC

_____

d. HBV

_____

e. HIV

_____

f. OSHA

_____

g. PPE

_____

h. TB

_____

i. RACE

_____

2. List four categories of events that require an incident report.

a. _____

b. _____

c. _____

d. _____

3. Describe the duties of an HUC during a fire drill.

_____

_____

4. List six guidelines that should be followed to ensure electrical safety:

a. _____

b. _____

c. _____

d. _____

e. _____

f. _____

5. Name three pathogenic microorganisms that are frequently responsible for hospital-acquired infection.

a. _____

b. _____

c. _____

6. Define the following:

a. Centers for Disease Control and Prevention

_____

b. reverse isolation

_____

c. respiratory arrest

_____

d. protective care

_____

e. pathogenic microorganisms

_____

f. medical emergency

_____

g. isolation

_____

h. incident

_____

i. communicable disease

_____

j. material safety data sheet

_____

k. cardiac arrest

_____

l. disaster procedure

_____

m. nosocomial infections

_____

n. standard precautions

_____

o. risk management

_____

p. airborne precautions

_____

7. List nine tasks that the HUC may perform during a medical emergency.

a. _____

b. _____

c. _____

d. _____

e. _____

f. _____

g. _____

h. _____

i. _____

8. What health precaution should the HUC take when handling or transporting specimens?

_____

_____

9. Why is it important to complete an incident report for events such as a nurse receiving a needle stick?

_____

_____

10. List six components that constitute the chain of infection.

a. _____

b. _____

c. _____

d. _____

e. _____

f. _____

11. Three methods by which bacteria may be transmitted include the following:

a. _____

b. _____

c. _____

12. Name three conditions that may cause a patient to become immunocompromised.

a. _____

b. _____

c. _____

13. List four types of PPE that are used with standard precautions.

a. _____

b. _____

c. _____

d. _____

14. In AIDS, what is meant by an "opportunistic infection"?

_____

15. Name the two opportunistic diseases related to AIDS.

a. _____

b. _____

16. Describe the process for acceptance and delivery of:

a. patient mail

_____

b. patient flowers

_____

THINK ABOUT...

1. Discuss the importance of fire and disaster drills.
2. Discuss the consequences of not using good hand washing technique and not adhering to standard precautions.

Websites of Interest

Centers for Disease Control and Prevention: www.cdc.gov

OSHA: www.osha-slc.gov

CHAPTER 23

Medical Terminology, Basic Human Structure, Diseases, and Disorders

UNIT 1
Medical Terminology: Word Parts, Analyzing, and Word Building

OUTLINE

UNIT OBJECTIVES

Upon completion of this unit, you will be able to:

1. Identify the three main origins of medical terms.
2. Name and define the four word parts that are commonly used in building medical terms.
3. List three guidelines to follow when connecting word parts to form a medical term.
4. Define *analysis of medical terms* and *synthesis of medical terms*.
5. Given a list of medical terms and a list of word parts, divide the medical terms into their component parts—that is, word roots, prefixes, suffixes, and combining vowels—and identify the types of word parts present in each term by name.
6. Given a description of the medical condition and a list of word parts—that is, word roots, prefixes, suffixes, and combining vowels—write out the medical term that represents a stated medical condition.

INTRODUCTION TO MEDICAL TERMS

Most medical terms are made up of Greek (e.g., *nephrology*) and Latin (e.g., *maternal*) words; however, some terms, such as *triage* and *lavage*, have been adapted from modern languages such as French. Two other sources of medical terms include acronyms and eponyms. An acronym is a word formed from the first letters of major terms in a descriptive phrase, such as laser (*l*ight *a*mplification by *s*timulated *e*mission of *r*adiation). An eponym is a name given to something that was discovered by or is identified with an individual. The Pap smear (Dr. Papanicolaou) and Lou Gehrig's disease (amyotrophic lateral sclerosis) are two examples of eponyms.

Although a background of Greek or Latin is not necessary to learn the meaning of medical terms, it is necessary to learn the English translation of the Greek or Latin word parts. In this course of study, the parts of the word are memorized rather than the whole word. By learning word parts, one will be able to build words according to a given definition and break down words into word parts to determine their meaning. For example, in the medical term

nephr / ectomy

nephr- is the word part that means "kidney" and *-ectomy* is the word part meaning "surgical removal." Thus, *nephrectomy* means "surgical removal of the kidney." Once one has memorized the meanings of the word parts (*nephr-* and *-ectomy*), one will know their meanings when they appear in other medical terms.

In the preceding example, one can define the term by literally translating it. However, a few medical terms have implied meanings.

For example, the word

an / emia

literally translated, means "without" (*an-*) "blood condition" (*-emia*). However, the correct interpretation of anemia—an implied meaning—is a deficiency of red blood cells (RBCs). Knowledge of the meanings of the word parts for a medical term with an implied meaning takes one almost, but not quite, to the exact meaning of the term.

Medical terms are used instead of English words because one medical word says what it would take many English words to say. For example, nephrectomy means "surgical removal of the kidney." Medical terms are efficient and factual, they save space, and they often describe a situation or procedure more exactly.

Pronunciation of medical terms varies. What is acceptable pronunciation in one part of the country may not be used in another part of the country; therefore, flexibility is necessary in the pronunciation of medical terms.

Correct spelling is absolutely necessary to avoid the incorrect use of a term. *Ileum* (portion of small intestine) and *ilium* (one of the bones of the hip) are two examples of terms close in spelling, yet anatomically diverse in meaning.

As you begin working with medical terminology, you may feel overwhelmed at the task of learning this new language. However, repeated use of the word parts will assist you in building your vocabulary, and soon you will be using medical terms fluently in your everyday speech. Many students employ the use of mnemonics (memory-aiding devices) to remember the word parts. For example, *entero* is the word part for "intestine." One might think of "digested food *entering* the intestine" and more easily recall the meaning of *entero*. Similarly, *ileum* of the small intestine is spelled with an *e* and one might associate "*eating*" with the intestine and not mistake this term with *ilium*, the bone in the hip.

This unit deals with word parts and how they are used together to form medical terms. *Remember:* It is important for you to master Unit 1 before proceeding to Unit 2, and so forth, because each unit is a continuation of the previously studied units.

WORD PARTS

In this course of study, the development of a medical vocabulary is based on memorizing parts of words rather than whole words. *Word part* is the term that will be used to describe the components of words. To build or analyze (divide into parts) medical terms, you first must learn the following four word parts:

1. Word root
2. Prefix
3. Suffix
4. Combining vowel

Word Root

The word root is the basic part of the word; it expresses the principal meaning of the word. For example, in the medical term

gastr / ic

gastr (stomach) is the word root.

Prefix

The prefix is the part of the word that is placed before the word root to alter its meaning. For example, in the medical term

intra / gastr / ic

intra- (within) is the prefix.

Suffix

The suffix is the part of the word that is added after the word root to alter its meaning. For example, in the medical term

gastr / ic

-ic (pertaining to) is the suffix.

Combining Vowel

The combining vowel, usually an *o*, is used between two word roots or between a word root and a suffix to ease pronunciation. Three guidelines are followed in using a combining vowel.

1. When a word root is connected to a suffix, a combining vowel usually is not used if the suffix begins with a vowel. For example, in the word [gastr / ectomy], *ectomy* (surgical removal) begins with the vowel *e*; thus, the combining vowel *o* is not used.
2. When two word roots are connected, the combining vowel is usually used even if the second root begins with a vowel. For example, in the word [gastr / o / enter / itis], the second word root *enter* (intestine) begins with the vowel *e*, but the combining vowel *o* is still used.
3. A combining vowel is not used when a prefix and a word root are connected. For example, in the medical term [sub / hepat / ic], a combining vowel is not used between the prefix, *sub-*, and the word root, *hepat*.

Note: A combining form, not a true word part, is simply the word root separated from its combining vowel with a slash mark. For example, gastr /o is a combining form. Although *o* is the most commonly used combining vowel, *a*, *e*, and *i* also may be used. Throughout this chapter, the word roots are listed in combining forms.

Word Root	Meaning
cardi / o	heart
cyt / o	cell
electr / o	electricity, electrical activity
enter / o	intestine
gastr / o	stomach
hepat / o	liver
nephr / o	kidney

Prefixes	Meaning
intra-	within
sub-	under, below
trans-	through, across, beyond

Suffixes	Meaning
-ectomy	excision, surgical removal
-gram	record, x-ray image
-ic	pertaining to
-itis	inflammation
-logy	study of

ANALYZING MEDICAL TERMS

To analyze medical terms, divide the term into word parts with the use of vertical slashes and identify the word part by labeling it as follows:

P	prefix
WR	word root
S	suffix
CV	combining vowel

After labeling and identifying, simply define the medical term according to the definitions of the word parts.

EXERCISE 1

Analyzing Medical Terms: Analyze the following medical terms by dividing each into word parts and writing *P, WR, S,* or *CV* above the appropriate part, as in the following examples. Use the list above to help you identify word parts.

Example 1: gastroenteritis

WR	CV		WR		S
gastr	/ o	/	enter	/	itis
stomach			intestine		inflammation of

Example 2: intragastric

P		WR		S
intra	/	gastr	/	ic
within		stomach		pertaining to

1. cytology _____

2. gastrectomy _____

3. subhepatic _____

4. electrocardiogram _____

5. cardiology _____

6. transhepatic _____

SYNTHESIS OF MEDICAL TERMS (WORD BUILDING)

Synthesis is the process of creating a medical term by using word parts. In building medical terms from a given definition, keep in mind that the beginning of the definition usually indicates the suffix that is needed to build the term.

EXERCISE 2

Synthesis: Build medical terms from the following definitions. Use the above list to assist you.

Example: study of the kidney—<u>nephrology</u>

1. study of the heart _____

2. study of cells _____

3. surgical removal of the stomach _____

4. inflammation of the stomach and intestines _____

5. pertaining to the stomach _____

6. pertaining to within the stomach _____

7. surgical removal of the kidney _____

REVIEW QUESTIONS

1. Name the three main origins of medical terms and give an example for each.

a. _____

b. _____

c. _____

2. List the four word parts. Define and give an example of each.

a. _____

Example: _____

b. _____

Example: _____

c. _____

Example: _____

d. _____

Example: _____

3. List the guidelines followed in connecting

   a. prefix and word root

   _____

   b. word root and word root

   _____

   c. word root and suffix

   _____

4. Define:

   a. analysis of medical terms

   _____

   b. synthesis of medical terms

   _____

UNIT 2
Body Structure, Integumentary System, and Oncology

OUTLINE

Unit Objectives
Body Structure (Anatomy) and Function (Physiology)
  Body Cells
  Body Tissues
  Body Organs
  Body Systems
  Body Cavities
  Body Directional Terms
Integumentary System
Diseases and Conditions of the Skin and Body Cells
  Cancer
  Burns
  Abscesses
  Lacerations and Abrasions

  Gangrene
  Infection
  Decubitus Ulcer
Review Questions
Medical Terminology Related to Body Structure, Integumentary System, and Oncology
  Word Parts
  Exercise 1
  Exercise 2
  Exercise 3
Medical Terms Related to Body Structure and Skin
  Exercise 4
  Exercise 5
  Exercise 6
Abbreviations
  Exercise 7

UNIT OBJECTIVES

Upon completion of this unit, you will be able to:

1. Define the terms *cell, tissue, organ,* and *system.*
2. Briefly describe the structure of the living cell.
3. Name four types of tissue.
4. List five body cavities and name a body organ contained in each.
5. List the four quadrants and nine regions of the abdominopelvic cavity.
6. Define *anatomical position* and the directional terms outlined in this unit.
7. Describe the structure and function of skin.
8. Describe cancer, burns, abscess, laceration, abrasion, gangrene, infection, and decubitus ulcer.
9. Define the unit abbreviations.

BODY STRUCTURE (ANATOMY) AND FUNCTION (PHYSIOLOGY)

Body Cells

The cell is the basic unit of all living things (Fig. 23-1). The human body is made up of trillions of cells. Cells perform specific functions, and their size and shape vary according to function. Bones, muscles, skin, and blood are all made up of different types of cells. Body cells are microscopic; approximately 2000 are needed to make an inch (although a single nerve cell may be several feet long). Cells are constantly growing and reproducing. Such growth is responsible for the development of an embryo into a child and a child into an adult. This growth is also responsible for the replacement of cells that have a relatively short life span and cells that are injured, diseased, or worn out.

To visualize the structure of a cell, we can diagrammatically compare the three main parts of the cell with the three parts of an egg: the egg shell, the egg white, and the egg yolk.

Cell Membrane

The cell membrane (egg shell), the boundary of the cell, is porous, flexible, and elastic. The protective cell membrane actively or passively regulates the movement of a substance into and out of the cell. The cell membrane keeps the cell intact. The cell dies if the cell membrane can no longer carry out these functions.

Cytoplasm

Cytoplasm (egg white) is the main body of the cell in which are found various organelles, such as the mitochondria, which are specialized structures that carry out activities necessary for the cell's survival. For example, in the muscle cell, basic contracting is done by the sarcomere within its cytoplasm, called *sarcoplasm.*

Nucleus

The nucleus (egg yolk), a small structure, is located near the center of the cell. It is the control center of the cell and plays an important role in reproduction. Chromosomes located in the nucleus contain the genes that determine hereditary characteristics. Not all cells contain a nucleus, such as the mature RBC. Some other cells, such as certain bone cells and skeletal muscle cells, contain several nuclei.

Body Tissues

A tissue is made up of a group of similar cells that work together to perform particular functions (Fig. 23-2). Tissues may be categorized into the following types:

- **Epithelial tissue:** Epithelial tissue forms a protective covering (skin) or lines body cavities (e.g., digestive, respiratory, and urinary tracts).
- **Connective tissue:** The main functions of connective tissue are to connect and hold tissues together, to transport substances, and to protect against foreign invaders. Connective tissue forms and protects bones, fat, blood cells, and cartilage and provides immunity.
- **Muscle tissue:** Muscle tissue makes up the muscles of the body that contract and relax to produce movement.
- **Nerve tissue:** Nerve tissue forms parts of the nervous system, which conducts electrochemical impulses and helps to coordinate body activities.

Body Organs

An organ is made up of two or more types of tissues that perform one or more common functions. The stomach is an organ that is made up of muscle, nerve, connective, and epithelial tissue.

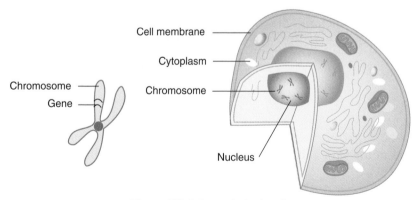

Figure 23-1 Parts of a body cell.

Body Systems

A *system* is a group of organs that work closely together in a common purpose to perform complex body functions (Fig. 23-3). For example, the urinary system is made up of the following organs: kidneys, ureters, urinary bladder, and urethra. Its main function is to remove wastes from the blood and eliminate them from the body. Other body systems include the digestive, musculoskeletal, nervous, reproductive, endocrine, circulatory, respiratory, sensory, and integumentary systems. Some organs are a part of more than one system. The pharynx, for example, is part of both the digestive and respiratory systems. In the digestive system, the pharynx allows for the passage of food; in the respiratory system, it allows for the passage of air.

Homeostasis is the maintenance of a stable, relatively constant environment within body cells and tissues. Stability of the body's normal volume, temperature, and chemicals is effected by the successful harmony of the organ systems and is regulated by the nervous and endocrine systems. Failure to keep the body systems in homeostasis results in disease.

Body Cavities

Large spaces within the body that contain internal organs, or viscera, are called *body cavities* (Fig. 23-4). The two major body cavities are the *dorsal cavity* (near the back) and the *ventral cavity* (near the front).

Dorsal Cavity

The dorsal cavity is composed of the cranial cavity and the spinal cavity, which form a continuous space.

- **Cranial cavity:** Space in the skull that contains the brain
- **Spinal cavity:** Space in the spinal column that contains the spinal cord

Ventral Cavity

The ventral cavity is composed of the thoracic (or chest) cavity and the abdominopelvic cavity.

- **Thoracic cavity:** The chest cavity contains additional spaces, including right and left pleural cavities and the mediastinum. Organs within the thoracic cavity include the heart, lungs, trachea, esophagus, thymus gland, and major blood vessels.
- **Right and left pleural cavities:** Double-walled sacs that create spaces that surround the lungs.
- **Mediastinum:** Space that contains the heart, trachea, esophagus, thymus gland, and major blood vessels.
- **Abdominopelvic cavity:** This space is divided into the abdominal cavity and the pelvic cavity.
- **Abdominal cavity:** Upper portion of the abdominopelvic cavity. This space contains the stomach; most of the intestines; and the kidneys, ureters, liver, pancreas, gallbladder, and spleen. The abdominal cavity is separated from the thoracic cavity by a muscle called the *diaphragm.*
- **Pelvic cavity:** Lower portion of the abdominopelvic cavity. This space contains the bladder, urethra, reproductive organs, part of the large intestine (sigmoid colon), and the rectum. The abdominopelvic cavity is divided into four quadrants and nine regions (Fig. 23-5). You will frequently encounter these descriptive terms during your health care employment.

Body Directional Terms

Directional terms, which are used to describe a location on or within the body, refer to the patient in the *anatomical position.* Anatomical position is the point of reference that ensures proper description: body erect, face and feet forward, arms at side, and palms facing forward. In Figure 23-11 (in Unit 3 of this chapter, page 451), the skeletal orientation is in the anatomical position.

- **Superior (cranial):** Pertaining to *above.* (The eye is located superior to the mouth.)
- **Inferior (caudal):** Pertaining to *below.* (The mouth is located inferior to the nose.)
- **Anterior (ventral):** Pertaining to *in front of.* (The eyes are located on the anterior of the head.)
- **Anteroposterior (AP):** Pertaining to *front to back.* (Directionally moving from the front to the back.)
- **Posterior (dorsal):** Pertaining to *in back of.* (The gluteus maximus is posterior to the navel.)
- **Posteroanterior (PA):** Pertaining to *back to front.* (Directionally moving from the back to the front.)
- **Lateral (lat):** Pertaining to the *side.* (The little toe is lateral to the big toe.)
- **Bilateral (bilat):** Pertaining to *two (both) sides.* (Bilateral otitis media [ear infections].)
- **Medial:** Pertaining to the *middle.* (The nose is medial to the ears.)
- **Abduction:** Pertaining to *away from.* (Spreading the fingers wide apart is an example of abduction.)
- **Adduction:** Pertaining to *toward.* (Bringing the fingers together from being spread out shows adduction.)
- **Proximal:** Pertaining to *closer than* another structure to the point of attachment. (The elbow is proximal to the wrist.)
- **Distal:** Pertaining to *farther than* another structure from the point of attachment. (The fingers are distal to the elbow.)
- **Superficial:** Toward the surface. (Hair follicles are superficial structures.)
- **Deep:** Farther from the surface. (The femur is deep to the skin.)
- **Prone:** Lying with the face downward. (The patient is placed in a prone position for suturing of the back of her head.)
- **Supine:** Lying on the back. (Supine positioning was required for his sternal puncture.)

INTEGUMENTARY SYSTEM

The integumentary system consists of the skin (the largest organ of the body) and accessory structures (hair, nails, and sweat and oil glands) (Fig. 23-6). The skin of an adult may weigh 20 pounds or more. The skin has many functions. The main one is to protect underlying tissues from

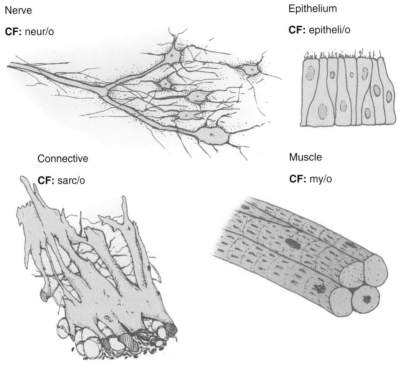

Nerve
CF: neur/o

Epithelium
CF: epitheli/o

Connective
CF: sarc/o

Muscle
CF: my/o

Figure 23-2 Types of tissues.

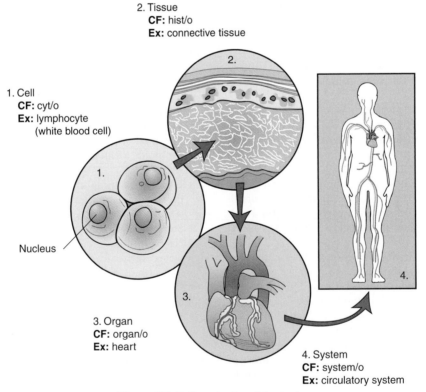

2. Tissue
  CF: hist/o
  Ex: connective tissue

1. Cell
  CF: cyt/o
  Ex: lymphocyte
    (white blood cell)

Nucleus

3. Organ
CF: organ/o
Ex: heart

4. System
CF: system/o
Ex: circulatory system

Figure 23-3 Organization of the body.

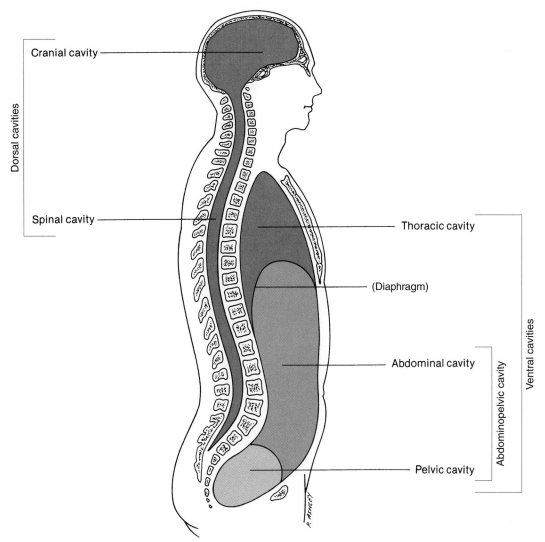

Figure 23-4 The body cavities.

pathogenic (disease-causing) microorganisms and other environmental hazards. The skin also assists in the regulation of body temperature and the synthesis of vitamin D. As a sensory organ, the specialized receptors of the skin pass messages of pain, temperature, pressure, and touch to the brain.

The thin outer layer of skin is called the *epidermis* and is composed of epithelial tissue. The cells of the innermost layer produce themselves. As they move toward the surface, the outermost cells are shed. Millions of cells are produced and shed each day. The epidermis contains no blood vessels.

The thick layer directly below the epidermis is called the *dermis*, or *true skin*. It is made up of connective tissue and contains blood vessels, nerve endings, hair follicles, and sweat and oil glands.

The subcutaneous tissue (or *hypodermis*), a thick, fat-containing tissue located below the dermis, serves to connect the skin to underlying muscles, bone, and organs.

Hair provides a protective function, for example, nasal hairs trap foreign particles to prevent them from being inhaled into the lungs. The hair follicle is a pouch-like depression in the skin from which the hair grows to extend above the skin surface. Oil glands (sebaceous glands) connect to the hair follicle through tiny ducts. Each sebaceous gland produces oil (sebum), which lubricates the hair and skin and inhibits bacterial growth.

The *sweat glands* (sudoriferous glands) are coiled, tube-like structures that are located mainly in the dermis. Each extends to the surface in the form of a tiny opening called a *pore*. Approximately 3000 pores can be found in the palm of a hand and 2,000,000 on the body surface. Sweat, a saline fluid, is produced by the sweat glands. As sweat evaporates on the body surface, it cools the body.

Skin color is determined by the amount of melanin in the epidermis of the skin. Skin color varies from pale yellow to black. A condition called *albinism* results when melanin cannot be formed by melanocytes. An albino can be recognized

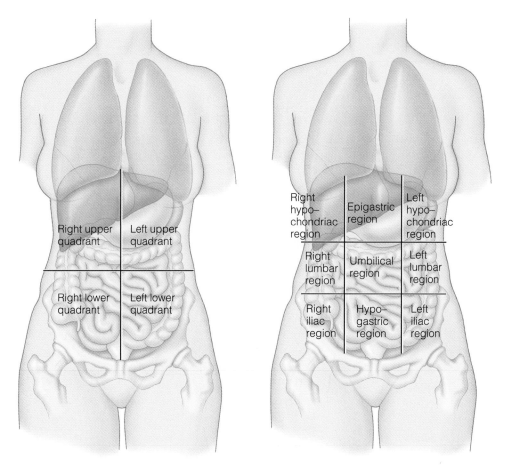

Figure 23-5 Division of the abdominopelvic cavity into four quadrants and nine regions.

by the characteristic absence of pigment in the hair, eyes, and skin.

DISEASES AND CONDITIONS OF THE SKIN AND BODY CELLS

Cancer

Cancer (often abbreviated as *Ca*) is a disease in which unregulated new growth of abnormal cells occurs. It is normal for worn-out body cells to be replaced by new cell growth and also for new cells to form to repair tissue damage. Normal cell growth is regulated; in cancer, cell division is unregulated, and cells continue to reproduce until a mass known as a *tumor*, or *neoplasm*, forms. Skin cancer arises from cell changes in the epidermis and is the most common form of human cancer. Exposure to broad-spectrum ultraviolet (UV) rays of the sun and artificial sources is thought to be an important factor in the development of skin cancer. Basal cell carcinoma and squamous cell carcinoma, two major types of skin cancers, both are very responsive to treatment and seldom metastasize (spread) to other body systems.

Cancerous tumors are malignant, which means they become progressively worse, whereas noncancerous tumors are benign or nonrecurrent. Malignant tumors grow in a disorganized fashion, interrupting body function and interfering with the food and blood supply to normal cells. Malignant cells may metastasize from one organ to another through the bloodstream or the lymphatic system.

Cancer consists of many different diseases, and a single cause of this abnormal cell division cannot be pinpointed. Genetic factors, steroidal estrogens, cigarette smoking, exposure to carcinogenic substances, and UV rays are believed to be among the causes of cancer.

Detection of cancer requires self-examination, x-ray imaging, blood tests, and microscopic tissue examination. Treatments for patients with cancer include surgery, chemotherapy, and radiation therapy.

Cancer's Seven Warning Signals

The seven warning signals of cancer may be recalled easily by the mnemonic CAUTION.

  <u>C</u>hange in bowel or bladder habits
  <u>A</u> sore that does not heal
  <u>U</u>nusual bleeding or discharge
  <u>T</u>hickening or lump in the breast, testes, or elsewhere
  <u>I</u>ndigestion or difficulty in swallowing
  <u>O</u>bvious change in a wart or mole
  <u>N</u>agging cough or hoarseness

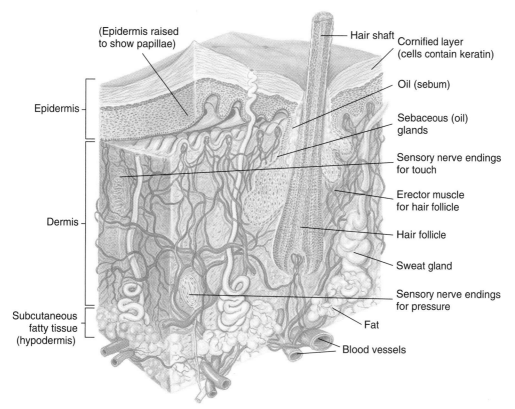

(Epidermis raised to show papillae)

Hair shaft

Cornified layer (cells contain keratin)

Oil (sebum)

Epidermis

Sebaceous (oil) glands

Sensory nerve endings for touch

Erector muscle for hair follicle

Dermis

Hair follicle

Sweat gland

Sensory nerve endings for pressure

Subcutaneous fatty tissue (hypodermis)

Fat

Blood vessels

Figure 23-6 The skin.

Burns

All burns are dangerous if they are not treated properly because infection can occur, and because shock is possible in more serious burns as a result of fluid loss from the skin. Burns are classified according to degree of severity, which reflects the depth of the burn (full or partial thickness) (Fig. 23-7) and the extent of surface area involvement (Fig. 23-8).

1. *First-degree burns* damage the epidermis. Also called a *partial-thickness* burn, sunburn is an example of a first-degree burn in which redness, minor discomfort, and slight edema may be present.
2. *Second-degree burns* damage the epidermis and the dermis. Also called *partial-thickness burns,* second-degree burns account for symptoms such as redness, pain, edema, and blisters.
3. *Third-degree* burns destroy the epidermis, dermis, and subcutaneous tissue. They are also called *full-thickness burns.* No pain occurs because the skin's sensory receptors are destroyed. Third-degree burns heal only from the edges, and debridement (removal of dead skin) and skin grafts are necessary.

Abscesses

An *abscess* is a cavity that contains pus. Abscesses usually are caused by pathogenic microorganisms that invade the tissue through a break in the skin. As the microorganisms destroy the tissue, an increased blood supply is rushed to the area, causing inflammation in the surrounding tissue. Abscesses are formed by the body to wall off the pathogenic microorganisms and keep them from spreading throughout the body.

Lacerations and Abrasions

A *laceration* is a wound that is produced by tearing of body tissue. An *abrasion* is a scraping away of the skin. Keeping lacerations and abrasions clean is important because of the danger of infection. Suturing may be required to repair lacerations.

Gangrene

Gangrene, a serious medical condition, is the death of body tissue caused by lack of blood supply to an area of the body; often, it is the result of infection or injury. Symptoms include fever, pain, darkening of the skin, and an unpleasant odor. Treatment, depending on the underlying cause, includes surgical debridement (removal with a sharp instrument) of necrotic tissue or amputation, administration of intravenous (IV) antibiotics, and the use of hyperbaric oxygen therapy to help kill the bacteria.

Infection

Infection is the invasion of the body by pathogenic microorganisms that reproduce and multiply, causing disease. Infections may be caused by streptococcal, staphylococcal, or *Pseudomonas* bacteria; by viruses; or by other organisms. Bacterial infections are treated with antibiotic therapy. Methicillin-resistant *Staphylococcus aureus* (MRSA) has become a widespread nosocomial (hospital- or health care setting–acquired) pathogen. The main mode of transmission of MRSA

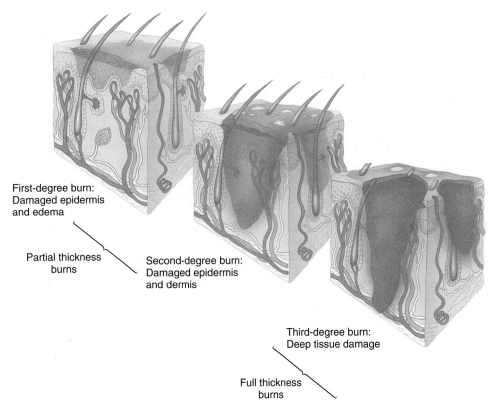

First-degree burn:
Damaged epidermis
and edema

Partial thickness
burns

Second-degree burn:
Damaged epidermis
and dermis

Third-degree burn:
Deep tissue damage

Full thickness
burns

Figure 23-7 First-degree burns damage the epidermis; second-degree burns damage the epidermis and the dermis; third-degree burns damage the epidermis, the dermis, and the subcutaneous tissue.

in the clinical setting is through the hands of health care workers. MRSA can be found on the skin, in the nose, and in blood and urine. Proper hand cleansing techniques should be reviewed with new employees by the Infection Control Department of the clinical setting to avoid transmission of MRSA.

Decubitus Ulcer

Decubitus ulcer, also known as *bedsore* or *pressure sore,* is a vascular condition that arises in patients who sit or lie in one position for long periods of time. The weight of the body, typically over bony projections such as the hips, heels, and ankles, slows blood flow, causing ulcers to form, and infection may develop when microorganisms enter the affected area. The decubitus ulcer, similar to the burn, is categorized according to severity in terms of stages (stage I to stage IV). Beginning as a reddened, sensitive, unbroken patch of skin categorized as *stage I,* the pressure sore may progress to an open sore (ulcer) for which strict attention to wound care is required. In stage IV, the patient may experience full-thickness skin loss with damage to muscle, bone, or other body structures. Periodic body position changes and soft support cushions may help to prevent the onset of pressure sores.

REVIEW QUESTIONS

1. Define the following terms:

a. cell: _____

b. tissue: _____

c. organ: _____

d. system: _____

2. Name four types of tissue.

a. _____

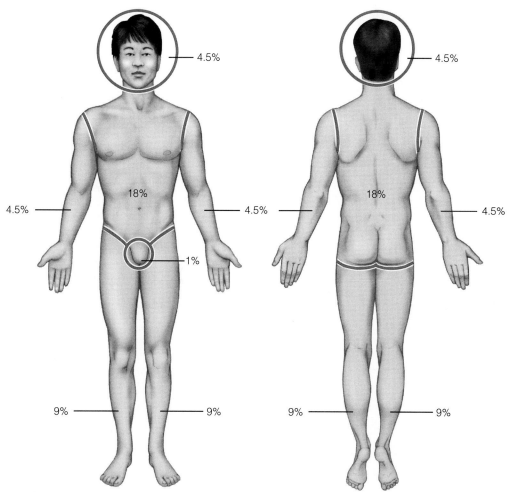

Figure 23-8 Surface area involvement of burns. The *rule of nines* is one method used to estimate the total body surface area (TBSA) burned in an adult. This method divides the TBSA into multiples of 9% (1% for the groin). The Lund-Browder Chart is used for infants and children because the surface area of the head and neck is greater than for adults, and the limbs are smaller.

b. _____

c. _____

d. _____

3. List five body cavities and name one internal organ contained in each.

a. _____

b. _____

c. _____

d. _____

e. _____

4. Match each directional term in Column 1 with its correct meaning in Column 2.

Column 1
a. superior
b. inferior
c. lateral
d. medial
e. anterior
f. posterior
g. adduction
h. abduction
i. proximal
j. distal
k. deep
l. superficial
m. supine
n. prone
o. anteroposterior
p. posteroanterior

Column 2
_____ 1. in front of
_____ 2. pertaining to the middle
_____ 3. pertaining to away from
_____ 4. pertaining to the side
_____ 5. above
_____ 6. below
_____ 7. pertaining to toward
_____ 8. in back of
_____ 9. farther from the surface
_____ 10. nearer (point of reference)
_____ 11. closer to the surface
_____ 12. farther from (point of reference)
_____ 13. lying with face downward
_____ 14. lying on the back
_____ 15. from back to front
_____ 16. from front to back

5. List four functions of the skin.

a. _____

b. _____

c. _____

d. _____

6. The thin outermost layer of the skin is called the _____. The thick layer of skin directly below this layer is called the _____. The innermost layer of fat-containing tissue is called the _____ tissue.

7. Skin color is determined by the amount of _____ in the skin. Absence of this results in _____.

8. _____ glands produce oil that lubricates the skin and hair.

9. _____ open to the surface of the skin in tiny openings called *pores.*

10. Describe the three main structures of a living cell.

_____

11. Match the terms in Column 1 with the phrases in Column 2.

Column 1
a. burns
b. abscess
c. laceration

d. gangrene
e. infection
f. cancer
g. abrasion
h. decubitus ulcer

Column 2
_____ 1. cavity that contains pus
_____ 2. classified according to degree of severity
_____ 3. invasion of the body by pathogenic microorganisms
_____ 4. new growth of abnormal cells
_____ 5. death of body tissue
_____ 6. wound produced by tearing
_____ 7. pressure sore
_____ 8. scraping away of skin

MEDICAL TERMINOLOGY RELATED TO BODY STRUCTURE, INTEGUMENTARY SYSTEM, AND ONCOLOGY

Upon mastery of medical terminology for this unit, you will be able to:

1. Define, spell, and pronounce the medical terms listed in this unit.
2. Analyze the medical terms that are built from word parts.
3. Given the meaning of a medical condition, build the corresponding medical terms, using word parts.

Word Parts

Listed below are the word parts you will be working with in this unit. You will need to memorize each one because you will continue to use them in this chapter and in your work environment. The exercises that follow these lists will assist you in this task. Practice pronouncing each word part aloud.

To review, a word root is the basic part of the word; a combining form is the word root plus a combining vowel (generally an *o*); a prefix is the modifying word part added to the beginning of a word, and a suffix is the modifying word part added to the end of a word root.

Word Roots/Combining Forms	Meaning
cancer / o, carcin / o (kăn-sĕr-ō) (kar′-sĭn-ō),	cancer
cutane/ o (kyū-tā′-nē-ō),	skin
cyt / o (sĭ′-to)	cell
dermat / o (dĕr′-mĕ-tō)	
derm / o (dĕr′-mō)	
epitheli / o (ĕp-ī-thē′-lē-ō)	epithelium
hist /o (hĭs′-to)	tissue
lip / o (lĭp′-ō)	fat
onc / o (ŏn′-kō)	
path / o (păth′-ō)	disease
sarc / o (sar′-cō)	connective tissue, flesh
trich / o (trĭk′-ō)	hair
ungu / o (ŭng′-ŭ-ō)	nail
viscer / o (vĭs′-ĕr-ō)	internal organs

Many of the suffixes presented in this course of study are made up of word roots and suffixes. For example, the suffix *-logy* (or *-ology*) is built from *log* (word root for "study") plus *-y* (suffix). For learning purposes, these will be studied as suffixes and analyzed as a single word part.

Prefixes	Meaning
sub-	under, below
trans- (trăns)	through, across, beyond

Suffixes	Meaning
-al, -ous	pertaining to
-genic (jĕn′-ĭk)	producing, originating, causing
-itis (ī′-tĭs)	inflammation
-oid (oyd)	resembling
-ologist (ŏl′-o-jĭst)	one who specializes in the diagnosis and treatment of (doctor)
-ology (ŏl′-o-jē)	study of
-oma (ō′-mah)	tumor

EXERCISE 1

Define each combining form listed below.

1. viscer / o

   _____

2. dermat / o

   _____

3. cyt / o

   _____

4. hist / o

   _____

5. derm / o

   _____

6. trich / o

   _____

7. path / o

   _____

8. carcin / o

   _____

9. sarc /o

   _____

10. epitheli / o

   _____

11. lip / o

_____

12. onc / o

_____

13. cutane / o

_____

14. cancer / o

_____

15. ungu / o

_____

EXERCISE 2

Define each suffix and prefix listed below.

1. -al

_____

2. -logy

_____

3. -logist

_____

4. -oid

_____

5. -itis

_____

6. -oma

_____

7. -genic

_____

8. trans-

_____

9. -ous

_____

10. sub-

_____

EXERCISE 3

Write the word parts for each definition below. Indicate which word parts are suffixes by writing S _in the space provided, indicate which word parts are word roots or combining forms by writing_ WR _in the space provided, and indicate which word parts are prefixes by writing_ P _in the space provided._

Meaning	Word Part	Type of Word Part
Example: inflammation	-itis	S
1. cell	_____	_____
2. skin		
a.	_____	_____
b.	_____	_____
c.	_____	_____
3. specialist	_____	_____
4. resembling	_____	_____
5. internal organs	_____	_____
6. tissues	_____	_____
7. pertaining to		
a.	_____	_____
b.	_____	_____
8. study of	_____	_____
9. through, across, beyond	_____	_____
10. cancer		
a.	_____	_____
b.	_____	_____
c.	_____	_____
11. under, below	_____	_____

MEDICAL TERMS RELATED TO BODY STRUCTURE AND SKIN

Listed below are the medical terms you need to know for this unit. Practice pronouncing these words aloud. Following the list are exercises that will assist you in learning these terms.

General Terms	Meaning
carcinogenic (kar′-sĭn-ō-jēn′-ik)	producing cancer
cytoid (sī′-toyd)	resembling a cell
cytology (sī-tŏl′-o-jē)	study of cells
dermal (dēr′-mal)	pertaining to the skin (may also use the term _cutaneous_)
dermatoid (dēr′-măh-toyd)	resembling skin
dermatologist (dēr-măh-tŏl′-o-jĭst)	one who specializes in the diagnosis and treatment of skin (diseases)

General Terms	Meaning
dermatology (dĕr-măh-tŏl′-o-je)	study of skin (branch of medicine that deals with diagnosis and treatment of skin disease)
dermoid (dĕrm′-ōid)	resembling skin
epithelial (ĕp-ĭ-thē′-lē-al)	pertaining to epithelium
histology (hĭs-tŏl′-o-jē)	study of tissues
oncology (ŏn-kol′-o-jē)	study of cancer
pathogenic (păth-ö-jĕn′-ĭk)	producing disease
pathologist (pă-thŏl′-o-jĭst)	one who specializes in the diagnosis and treatment of disease (body changes caused by disease)
pathology (pă-thŏl′-o-jē)	the study of disease
subcutaneous (sŭb-cŭ-tān′-ē-ŭs)	pertaining to under the skin
subungual (sŭb-ŭng′-ŭăl)	pertaining to under the nail
transdermal (trăns-dĕr′-mal), or transcutaneous	pertaining to (entering) through the skin
trichoid (trĭk′-oyd)	resembling hair
visceral (vĭs′-er-al)	pertaining to internal organs

Diagnostic Terms	Meaning
carcinoma (kăr-sĭ-nō′-mah)	cancerous tumor (malignant)
dermatitis (dĕr-mah-tī′-tĭs)	inflammation of the skin
epithelioma (ĕp-ĭ-thē-lē-ō′-mah)	tumor (composed of) epithelial cells
lipoma (li-pō′-mah)	tumor (containing) fat
sarcoma (sar-kō′-mah)	tumor (composed of) connective tissue (highly malignant)

EXERCISE 4

Analyze and define each term listed below.

Example: pathologist
Analyze:

WR	/	CV	/	S
path	/	o	/	logist

Define:
Specialist in the diagnosis and treatment of disease

1. cytology

_____

_____

2. trichoid

_____

_____

3. pathology

_____

_____

4. pathogenic

_____

_____

5. dermal

_____

_____

6. cytoid

_____

_____

7. visceral

_____

_____

8. histology

_____

_____

9. dermatologist

_____

_____

10. dermatitis

_____

_____

11. carcinogenic

_____

_____

12. epithelial

_____

_____

13. carcinoma

_____

_____

14. epithelioma

_____

_____

15. sarcoma

_____

_____

16. lipoma

_____

_____

17. pathologist

_____

_____

18. dermatoid

_____

_____

19. dermatology

_____

_____

20. transdermal

_____

_____

21. oncology

_____

_____

22. subungual

_____

_____

23. subcutaneous

_____

_____

EXERCISE 5

Build the medical terms that correspond with the definitions listed here. Remember that the beginning of the definition usually indicates the suffix that is needed to build the term.

1. resembling a cell

_____

2. resembling hair

_____

3. resembling skin

a. _____

b. _____

4. one who specializes in the diagnosis and treatment of disease (body changes caused by disease)

_____

5. one who specializes in the diagnosis and treatment of skin (diseases)

_____

6. pertaining to the skin

a. _____

b. _____

7. pertaining to the internal organs

_____

8. study of tissues

_____

9. study of disease

_____

10. study of skin

_____

11. producing disease

_____

12. study of cells

_____

13. inflammation of the skin

_____

14. tumor containing fat

_____

15. tumor composed of epithelial cells

_____

16. pertaining to epithelium

_____

17. producing cancer

_____

18. a tumor composed of connective tissue

_____

19. cancerous tumor

_____

20. pertaining to through the skin

_____

21. study of cancer

_____

22. pertaining to under the nail

_____

23. pertaining to under the skin

_____

EXERCISE 6

Write each medical term studied in this unit by having some-one dictate all terms to you.

1. _____

2. _____

3. _____

4. _____

5. _____

6. _____

7. _____

8. _____

9. _____

10. _____

11. _____

12. _____

13. _____

14. _____

15. _____

16. _____

17. _____

18. _____

19. _____

20. _____

21. _____

22. _____

23. _____

24. _____

25. _____

ABBREVIATIONS

Abbreviation	Meaning
AP	anteroposterior
Ca	cancer
Lat	lateral
LLQ	left lower quadrant
LUQ	left upper quadrant
PA	posteroanterior
RLQ	right lower quadrant
RUQ	right upper quadrant
SQ	subcutaneous

EXERCISE 7

Define the following abbreviations.

1. PA

   _____

2. RUQ

   _____

3. AP

   _____

4. RLQ

   _____

5. SQ

   _____

6. Lat

   _____

7. Ca

   _____

8. LLQ

   _____

9. LUQ

   _____

UNIT 3
The Musculoskeletal System

OUTLINE

UNIT OBJECTIVES

Upon completion of this unit, you will be able to:

1. Describe five functions of the skeletal system.
2. Describe bone structure.
3. Name, number, and spell correctly the bones of the body.
4. Distinguish between the axial skeleton and the appendicular skeleton.
5. Define joint, ligament, and tendon.
6. Describe the four main functions of the muscular system.
7. Describe three types of muscles.
8. Describe arthritis, herniated disk, osteoporosis, Paget's disease, types of fractures, and joint replacement.
9. Define the unit abbreviations.

THE SKELETAL SYSTEM

Organs of the Skeletal System

An adult skeleton has 206 bones.

Functions of the Skeletal System

- **Protection:** To protect the internal organs from injury
- **Support:** To provide a framework for the body
- **Movement:** To act with the muscles to produce body movement
- **Blood cell production:** To produce blood cells (hematopoiesis) in the red marrow of certain bones
- **Mineral storage:** To store calcium and phosphorus—minerals essential for cellular activities

Bone Structure

- There are four types of bones: long, short, flat, and irregular.
- Bones have their own system of blood vessels and nerves.
- Bones contain *red bone marrow* (produces red blood cells, white blood cells, and platelets) and *yellow bone marrow* (consists mostly of adipose tissue, or fat).
- Bones are covered with a thin membrane called *periosteum*, which is necessary for growth and repair and is the attachment point for ligaments and tendons.

Axial Skeleton

The axial skeleton (80 bones) consists of skull, hyoid bone, vertebral column, and rib cage and is so named because the bones revolve around the vertical *axis* of the skeleton.

Bone Framework of the Head

(Fig. 23-9)

Skull/Cranium (8 Bones):
- **Frontal bone (1):** Framework of the forehead and roof of the eye socket
- **Parietal bones (2):** Form the upper sides of the cranium
- **Temporal bones (2):** Form the lower sides of the cranium and contain parts of the ear
- **Ethmoid bone (1):** Forms part of the cranial floor and part of the nasal cavity
- **Sphenoid bone (1):** Bat-shaped bone that extends behind the eyes and forms part of the base of the skull
- **Occipital bone (1):** Composes the back and most of the base of the skull. It connects with the parietal and temporal bones

Facial Bones (14 Bones):
- **Maxillary bones (2):** Upper jaw bones
- **Mandible (1):** Lower jaw bone; the only movable bone in the skull
- **Nasal bones (2):** Support the bridge of the nose
- **Lacrimal bones (2):** Corners of the eye sockets
- **Zygomatic bones (2):** Cheekbones
- **Vomer (1):** Lower portion of the nasal septum
- **Inferior nasal concha (2):** Lateral walls of the nasal cavity

- **Palatine (2):** Hard palate and part of nasal cavities and orbit walls
- **Hyoid bone (1):** U-shaped bone in the throat; anchors the tongue
- **Auditory ossicles (6):** In the middle ear; transmit sound
- **Malleus (2):** Hammer
- **Incus (2):** Anvil
- **Stapes (2):** Stirrup

Vertebral Column (26 Vertebrae)

(Fig. 23-10)

- **Cervical (7):** The first seven vertebrae; form the neck
- **Thoracic (12):** The next 12 vertebrae; form the outward curve of the spine and join with 12 pairs of ribs
- **Lumbar (5):** The next five vertebrae, the largest and strongest; form the inward curvature of the spine
- **Sacrum (1):** The next five vertebrae; fuse together to form one sacrum in the adult
- **Coccyx (1):** The last three to five vertebrae; in the adult, these fuse together to form one coccyx

The vertebrae form the spinal column. Openings in the vertebrae provide a continuous space through which the spinal cord travels. The vertebrae are separated by disks (plates of cartilage). The central portion of the disk is filled with a pulpy elastic substance called *nucleus pulposus*. The disks allow for flexibility and absorb shock. The lamina is located on the posterior arch of the vertebra.

Rib Cage (24 Bones)

(Fig. 23-11)

All 24 ribs (12 pairs) are attached posteriorly to the thoracic vertebrae. The first seven pairs of ribs *(true ribs)* attach anteriorly to the sternum; the next three pairs converge and join the seventh rib anteriorly; the last two pairs remain free at the anterior ends. The last five pairs of ribs are called *false ribs* because they do not attach directly to the sternum. The last two pairs are often referred to as *free* or *floating ribs*.

Sternum (1 Bone)

The sternum is the breastbone.

Appendicular Skeleton (126 Bones)

The appendicular skeleton consists of the limbs that have been appended to the axial skeleton.

Upper Extremities (64 Bones)

- **Clavicle (2):** Collar bone
- **Scapula (2):** Shoulder blade

  Arm and Hand Bones (60 Bones):
  - **Humerus (2):** Upper arm bone
  - **Ulna (2):** Smaller lower arm bone, small finger side
  - **Radius (2):** Larger lower arm bone, thumb side
  - **Carpals (16):** Wrist bones
  - **Metacarpals (10):** Bones of the hand
  - **Phalanges (28):** Three bones in each finger and two bones in each thumb

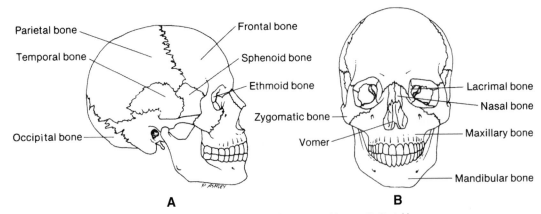

Figure 23-9 The bones of the skull. **A,** Cranial bones. **B,** Facial bones.

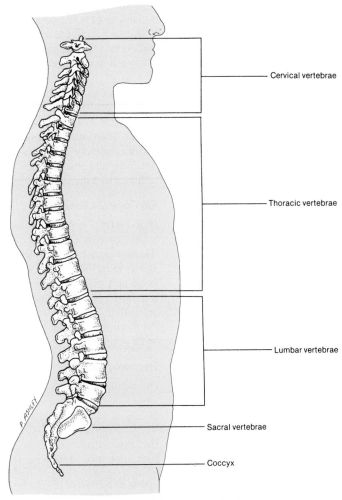

Figure 23-10 The vertebral column.

Lower Extremities (62 Bones)

In the child, the pelvic girdle consists of three pairs of separate bones: a superior element (the ilium) and two inferior elements (the ischium posteriorly and the pubis anteriorly). These bones fuse during adolescence and form the single pelvic bone on either side, characteristic of the adult.

Pelvic or Hip Bones (Fused):
- **Ilium (2):** Upper hip bones
- **Ischium (2):** Lower (sitting) hip bones
- **Pubis (2):** Front hip bones

Leg and Foot Bones:
- **Femur (2):** Thigh bone; largest bone in the body
- **Patella (2):** Kneecap

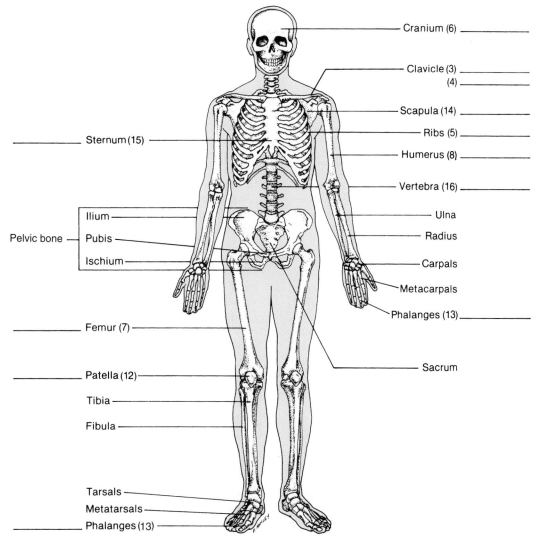

Figure 23-11 The skeleton.

- **Tibia (2):** Larger, inner lower leg bone (shin bone)
- **Fibula (2):** Smaller, outer lower leg bone
- **Tarsals (14):** Instep bones; form heel and back portion of foot
- **Metatarsals (10):** Bones of the foot
- **Phalanges (28):** Three bones in each toe, except for two in each big toe

Joints

A joint is that place in the skeleton where two or more bones meet. Joints allow for movement and hold bones together. Immovable joints, which are found only in the skull, are called *sutures*. In the newborn, the sutures are not yet entirely closed; these fontanels or soft spots allow for "give" in the skull during the birth process. Ligaments are tough bands of tissue that connect one bone with another bone at a joint.

THE MUSCULAR SYSTEM

Organs of the Muscular System

Muscles: More than 600 muscles are included in the human body.

Muscular Function

Muscles enable movement of body parts (including blood through blood vessels, food through the digestive system, and glandular secretions through ducts), maintain posture, stabilize joints, and generate heat. Supplies of oxygen and nerves to the muscle are necessary for adequate muscle function.

Types of Muscles

- **Skeletal muscle:** Skeletal muscles enable the body to move. These muscles are attached to the bones by tendons. Motion is produced by the contraction of muscles, and the muscles often work in pairs. Skeletal muscle is a voluntary muscle in that it is controlled by the conscious portion of the brain.
- **Smooth muscle:** Smooth muscles generally make up the walls of hollow organs and serve to propel substances through body passageways and to adjust the pupil. Smooth muscles, which are involuntary muscles, may be found in the walls of blood vessels, in the eye, and in the digestive, urinary, and reproductive tracts.

- **Cardiac muscle:** Cardiac muscle, which is found only in the heart, is an involuntary muscle because it is not under the control of the conscious part of the brain, but it does respond to impulses from the autonomic nerves. It is especially conductive and contractile.

DISEASES AND CONDITIONS OF THE MUSCULOSKELETAL SYSTEM

Arthritis

More than 100 types of joint diseases are known; the two most common types are rheumatoid arthritis and osteoarthritis. Much is still unknown about the causes of arthritis; however, it has been observed that emotional upset can aggravate the disease.

Rheumatoid Arthritis

Rheumatoid arthritis, which is thought to be an autoimmune disease, usually occurs between the ages of 35 and 50 years, more commonly in women. The onset of symptoms, which include malaise, fever, weight loss, and stiffness of the joints, is gradual. The symptoms come and go. If the disease becomes chronic, degeneration of the joints, with permanent damage, occurs. Treatment consists of heat and drugs such as aspirin, nonsteroidal anti-inflammatory drugs (NSAIDs), and corticosteroids, given to reduce inflammation and pain.

Osteoarthritis

Osteoarthritis, the most common form of arthritis, usually occurs in weight-bearing joints, such as the hips or knees, as chronic inflammation of the bone and joints caused by degenerative changes in the cartilage covering the surfaces of the joints. It occurs most often in older individuals. Treatment consists of drugs to reduce pain and inflammation and physical therapy to loosen the impaired joints.

Ruptured Disk

A *ruptured disk* also may be referred to as a slipped or herniated disk or as a herniated nucleus pulposus (HNP). It is the abnormal protrusion of the soft, gelatinous core of an intervertebral disk (nucleus pulposus) into the neural canal that causes pressure on the spinal cord. Such herniation generally occurs in the lumbar spine (lower back). Treatment consists of bed rest, physical therapy, and analgesics. A laminectomy may be performed to remove a portion of the vertebra, creating more room for the protruding portion of the disk, or a diskectomy may be performed, in which the disk is removed and two or more vertebrae are fused together (Fig. 23-12).

Osteoporosis

Osteoporosis, an abnormal decrease in bone mass, is the leading cause of fractures because the bone tissue becomes porous, thin, and brittle. It is the most prevalent bone disease in the world. More than 20 million people in the United States have osteoporosis. Postmenopausal estrogen-deficient women are most likely to be affected. Age-related osteoporosis affects men and women equally. Osteoporosis is known as the "silent crippler," which results in a virtually symptomless process.

Symptoms occur after the disease has progressed. The most common symptoms are pain and loss of height due to the bent-over position that the person assumes. The disease can cause up to an 8-inch loss in height. Fractures can occur in all parts of the skeletal system.

Osteoporosis is diagnosed by radiologic and laboratory studies performed to measure bone density and serum calcium levels. Because onset of the disease is virtually symptom free, the focus is on prevention to minimize bone loss. Preventive and therapeutic measures, aimed at improving bone density, include taking calcium supplements and vitamin D, weight-bearing exercise, hormone replacement therapy (if appropriate), and attention to correct posture. Bisphosphonates and calcitonin, drugs that slow down the dissolving process of the osteoclasts, are also useful in treating osteoporosis.

Paget's Disease (Osteitis Deformans)

Paget's disease, the second most common bone disease in the world, causes bones to become extremely weak. Affected individuals are generally older than 40 years of age. The bone may fracture with a very slight blow. If the vertebrae are involved, they may collapse. Bones are living substances that are involved in a constant process of dissolving and rebuilding. Osteoblasts are the cells that rebuild bone, and osteoclasts are the cells that dissolve bone. An imbalance of this dissolving and rebuilding process results in weak areas or lesions of the bone.

The symptoms of Paget's disease depend on the bones that are affected. Lesions in long bones cause pain, bowing, and arthritic changes in the extremities. When the disease affects the skull, the patient may have headaches, ringing in the ears, hearing loss, and dizziness. If skull involvement affects the occipital region, pressure is placed on the cerebellum that may compress the spinal cord. Pressure on the spinal cord causes neurologic changes such as muscle weakness, loss of coordination, and ataxia.

Diagnosis is confirmed by abnormal radiologic studies characteristic of Paget's disease and by elevated laboratory values for serum alkaline phosphatase, an enzyme produced by the osteoblasts during bone formation. Treatment for Paget's disease includes use of a bisphosphonate or calcitonin to slow down the dissolving process of the osteoclasts.

Fractures

Fracture, the medical term for break (often abbreviated *Fx*), is an injury to a bone in which the bone is broken (Fig. 23-13). A fracture is classified by the bone that is injured, such as fractured radius. Some types of fractures are listed here:

- **Closed (simple):** A broken bone with no open wound
- **Open (compound):** A broken bone with an open wound in the skin
- **Greenstick (incomplete):** A partially bent and partially broken bone; this is more commonly seen in children in whom the bone is more pliable than in an adult
- **Comminuted:** Splintered or crushed bone
- **Spiral:** A bone that has been twisted apart
- **Compression:** Occurs when the vertebrae collapse through trauma or pathology

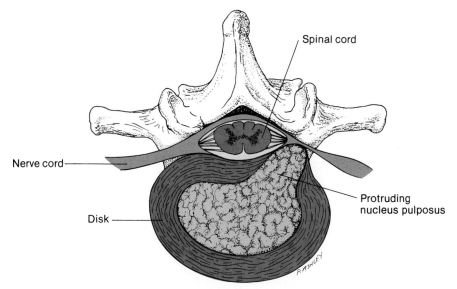

Figure 23-12 Ruptured disk.

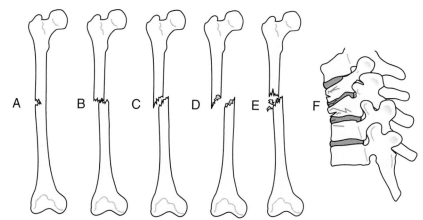

Figure 23-13 Types of fractures. **A,** Greenstick. **B,** Transverse. **C,** Oblique. **D,** Spiral. **E,** Comminuted. **F,** Compression.

An *open* or *closed reduction* is used to correct a displaced fracture to restore the fractured ends into normal alignment. In a closed reduction, the bone is realigned through manipulation and/or traction without an incision, whereas an open reduction with internal fixation (ORIF) is performed after an incision is made into the fracture site. Internal or external devices (plates, nails, screws, or rods) may be applied to maintain proper alignment of the bone during healing.

Joint Replacement

Joint replacement, a surgical procedure known as *arthroplasty*, is performed to replace an arthritic or damaged joint. An artificial joint, or *prosthesis*, is used to replace the patient's hip or knee joint. With total or partial arthroplasty, hip and knee joints and, less commonly, ankle, elbow, shoulder, wrist, and finger joints are replaced in cases of advanced osteoarthritis and improperly healed fracture, or to relieve a chronically painful or stiff joint.

REVIEW QUESTIONS

1. List five functions of the skeletal system.

a. _____

b. _____

c. _____

d. _____

e. _____

2. _____ is a thin membrane that covers bones.

3. Write the names of the bones that make up the cranium and the face. Indicate the number of each.

Cranium

a. _____

b. _____

c. _____

d. _____

e. _____

f. _____

Face

a. _____

b. _____

c. _____

d. _____

e. _____

f. _____

g. _____

h. _____

4. Name the bone in the throat that anchors the tongue.

_____

5. Name the middle ear bones and indicate the number of each.

a. _____

b. _____

c. _____

6. List the five regions of the vertebral column and indicate the number of vertebrae in each region.

a. _____

b. _____

c. _____

d. _____

e. _____

7. Write the name of the bone to match the definitions written below.

a. shoulder blade _____

b. collarbone _____

c. upper arm bone _____

d. lower arm bone, thumb side _____

e. lower arm bone, finger side _____

f. wrist bones _____

g. bones of the hand _____

h. finger bones _____

8. Write the names of three pairs of bones that are fused together to form the pelvis.

a. _____

b. _____

c. _____

9. List the bones of the leg and foot.

a. _____

b. _____

c. _____

d. _____

e. _____

f. _____

g. _____

10. Name the three types of muscles and give an example of each. Note whether the muscle type is voluntary or involuntary.

a. _____

b. _____

c. _____

11. Define:

a. joint

_____

b. tendon

_____

    c. ligament

    _____

12. Two types of arthritis are:

    a. _____

    b. _____

13. Two operations that may be performed for a herniated disk are:

    a. _____

    b. _____

14. Define:

    a. closed fracture

    _____

    b. open fracture

    _____

    c. spiral fracture

    _____

    d. comminuted fracture

    _____

    e. greenstick fracture

    _____

    f. compression fracture

    _____

15. Joint replacement is also called _____.

16. Cells that dissolve bone are called _____, and cells that rebuild bone are called _____.

17. When Paget's disease affects the skull, symptoms include the following:

    a. _____

    b. _____

    c. _____

    d. _____

18. An abnormal decrease in the amount of bone mass is called _____.

19. In osteoporosis, preventive interventions include:

a. _____

b. _____

c. _____

d. _____

e. _____

MEDICAL TERMINOLOGY RELATED TO THE MUSCULOSKELETAL SYSTEM—PREFIXES AND SUFFIXES

Upon mastery of the medical terminology for this unit, you will be able to:

1. Define and spell the word parts and medical terms presented in this unit of study.
2. Analyze the medical terms built from word parts.
3. Given the meaning of a medical condition related to the musculoskeletal system, build with word parts the corresponding medical term.
4. Given descriptions of hospital situations in which the health unit coordinator (HUC) may encounter medical terminology, apply the correct medical terms to the situations.

Word Parts

Listed below are the word parts related to the skeletal system that you need to memorize. The exercises included in this unit will help you with this task. You will continue to use these word parts throughout the course and during employment. Practice pronouncing each word element aloud.

Skeletal System	Meaning
1. arthr / o (ar'-thrō)	joint
2. chondr / o (kŏn'-drō)	cartilage
3. clavic / o (klăv'-ĭ-kō)	clavicle (collarbone)
4. clavicul / o (klah-vĭk'-ū-lō)	clavicle (collarbone)
5. cost / o (kŏs'-tō)	rib
6. crani / o (krā'-nē-ō)	cranium (skull)
7. femor / o (fĕm'-or-ō)	femur (thigh bone)
8. humer / o (hūm'-er-ō)	humerus (upper arm bone)
9. lamin / o (lăm'-ĭ-nō)	lamina (bony arch of the vertebrae)
10. menisc / o (mĕ-nĭs'-kō)	meniscus (cartilage of the knee joint)
11. oste / o (ōs'-tē-ō)	bone
12. patell / o (pah-tĕl'-ō)	patella (kneecap)
13. phalang / o (fah-lăn'-jō)	phalange (finger or toe bone)
14. scapul / o (skăp'-ū-lō)	scapula (shoulder blade)
15. stern / o (ster'-nō)	sternum (breastbone)
16. vertebr / o (ver'-tĕ-brō)	vertebra (s), vertebrae (pl) (bones of the spine)

Muscular System	Meaning
my / o (mī'-ō)	muscle
myos / o (mī'-ō-sō)	muscle

Other	Meaning
electr / o (ē-lĕk'-trō)	electricity, electrical activity
scoli / o (skō'-lē-ō)	crooked, curved (lateral)

EXERCISE 1

Write the combining forms for the skeletal system in the spaces provided on the diagram in Figure 23-11 (page 451). The number preceding the combining form in the list above matches the number of the body part(s) in the diagram.

EXERCISE 2

Define each combining form listed below.

1. arthr / o

_____

2. oste / o

_____

3. cost / o

_____

4. crani / o

_____

5. femor / o

_____

6. my / o

_____

7. humer / o

_____

8. patell / o

_____

9. stern / o

_____

10. clavicul / o

_____

11. scapul / o

_____

12. phalang / o

_____

13. vertebr / o

_____

14. clavic / o

_____

15. electr / o

_____

16. lamin / o

_____

17. chondr / o

_____

18. menisc / o

_____

19. scoli / o

_____

EXERCISE 3

Write the combining form for each part of the body listed below.

1. finger bone   _____

2. joint   _____

3. bone   _____

4. thigh bone   _____

5. kneecap   _____

6. shoulder blade   _____

7. bones of the spine _____

8. collarbone   _____

   a. _____

   b. _____

9. skull   _____

10. breastbone   _____

11. upper arm bone   _____

12. rib   _____

13. muscle   _____

14. lamina   _____

15. cartilage   _____

16. meniscus   _____

Recall from Units 1 and 2 that suffixes are letters that may be added to the end of a word root. Listed below are the suffixes that you need to know for this unit. Continue to use these throughout the chapter. The exercises will assist you in learning each suffix.

Suffix	Meaning
-algia (ăl′-ja)	pain
-ar, -ic	pertaining to (Recall you have already learned -al, -ous)
-centesis (sĕn-tē′-sĭs)	surgical puncture to aspirate fluid
-ectomy (ĕk′-to-mē)	surgical removal or excision
-gram	record, x-ray image, picture
-graph	instrument used to record
-graphy	process of recording, x-ray imaging, taking a picture
-osis (ŏ′-sĭs)	abnormal condition
-pathy (păthē)	disease of
-plasty (plăs′-tē)	surgical repair
-scope (skōp)	instrument used for visual examination
-scopy (skōp′-ē)	visual examination
-tomy (ŏt′-o-mē)	surgical incision, or to cut into
-trophy (trōf′-ē) (also may be used as a word root)	development, nourishment

---

EXERCISE 4

Write the suffix for each term listed below.

1. surgical repair   _____

2. pain   _____

3. pertaining to _____

    a. _____

    b. _____

    c. _____

    d. _____

4. surgical incision _____

5. surgical removal _____

6. instrument used to record _____

7. process of recording _____

8. record, x-ray image, picture _____

9. development, nourishment _____

10. abnormal condition _____

11. instrument used for visual
    examination _____

12. visual examination _____

13. surgical puncture to aspirate
    fluid _____

14. disease of _____

EXERCISE 5

Write the definition for each suffix listed below.

1. -algia

_____

2. -graph

_____

3. -gram

_____

4. -graphy

_____

5. -tomy

_____

6. -trophy

_____

7. -ic

_____

8. -plasty

_____

9. -ectomy

_____

10. -ar

_____

11. -osis

_____

12. -scopy

_____

13. -scope

_____

14. -centesis

_____

15. -pathy

_____

Recall from Unit 1 that prefixes are letters that may be added to the beginning of a word root to modify its meaning. Listed below are six prefixes that you need to memorize in this unit.

Prefix	Meaning
a-, an-	without or absence of (if used with a word root that begins with a vowel, use *an*; if used with a word root that begins with a consonant, use *a*)
dys- (dĭs)	difficult, painful, labored, abnormal
inter-	between
intra-	within
supra-	above

EXERCISE 6

Write the prefix for each term listed below.

1. within _____

2. painful _____

3. under _____

4. without _____

a. _____

b. _____

5. between _____

6. above _____

EXERCISE 7

Write the definition for each prefix listed below. You may be asked to recall a prefix from previous study.

1. intra- _____

2. supra- _____

3. sub- _____

4. dys- _____

5. a-, an- _____

6. inter- _____

MEDICAL TERMS RELATED TO THE MUSCULOSKELETAL SYSTEM

Listed below are the medical terms for the musculoskeletal system that you need to know. Most are made up of the word roots, prefixes, and suffixes you have been working with; however, some words that relate to the musculoskeletal system are not made up of the word parts you have studied thus far. These are also included in the list. Following the list are exercises that will assist you in learning the meaning and spelling of each word. Practice pronouncing each word aloud.

General Terms	Meaning
atrophy (ăt'-rō-fē)	without development (a decrease in the size of a normally developed organ)
chondrogenic (kŏn-drō-jĕn'-ĭk)	producing cartilage
cranial (krā'-nē-al)	pertaining to the cranium
dystrophy (dĭs'-trō-fē)	abnormal development
femoral (fĕm'-ō-ral)	pertaining to the femur (or thigh bone)
humeral (hū'-mĕr-al)	pertaining to the humerus
intervertebral (ĭn-tĕr-vĕr'-tĕ-bral)	pertaining to between the vertebrae
intracranial (ĭn-trah-krā'-nē-al)	pertaining to within the cranium
orthopedics (or-thō-pē'-dĭks)	branch of medicine that deals with the diagnosis and treatment of disease, abnormalities, or fractures of the musculoskeletal system
orthopedist (or-thō-pē'-dist)	a doctor who specializes in orthopedics

General Terms	Meaning
osteoma (ŏs-tē-ō'-mah)	a tumor (composed of) bone
sternal (stĕr'-nal)	pertaining to the sternum
sternoclavicular (stĕr'-nō-klah-vĭk'-ū-lar)	pertaining to the sternum and clavicle
sternocostal (stĕr-nō-kŏs'-tal)	pertaining to the sternum and ribs
sternoid (stĕr'-noyd)	resembling the sternum
subcostal (sŭb-kŏs'-tal)	pertaining to below a rib or ribs
subscapular (sŭb-skăp'-ū-lar)	pertaining to below the scapula
suprascapular (soo-prah-skăp'-ū-lar)	pertaining to above the scapula
vertebrocostal (vĕr'-tĕ-brō-kŏs'-tal)	pertaining to the vertebrae and ribs

Surgical Terms	Meaning
arthroplasty (ar'-thrō-plăs'-tē)	surgical repair of a joint
arthrotomy (ar-thrŏt'-o-mē)	surgical incision of a joint
chondrectomy (kŏn-drĕk'-to-mē)	excision of a cartilage
clavicotomy (klăv-ĭ-kŏt'-o-mē)	surgical incision into the clavicle
costectomy (kŏs-tĕk'-to-mē)	excision of a rib
cranioplasty (krā-nē-ō-plăs'-tē)	surgical repair of the cranium
craniotomy (krā-nē-ŏt'-o-mē)	surgical incision into the cranium
laminectomy (lăm-ĭ-nĕk'-to-mē)	surgical removal of lamina (often performed to relieve symptoms of a ruptured [slipped] disk)
meniscectomy (mĕn-ĭ-sĕk'-to-mē)	excision of the meniscus (of the knee joint)
patellectomy (păt-ĕ-lĕk'-to-mē)	excision of the patella
vertebrectomy (vĕr-tĕ-brĕk'-to-mē)	excision of a vertebra

Diagnostic Terms	Meaning
arthralgia (ar-thrăl'-ja)	pain in a joint
arthritis (ar-thrī'-tĭs)	inflammation of a joint
arthrosis (ar-thrŏ'-sĭs)	abnormal condition of a joint
chondritis (krŏn-drī'-tĭs)	inflammation of the cartilage
meniscitis (mĕn-ĭ-sī'-tĭs)	inflammation of the meniscus (of the knee joint)
muscular dystrophy (mŭs'-kū-lar) (dĭs'-trō-fē)	a number of muscle disorders characterized by a progressive, degenerative disease of the muscles
myoma (mī-ō'-mah)	a tumor (formed) of muscle (tissue)
myositis (mī-ō-sī'-tĭs)	inflammation of the muscles
scoliosis (skō-lē-ō'-sĭs)	abnormal condition of a (lateral) curve (of the spine)

**Terms Related to
Diagnostic Procedures** | **Meaning**

Terms Related to Diagnostic Procedures	Meaning
arthrocentesis (ar-thrō-sĕn-tē′-sĭs)	surgical puncture to aspirate a joint
arthrogram (ar′-thrō-grăm)	x-ray image of a joint (contrast medium, dye, or air is used)
arthroscope (ar′-thrō-scōpe)	instrument used to visualize a joint (commonly the knee and shoulder)
arthroscopy (ar-thrŏs′-ko-pē)	visual examination of a joint (for diagnosing, identifying, and correcting problems)
electromyogram (ē-lĕk′-trō-mī′-ō-grăm) (EMG)	record of electrical activity of a muscle
electromyograph (ē-lĕk′-trō-mī′-ō-grăph)	instrument used to record the electrical activity of a muscle
electromyography (ē-lĕk′-trō-mī-ŏg′-rah-fē)	process of recording the electrical activity of muscle
sternal puncture (stĕr′-nal) (pŭngk′-chŭr)	insertion of a hollow needle into the sternum to obtain a sample of bone marrow to be studied in the laboratory (Fig. 23-14) (used for diagnosing blood disorders such as anemia and leukemia)

Figure 23-14 Sternal puncture. (From LaFleur M, Starr W: *Exploring medical language,* St. Louis, 1985, Mosby, with permission.)

EXERCISE 8

Analyze and define each medical term listed below.

1. electromyogram

   _____

2. myoma

   _____

3. sternoclavicular

   _____

4. cranial

   _____

5. vertebrocostal

   _____

6. arthritis

   _____

7. intervertebral

   _____

8. humeral

   _____

9. dystrophy

   _____

10. subscapular

    _____

11. arthrosis

    _____

12. electromyography

    _____

13. arthrogram

    _____

14. electromyograph

    _____

15. sternocostal

    _____

16. arthralgia

    _____

17. subcostal

    _____

18. femoral

    _____

19. clavicotomy

    _____

20. arthrotomy

_____

21. intracranial

_____

22. atrophy

_____

23. arthroplasty

_____

24. osteoma

_____

25. costectomy

_____

26. cranioplasty

_____

27. patellectomy

_____

28. vertebrectomy

_____

29. craniotomy

_____

30. suprascapular

_____

31. myositis

_____

32. chondrogenic

_____

33. arthroscopy

_____

34. chondritis

_____

35. arthroscope

_____

36. chondrectomy

_____

37. laminectomy

_____

38. sternal

_____

39. meniscectomy

_____

40. arthrocentesis

_____

41. meniscitis

_____

EXERCISE 9

Using word roots, prefixes, suffixes, and combining vowels as needed, build a medical term from each definition listed below.

1. pertaining to the cranium   _____

2. inflammation of muscle   _____

3. pertaining to below the scapula   _____

4. pertaining to the femur   _____

5. surgical incision into a joint   _____

6. excision of a cartilage   _____

7. pain in a joint   _____

8. inflammation in a joint   _____

9. abnormal condition of a joint   _____

10. pertaining to the humerus   _____

11. without development   _____

12. pertaining to the vertebrae and ribs   _____

13. surgical incision into the cranium   _____

14. surgical removal of a rib   _____

15. pertaining to below the rib   _____

16. x-ray image of a joint   _____

17. surgical removal of a vertebra   _____

18. record of the electrical activity
 of a muscle _____

19. surgical incision into the clavicle _____

20. process of recording electrical
 activity of a muscle _____

21. abnormal development _____

22. a tumor (formed) of muscle (tissue) _____

23. machine used to record electrical
 activity of a muscle _____

24. pertaining to the sternum and
 clavicle _____

25. pertaining to between the vertebrae _____

26. pertaining to within the cranium _____

27. pertaining to the sternum and rib _____

28. surgical removal of the patella _____

29. surgical repair of the cranium _____

30. a tumor composed of bone _____

31. surgical incision into the clavicle _____

32. producing cartilage _____

33. visual examination of a joint _____

34. instrument used for visual
 examination of a joint _____

35. inflammation of cartilage _____

36. excision of cartilage _____

37. surgical removal of the lamina _____

38. pertaining to the sternum _____

39. puncture and aspiration of
 a joint _____

40. excision of the meniscus _____

41. inflammation of the meniscus _____

EXERCISE 10

Define each medical term listed below.

1. orthopedics

_____

2. orthopedist

_____

3. muscular dystrophy

_____

4. sternal puncture

_____

EXERCISE 11

Spell each medical term studied in this unit by having someone dictate the terms to you.

1. _____

2. _____

3. _____

4. _____

5. _____

6. _____

7. _____

8. _____

9. _____

10. _____

11. _____

12. _____

13. _____

14. _____

15. _____

16. _____

17. _____

18. _____

19. _____

20. _____

21. _____

22. _____

23. _____

24. _____

25. _____

26. _____

27. _____

28. _____

29. _____

30. _____

31. _____

32. _____

33. _____

34. _____

35. _____

36. _____

37. _____

38. _____

39. _____

40. _____

41. _____

42. _____

43. _____

44. _____

45. _____

EXERCISE 12

Answer the following questions.

1. _____ is the name of the nursing unit in the hospital that cares for patients with *fractures, abnormalities,* or *diseases of the bone.* _____ is the name of the doctor who specializes in this area of medicine.

2. A _____ tray is used by the doctor to obtain a *sample of bone marrow from the sternum.* The tray is named after the procedure.

3. The doctor ordered a procedure to determine the *electrical activity of a muscle.* This procedure is called a(n) _____.

---

4. Following is a list of diagnostic phrases. In the space provided, write the name of the fractured bone.

   Example: fractured femur thigh bone

   a. fractured tibia   a. _____
   b. fractured humerus   b. _____
   c. fractured cervical 6 (C6) c. _____
   d. fractured ilium   d. _____
   e. fractured clavicle   e. _____
   f. fractured radius   f. _____

5. A surgery schedule is a list of operations to be performed on a given day in the hospital. Following are the types of operations recorded on the surgery schedule. Indicate the terms that are incorrectly spelled by rewriting the term correctly in the space provided.

   a. castectomy   _____

   b. craniotomy   _____

   c. lamonectomy   _____

   d. clavictamy   _____

   e. cranioplasty   _____

   f. patelectomy   _____

   g. ostoarthrotomy   _____

   h. meniscectomy   _____

6. The doctor ordered a procedure to x-ray a joint that requires the use of contrast medium. This procedure is called a(n) _____. Puncture and aspiration of a joint is called _____.

ABBREVIATIONS

Abbreviation	Meaning
AKA	above the knee amputation
BKA	below the knee amputation
EMG	electromyogram
Fx	fracture
HNP	herniated nucleus pulposus
NSAID	nonsteroidal anti-inflammmatory drugs
ORIF	open reduction, internal fixation
THA	total hip arthroplasty
THR	total hip replacement

EXERCISE 13

Define the following abbreviations.

1. AKA

_____

2. BKA

_____

3. Fx

_____

4. ORIF

_____

5. HNP

_____

6. NSAID

_____

7. EMG

_____

8. THA

_____

9. THR

_____

UNIT 4
The Nervous System

OUTLINE

UNIT OBJECTIVES

Upon completion of this unit, you will be able to:

1. Name the organs of the nervous system.
2. Describe the overall function of the nervous system.
3. List and describe the organs of the nervous system covered in this unit.
4. Describe the functions of the meninges and locate and name the three layers of tissue that make up the meninges.
5. Describe cerebrovascular accident, Parkinson's disease, transient ischemic attack, Alzheimer's disease, and epilepsy.
6. Define the unit abbreviations.

THE NERVOUS SYSTEM

Organs of the Nervous System

- Nerves
- Brain
- Spinal cord

The nervous system is commonly divided into two parts:

1. The central nervous system (CNS) consists of the brain and spinal cord.
2. The peripheral nervous system (PNS) consists of the nerves of the body (12 pairs of cranial nerves and 31 pairs

of spinal nerves). The autonomic (involuntary) and somatic (voluntary) nervous systems are subdivisions of the PNS. The autonomic nervous system is further divided into the sympathetic (fight or flight) and parasympathetic (tranquil: rest and digestion) nervous systems.

Functions of the Nervous System

All body parts and systems must work together to maintain a healthy body. The nervous system monitors, regulates, and controls the functions of body organs and body systems by using nerve impulses to transmit information from one part of the body to another (Fig. 23-15). The nervous system works in concert with the endocrine system to maintain homeostasis, a constant internal environment, by inhibiting or stimulating the release of hormones.

Nerves

A *nerve* is a cord-like structure that is located outside the CNS. It contains nerve cells called *neurons*. The neuron transmits nerve impulses from one part of the body to another. Two types of neurons are:

1. Sensory neurons, which transmit impulses to the brain and spinal cord
2. Motor neurons, which transmit impulses from the brain and spinal cord to the muscles or glands

Brain

The brain is located within the cranial cavity and is the main center for coordinating body activities. The brain is divided into three parts: the cerebrum, the cerebellum, and the brainstem. Each part of the brain is responsible for controlling certain body functions.

The *cerebrum* is the largest part of the brain. It is located in the upper portion of the cranium. The cerebrum is divided into right and left hemispheres, which are connected only at the lower middle portion. The cerebrum contains the sensory, motor, sight, and hearing centers. Memory, intellect, judgment, and emotional reactions also take place in the cerebrum.

Four spaces within the brain, called *ventricles*, produce a watery fluid known as *cerebrospinal fluid (CSF)*. This cushion of fluid surrounds the brain and spinal cord. Its functions are to absorb shocks that may occur to the spinal cord or brain and to nourish and remove waste from the nervous tissue. The *cerebellum*, or "little brain," is situated below the posterior portion of the cerebrum. Its functions are to assist in the coordination of voluntary muscles and to maintain balance. The *brainstem* has three main parts: the midbrain, pons, and medulla oblongata. It contains the nerve fibers that form the connecting links between the different parts of the brain and the centers that control three vital functions: blood pressure, respiration, and heartbeat.

Spinal Cord

The spinal cord extends from the brainstem and passes through the spinal cavity to between the first and second lumbar vertebrae (see Fig. 23-17, *A,* page 473). The spinal cord is the pathway for conducting *sensory impulses* up to the brain and *motor impulses* down from the brain. Injury to the spinal cord can result in paralysis, the loss of voluntary muscle function.

Meninges

The meninges are made up of three layers of connective tissue that completely surround and protect the spinal cord and brain. The outer tough layer is called the *dura mater.* The middle layer is the *arachnoid (mater)*, a web-like structure. The inner thin, tender layer, the *pia mater,* carries blood vessels that provide nourishment to the nervous tissue. Cerebrospinal fluid flows through a space between the arachnoid and the pia mater called the *subarachnoid space* (see Fig. 23-17, *C,* page 473).

DISEASES AND CONDITIONS OF THE NERVOUS SYSTEM

Cerebrovascular Accident

Cerebrovascular accident (CVA), also called a *stroke,* is the interference of blood flow to the brain, which reduces the supply of oxygen and nutrients, causing damage to brain tissue. The major causes of CVA are embolism, thrombosis, and hemorrhage (Fig. 23-16). Strokes affect about 700,000 people each year, causing death in one quarter of them.

Damage to the brain tissue varies according to the artery affected. Paralysis is a result of the damage, and it may range from slight to complete hemiplegia (paralysis of one side of the body). CVA of the left hemisphere of the brain produces symptoms on the right side of the body, and CVA of the right side of the brain produces symptoms on the left side of the body. The more quickly the circulation returns, the better the chance for recovery.

Transient Ischemic Attack

Transient ischemic attacks (TIAs) are recurrent episodes of decreased neurologic function that occur as double vision, slurred speech, weakness in the legs, and dizziness lasting from seconds to 24 hours, then clearing. TIAs are considered warning signs for strokes. TIAs are caused by small emboli that temporarily interrupt blood flow to the brain. Treatment includes administration of aspirin and anticoagulants to minimize thrombosis in the hope of preventing a CVA. Preventive treatment may include a *carotid endarterectomy,* a surgical procedure that is performed to remove the thickened inner area of the carotid artery.

Parkinson's Disease

Parkinson's disease, also called *shaking palsy, parkinsonism,* and *paralysis agitans,* is one of the most common crippling diseases in the United States. Parkinson's disease, a gradual progressive disorder of the CNS, occurs with degeneration of the dopamine-releasing neurons in the *substantia nigra,* an area of the brain. Dopamine, one of the chemical messengers *(neurotransmitters)* responsible for transmitting signals within the brain, initiates and controls movement and balance. The cause of Parkinson's disease is

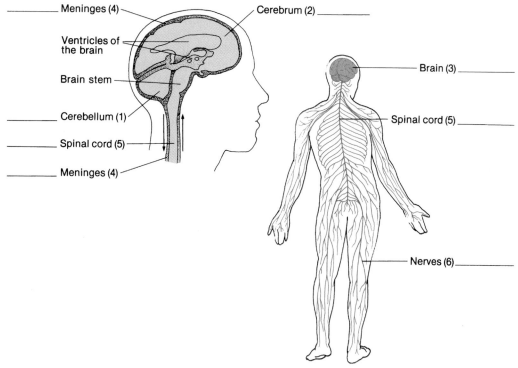

Figure 23-15 The nervous system.

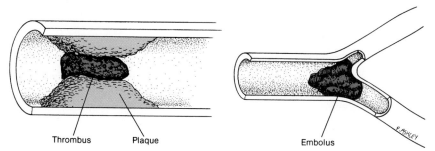

Figure 23-16 Thrombus (blood clot) or embolus (floating mass that blocks a vessel) in a cerebral artery can cause a cerebrovascular accident (CVA).

most often unknown, but it is thought to result from genetic factors, viral infection, exposure to toxins, or cerebral arteriosclerosis. Symptoms include muscle rigidity, tremors, and a shifting gait. Deterioration is progressive. No cure is known; treatment is aimed at relieving symptoms and promoting function for as long as possible. Parkinson's disease does not impair intellect.

Alzheimer's Disease

Alzheimer's disease, also called *presenile dementia*, is characterized by confusion, mental deterioration (dementia), restlessness, hallucinations, and the inability to carry out purposeful speech and movement. The patient may lose bowel and bladder control and refuse to eat. The disease is progressive and usually begins in later midlife. Because the precise cause of Alzheimer's disease has not been identified, definitive treatment has not been established. Care of the patient generally includes maintaining proper hygiene,

providing appropriate nutrition, preventing injury, and promoting purposeful activity.

Epilepsy

Epilepsy, a group of chronic disorders of the CNS, is the result of abnormal electrical (neuron) activity in the brain. It is common to hear epilepsy and seizure used synonymously; the difference is that epilepsy is the disease and seizure is the result of the disease. Epilepsy usually occurs in childhood or after age 50. The disease can be classified as idiopathic (origin unknown) or acquired. Some of the known causes of acquired epilepsy are brain tumors, brain injury, and endocrine disorders. Seizures that result from fever, otitis media, or drug toxicity are usually isolated incidents and do not warrant the diagnosis of epilepsy.

Seizures are classified according to the origin of the abnormal brain signals. Involvement of the entire brain is known as *generalized seizure*, whereas a *partial seizure* is one in which abnormal electrical activity occurs in a particular region of the brain.

Seizure activity is divided into three stages: (1) during the *preictal* stage, the patient may experience abnormal somatic and psychic sensations, including strange sounds, tastes, and smells. These sensations are called an *aura;* (2) the second stage is called *interictal* and includes violent jerking of some parts of or the total body. The patient may experience a grand mal seizure characterized by incontinence of urine and stool, foaming or frothing from the mouth, changes in skin color, tongue biting, arching of the back, and turning of the head to one side; and (3) the period immediately after the seizure is called the *postictal* stage. During this stage, the patient may become confused and lethargic and may report headache and sore muscles. The petit mal seizure, another form of generalized seizure, is marked by a brief loss of consciousness along with unresponsive behaviors.

Diagnosis is confirmed by observation of the seizure activity, blood testing to rule out other ailments, and magnetic resonance imaging (MRI) or computed tomography scan (CT) of the brain to look for a lesion. An electroencephalogram (EEG) also may locate the site and possible cause of the disorder. Additional studies include EP (evoked potential), which is a group of tests that measure brain wave changes in response to various stimuli, and positron emission tomography, or PET scanning, a nuclear medicine test that more closely studies brain function and metabolism.

Treatment requires stabilization on anticonvulsant drugs (see Chapter 13 for a list of these drugs); 95% of the population responds to drug therapy. The other 5% is treated surgically to remove affected brain tissue. Patient education is included in the treatment regimen. Information about seizure triggers and how to avoid those triggers is an important part of patient education. A national association (National Association of Epilepsy Centers; http://www.naec-epilepsy.org) has been formed to help the patient deal with self-esteem issues and the stigma that is still attached to epilepsy. Because of stigmatization, many people who have epilepsy will not wear an identification bracelet and will not inform others of their illness.

🖉 TAKE NOTE

Patients who are experiencing a seizure need to be protected from injury, especially head injury. Remove any furniture or other objects that the patient may strike. If possible, put a pillow under the patient's head. Call for help. *Do not try to restrain the movements of the patient.* Protect the patient's privacy. Ask those who are uninvolved with the care of patients to please leave the area.

REVIEW QUESTIONS

1. Name the organs of the nervous system. Write the function of each organ.

a. _____

b. _____

c. _____

2. A nerve cell is called a(n) _____. The two types of nerve cells are _____ and

_____.

3. Name three parts of the brain and describe the functions of each.

a. _____

b. _____

c. _____

4. Describe the location and function of the spinal cord.

_____

5. The meninges are made up of three layers of tissue. The tough outer layer is called the _____; the middle layer is called the _____; and the inner layer is called the _____.

6. Match the terms in Column 1 with the appropriate phrases in Column 2.

Column 1	Column 2
a. Parkinson's disease	_____ 1. also called shaking palsy
b. Alzheimer's disease	_____ 2. may be idiopathic or acquired
c. transient ischemic attack	_____ 3. may result in hemiplegia
d. cerebrovascular accident	_____ 4. warning sign for strokes
e. cerebral palsy	_____ 5. symptoms include confusion and
f. epilepsy	hallucinations

7. Name the three stages of a seizure.

a. _____

b. _____

c. _____

MEDICAL TERMINOLOGY RELATED TO THE NERVOUS SYSTEM AND PSYCHOLOGY

Upon mastery of the medical terminology for this unit, you will be able to:

1. Spell and define the word parts and medical terms that relate to the nervous system.
2. Analyze the medical terms related to the nervous system that are built from word parts.
3. Given the meaning of a medical condition related to the nervous system, build with word parts the corresponding medical term.
4. Spell and use in sentence form the psychology terminology presented in this unit.
5. Given descriptions of hospital situations in which the HUC may encounter medical terminology, apply the correct medical terms to the situations.

Word Parts

Listed below are the word parts related to the nervous system that you need to memorize. The exercises included in this unit will help you with this task. You will continue to use these word parts throughout the course and during employment. Practice pronouncing each word element aloud.

Word Roots/ Combining Forms	Meaning
1. cerebell / o (sĕr-ĕ-bĕl′-ō)	cerebellum (little brain)
2. cerebr/ o (sĕr′-ē-brō)	cerebrum (main portion of the brain)
3. dur / o (dū′-rō)	dura mater (outer meningeal layer)
4. encephal / o (ĕn-sĕf′-ah-lō)	brain
5. mening / o (mĕ-nĭng′-gō)	meninges (spinal cord covering)
6. myel / o (mī′-ĕl-ō)	spinal cord (also means *bone marrow*)
7. neur / o (nū′-rō)	nerve
8. phas / o (fāz′-ō)	speech
9. psych / o (sī′-kō)	mind

Other Word Roots/ Combining	Meaning
poli / o (pō′-lē-ō)	gray matter

Suffixes	Meaning
-cele (sēl)	herniation or protrusion
-ia	abnormal condition of
-plegia (plē′-ja)	paralysis, stroke

Word Roots/ Combining Forms	Meaning
-rrhagia (rah′-ja)	rapid flow of blood
-rrhaphy (rah′-fē)	to suture (surgical), repair
-rrhea (rē′-ah)	excessive discharge, flow

EXERCISE 1

Write in the spaces provided the combining forms for the parts of the nervous system shown on the diagram in Figure 23-15 (page 467). The number preceding the combining form in the list above matches the number of the body part on the diagram.

EXERCISE 2

Define each combining form listed below.

1. cerebr / o

   _____

2. encephal / o

   _____

3. neur / o

   _____

4. poli / o

   _____

5. mening / o

   _____

6. dur / o

   _____

7. myel / o

   _____

8. cerebell / o

   _____

9. phas / o

   _____

10. psych / o

_____

15. abnormal condition of   _____

EXERCISE 3

Write the combining forms for each term listed below.

1. nerve   _____

2. cerebrum   _____

3. meninges   _____

4. spinal cord   _____

5. cerebellum   _____

6. brain   _____

7. dura mater   _____

8. gray matter   _____

9. speech   _____

10. mind   _____

EXERCISE 4

Write the suffix(es) that match each definition written below.
(Note: This exercise includes suffixes from this unit and from
previous units. Refer back as needed.)

1. tumor   _____

2. surgical repair _____

3. pertaining to   _____

4. to suture   _____

5. excessive discharge _____

6. inflammation   _____

7. specialist   _____

8. record, x-ray image,
   picture   _____

9. study of   _____

10. rapid discharge _____

11. herniation   _____

12. surgical removal _____

13. incision   _____

14. pain   _____

EXERCISE 5

Write the definition for each suffix listed below. (Note: This
exercise includes suffixes from this unit and from previous units.
Refer back as needed.)

1. -gram

_____

2. -itis

_____

3. -logy

_____

4. -rrhea

_____

5. -rrhagia

_____

6. -rrhaphy

_____

7. -cele

_____

8. -ar

_____

9. -ectomy

_____

10. -plasty

_____

11. -tomy

_____

12. -algia

_____

13. -osis

_____

14. -ia

_____

✎ *TAKE NOTE*

Cerebrovascular Accident (Stroke) Warning Signs and Treatment

Warning Signs

- Sudden numbness, weakness, or paralysis of the face, arm, or leg, especially on one side of the body
- Sudden confusion; problems with memory or perception
- Sudden loss of speech; difficulty speaking or understanding
- Sudden trouble seeing out of one or both eyes; blurred or double vision
- Sudden difficulty walking, dizziness, or loss of balance or coordination
- Sudden, severe headache with no known cause

Thrombolytic Treatment

Tissue plasminogen activator (tPA) is a thrombolytic agent (clot-busting drug) approved for use in certain patients who are having a heart attack or stroke caused by blood clots that block blood flow. This class of drugs may dissolve blood clots, which cause most heart attacks and ischemic strokes, if given within 3 hours of the onset of symptoms. Administered by hospital personnel through an IV line, tPA can reduce significantly the effects of a stroke caused by a clot, including permanent disability.

MEDICAL TERMS RELATED TO THE NERVOUS SYSTEM

Listed below are medical terms related to the nervous system that you will need to know. Exercises following this list will assist you in learning these terms. Practice pronouncing these terms aloud.

General Terms	Meaning
aphasia (ah-fā′-zha)	abnormal condition characterized by no speech (loss of expression or understanding of speech or writing)
cerebrospinal (ser′-ē-brō-spī′-nal)	pertaining to the brain and spine
hemiplegia (hĕm-ĭ-plē′-ja)	paralysis of the right or left side of the body (usually caused by a stroke)
myelorrhagia (mī-ĕ-lō-rā′-ja)	rapid flow of blood into the spinal cord
neurologist (nū-rŏl′-o-jĭst)	one who specializes in the diagnosis and treatment of disorders of the nerves
neurology (nū-rŏl′-o-jē)	the study of nerves (the branch of medicine that deals with the diagnosis and treatment of disorders or diseases of the nervous system)

General Terms	Meaning
paraplegia (păr-ăh-plē′-ja)	paralysis of the legs and sometimes the lower part of the body, usually caused by injury to the spinal cord
quadriplegia (kwăd-rĕ-plē′-ja)	paralysis that affects all four limbs

Surgical Terms	Meaning
neuroplasty (nū′-rō-plăs′-tē)	surgical repair of a nerve
neurorrhaphy (nū-rŏr′-ah-fē)	suturing of a nerve

Diagnostic Terms	Meaning
cephalalgia (sĕf-ah-lăl′-ja)	pain in the head (headache)
cerebellitis (ser-ĕ-bĕl-ī′-tĭs)	inflammation of the cerebellum
cerebral palsy (ser′-ē-bral) (paul′-zē)	partial paralysis and lack of muscle coordination that results from a defect, injury, or disease of the brain that is present at birth or shortly thereafter
cerebrosis (ser-ĕ-brō′-sĭs)	abnormal condition of the cerebrum (of the brain)
cerebrovascular (ser′-ĕ-brō-văs′-kŭ-lăr) accident (CVA)	impaired blood supply to parts of the brain; also called a *stroke*
encephalitis (ĕn-sĕf-ah-lī′-tĭs)	inflammation of the brain
encephalocele (ĕn-sĕf′-ah-lō-sēl)	herniation of brain (tissue through a gap in the skull)
epilepsy (ĕp′-ĭ-lĕp-sē)	convulsive disorder of the nervous system characterized by chronic or recurrent seizures

General Terms	Meaning
meningitis (mĕn-ĭn-jī′-tĭs)	inflammation of the meninges
meningomyelocele (mĕ-nĭng-gō-mī′-ĕ-lō-sēl)	protrusion of the spinal cord and meninges (through the vertebral column)
multiple sclerosis (mŭl′-tĭ-pl) (sklĕ-rō′-sĭs) (MS)	a degenerative disease of the nerves that control the muscles, characterized by hardening patches along the brain and spinal cord
neuralgia (nū-răl′-ja)	pain in a nerve
neuritis (nū-rī′-tĭs)	inflammation of a nerve
neuroma (nū-rō′-mah)	a tumor made up of nerve (cells)
poliomyelitis (pō′-lē-ō-mī-ĕ-lī′-tĭs)	inflammation of the gray matter of the spinal cord (virally caused disease, commonly known as polio)

General Terms	Meaning
subdural hematoma (sŭb-dū′-ral) (hēm-ah-tō′-mah)	blood tumor that pertains to the area below the dura mater (accumulation of blood in the subdural space)

Terms Related to Diagnostic Procedures	Meaning
CT scan (computed tomography)	use of radiologic imaging that produces images of blood-less "slices" of the body; CT scanning can detect hemorrhages, tumors, and brain abnormalities
electroencephalogram (ē-lĕk′-trō-ĕn-sĕf′-ăh-lō-grăm) (EEG)	record of the electrical activity of the brain
lumbar puncture (lŭm′-băr) (pŭngk′-chŭr) (LP)	removal of cerebrospinal fluid (CSF) for diagnostic and therapeutic purposes; a hollow needle is inserted into the subarachnoid space between the third and fourth lumbar vertebrae (Fig. 23-17)
magnetic resonance imaging (MRI)	noninvasive procedure for imaging tissues that cannot be seen through other radiologic techniques; the advantage of this diagnostic procedure is not only the avoidance of harmful radiation through its use of magnetic fields and radiofrequencies, but also the ability to detect small brain abnormalities; patients with pacemakers or any metallic foreign bodies generally cannot undergo this procedure
myelogram (mī′-ĕ-lō-grăm)	x-ray image of the spinal cord (injected dye is used as the contrast medium)

EXERCISE 6

Analyze and define each medical term listed below.

1. neurology

———————————————————

2. cerebrospinal

———————————————————

3. neuralgia

———————————————————

4. poliomyelitis

———————————————————

5. neuroplasty

———————————————————

6. encephalitis

———————————————————

7. meningitis

———————————————————

8. neuropathy

———————————————————

9. neurologist

———————————————————

10. encephalocele

———————————————————

11. electroencephalogram

———————————————————

12. meningomyelocele

———————————————————

13. cerebellitis

———————————————————

14. cerebrosis

———————————————————

15. neuroma

———————————————————

16. myelorrhagia

———————————————————

17. myelogram

———————————————————

18. neuritis

———————————————————

EXERCISE 7

Define each medical term listed below.

1. multiple sclerosis

———————————————————

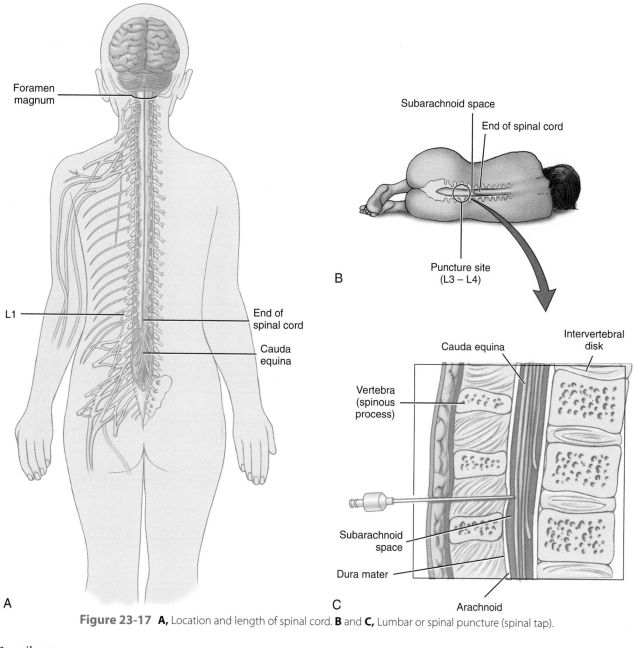

Foramen magnum

L1

End of spinal cord

Cauda equina

A

Subarachnoid space

End of spinal cord

Puncture site (L3 – L4)

B

Cauda equina

Intervertebral disk

Vertebra (spinous process)

Subarachnoid space

Dura mater

Arachnoid

C

Figure 23-17 A, Location and length of spinal cord. **B** and **C,** Lumbar or spinal puncture (spinal tap).

2. epilepsy

_____

3. cerebral palsy

_____

4. cerebrovascular accident

_____

5. echoencephalography

_____

6. hemiplegia

_____

7. paraplegia

_____

8. quadriplegia

_____

9. lumbar puncture

_____

10. subdural hematoma

_____

11. CT scan

_____

12. MRI

_____

13. aphasia

_____

EXERCISE 8

Using the word elements studied in this unit and in previous units, build a medical term from each of the definitions listed below.

1. inflammation of a nerve   _____

2. inflammation of the brain   _____

3. inflammation of the meninges   _____

4. surgical repair of a nerve   _____

5. one who specializes in the diagnosis and treatment of nerves   _____

6. disease of a nerve   _____

7. tumor made of nerve cells   _____

8. pain in a nerve   _____

9. pertaining to the cerebrum and spine   _____

10. herniation of the meninges and spinal cord (through the vertebral column)   _____

11. inflammation of the cerebellum   _____

12. herniation of the brain (through a gap in the skull)   _____

13. rapid flow of blood into the spinal cord   _____

14. record of the electrical activity of the brain   _____

15. x-ray image of the spinal cord   _____

EXERCISE 9

Spell each medical term studied in this unit by having someone dictate the terms to you.

1. _____

2. _____

3. _____

4. _____

5. _____

6. _____

7. _____

8. _____

9. _____

10. _____

11. _____

12. _____

13. _____

14. _____

15. _____

16. _____

17. _____

18. _____

19. _____

20. _____

21. _____

22. _____

23. _____

24. _____

25. _____

26. _____

27. _____

28. _____

29. _____

30. _____

31. _____

32. _____

33. _____

TERMS RELATED TO PSYCHOLOGY

An extensive knowledge of psychology vocabulary is not necessary for general hospital employment; therefore, we will discuss only those terms that you as an HUC may encounter in general medical and surgical areas of employment.

Psych / o is a combining form meaning "mind." The following words are developed from the word root *psych* and suffixes, most of which you have already studied.

Psychology Terms	Meaning
psychiatrist (sī-kī′-ah-trĭst)	a doctor who specializes in the mind
psychiatry (sī-kī′-ah-trē)	treatment of the mind (a branch of medicine that deals with the study, treatment, and prevention of mental illness)
psychologist (sī-kŏl′-ō-jĭst)	one who specializes in the diagnosis and treatment of the mind (a person trained to perform psychological analysis, therapy, or research, generally at a master's level of education or PhD)
psychology (sī-kŏl′-ō-jē)	study of the mind (behavior)
psychosis (sī-kō′-sĭs)	abnormal condition of the mind

Psychology Terms	Meaning
neur / o (nŭ′-rō)	the combining form that means "nerve"; it may be used to describe certain psychiatric disorders, as in the following terms
neurosis (nŭ-rō′-sĭs)	an emotional disorder considered less serious than a psychosis
neurotic (nŭ-rŏt′-ĭk)	having a neurosis
psychosomatic (sī′-kō-sō-măt′-ĭk)	pertaining to the mind and body (relationship)

EXERCISE 10

Spell each psychology term studied in this unit by having someone dictate the terms to you.

1. _____

2. _____

3. _____

4. _____

5. _____

6. _____

7. _____

8. _____

EXERCISE 11

Fill in the blanks below.

1. _____ is the name of the nursing unit in the hospital that cares for patients with disorders of the nervous system. _____ is the name of the doctor who specializes in this area of medicine.

2. The patient is admitted to the hospital with the admitting diagnosis of stroke or _____ _____. The abbreviation for this term is _____. The patient is paralyzed on the left side of her body. She has _____.

3. A child is diagnosed as having an inflammation of the meninges or _____. The doctor performs a procedure to obtain cerebrospinal fluid for diagnostic study. The procedure is called _____ _____. To perform this procedure, the doctor uses a special tray named after the procedure. It is called a _____ _____ tray.

4. Name four diagnostic procedures that end in the suffix *-gram* that the doctor may order to gather information about the nervous system organs or about their functions:

   a. _____

   b. _____

   c. _____

   d. _____

ABBREVIATIONS

Abbreviation	Meaning
CNS	central nervous system
CSF	cerebrospinal fluid
CT	computed tomography
CVA	cerebrovascular accident (stroke)
EEG	electroencephalogram
EP	evoked potentials
LP	lumbar puncture
MRI	magnetic resonance imaging
MS	multiple sclerosis
PET	positron emission tomography
PNS	peripheral nervous system
TIA	transient ischemic attack

EXERCISE 12

Define the following abbreviations.

1. CNS

   _____

2. CSF

   _____

3. CT

   _____

4. CVA

   _____

5. EEG

   _____

6. EP

   _____

7. LP

   _____

8. MS

   _____

9. PNS

   _____

10. PET

   _____

11. MRI

   _____

12. TIA

   _____

UNIT 5
The Eye and the Ear

OUTLINE

UNIT OBJECTIVES

Upon completion of this unit, you will be able to:

1. Name and locate the parts and accessory structures of the eye and briefly describe the function of each part.
2. Describe how the eye is protected.
3. Trace the pathway of light from the outside environment to the cerebrum.
4. Name and describe the functions of the two types of nerve cells located in the retina.
5. Name and locate the parts of the ear.
6. Trace the travel of sound waves from the outside environment to the brain.
7. Describe cataract, glaucoma, retinal detachment, and tinnitus.
8. Define the unit abbreviations.

THE EYE

The eye (Fig. 23-18) is the organ of vision. The eye receives light waves that are focused on the retina and produces visual nerve impulses that are transmitted to the visual area of the brain by the optic nerve. The eye is divided into three layers: sclera, choroid, and retina.

The eye, a spherical, delicate structure, is protected by the skull bones and its accessory organs: eyelashes (close eyelids when disturbed), eyelids (protect and shade), lacrimal apparatus (glands secrete lubricating tears), and conjunctiva (protective membrane). The *conjunctiva* is a transparent membrane that lines the upper and lower eyelids and the anterior portion of the eye. It helps protect the eye from harmful bacteria.

The *sclera,* the outer protective layer of the eye, helps maintain the shape of the eyeball and is the site for muscle attachment. We can see the anterior portion of the sclera. It is often referred to as the white of the eye. The *cornea* is the transparent, avascular part of the sclera that lies over the iris of the eye and allows light rays to enter.

The middle layer of the eye is called the *choroid.* The choroid contains blood vessels that supply nutrients to the eye. The *iris* and the *ciliary muscle* make up the anterior middle portion of the choroid. The iris, the colored portion of the eye, has an opening in the center called the *pupil.* Muscles of the iris regulate the amount of light entering the eye through dilatation and contraction of the pupil.

✐ TAKE NOTE

The eye examination during the history and physical (H&P) may include the acronym *PERRLA,* meaning *pupils equal, round, reactive to light and accommodation.*

The *lens,* located directly behind the pupil, focuses light rays on the retina. The ciliary muscle regulates the shape of the lens to make this possible through a process known as *accommodation.*

The inner layer of the eye is called the *retina.* Two different sets of nerve cells, or photoreceptor neurons, called *rods* and *cones,* are responsible for the adaptation to light. The cones are sensitive to bright light and are responsible for color vision. The rods, far more numerous than cones, adapt to provide both peripheral vision and vision in dim light. The rods and cones transmit impulses to the optic nerve. The optic nerve carries these impulses to the vision center in the cerebrum, where they are registered as visual sensations.

The anterior and posterior cavities inside the eyeball are filled with fluid. The small anterior cavity in front of the lens is divided into an anterior and a posterior chamber. These chambers are filled with a watery substance called *aqueous humor,* which is constantly formed and drained. The large posterior cavity behind the lens is filled with a jelly-like substance called *vitreous humor,* which remains relatively constant. The functions of these fluids are to maintain the shape of the eyeball with proper intraocular pressure and to assist in bending the light rays to focus on the retina.

✐ TAKE NOTE

Pathway of Light Rays

conjunctiva → cornea → aqueous humor → pupil → lens → vitreous humor → retina → optic nerve (converted to nerve impulses) → cerebrum

Diseases of the Eye
Cataract

Cataracts represent the gradual development of cloudiness of the lens of the eyes; they usually occur in both eyes. Most cataracts develop after a person is 50 years of age and are caused by degenerative changes. At first, vision is blurred; if not treated, cataracts eventually lead to loss of eyesight. Treatment consists of surgical removal of the lens followed by correction of the visual defects. Two types of surgery used to remove cataracts are extraction of the entire lens and *phacoemulsification,* which is the use of ultrasonic vibrations to break the lens into pieces, followed by *aspiration,* or sucking out of the pieces.

Correction of visual defects requires a lens implant. Following removal of the cataract, a synthetic lens is inserted into the eye through a corneal incision. Corrective eyeglasses or contact lens also may be used to correct the visual defect caused by cataract extraction.

Glaucoma

Glaucoma is the abnormal increase in intraocular (within the eye) pressure. It is the most preventable cause of blindness and yet is the cause of 15% of all cases of blindness in the United States. Pressure is caused by overproduction of aqueous humor or obstruction of its outflow, which causes damage to the retina that results in blindness.

Two forms of glaucoma exist: chronic and acute. Chronic glaucoma affects vision gradually and may not be diagnosed until after some loss of vision has occurred. The acute form causes severe pain and sudden dimming of vision.

Treatment varies, but glaucoma often is treated with drugs that help to reduce intraocular pressure. The patient has to understand that the medication must be taken for the rest of their life.

Retinal Detachment

Retinal detachment is the separation of the retina from the choroid in the back of the eye, which allows vitreous humor to leak between the choroid and the retina. Retinal detachment may be caused by trauma but is often the result of aging. *Photocoagulation, cryosurgery,* and *scleral buckling* are the surgical procedures that are used for treatment.

THE EAR

Two functions of the ear include hearing and equilibrium (sense of balance). The ear is divided into three main parts: the outer ear, the middle ear, and the inner ear (Fig. 23-19).

The Outer Ear

The outer ear is made up of two parts: the pinna, or auricle, and the auditory canal. The *pinna* is the appendage we see on each side of the head. The *auditory canal* is the tube that leads

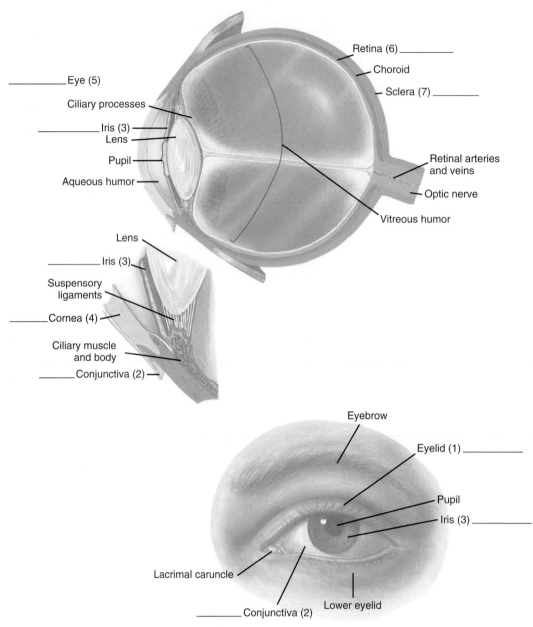

Retina (6) _____
Choroid
Eye (5) _____
Ciliary processes
Sclera (7) _____
Iris (3)
Lens
Pupil
Aqueous humor
Retinal arteries and veins
Optic nerve
Vitreous humor
Lens
Iris (3)
Suspensory ligaments
Cornea (4)
Ciliary muscle and body
Conjunctiva (2)
Eyebrow
Eyelid (1) _____
Pupil
Iris (3) _____
Lacrimal caruncle
Lower eyelid
Conjunctiva (2)

Figure 23-18 The eye.

from the outer ear to the middle ear through which sound waves pass.

The Middle Ear

The *tympanic membrane* (eardrum) separates the outer ear from the middle ear. Located just inside the eardrum are three small bones, or *ossicles*, called the *malleus*, the *incus*, and the *stapes*. These three small bones form a chain across the middle ear from the tympanic membrane (eardrum) to the oval window. They transfer vibrations of the eardrum to the inner ear. The middle ear also contains the *eustachian tube*, which leads from the middle ear to the pharynx (throat). The eustachian tube serves to equalize pressure on both sides of the tympanic membrane. Disease-causing bacteria, especially in children, may travel from the throat to the middle ear through the eustachian tube, resulting in middle ear infection.

The Inner Ear (or Labyrinth)

The *oval window* separates the middle ear from the inner ear. The structure next to the oval window in the inner ear is the *cochlea*, an organ that is shaped like a snail, with receptors for hearing. It contains special fluids that carry sound vibrations. The inner ear also contains the *semicircular canals*. The cerebellum interprets impulses from the semicircular canals to maintain balance and equilibrium.

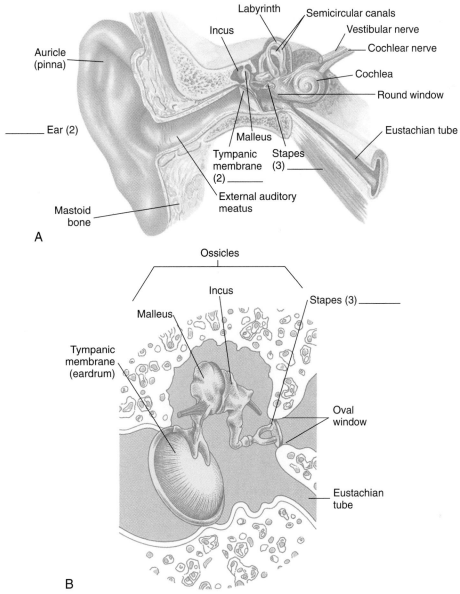

Figure 23-19 A, The ear. **B,** Enlarged view of inner ear.

Diseases and Disorders of the Ear

Tinnitus

Tinnitus, a symptom in most disorders of the ear, is described as a ringing, buzzing, or roaring noise in the ears. In some patients, this noise can be heard by others with the use of a stethoscope (objective tinnitus) and may be caused by muscle spasm or an abnormality in blood vessels. Common causes of tinnitus include chronic infection, head injury, prolonged exposure to loud environmental noise, hypertension, and cardiovascular disease. Another common cause of tinnitus is intake of drugs that are ototoxic. Ringing in the ears is a very common adverse effect of aspirin.

Persistent and severe noises in the ear can interfere with the person's ability to carry on normal activities such as resting and sleeping. Medical treatment begins with an audiologic and vascular examination that is performed to try to determine the underlying cause of the tinnitus. Many cases have been unresponsive to all conventional methods of treatment. One frequent approach to treatment is to try to mask ear noises by providing soft background music. Biofeedback has been marginally effective in cases caused by stress or hysteria. Because the condition is so prevalent, a national association has been established. (American Tinnitus Association—http://www.ata.org; or American Speech-Language-Hearing Association—http://www.asha.org). One of the primary goals of the association is management and study of the condition.

✐ *TAKE NOTE*

Pathway of Sound Waves Through the Ear
pinna → auditory canal → tympanic membrane → ossicles (malleus, incus, stapes) → oval window → cochlea → auditory nerve (converted to nerve impulses) → cerebrum

REVIEW QUESTIONS

1. Five body structures that help protect the eye in various ways are:

a. _____   d. _____
b. _____   e. _____
c. _____

2. Explain how sound waves (vibrations) travel from the pinna to the cerebrum (brain).

_____

3. Match the terms in Column 1 with the definitions in Column 2.

Column 1
a. choroid
b. pupil
c. stapes
d. retina
e. auditory nerve
f. cornea
g. cochlea
h. iris
i. sclera
j. lens
k. optic nerve

Column 2
_____ 1. anterior transparent part of the sclera
_____ 2. the colored portion of the eye
_____ 3. located directly behind the pupil
_____ 4. outer protective layer of the eye
_____ 5. the opening in the center of the iris
_____ 6. inner layer of the eye
_____ 7. transmits impulses from the retina to the brain
_____ 8. middle layer of the eye

4. List in order, beginning with the conjunctiva, the organs of the eye through which light rays travel to the retina.

a. _____   d. _____
b. _____   e. _____
c. _____   f. _____

5. Name and describe the functions of the two types of nerve cells located in the retina.

a. nerve cell: _____

function: _____

b. nerve cell: _____

function: _____

6. List the parts of:

a. the outer ear: _____

b. the middle ear: _____

c. the inner ear: _____

7. Describe the clinical presentation of cataracts.

_____

8. The physician's eye pressure examination for glaucoma will reveal

_____

9. List six factors that cause tinnitus.

a. _____   d. _____

b. _____   e. _____

c. _____   f. _____

10. List two treatments for tinnitus.

a. _____

b. _____

11. An examination in which retinal detachment is the diagnosis will show

_____ .

12. Three surgical procedures used to treat retinal detachment are:

a. _____

b. _____

c. _____

MEDICAL TERMINOLOGY RELATED TO THE EYE AND THE EAR

Upon mastery of the medical terminology for this unit, you will be able to:

1. Spell and define the word parts and medical terms for the eye and the ear.
2. Given the meaning of a medical condition related to the eye or the ear, build the corresponding medical term with word parts.
3. Analyze the medical terms that are built from word parts that relate to the eye and ear.
4. Given a description of hospital situations in which the HUC may encounter medical terminology, apply the correct medical terms to the situations.

Word Parts

Listed below are the combining forms for this unit. Memorize each combining form. Practice pronouncing each word part aloud.

Word Roots/ Combining Forms	Meaning
Eye	
1. blephar / o (blĕf′-ah-rō)	eyelid
2. conjunctiv / o (kŏn-jŭnk′-tĭv-ō)	conjunctiva (membrane covering the eye and lining of the eyelid)
3. irid / o (ĭ′-rĭd-ō)	iris (colored portion of the eye)
4. kerat / o (kĕr′-ah-tō)	cornea (clear anterior covering of the eye; also means "hard")
5. ophthalm / o (ŏf-thal′-mō)	eye

Word Roots/ Combining Forms	Meaning
6. retin / o (rĕt′-ĭn-ō)	retina (inner layer of eye)
7. scler / o (skleù′-rō)	sclera (white covering of the eye)
Ear	
1. myring / o (mĭ-rĭng′-gō)	tympanic membrane (eardrum)
2. ot / o (ŏ′-tō)	ear
3. staped / o (stā-pē′-dō)	stapes (in middle ear)

EXERCISE 1

1. *Write the combining forms for the eye in the spaces provided on the diagram in Figure 23-18. The number that precedes the combining form in the list above matches the number of the body part on the diagram.*

2. *Write the combining forms for the ear in the spaces provided on the diagram in Figure 23-19. The number preceding the combining form in the list above matches the number of the body part on the diagram.*

EXERCISE 2

Define each combining form listed below.

1. retin / o _____

2. kerat / o _____

3. scler / o _____

4. ophthalm / o _____

5. conjunctiv / o _____

6. ot / o _____

7. myring / o _____

8. blephar / o _____

9. irid / o _____

10. staped / o _____

EXERCISE 3

Write the word roots for each part of the body listed below.

1. eye

   _____

2. eyelid

   _____

3. retina

   _____

4. ear

   _____

5. eardrum

   _____

6. sclera

   _____

7. conjunctiva

   _____

8. iris

   _____

9. cornea

   _____

10. stapes

    _____

MEDICAL TERMS RELATED TO THE EYE AND THE EAR

The following list consists of medical terms related to the eye and the ear that you will need to know. Exercises following this list will assist you in learning these terms. Practice pronouncing these terms aloud.

General Terms	Meaning
ophthalmologist (ŏf′-thal-mŏl′-o-jĭst)	one who specializes in the diagnosis and treatment of the eye (doctor)
ophthalmology (ŏf′-thăl-mŏl′-o-jē)	study of the eye (and its diseases and disorders)
optometrist (ŏp-tŏm′-e-trĭst)	a professional person trained to examine the eyes and prescribe glasses
otorrhea (ō-tō-rē′-ah)	discharge from the ear

Surgical Terms	Meaning
blepharoplasty (blĕf′-ah-rō-plăs′-tē)	surgical repair of the eyelid
blepharorrhaphy (blĕf′-ah-rōr′-ah-fē)	suturing of an eyelid
cataract extraction (kăt′-ah-răkt) (ĕk-străk′-shŭn)	removal of the clouded lens of the eye
corneal (kor′-nē-al) transplant	transplantation of a donor cornea into the eye of the recipient
enucleation (ē-nū-klē-ā′-shŭn)	removal of an organ; often used to indicate surgical removal of the eyeball
iridectomy (īr-ĭ-dĕk′-to-mē)	excision of (a part of) the iris
iridosclerotomy (īr-ĭ-dō-sklĕ-rŏt′-o-mē)	incision into the iris and the sclera
keratectomy (kĕr-ah-tĕk′-to-mē)	procedure whereby an excimer laser is used to correct myopia; includes removal of part of the cornea (PRK, photorefractive keratectomy)
keratoplasty (kĕr-ah-to-plăs′-tē)	procedure in which the laser is used to correct myopia; involves reshaping corneal tissue below the surface (LASIK [laser-assisted in situ keratomileusis])
keratotomy (kĕr-ah-tot′-ō-mē)	incision into the cornea (RK, radial keratotomy, is an operation in which a series of incisions, in spoke-like fashion, are made in the cornea; done to correct myopia [nearsightedness])
myringoplasty (mĭ-rĭng′-gō-plăs′-tē)	surgical repair of the tympanic membrane
myringotomy (mĭ-rĭng-gŏt′-o-mē)	incision of the tympanic membrane
ophthalmectomy (ŏf-thal-mĕk′-to-mē)	excision of the eye
scleroplasty (sklŭ′-rō-plăs′-tē)	surgical repair of the sclera
sclerotomy (sklĕ-rŏt′-o-mē)	incision into the sclera
stapedectomy (stā-pē-dĕk′-to-mē)	excision of the stapes

Diagnostic Terms	Meaning
cataract (kăt′-ah-răkt)	cloudiness of the lens of the eye
conjunctivitis (kŏn-jŭnk-tī-vī′-tĭs)	inflammation of the conjunctiva (pinkeye)
glaucoma (glaw-kō′-mah)	an eye disease caused by increased pressure within the eye
keratocele (kĕr′-ah-tō-sĕl)	herniation (of a layer) of the cornea
keratoconjunctivitis (kĕr′-ah-tō-kŏn-jŭnk-tĭ-vī′-tĭs)	inflammation of the cornea and the conjunctiva
otitis media (ō-tī′-tĭs) (mē′-dē-ah) (OM)	inflammation of the middle ear
retinal detachment (rĕt′-ĭn-al) (dē-tăch′-mĕnt)	complete or partial separation of the retina from the choroid
strabismus (străh-bĭz′-mŭs)	weakness of the muscle of the eye that causes the eye to look in different directions (medical term for crossed eyes)

Terms Related to Diagnostic Procedures	Meaning
ophthalmoscope (ŏf-thal′-mō-skōp)	instrument used for visual examination of the eye
otoscope (ō′-tō-skōp)	instrument used for visual examination of the ear

8. blepharoplasty

_____

9. blepharorrhaphy

_____

10. keratoconjunctivitis

_____

11. keratocele

_____

12. conjunctivitis

_____

13. myringotomy

_____

14. myringoplasty

_____

15. keratotomy

_____

EXERCISE 4

Analyze and define each medical term listed below.

1. ophthalmoscope

_____

2. ophthalmologist

_____

3. ophthalmectomy

_____

4. otorrhea

_____

5. otoscope

_____

6. iridosclerotomy

_____

7. iridectomy

_____

EXERCISE 5

Build a medical term from each definition listed below.

1. inflammation of the middle ear

_____

2. instrument used for visual examination of the eye

_____

3. suturing of the eyelid

_____

4. discharge from the ear

_____

5. incision into the iris and the sclera

_____

6. surgical repair of the sclera

_____

7. excision of part of the iris

_____

8. herniation of the cornea

_____

9. instrument used for visual examination of the ear

_____

10. excision of the eye

_____

11. incision of the sclera

_____

12. surgical repair of the eyelid

_____

13. incision into the tympanic membrane

_____

14. surgical repair of the tympanic membrane

_____

15. inflammation of the cornea and the conjunctiva

_____

16. inflammation of the conjunctiva

_____

17. incision into the cornea

_____

EXERCISE 6

Define each medical term listed below.

1. cataract

_____

2. cataract extraction

_____

3. retinal detachment

_____

4. enucleation of the eye

_____

5. strabismus

_____

6. glaucoma

_____

7. optometrist

_____

8. corneal transplant

_____

EXERCISE 7

Spell each medical term studied in this unit by having someone dictate the terms to you.

1. _____

2. _____

3. _____

4. _____

5. _____

6. _____

7. _____

8. _____

9. _____

10. _____

11. _____

12. _____

13. _____

14. _____

15. _____

16. _____

17. _____

18. _____

19. _____

20. _____

21. _____

22. _____

23. _____

24. _____

25. _____

26. _____

27. _____

28. _____

EXERCISE 8

Answer the following questions.

1. Instruments used to examine the eye and the ear visually are usually part of the equipment stored at the nurses' station in the hospital. The instrument used to examine the eye is called a(n) _____ . The instrument used to examine the ear is called a(n) _____.

2. Children often develop inflammation of the middle ear, called _____ _____.
   Children who have had repeated middle ear infections may have a buildup of fluid in the middle ear. The doctor may surgically treat this condition by making an incision into the eardrum, known as _____, and inserting tiny tubes.

3. The patient is admitted to the hospital with a diagnosis of cloudiness of the lens of the right eye, or _____.
   She is scheduled for surgical removal of the diseased lens. The operation is called _____.

4. Two medical words are used to describe surgical removal of the eyeball. These words are _____ and _____.

5. _____ is the medical term for crossed eyes.

ABBREVIATIONS

Abbreviation	Meaning
OD	oculus dexter (right eye)
OM	otitis media (middle ear infection)
OS	oculus sinister (left eye)
OU	oculus uterque (both eyes)
PERRLA	pupils equal, round, reactive to light and accomodation
PRK	photorefractive keratectomy
RK	radial keratotomy

EXERCISE 9

Define the following abbreviations.

1. PERRLA

   _____

2. OM

   _____

3. PRK

   _____

4. RK

   _____

5. OD

   _____

6. OS

   _____

7. OU

   _____

UNIT 6
The Cardiovascular and Lymphatic Systems

OUTLINE

UNIT OBJECTIVES

Upon completion of this unit, you will be able to:

1. Name and describe the functions of the organs of the circulatory system.
2. Name and describe the structures of the heart and describe the circulation of blood through the heart.
3. Name three types of blood vessels and briefly describe the function of each.
4. Briefly describe the composition of blood and list and describe the functions of the three types of blood cells.
5. Name and describe the functions of the organs of the lymphatic system.
6. Describe two functions of the spleen.
7. Describe coronary artery disease, congestive heart failure, anemia, varicose veins, and acquired immunodeficiency syndrome.
8. Define the unit abbreviations.

THE CARDIOVASCULAR AND LYMPHATIC SYSTEMS

Organs of the Circulatory System

* Heart
* Blood vessels
* Blood

Functions of the Circulatory System

* **Transportation** of nutrients, oxygen, and hormones to cells, and removal of wastes

* **Protection** by white blood cells and antibodies to defend the body against foreign invaders
* **Regulation** of body temperature, fluids, and water volume of cells

All living cells, which are metabolically active structures, need constant nourishment and oxygen for life and for continuous removal of their waste products. The circulatory system provides the vital transportation service that carries nourishment (oxygen, nutrients, and hormones) to the cells of the body and carries the waste away (nitrogenous wastes, carbon dioxide, and heat). Blood is the tissue that is most frequently examined by clinicians to determine the state of health.

The heart pumps blood to the lungs and the body cells through a network of tubing called *blood vessels.* Blood is the carrying agent for food, oxygen, waste, and other materials needed for or produced by cell function.

THE HEART

The heart is located in the mediastinum, the cavity between the lungs that is situated behind the sternum. It is a four-chambered organ the size of a fist, and it weighs less than a pound. The heart performs the action of pumping the blood through the blood vessels to all parts of the body, circulating it in a one-way movement. The heart is surrounded by the *pericardium,* a loose-fitting double-layered sac. Serous membranes of the pericardium secrete a small amount of fluid to prevent irritation as the heart contracts.

Structure of the Heart

The heart wall is made up of three layers. The outer layer of the heart wall, the *epicardium,* is the visceral layer of the pericardium. The thickest, muscular middle layer is called the *myocardium.* The *endocardium,* the inner lining of the heart, also forms the heart valves.

The heart is divided into four cavities or chambers (Fig. 23-20), through which blood entering the heart travels. Each chamber has a valve (or one-way door) that prevents the blood from flowing backward into the chamber. The *septum* is a partition that divides the heart into a right and a left side. Each side is divided by halves into two upper chambers—the *right atrium* and the *left atrium*—and two lower chambers—the *right ventricle* and the *left ventricle.* The left atrium is separated from the left ventricle by the *bicuspid,* or *mitral, valve.* On the right side, the right atrium is separated from the right ventricle by the *tricuspid,* or *atrioventricular (AV), valve.* The *semilunar valves* (pulmonary and aortic) are located between the right ventricle and the pulmonary artery and between the left ventricle and the aorta.

Conduction System of the Heart

Regular and coordinated cardiac muscle contraction is conducted by electrical impulses that originate within the heart muscle; it is regulated by the central nervous system as well as by hormones. A normal heartbeat begins with an impulse from the sinoatrial (SA) node to the atrioventricular (AV) node, through the bundle branches, and finally through the Purkinje fibers to effect a complete heart contraction. The electrical impulses that generate the rhythm are measured by the electrocardiogram (EKG/ECG). (See Fig. 16-4, page 318, for an EKG/ECG.)

BLOOD VESSELS

Blood vessels are the tubular structures through which blood flows to and from the heart to the body parts (Fig. 23-21). Three major types of blood vessels are present: arteries, capillaries, and veins.

Arteries, except for the pulmonary artery, carry blood away from the heart. The pulmonary artery is the only artery in the body that carries blood with low levels of oxygen and a high concentration of carbon dioxide. All other arteries carry blood that is high in oxygen concentration from the heart to the body cells. *Arterial walls* are the thickest because they must withstand the pumping force of the heart. Within the walls are smooth muscles, whose contraction and relaxation affect blood pressure. Arteries branch into *arterioles,* tiny arteries that connect the arteries to capillaries. The aorta, the largest artery of the body, measures approximately 1 inch in diameter. It carries blood away from the left ventricle of the heart.

The *veins* are the vessels that carry blood from the capillary beds back to the heart. Venous blood, except that in the pulmonary veins, carries carbon dioxide and other waste products. Veins carry blood that is high in oxygen concentration from the lungs to the heart. Vein walls are thinner than arterial walls, and they contain tiny valves that help to prevent the backward flow of blood and to keep it moving in one direction. *Venules* are tiny veins that connect the capillaries with the veins. The *superior vena cava* and the *inferior vena cava* are large veins through which the blood returns from the body to the right atrium.

Capillaries are microscopic, thin-walled blood vessels. The exchange of substances takes place between the blood and the body cells while the blood is in the capillaries. The cells take in nutrients and oxygen from the blood and give off waste and carbon dioxide to the blood. Blood carries the waste to the organ that removes it from the body. Capillaries provide the links between arteries and veins.

Flow of Blood Through the Blood Vessels of the Body

Blood leaves the heart through the aorta. It travels first through the arteries and then through the arterioles to the capillaries, where the exchange of gases, nutrients, and waste takes place. The blood returns from the capillaries by first entering the venules and then flowing through the veins, finally entering the right atrium of the heart through the superior and inferior venae cavae. The superior vena cava returns blood to the heart from the upper part of the body, and the inferior vena cava returns blood to the heart from the lower part of the body.

Blood Pressure

Blood pressure (BP), measured in milliliters of mercury (mm Hg) (e.g., 120/70), records the forces created by circulating blood against the walls of the arteries, veins, and chambers of the heart. The upper number—systolic blood pressure—represents the pressure in the aorta and other large arteries during ventricular contraction. The lower number—diastolic blood pressure—represents the pressure during relaxation of the heart.

BLOOD

Blood is the carrying agent of the transportation system. It is a warm, sticky fluid that ranges in color from dark bluish-red to bright red, according to the amount of oxygen it is carrying. An adult has approximately 5.7 L (6 qt) of blood.

✎ *TAKE NOTE*

Pathway: blood saturated with carbon dioxide (CO_2) returns to the right side of the heart via the inferior and superior venae cavae → right atrium → tricuspid valve → right ventricle → pulmonary valve → pulmonary artery → to the lungs → (exchange of CO_2 and oxygen [O_2] takes place in the lungs) from the lungs saturated with O_2 → pulmonary veins → left atrium → bicuspid valve (mitral valve) → left ventricle → aortic valve → aorta

Function of Blood

The blood has three main functions: transportation, fighting of infection, and regulation.

Transportation

The blood carries oxygen from the lungs and nutrients from the digestive tract to the body cells. It carries waste products from the cells, carbon dioxide to the lungs, and other waste (urea) to the kidneys. The blood also transports hormones and other chemicals.

YOUR HEART AND HOW IT WORKS

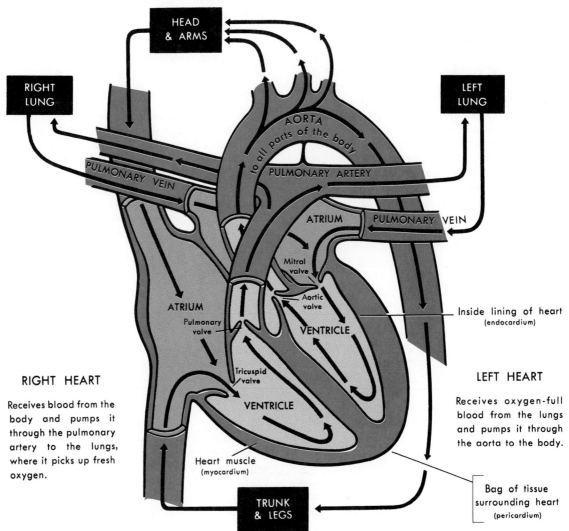

Figure 23-20 The heart. (Courtesy of the American Heart Association and its affiliates.)

Fighting Infection

Certain blood cells help the body to fight disease-causing organisms. White blood cells, or leukocytes, acting as the main line of defense against infection, respond when they encounter microbes or toxins. Certain leukocytes (e.g., B lymphocytes) produce proteins called *antibodies* (or immunoglobulins), which neutralize these foreign substances.

Regulation

The blood distributes hormones and other chemicals as needed, maintains body temperature through dilatation and constriction of blood vessels in the skin, and maintains the homeostatic balance of fluids necessary for survival.

Blood Composition

Blood is made up of plasma and cells.

Plasma

Plasma is the clear, fluid portion of the blood in which blood cells are suspended. Plasma consists of approximately 90%

water and contains more than 100 other constituents, such as glucose, fibrinogen, and protein. It makes up approximately 50% of the total amount of the blood. Plasma transports nutrients, waste material, hormones, and so forth, to and from the body cells. Fibrinogen in the plasma assists in the blood-clotting process.

Blood Cells, or Formed Elements

Three types of *blood cells* have been identified; each carries out certain functions.

- *Erythrocytes* (RBCs) are produced by the red bone marrow. Red bone marrow is found in the flat bones of the body, such as the sternum and the pelvic bones. A *sternal puncture* is a procedure that is performed to obtain bone marrow from the sternum. The bone marrow is then studied to determine its ability to produce RBCs. The function of RBCs is to carry oxygen (carbon dioxide is dissolved in the plasma). *Hemoglobin* is the oxygen-carrying protein of the erythrocyte that gives blood its color. The average RBC count is 4.5 to 5 million/mm^3 of blood. Erythrocytes exist

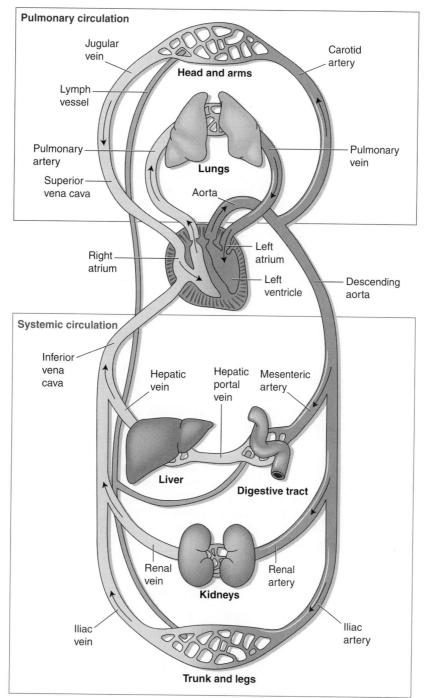

Figure 23-21 The blood vessels. (From Warekois RS, Robinson R: Phlebotomy: Worktext and Procedures Manual, 2nd ed. St. Louis: Saunders, 2007.)

for approximately 4 months. It is estimated that each erythrocyte travels approximately 700 miles during its lifetime.

- *Leukocytes* (white blood cells) are colorless cells that are produced by the spleen, bone marrow, and lymph nodes. Their chief function is to fight against pathogenic microorganisms (disease-causing bacteria). The normal white blood cell (WBC) count is 5000 to 9000/mm³ of blood. An elevated blood count may indicate the presence of infection in the body. Leukocytes last a very short time—approximately 14 hours or less.
- *Platelets* (thrombocytes) also are formed in the red bone marrow. Their prime function is to aid in the clotting of blood. A normal platelet count is about 250,000/mm³ of

blood. Platelets exist for a short time in the bloodstream and are replaced approximately every 4 days.

CIRCULATION OF BLOOD THROUGH THE HEART

Blood that carries the waste product carbon dioxide returns from circulating through the body and enters the right atrium of the heart through the superior vena cava and the inferior vena cava. Blood travels through the tricuspid valve to the right ventricle. The right ventricle pumps the blood through the *pulmonary arteries* to the lungs. (The pulmonary artery is the only artery that transports waste-carrying blood.) The blood, while in the lungs, gets rid of the carbon dioxide and takes on oxygen. This exchange changes the appearance of the blood from a bluish-red color to a bright red color. Oxygenated blood returns to the left atrium through the *pulmonary veins.*

The pulmonary vein is the only vein in the body that carries oxygenated blood. The blood passes through the bicuspid valve to the left ventricle. The left ventricle pumps the blood through the aorta and out to the body parts. Refer to Figure 23-20; the arrows indicate the passage of blood through the heart.

LYMPHATIC SYSTEM

The lymphatic system consists of the spleen, thymus gland, lymph nodes, a fluid called lymph, and the lymphatic vessels. The two principal functions of the lymphatic system involve the maintenance of fluid balance and immunity. Lymphatic vessels collect excessive tissue fluids and return them to the blood circulation.

Spleen

The *spleen,* the largest lymphatic organ, is located in the upper left abdomen and is protected by the lower ribs. Two important functions of the spleen are to destroy old RBCs, bacteria, and germs and to store blood for emergency use. The spleen produces RBCs in the fetus.

Thymus Gland

The *thymus gland,* one of the primary lymphatic organs, plays an important role in the development of the body's defenses against infection by promoting the maturation of cells that provide immune responses (T lymphocytes).

DISEASES AND DISORDERS OF THE CIRCULATORY SYSTEM

Coronary Artery Disease

Coronary artery disease (CAD) usually is caused by occlusion, or narrowing, of the arteries caused by the buildup of plaque on the arterial walls, a condition called *atherosclerosis. Angina pectoris* is a condition that is caused by lack of oxygen to the myocardium as a result of atherosclerosis of the coronary arteries. Atherosclerosis can block the artery completely, creating a condition called *coronary occlusion,* or a *thrombus* (blood clot) can develop on segments of the artery that contain plaque, causing a blockage. This condition is referred to as *coronary thrombosis.* Both conditions may lead to *myocardial infarction (MI)* (heart attack) because they reduce the flow of blood to the heart, which denies the myocardium the oxygen

and nutrients it needs. A symptom of an MI is sudden *onset* of chest pain, sometimes radiating to the arms. The severity of the heart attack depends on which artery is blocked and to what extent it is blocked.

Coronary artery bypass graft surgery (CABG) may be performed in coronary artery disease to improve the blood supply to the myocardium. This type of surgery consists of using a vein from the leg that is grafted to the aorta and the clogged coronary artery to form an alternative route for the flow of blood.

Angioplasty, surgical repair of a blood vessel, refers to various techniques such as the use of surgery, lasers, or tiny balloons at the tip of a catheter to repair or replace damaged blood vessels. *Percutaneous transluminal coronary angioplasty (PTCA)* is a cardiac procedure in which fatty plaques in the blood vessels are flattened against vessel walls by passage of a balloon within a catheter through the affected blood vessels. A coronary stent, a wire mesh tube, is commonly placed in the cleared artery to maintain its patency. *Laser angioplasty* makes use of light amplification through stimulated emission of radiation (laser beam) through a fiberoptic probe to open blocked arteries.

Congestive Heart Failure

Congestive heart failure (CHF) occurs when the heart is unable to pump the required amount of blood, resulting in accumulation of blood in the lungs and the liver. CHF develops gradually. Symptoms include fatigue, dyspnea (shortness of breath), and peripheral edema. Diagnostic testing includes chest x-ray, EKG, echocardiogram, angiogram, and blood tests. Treatment consists of dietary changes (i.e., restricted sodium, fats, cholesterol, fluids) and administration of medications such as angiotensin-converting enzyme (ACE) inhibitors, beta blockers, digoxin, and diuretics. Surgical options that may be used to correct the underlying cardiac problem include coronary bypass surgery, valve repair or replacement, cardiac resynchronization therapy, ventricular remodeling, and heart transplantation.

Anemia

Anemia is a disorder that is characterized by an abnormally low level of hemoglobin in the blood, or inadequate numbers of RBCs. It may result from decreased RBC production, from increased RBC destruction, or from blood loss. Treatment varies according to the cause. The anemic person becomes easily fatigued. Pallor also may indicate anemia. Sternal puncture to obtain bone marrow for study and blood tests are used to diagnose anemia.

Varicose Veins

Varicose veins are swollen, distended, and knotted veins that usually are found among the superficial veins of the leg. One-way valves in the veins assist in moving the blood upward to the heart. Standing or sitting for prolonged periods causes the valves to dilate from the weight of pooled blood and can result in loss of elasticity of the valves. Other causes of varicose veins include pregnancy, obesity, illness, injury, and heredity. Elevation of the leg and the use of elastic stockings are used to reduce blood pooling in the great saphenous vein, the largest superficial vein. Minimally invasive surgery, in which the affected veins are pulled out, called *ambulatory phlebectomy,* may be required in more severe cases. Hemorrhoids are internal or external varicose veins in the rectal area.

Acquired Immunodeficiency Syndrome

In *acquired immunodeficiency syndrome (AIDS),* which manifests as the destruction of patients' immune systems, carriers are highly susceptible to infection. AIDS is caused by the human immunodeficiency virus (HIV), which infects certain WBCs of the body's immune system and gradually destroys the body's ability to fight infection. Many infected persons develop previously rare types of pneumonia (*Pneumocystis carinii* pneumonia) and a form of skin cancer (Kaposi's sarcoma).

HIV has been isolated from semen and blood and is transmitted via direct or intimate contact involving the mucous membranes or breaks in the skin, across the placenta from mother to fetus, or before or during birth. The sharing of hypodermic needles among IV drug users, blood transfusions, and needle sticks are other ways by which infection is spread. The virus cannot penetrate intact skin. AIDS has become one of the deadliest epidemic diseases of modern times and will remain a major global health concern until more definitive treatment can be provided.

REVIEW QUESTIONS

1. Label the following diagram of the heart, including the blood vessels through which the blood enters and leaves the heart. Include the following parts:

endocardium	pulmonary artery	right atrium
myocardium	pulmonary vein	left atrium
pericardium	aorta	right ventricle
bicuspid valve	superior vena cava	left ventricle
tricuspid valve	inferior vena cava	

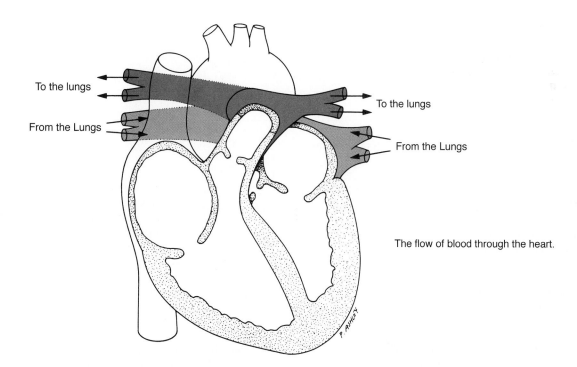

To the lungs

From the Lungs

To the lungs

From the Lungs

The flow of blood through the heart.

2. Using arrows, trace on the same diagram the circulation of blood from the superior and inferior venae cavae to the aorta.

3. Blood travels through a network of tubes called *blood vessels.* Name, in sequence, the types of blood vessels through which the blood travels when it leaves the heart until reentry, and describe the function of each.

a. _____

b. _____

c. _____

d. _____

e. _____

4. The fluid portion of the blood is called the _____. Its functions are:

a. _____

b. _____

c. _____

5. List three types of blood cells (formed elements) and briefly describe the function of each.

a. _____

b. _____

c. _____

6. Name the four blood types.

a. _____

b. _____

c. _____

d. _____

7. Two functions of the spleen are:

a. _____

b. _____

8. Match the terms in Column 1 with the phrases in Column 2.

Column 1
a. anemia
b. CHF
c. CAD
d. coronary thrombosis
e. myocardial infarction
f. bypass
g. angina pectoris
h. ambulatory phlebectomy
i. AIDS

Column 2
_____ 1. caused by lack of oxygen to the myocardium
_____ 2. the heart is unable to efficiently pump blood
_____ 3. narrowing of arteries
_____ 4. below normal level of hemoglobin
_____ 5. causes occlusion of an artery
_____ 6. surgery for varicose veins
_____ 7. damage to the heart muscle
_____ 8. caused by HIV

MEDICAL TERMINOLOGY RELATED TO THE CIRCULATORY SYSTEM

Upon mastery of the medical terminology for this unit, you will be able to:

1. Spell and define the word parts and the medical terms for the circulatory system.

2. Given the meaning of a medical condition related to the circulatory system, build with word parts the corresponding medical term.

3. Analyze the medical terms that are built from word parts that relate to the circulatory system.

4. Given a list of word parts, identify them as word roots, suffixes, or prefixes.

5. Given descriptions of hospital situations in which the HUC may encounter medical terminology, apply the correct medical terms to the situations.

Word Parts

The list below contains the word parts related to the circulatory system that you need to memorize. The exercises included in this unit will help you with this task. You will continue to use these word parts throughout this course and during your employment. Practice pronouncing each word part aloud.

Word Roots/Forms	Combining Meaning
angi / o (ăn′-jē-ō)	blood vessel
aort / o (ā-ŏr′-tō)	aorta
arteri / o (ar-tē′-rē-ō)	artery
cardi / o (kar′-dē-ō)	heart
hem / o (hē′-mō); hemat / o (hēm′-ah-tō)	blood
phleb / o (flĕb′-ō); ven / o (vē′-nō)	vein
splen / o (splē′-nō)	spleen
thromb / o (thrŏm′-bō)	clot

Color Word Roots/ Combining Forms	Meaning
cyan / o (sī′-ah-nō)	blue
erythr / o (ĕ-rĭth′-rō)	red
leuk / o (loo′-kō)	white

Prefixes	Meaning
brady- (bră′-dee)	slow
endo- (ĕn′-dō)	inside
hyper- (hī′-per)	above normal
hypo- (hī′-pō)	below normal
peri- (pĕr′-ē)	surrounding (outer)
tachy- (tăk′-kē)	fast, rapid

Suffixes	Meaning
-emia (ē′-mē-ah) (also may be used as a word root)	condition of the blood
-megaly (mĕg′-ah-lē)	enlargement
-pexy (pĕk′-sē)	surgical fixation (suspension)
-sclerosis (sklĕ-rō′-sĭs)	hardening (also may be used as a word root)
-stenosis (stĕ-nō′-sĭs)	narrowing (also may be used as a word root)

EXERCISE 1

Identify each word part listed here by writing P for prefix, S for suffix, or WR for word root in the space provided. Then define each word part in the space provided. Word parts studied in previous units are also included in this exercise.

Word Part	Type	Meaning
Example: pexy	S	surgical fixation
1. hypo	_____	_____
2. a, an	_____	_____

Word Part	Type	Meaning
3. hem	_____	_____
4. spleen	_____	_____
5. cyt	_____	_____
6. stenosis	_____	_____
7. endo	_____	_____
8. leuk	_____	_____
9. erythr	_____	_____
10. angi	_____	_____
11. cardi	_____	_____
12. arteri	_____	_____
13. peri	_____	_____
14. inter	_____	_____
15. intra	_____	_____
16. sclerosis	_____	_____
17. emia	_____	_____
18. megaly	_____	_____
19. phleb	_____	_____
20. aort	_____	_____
21. thromb	_____	_____
22. hyper	_____	_____
23. tachy	_____	_____
24. brady	_____	_____

EXERCISE 2

Write the word parts for the meanings listed on the following page. Identify each word part that you write in the answer column. Use P for prefix, S for suffix, and WR for word root or combining form. For review purposes, word parts from previous units are included in this exercise.

Meaning	Type	Word Parts
1. aorta	_____	_____
2. enlargement	_____	_____
3. hardening	_____	_____
4. between	_____	_____
5. artery	_____	_____
6. blood vessel	_____	_____
7. white	_____	_____
8. narrowing	_____	_____
9. spleen	_____	_____
10. without	_____	_____
11. surgical fixation	_____	_____
12. inside	_____	_____
13. blood	_____	_____
14. cell	_____	_____
15. below normal	_____	_____
16. redī	_____	_____
17. heartī	_____	_____
18. surrounding (outer)	_____	_____
19. blood condition	_____	_____
20. veinī	_____	_____
21. clotī	_____	_____
22. fast, rapid	_____	_____
23. slow	_____	_____

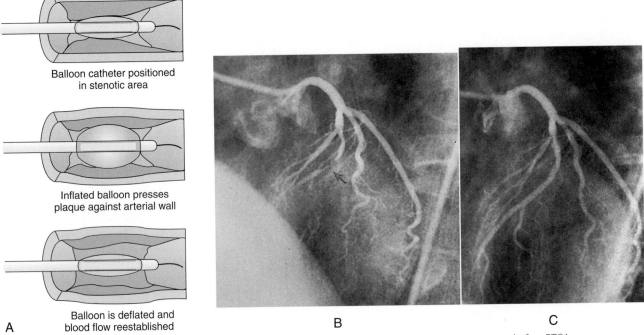

Balloon catheter positioned
in stenotic area

Inflated balloon presses
plaque against arterial wall

Balloon is deflated and
blood flow reestablished

A   B   C

Figure 23-22 A, Percutaneous transluminal coronary angioplasty (PTCA). **B,** Coronary artery before PTCA. *Arrow* indicates a stenotic area, estimated at 95% minimum blood flow distal to the lesion. **C,** Coronary arteriogram after PTCA in the same patient. Blood flow is estimated to be 100%.

MEDICAL TERMS RELATED TO THE CIRCULATORY SYSTEM

The following list is made up of medical terms for the circulatory system that you will need to know. Exercises following this list will assist you in learning these terms. Practice the pronunciation of these terms out loud.

General Terms	Meaning
aortic (ā-or′-tĭk)	pertaining to the aorta
arrhythmia (ah-rĭth′-mē-ah)	variation from a normal rhythm, especially of the heartbeat (also called *dysrhythmia*)
bradycardia (brā-dy-căr′-dĭă)	condition of slow heart (rate)
cardiac arrest (kar′-dē-ăk) (ah-rĕst′)	sudden and often unexpected stoppage of the heartbeat
cardiologist (kar-dē-ŏl′-o-jĭst)	one who specializes in the diagnosis and treatment of the heart (doctor)
cardiology (kar-dē-ŏl′-o-jē)	the study of the heart (and its functions and diseases)
cardiomegaly (kar′-dē-ō-mĕg′-ah-lē)	enlargement of the heart
cardiovascular (kar′-dē-ō-văs′-kū-lar)	pertaining to the heart and blood vessels
coronary (kŏr′-ō-nā-rē)	a term used to describe blood vessels that supply blood to the heart
endocardial (ĕn-dō-kar′-dē-al)	pertaining to within the heart
erythrocyte (ĕ-rĭth′-rō-sīt)	red blood cell (RBC)
hemorrhage (hĕm′-ō-rĭj)	the rapid flow of blood (from a blood vessel)

General Terms	General Terms
hypertension (hī-per-tĕn′-shŭn) (HTN)	high blood pressure
hypotension (hī-pō-tĕn′-shŭn)	low blood pressure
intravenous (ĭn-trah-vē′-nŭs)	within a vein
leukocyte (loo′-kō-sīt)	white blood cell (WBC)
phlebotomy (flĕ-bŏt′-ō-mē)	incision into the vein (to withdraw blood)
splenomegaly (splē-nō-mĕg′-ah-lē)	enlargement of the spleen
tachycardia (tăk-ē-kar′-dē-ah)	condition of rapid heart (rate)
thrombosis (thrōm-bō′-sĭs)	abnormal formation of a blood clot

Surgical Terms	Meaning
angioplasty (ăn′-jē-ō-plăs′-tē)	surgical repair of a blood vessel (Fig. 23-22)
angiorrhaphy (ăn-jē-ōr′-ah-fē)	suturing of a blood vessel
hemorrhoidectomy (hĕm-ō-roi-dĕk′-tō-mē)	excision of hemorrhoids
splenectomy (splē-nĕk′-tō-mē)	excision of the spleen
splenopexy (splē′-nō-pĕk-sē)	surgical fixation of the spleen

Diagnostic Terms	Meaning
anemia (ah-nē′-mē-ah)	condition of blood without (deficiency in the number of erythrocytes [RBCs])
aneurysm (ăn′-ū-rĭzm)	dilatation of a weak area of the arterial wall
arteriosclerosis (ar-tē′-rē-ō-sclĕ-rō′-sĭs)	abnormal condition of hardening of the arteries

Diagnostic Terms	Meaning
arteriostenosis (ar-tē′-rē-ō-stĕ-nō′-sĭs)	abnormal condition of narrowing of an artery
congestive heart failure (CHF)	inability of the heart to pump sufficient amounts of blood to the body parts
coronary occlusion (kŏr′-ŏ-nā-rē) (ō-kloo′-zhŭn)	the closing off of a coronary artery; which usually results in damage to the heart muscle; commonly referred to as a heart attack
coronary thrombosis (kŏr′-ŏ-nā-rē) (thrŏm-bō′-sĭs)	the blocking of a coronary artery by a blood clot; commonly referred to as a heart attack
edema (ĕ-dē′-mah)	an abnormal accumulation of fluid in the intercellular spaces of the body
embolism (ĕm′-bō-lĭzm)	a floating mass that blocks a vessel
endocarditis (ĕn-dō-kar-dī′-tĭs)	inflammation of the inner (lining) of the heart
hematology (hē-mah-tŏl′-o-jē)	study of the blood (also, a diagnostic division within a hospital laboratory that performs diagnostic tests on blood components)
hematoma (hē-mah-tō′-mah)	a tumor-like mass formed from blood (in the tissues)
hemophilia (hē-mō-fĭl′-ē-ah)	a congenital disorder characterized by excessive bleeding
hemorrhoid (hĕm′-ōrr-oyd)	enlarged veins in the rectal area
leukemia (loo-kē′-mē-ah)	a type of cancer characterized by rapid abnormal production of white blood cells
myocardial infarction (mī-ō-kar′-dē-al) (ĭn-fark′-shŭn) (MI)	damage to the heart muscle caused by insufficient blood supply to the area; a condition the layperson refers to as a heart attack
pericarditis (pĕr-ĭ-kar-dī′-tĭs)	inflammation of the outer (sac) of the heart (or pericardium)
thrombophlebitis (thrŏm′-bō-flĕ-bī′-tĭs)	inflammation of a vein (as the result of a clot)
ventricular fibrillation (VFib)	life-threatening uncoordinated contractions of the ventricles; immediate application of an electrical shock with a defibrillator is necessary treatment

Terms Related to Diagnostic Procedures	Meaning
angiogram (ăn′-jē-ō-grăm)	an x-ray image of a blood vessel (using dye as a contrast medium)
aortogram (ā-ōr′-tō-grăm)	an x-ray image of the aorta (using dye as a contrast medium)

Terms Related to Diagnostic Procedures	Meaning
arteriogram (ar-tē′-rē-ō-grăm)	an x-ray image of an artery (using dye as a contrast medium)
cardiac catheterization (kar-dē-ăk) (kăth′-ē-ter-ĭ-zā′-shŭn)	a diagnostic procedure used to visualize the heart to determine the presence of heart disease or heart defects; a long catheter is threaded from a blood vessel to the heart cavities and vessels; if arteriograms are done, contrast medium (dye) is injected into the blood vessels for the purpose of taking real-time x-rays (fluoroscopy)
electrocardiogram (ē-lĕk′-trō-kar′-dē-ō-grăm) (EKG/ECG)	a record of the electrical activity of the heart
electrocardiograph (ē-lĕk′-trō-kar′-dē-ō-grăf)	an instrument used to record electrical activity of the heart
electrocardiography (ē-lĕk′-trō-kar-dē-ōg′-rah-fē)	the process of recording the electrical activity of the heart
hematocrit (hē-măt′-ō-krĭt)	hematocrit, which means "to separate blood," is a laboratory test that measures the volume percentage of RBCs in whole blood
hemoglobin (hē′-mō-glō′-bĭn)	the oxygen-carrying protein of the RBCs

---

EXERCISE 3

Analyze and define each medical term listed below.

1. aortic

   _____

2. splenomegaly

   _____

3. hemorrhage

   _____

4. thrombosis

   _____

5. leukocyte

   _____

6. erythrocyte

   _____

7. cardiologist

_____

8. cardiomegaly

_____

9. phlebotomy

_____

10. angiorrhaphy

_____

11. splenectomy

_____

12. splenopexy

_____

13. endocarditis

_____

14. arteriosclerosis

_____

15. arteriostenosis

_____

16. thrombophlebitis

_____

17. hematoma

_____

18. hematology

_____

19. leukemia

_____

20. anemia

_____

21. electrocardiogram

_____

22. electrocardiograph

_____

23. electrocardiography

_____

24. angiogram

_____

25. arteriogram

_____

26. aortogram

_____

27. pericarditis

_____

28. tachycardia

_____

29. bradycardia

_____

30. angioplasty

_____

EXERCISE 4

Using the word elements you have studied in this unit and in previous units, build a medical term from each definition listed below.

1. x-ray image of the aorta _____

2. x-ray image of an artery _____

3. x-ray image of a blood vessel _____

4. a record of the electrical activity of the heart _____

5. inflammation of the inner lining of the heart _____

6. hardening of the arteries _____

7. inflammation of a vein due to blood clot formation _____

8. study of the blood _____

9. study of the heart _____

10. one who specializes in the diagnosis and treatment of the heart _____

11. enlarged heart _____

12. incision into a vein   _____

13. excision of the spleen   _____

14. surgical fixation of the spleen   _____

15. rapid discharge of blood   _____

16. white blood cell   _____

17. red blood cell   _____

18. inflammation of the outer (sac)
    of the heart   _____

EXERCISE 5

Define each medical term listed below.

1. hematocrit

   _____

2. hemoglobin

   _____

3. cardiac arrest

   _____

4. cardiovascular

   _____

5. hemorrhoidectomy

   _____

6. myocardial infarction

   _____

7. hemorrhoid

   _____

8. intravenous

   _____

9. cardiac catheterization

   _____

10. aneurysm

    _____

11. embolism

    _____

12. hypertension

    _____

13. hypotension

    _____

14. congestive heart failure

    _____

15. coronary

    _____

16. edema

    _____

17. arrhythmia

    _____

18. tachycardia

    _____

EXERCISE 6

Spell each medical term studied in this unit by having someone dictate the terms to you.

1. _____

2. _____

3. _____

4. _____

5. _____

6. _____

7. _____

8. _____

9. _____

10. _____

11. _____

12. _____

13. _____

14. _____

15. _____

16. _____

17. _____

18. _____

19. _____

20. _____

21. _____

22. _____

23. _____

24. _____

25. _____

26. _____

27. _____

28. _____

29. _____

30. _____

31. _____

32. _____

33. _____

34. _____

35. _____

36. _____

37. _____

38. _____

39. _____

40. _____

41. _____

42. _____

43. _____

44. _____

45. _____

46. _____

47. _____

48. _____

49. _____

50. _____

51. _____

52. _____

53. _____

EXERCISE 7

Fill in the following blanks with the requested information.

1. _____ is a division within the laboratory that performs diagnostic tests on blood components. _____ and _____ are two tests performed in this laboratory division whose results yield RBC information.

2. The coronary care unit (CCU) in the hospital is an intensive care unit that is set up to care for patients who have had heart attacks. The admitting diagnoses of these patients may be:

   a. _____

   b. _____

   c. _____

3. Below is a list of medical terms. Circle the terms that may be found on the surgical schedule. Underline the part of the word that makes it a surgical procedure.

   cardiology   hemorrhoidectomy

   electroencephalogram   hypertension

   endocarditis   splenectomy

4. A doctor who performs surgery on the heart or blood vessels may be called a _____ surgeon.

5. A patient is having symptoms that suggest the presence of a disease or a complication involving the circulatory system. The attending doctor is a good practitioner. He wishes the patient to see a heart specialist. He will contact a _____.

6. Each hospital has a team of people to call for emergency conditions such as sudden stoppage of the heart or _____. This team may be called the _____ team.

7. The doctor orders a diagnostic procedure to record the electrical activity of the heart called a(n) _____. The technician brings a(n) _____ (machine) to the patient's bedside to perform this test.

8. The patient is scheduled for an x-ray image of the blood vessels to be visualized through the use of dye as a contrast medium. The patient is scheduled for a(n) _____.

9. The patient is scheduled for a diagnostic test that uses dye as a contrast medium to visualize parts of the heart. A long catheter is threaded from a blood vessel to the heart. _____is the name of this test.

10. Below are listed three types of blood cells. Look under "Doctors' Orders for Hematology Studies." Write the name of the laboratory test used to study each cell listed below:

   a. leukocyte _____

   b. erythrocyte _____

   c. platelet _____

11. _____ is the clear, fluid portion of the blood that may be ordered by the doctor to be administered intravenously to the patient.

ABBREVIATIONS

Abbreviation	Meaning
ASHD	atherosclerotic heart disease
BP	blood pressure
CABG	coronary artery bypass graft
CAD	coronary artery disease
CHF	congestive heart failure
DVT	deep vein thrombosis
ECG	electrocardiogram
EchoCG	echocardiogram
EKG	electrocardiogram
HIV	human immunodeficiency virus
HTN	hypertension (high blood pressure)
PTCA	percutaneous transluminal coronary angioplasty
PVD	peripheral vascular disease
RBC	red blood cell (erythrocyte)
Vfib	ventricular fibrillation
WBC	white blood cell (leukocyte)

EXERCISE 8

Define the following abbreviations.

1. BP

   _____

2. ASHD

   _____

3. CABG

   _____

4. CAD

   _____

5. CHF

   _____

6. ECG

   _____

7. EchoCG

   _____

8. EKG

   _____

9. HIV

   _____

10. HTN

   _____

11. Vfib

   _____

12. MI

   _____

13. PTCA

   _____

14. PVD

   _____

15. RBC

   _____

16. WBC

   _____

17. DVT

   _____

UNIT 7
The Digestive System

OUTLINE

UNIT OBJECTIVES

Upon completion of this unit, you will be able to:

1. Define the overall functions of the digestive system.
2. Name and describe the functions of the organs of the digestive system.
3. Name the digestive enzymes.
4. Trace the passage of food through the digestive tract.
5. Name the five sphincters of the digestive tract.
6. List the accessory organs to the digestive tract and tell how each contributes to the digestive process.
7. Describe peptic ulcer, diverticular disease, gallstones, and pyloric stenosis.
8. Define the unit abbreviations.

ORGANS OF THE DIGESTIVE SYSTEM

Digestive Tract

- Mouth
- Pharynx
- Digestive sphincter muscles
- Esophagus
- Stomach
- Small intestine
- Large intestine

Accessory Organs

- Salivary glands
- Teeth and tongue
- Liver
- Gallbladder
- Pancreas

The accessory organs play a vital role in the digestive process. Although food does not pass through the salivary glands, liver, gallbladder, or pancreas, these organs provide secretions necessary for the chemical digestion of food.

Functions of the Digestive System

- **Ingestion:** Taking nutrients into the digestive tract through the mouth
- **Digestion:** The mechanical and chemical breakdown of food for use by body cells
- **Absorption:** The transfer of digested food from the small intestine to the bloodstream
- **Elimination:** The removal of solid waste from the body

Food passes through a long tubular structure called the *digestive tract* (also called the *alimentary canal* and the *gastrointestinal [GI] tract*), which extends from the mouth to the rectum. Along the way, food is prepared for absorption by the organs of the digestive tract and the accessory organs. Waste material—that material that is not transferred to the bloodstream during absorption—is eliminated from the body. Ingestion, digestion, absorption, and elimination are the main functions of the digestive system.

THE DIGESTIVE TRACT

Mouth

In the mouth, the chewing of food, or *mastication*, starts the mechanical breakdown of food necessary for *metabolism*, the utilization of digested food by body cells. The tongue helps guide the food to the teeth, where mechanical digestion begins. The salivary glands (Fig. 23-23) produce saliva that contains the enzyme amylase. This enzyme starts the chemical breakdown of carbohydrates (starches and sugars). The three pairs of salivary glands are:

1. **Parotid:** The largest, located near the ear
2. **Submandibular:** Located near the lower jaw
3. **Sublingual:** The smallest, located under the tongue

Each salivary gland has a duct (canal) that opens into the mouth to allow for the flow of saliva.

Pharynx

The *pharynx* (throat) allows for the passage of food from the mouth to the esophagus and is about 5 inches long (12.5 cm). The pharynx is shared with the respiratory tract because it is also used for the passage of air. The epiglottis, a flexible flap of cartilage, prevents food from entering the respiratory system.

Digestive Sphincter Muscles

Sphincters, circular muscles that close or open a natural body opening, regulate the passage of substances. The arrangement of the circular fibers creates a central opening when relaxed and closure when they are contracted. Five sphincter muscles are located along the digestive tract. These digestive sphincters are called *upper esophageal, lower esophageal (cardiac), pyloric, ileocecal,* and *anal* sphincters.

Esophagus

The *esophagus* is a muscular tube that extends from the pharynx to the stomach. It passes through the thoracic cavity, behind the heart, to the abdominal cavity. The esophagus is approximately 9 inches (22.5 cm) long. Its function is simply the passage of food, which is propelled along by involuntary wave-like movements; this action is called *peristalsis.* The movement of food into and out of the esophagus is regulated by an upper esophageal sphincter and the lower esophageal (cardiac) sphincter, located between the esophagus and the stomach.

Stomach

The stomach is located in the upper left portion of the abdomen, below the diaphragm. It is a container for food during part of the digestive process. Gastric glands located in the mucous membrane lining of the stomach secrete enzymes (lipase and pepsin) and hydrochloric acid. These secretions continue the chemical breakdown of food. The smooth muscles of the stomach are circular, diagonal, and longitudinal. This muscular construction of the stomach makes the organ very strong (Fig. 23-24). The function of the stomach is to secrete the enzymes and mix and churn the food to a liquid consistency. This process of mixing and churning continues the mechanical breakdown of food. When the food is liquefied, it is referred to as *chyme.*

After about 30 minutes, the food begins to leave the stomach at 30-minute intervals. It passes through the pyloric sphincter muscle into the duodenum, which is the first part of the small intestine. It takes 2 to 4 hours for the stomach to empty completely.

Small Intestine

The small intestine, so called because it is smaller in diameter than the large intestine, is approximately 20 feet long. It extends from the stomach to the large intestine (Fig. 23-25). The first part of the small intestine is called the *duodenum.* Two accessory organs, the *pancreas* and the *gallbladder,* secrete into the duodenum through tiny tubes called *ducts.* The pancreas secretes many enzymes necessary for digestion. The gallbladder

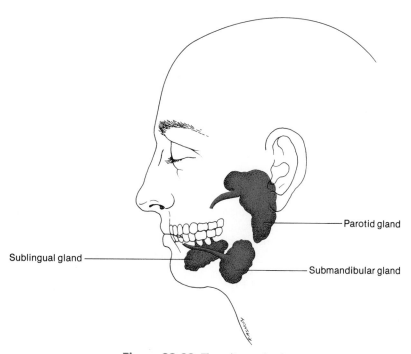

Figure 23-23 The salivary glands.

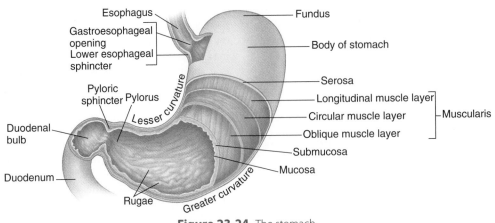

Figure 23-24 The stomach.

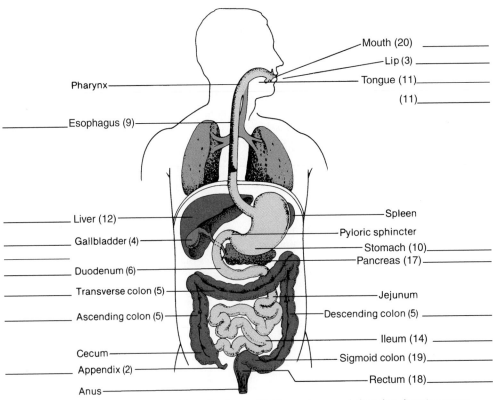

Figure 23-25 The digestive system. (From Applegate EJ: *The anatomy and physiology learning system*, Philadelphia, 1995, WB Saunders, with permission.)

secretes bile that has been produced by the liver and stored in the gallbladder. The *jejunum*, followed by the *ileum*, forms the remainder of the small intestine. (The *ilium*, one of the pelvic bones studied in the musculoskeletal system, has the same pronunciation as *ileum*. Correct spelling of the word to communicate the proper meaning is absolutely essential.) The mucosal cells located in the lining of the small intestine secrete enzymes that continue the chemical breakdown of food. These enzymes include sucrase, maltase, lipase, peptidase, and lactase. Digestion is completed in the small intestine and absorption takes place here.

✏ TAKE NOTE

Pathway: food ingestion → mouth → esophagus → cardiac sphincter → stomach → pyloric sphincter → small intestine (duodenum, jejunum, ileum) → nutrients absorption by the blood and carried to all cells for metabolic waste → ileocecal sphincter → large intestine (cecum, ascending colon, transverse colon, descending colon, sigmoid colon, rectum) → anal sphincter → elimination

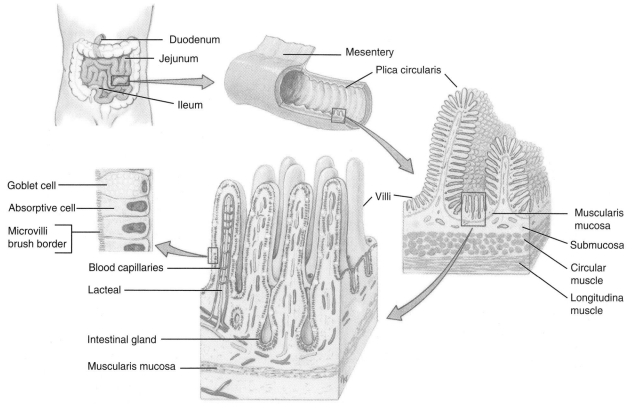

Figure 23-26 Intestinal villi. (From Applegate EJ: *The anatomy and physiology learning system*, Philadelphia, 1995, WB Saunders, with permission.)

Absorption is the passage of the end products of digestion from the small intestine into the bloodstream. The passage of nutrients from the small intestine to the bloodstream is facilitated through the capillary walls of the villi, which have a surface area of approximately 100 square feet. The *villi*, which are tiny, finger-like projections that line the walls of the small intestine (Fig. 23-26), increase the surface area of the small intestine to make it the main site of digestion and absorption. The blood carries the nutrients to all body cells, where they are used according to need. The process of cell utilization of nutrients is called *metabolism.*

The food substance (waste) that is not absorbed continues to move by peristalsis through the ileocecal sphincter into the large intestine.

Large Intestine

The large intestine is approximately 5 feet long. Peristalsis continues into the large intestine. The large intestine extends from the ileum to the *anus,* the opening at the end of the rectum to the outside. The large intestine is divided into the following parts, listed in sequence extending from the ileum: the *cecum;* the *colon,* which is divided into four parts—the ascending colon, the transverse colon, the descending colon, and the sigmoid colon; and the *rectum.* The function of the large intestine is the absorption of water and the elimination of solid waste products of digestion from the body.

The appendix is a small blind tube attached to the cecum. It has no function.

Accessory Organs: Liver, Gallbladder, and Pancreas

The liver, the largest gland in the body, is located in the upper right portion of the abdominal cavity. Although it has many important functions, we will discuss only one, the production of bile. The liver secretes bile, which aids in the digestion of fats. Bile is stored in the gallbladder, a small sac located under the liver. The gallbladder concentrates the bile by reabsorbing water. When food (especially food that contains fat) enters the duodenum from the stomach, the gallbladder is stimulated to contract and release bile into the duodenum.

The pancreas is located behind the stomach. Part of its function is to secrete the enzymes lipase, protease, amylase, and bicarbonate into the duodenum. These enzymes continue the digestion process by chemically breaking down food particles. The islets of Langerhans are contained in the pancreas. They secrete two hormones—glucagon and insulin—that are released directly into the bloodstream. Insulin is necessary for the metabolism of carbohydrates in the body, and it decreases blood glucose levels. Glucagon, also instrumental in digestion, increases blood glucose.

DISEASES AND CONDITIONS OF THE DIGESTIVE SYSTEM

Gastritis and Peptic Ulcer Disease

A peptic ulcer is a lesion, or sore, of the mucous membrane of the stomach (gastric ulcer) or duodenum (duodenal ulcer) (Fig. 23-27). A combination of factors cause peptic ulcer disease (PUD), including excessive secretion of gastric

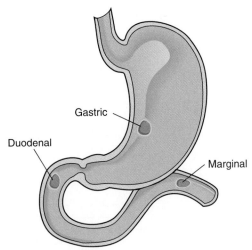

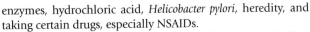

Figure 23-27 Types of ulcers.

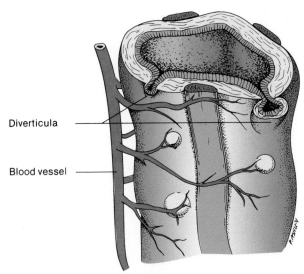

Figure 23-28 Diverticula.

enzymes, hydrochloric acid, *Helicobacter pylori*, heredity, and taking certain drugs, especially NSAIDs.

Symptoms include pain 1 to 3 hours after eating, which is usually relieved by eating or taking antacids. Also, a gnawing sensation in the epigastric region is experienced. If untreated, bleeding, hemorrhage, or perforation may occur. Perforation allows the contents of the stomach or the small intestine to escape into the peritoneal cavity. The GI series, gastroscopy, and gastric analysis are used for diagnosing peptic ulcers. Because symptoms of peptic ulcer are similar to symptoms of stomach or duodenal cancer, early diagnosis is important. Early treatment includes diet control, medication, and, if present, eradication of *H pylori* bacteria with antibiotics. Surgery may be indicated when scarring, recurrent bleeding, or perforation occurs.

Diverticular Disease

Diverticular disease is caused by the formation of small pouches, called *diverticula*, on the wall of the large intestine, generally the colon (Fig. 23-28). Two forms of diverticular disease may occur: diverticulosis and diverticulitis. In diverticulosis, diverticula are present but for most people cause no symptoms. In diverticulitis, diverticula are inflamed or infected and may cause obstruction, infection, or hemorrhage.

Symptoms include cramping in the abdomen and muscle spasms. Medical treatment includes eating a high-fiber or restricted diet and taking antibiotics to treat infection. Severe cases may require surgical removal of the involved segment of the intestine and a temporary colostomy (surgical opening between the colon and the body surface).

Cholelithiasis and Choledocholithiasis

Cholelithiasis (or *gallstones*), a condition that affects 20% of the population older than 40 years of age, is more common in women than in men (Fig. 23-29). The stones form because of changes in bile content. Gallstones can lodge in the common bile duct, which leads to the duodenum. This condition is called *choledocholithiasis*. Pain is caused by buildup of pressure in the gallbladder.

Symptoms of a typical gallbladder attack include acute abdominal pain after eating a fatty meal. Sometimes, the pain is so severe that the patient may seek emergency treatment. Other symptoms involve digestive disturbances, such as belching and flatulence. MRI, CT scan, cholecystogram, or abdominal ultrasound may be used for diagnosing gallstones. Treatment includes laparoscopic cholecystectomy and choledocholithotomy.

Pyloric Stenosis

Pyloric stenosis is an obstruction that is caused by narrowing of the pyloric sphincter muscle. The condition may be congenital or acquired. In adults, the condition most often is caused by peptic ulceration or tumors that may be cancerous. Symptoms include vomiting that becomes progressively more frequent and forceful. Infants with pyloric stenosis may be diagnosed at first with failure to thrive. Adults experience a gradual weight loss.

Diagnosis is confirmed by an upper gastrointestinal examination in which barium is used as a contrast medium. Treatment is usually surgical. In infants, a formula that is thickened with cereal may be sufficient to stretch out the sphincter muscle if stenosis is not severe.

REVIEW QUESTIONS

1. Define the following:

a. ingestion

_____

b. digestion

_____

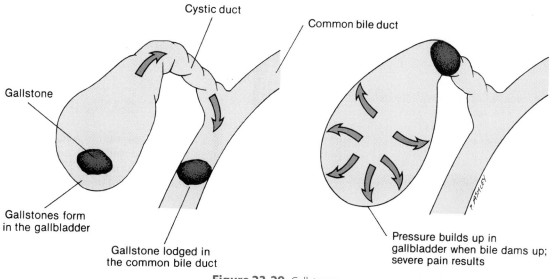

Figure 23-29 Gallstones.

c. absorption

_____

d. elimination

_____

2. Describe the overall function of the digestive system.

_____

3. Beginning with the mouth, list in order the organs through which food passes during ingestion, digestion, and elimination. Include the names of the parts of the small intestine, large intestine, and sphincter muscles.

_____

4. List the digestive chemicals and enzymes, the organs that secrete them, and the digestive organ in which they perform their functions.

Name of Digestive Chemical or Enzyme	**Organ of Secretion**	**Organ of Function**
a. _____	_____	_____
b. _____	_____	_____
c. _____	_____	_____
d. _____	_____	_____
e. _____	_____	_____

5. Name the six accessory organs of digestion.

a. _____   d. _____

b. _____   e. _____

c. _____   f. _____

6. A narrowing of the opening between the stomach and the small intestine is called _____.

7. Describe the function of the following organs in the digestive process:

a. mouth _____

b. stomach _____

c. small intestine _____

d. large intestine _____

e. gallbladder _____

8. Match the terms in Column 1 with the definitions in Column 2.

Column 1
a. diverticulitis
b. cholelithiasis
c. cholecystectomy
d. diverticulosis
e. peptic ulcer
f. choledocholithiasis

Column 2
_____ 1. lesion of the mucous membrane of the stomach
_____ 2. inflamed diverticula
_____ 3. stones in the gallbladder
_____ 4. stone in the common bile duct
_____ 5. diverticula with no symptoms

MEDICAL TERMINOLOGY RELATED TO THE DIGESTIVE SYSTEM

Upon mastery of the medical terminology for this unit, you will be able to:

1. Spell and define the word parts and medical terms related to the digestive system.
2. Given the meaning of a medical condition related to the digestive tract, build with word parts the corresponding medical term.
3. Given a list of medical terms, identify those that are surgical procedures and those that are diagnostic studies.
4. Compare the three *-tomy* suffixes.
5. Analyze and define medical terms built from word parts that relate to the digestive system.
6. Given a description of hospital situations in which the HUC may encounter medical terminology, apply the correct medical terms to the situations.

Word Parts

The list below contains the word parts related to the digestive system that you need to memorize. The exercises included in this unit will help you with this task. You will continue to use these word parts throughout this course and during your employment. Practice pronouncing each part aloud.

Word Roots/ Combining Forms	Meaning
1. abdomin / o (ăb-dŏm′-ĭ-nō)	abdomen
2. appendic / o (ăp-ĕn-dĕk′-ō)	appendix
3. cheil / o (kī′-lō)	lip
4. chol / o (kō′-lō) or chol / e (kō′-lē)	bile, gall
5. col / o (kō′-lō)	colon
6. colon / o (kō′-lŏ- nō)	colon
7. cyst / o (sĭs′-tō)	bladder (urinary unless otherwise used)

Word Roots/ Combining Forms	Meaning
8. duoden / o (doo-ō-dē′-nō)	duodenum
9. enter / o (ĕn′-ter-ō)	intestine
10. esophag / o (ĕ-sŏf′-ah-gō)	esophagus
11. gastr / o (găs′-trō)	stomach
12. gloss / o (glŏss′-ō); lingu / o (lĭng′-gwō)	tongue
13. hepat / o (hĕp′-a-tō)	liver
14. herni / o (her′-nē-ō)	protrusion of a body part
15. ile / o (ĭl′-ē-ō)	ileum
16. lapar / o (lăp′-ah-rō)	abdomen
17. lith / o (lĭth′-ō)	stone or calculus
18. pancreat / o (păn′-krē-ă-tō)	pancreas
19. proct / o (prŏk′-tō)	rectum
20. sigmoid / o (sĭg′-moy-dō)	sigmoid colon (part of the colon)
21. stomat / o (stō′-mah-tō)	mouth

Suffixes	Meaning
-iasis (ĭ′-ah-sĭs)	condition of
-stomy (ŏs′-to-mē)	creation of an artificial opening into

-tomy Suffixes

You are already familiar with two *-tomy* suffixes that are used to describe surgical procedures. These include *-tomy*, which means an incision into a part of the body, and *-ectomy*, which means surgical removal of a part of the body. The third *-tomy* suffix you will study in this unit is *-stomy*, which describes a surgical procedure that is performed to create an artificial opening into a part of the body. For example, in the medical term *colostomy* (col / o is the combining form for colon), a portion of the colon is attached to the surface of the abdomen, which creates an artificial opening between the colon and the abdominal surface (Fig. 23-30). This artificial opening is used for the passage of stools.

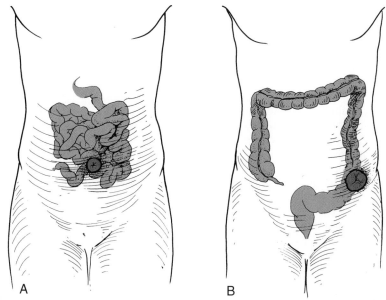

Figure 23-30 A, Ileostomy. **B,** Colostomy. (From LaFleur M: *Exploring medical language,* ed 5, St. Louis, 2002, Mosby, p. 399.)

EXERCISE 1

Write the combining forms for the digestive system in the spaces provided on the diagram in Figure 23-25 (page 502). The number preceding the combining form in the preceding list matches the number of the body part in the diagram.

EXERCISE 2

Define the word parts listed below. Indicate the word parts that are suffixes by writing S after each in the space provided.

Word Parts	Definition	Suffix?
1. stomat		
2. gloss		
3. gastr		
4. proct		
5. pancreat		
6. enter		
7. hepat		
8. cheil		
9. esophag		
10. iasis		
11. chol		
12. cyst		
13. duoden		
14. col		
15. ile		
16. abdomin		
17. appendic		
18. lapar		
19. lith		
20. stomy		
21. herni		
22. sigmoid		

EXERCISE 3

Define the three -tomy suffixes. Build a medical term using each suffix and write the meaning of each term you have built.

1. -tomy

2. -ectomy

3. -stomy

MEDICAL TERMS RELATED TO THE DIGESTIVE SYSTEM

Following is a list of medical terms related to the digestive system that you will need to know. Exercises following this list will assist you in learning these terms. Practice pronouncing each term aloud.

General Terms	Meaning
abdominal (ăb-dŏm′-ĭn-al)	pertaining to the abdomen
diarrhea (dīī′-ah-rē′-ah)	frequent discharge of watery stool
duodenal (doo-ō-dē′-nal)	pertaining to the duodenum
dysentery (dĭs′-ĕn-tĕr-ē)	condition of bad or painful intestines accompanied by diarrhea

General Terms	Meaning
glossoplegia (glŏss-ō-plē′-ja)	paralysis of the tongue
hepatoma (hĕp-ah-tō′-mah)	a tumor of the liver
hepatomegaly (hĕp′-ah-tō-mĕg′-ah-lē)	enlargement of the liver
hernia (her′-nē-ah)	an abnormal protrusion of a body part through the containing structure
jaundice (jawn′-dĭs)	yellowness of the skin and eyes; a symptom of hepatitis
pancreatic (păn-krē-ăt′-ĭk)	pertaining to the pancreas
proctorrhea (prŏk-tō-rē′-ah)	excessive discharge from the rectum
stomatogastric (stō′-mah-tō-găs′-trĭk)	pertaining to the mouth and stomach
sublingual (sŭb-lĭng′-gwal)	pertaining to under the tongue
ulcer (ŭl′-ser)	a sore of the skin or mucous membrane

Surgical Terms	Meaning
abdominal herniorrhaphy (ăb-dŏm′-ĭn-al) (her-nē-ōr′-ah-fē)	suturing of a weak spot or opening in the abdominal wall to prevent protrusion of organs
appendectomy (ăp-ĕn-dĕk′-to-mē)	excision of the appendix
cheiloplasty (kī′-lō-plăs′-tē)	surgical repair of the lip
cholecystectomy (kō-lē-sĭs-tĕk′-to-mē) Note: e is used as the combining vowel between the word roots chol and cyst.	excision of the gallbladder
colectomy (kō-lĕk′-to-mē)	excision of the colon
colostomy (kō-lŏs′-to-mē)	creation of an artificial opening into the colon; a portion of the colon is attached to the surface of the abdomen for the passage of stools
esophagoenterostomy (ē-sŏf′-ah-gō-ĕn-ter-ŏs′-to-mē)	creation of an artificial opening between the esophagus and the intestine
gastrectomy (găs-trĕk′-to-mē); pyloroplasty (pī-lōr′-ō-plăs′-tē); and vagotomy (vă-gŏt′-o-mē)	surgical procedures performed for treatment of ulcers; gastrectomy is the removal of the stomach; pyloroplasty is the plastic repair of the pyloric sphincter, located at the lower end of the stomach; vagotomy is an incision into the vagus nerve, performed to reduce the quantity of gastric juices in the stomach

Surgical Terms	Meaning
gastric bypass—malabsorptive	surgical procedure for obesity in which a small pouch is created at the top of the stomach to restrict food intake
gastrostomy (găs-trŏs′-to-mē)	creation of an artificial opening into the stomach (for feeding purposes)
glossorrhaphy (glŏ-sŏr′-ah-fē)	suturing of the tongue
herniorrhaphy (her-nē-ōr′-ah-fē)	surgical repair of a hernia (suturing of the containing structure, e.g., the abdominal wall)
ileostomy (ĭl-ē-ŏs′-to-mē)	creation of artificial opening into the ileum; a portion of the ileum is attached to the surface of the abdomen for passage of stools
laparoscopy (lăp-ah-rŏs′-ko-pē)	visual examination of the abdomen (with instruments introduced through incisions, often done in order to perform minimally invasive surgery)
laparotomy (lăp-ah-rŏt′-o-mē)	incision into the abdominal wall

Diagnostic Terms	Meaning
appendicitis (ah-pĕn-dĭ-sī′-tĭs)	inflammation of the appendix
cholecystitis (kō-lē-sĭs-tī′-tĭs)	inflammation of the gallbladder
cholelithiasis (kō-lē-lĭ-thī′-ah-sĭs) Note: e is used as the combining vowel between the word roots chol and lith.	a condition of gallstones
Crohn's (krōnz) disease	chronic inflammatory disease that can affect any part of the bowel, most often the lower small intestine
diverticulitis (dī-ver-tĭk-ū-lī′-tĭs)	inflammation of the diverticula (small pouches in the intestinal wall)
duodenal ulcer (dū-ō-dē′-nal) (ŭl′-sĕr)	ulcer (sore open area) in the duodenum
gastric ulcer (găs′-trĭk) (ŭl′-ser)	ulcer pertaining to the stomach
gastritis (găs-trī′-tĭs)	inflammation of the stomach
hepatitis (hĕp-ah-tī′-tĭs)	inflammation of the liver
ileitis (ĭl-ē-ī′-tĭs)	inflammation of the ileum
infectious hepatitis (ĭn-fĕk′-shŭs) (hĕp-ah-tī′-tĭs)	inflammation of the liver (caused by a virus)

Diagnostic Terms	Meaning
pancreatitis (păn-krē-ah-tī′-tĭs)	inflammation of the pancreas
stomatitis (stŏ-mah-tī′-tĭs)	inflammation of the mouth
ulcerative colitis (ul′-sĕ-rā-tĭv) (kō-lī′-tĭs)	inflammation of the colon with the formation of ulcers

Terms Related to Diagnostic Procedures	Meaning
abdominocentesis (ăb-dŏm′-ĭ-nō-sĕn-tē′-sĭs)	aspiration of fluid from the abdominal cavity
barium enema (bă′-rē-ŭm) (ĕn′-ĕ-mah) (BE)	x-ray of the colon (fasting x-ray); barium is used as the contrast medium
cholangiogram (kō-lăn′-jē-ŏ-grăm)	x-ray image of the bile ducts (fasting x-ray), usually done after a cholecystectomy; dye is the contrast medium
cholecystogram (kō-lē-sĭs′-to-grăm)	x-ray image of the gallbladder (most commonly done intraoperatively); contrast medium is used
colonoscope (kō-lŏn′-ō-skōp)	instrument used for visual examination of the colon
colonoscopy (kō-lŏn-ŏs′-ko-pē)	visual examination of the colon
esophagogastroduodenoscopy (ĕ-sŏf′-ah-gō-gas-trō-doo-odd-ĕn-ŏs′-ko-pē) (EGD)	visual examination of the esophagus, stomach, and duodenum
esophagoscope (ĕ-sŏf′-ah-gō-skōp)	instrument used for visual examination of the esophagus
esophagoscopy (ĕ-sŏf′-ah-gŏs′-ko-pē)	visual examination of the esophagus
gastroscope (găs′-trō-skōp)	instrument used for visual examination of the stomach
gastroscopy (găs-trŏs′-ko-pē)	visual examination of the stomach
proctoscope (prŏk′-tō-skōp)	instrument used for visual examination of the rectum
proctoscopy (prŏk-tŏs′-ko-pē)	visual examination of the rectum
sigmoidoscopy (sĭg-mol-dŏs′-ko-pē)	visual examination of the sigmoid colon
upper gastrointestinal (găs′-trō-ĭn-tĕs′-tĭ-nal) (UGI)	x-ray of the esophagus and the stomach (fasting x-ray); barium is used as the contrast medium; UGI with small-bowel follow-through is an x-ray of the stomach and small intestines

---

EXERCISE 4

Analyze and define the terms listed below.

1. glossoplegia

   _____

2. appendectomy

   _____

3. cholecystectomy

   _____

4. gastrostomy

   _____

5. hepatomegaly

   _____

6. ileostomy

   _____

7. pyloroplasty

   _____

8. protorrhea

   _____

9. cholecystitis

   _____

10. gastritis

    _____

11. sublingual

    _____

12. ileitis

    _____

13. cholecystogram

    _____

14. sigmoidoscopy

    _____

15. gastrectomy

_____

16. gastroscopy

_____

17. gastroscope

_____

18. colitis

_____

19. hepatitis

_____

20. colostomy

_____

✎ TAKE NOTE

Scope It Out

Modern medical advances and surgical innovation have paved the way for a growing number of minimally invasive surgeries. In procedures that range from appendectomy and blepharoplasty (cosmetic repair of eyelids) to cardiac and foot surgery, the thin, flexible tube with a small video camera and a light on the end is able to penetrate organs, joints, and cavities; to diagnose and correct various conditions; and to record the episode at the same time. Local or general anesthesia may be used during the procedure. Frequently, conscious sedation is administered, with a combination of sedatives and pain relievers that achieve an altered state of consciousness. Most endoscopies are performed on an outpatient basis.

Expanding use of the fiberoptic endoscope beyond the digestive system is responsible for smaller incisions, shorter recovery time, and lower medical costs. Nearly all specialties are making use of endoscopy as a more efficient means of providing diagnostic and therapeutic interventions.

The endoscope, an instrument used for visual examination within a hollow organ or body cavity, is introduced through a small incision. Through a separate small incision, tiny folding surgical instruments (e.g., forceps, scissors, brushes, snares, baskets for tissue excision) are introduced and manipulated within the tissue.

- **Arthroscopy:** Examination of joints for diagnosis and treatment
- **Bronchoscopy:** Examination of the trachea and lung bronchial trees to diagnose abscesses, bronchitis, carcinoma, tumors, tuberculosis, alveolitis, infection, and inflammation
- **Colonoscopy:** Examination of the inside of the colon and large intestine to detect polyps, tumors, ulceration, inflammation, colitis diverticula, and Crohn's disease, and for discovery and removal of foreign bodies
- **Colposcopy:** Direct visualization of the vagina and cervix to detect cancer, inflammation, and other conditions
- **Cystoscopy:** Examination of the bladder, urethra, urinary tract, ureteral orifices, and prostate (men) performed with insertion of the endoscope through the urethra
- **Endoscopic biopsy:** Removal of tissue specimens for pathologic examination and analysis.
- **Endoscopic laser foraminoplasty:** With the use of an endoscope and a laser to create an opening through the foramen (itself an opening) into the epidural space, the endoscopic surgeon can visualize the nerves in the spinal column to repair ruptured or herniated disks.
- **Endoscopic retrograde cholangiopancreatography (ERCP):** Makes use of the endoscope for radiographic examination with contrast medium introduced through a catheter. The endoscopist visualizes the liver's biliary tree, the gallbladder, the pancreatic duct, and other nearby anatomy to check for stones, obstructions, and disease. Fluoroscopic x-ray images are taken to show any abnormality or blockage. If disease is detected, it sometimes can be treated at the same time, or biopsy can be performed to test for cancer or other pathologic conditions. ERCP may reveal biliary cirrhosis, cancer of the bile ducts, pancreatic cysts, pseudocysts, pancreatic tumors, chronic pancreatitis, and gallbladder stones.
- **Esophagogastroduodenoscopy (EGD):** Visual examination of the upper gastrointestinal (GI) tract (also referred to as gastroscopy) to diagnose hemorrhage, hiatal hernia, inflammation of the esophagus, and gastric ulcers
- **Gastroscopy:** Examination of the lining of the esophagus, stomach, and duodenum. Gastroscopy often is used to diagnose ulcers and other sources of bleeding and to guide the biopsy of suspect GI cancers.
- **Hysteroscopy:** Visual examination of the uterus
- **Laparoscopy:** Visual examination of the abdominal cavity: stomach, liver, and other abdominal organs, including the female reproductive organs (e.g., fallopian tubes, uterus, ovaries)
  - Laparoscopic adrenalectomy
  - Laparoscopic appendectomy
  - Laparoscopic cholecystectomy
  - Laparoscopic choledochoscopy and choledocholithotomy
  - Laparoscopic tubal ligation
- **Laryngoscopy:** Visual examination of the larynx (voice box)
- **Proctoscopy, proctosigmoidoscopy, sigmoidoscopy:** Visual examination of the rectum and sigmoid colon
- **Thoracoscopy:** Visual examination of the thorax (chest: pleura [sac that covers the lungs], pleural spaces, mediastinum, and pericardium)

21. herniorrhaphy

_____

22. colonoscope

_____

23. colonoscopy

_____

24. esophagogastroduodenoscopy

_____

EXERCISE 5

Using the word parts studied in this unit and in previous units, build medical terms from the definitions listed below. Also, identify which are surgical procedures by writing S in the space provided, and which are diagnostic studies by writing D in the space provided. Underline the word part that indicates that the word is a surgical procedure or a diagnostic study. (Note: Some words in the list will not fall into either of these categories.)

| Examples: | gastre<u>ctomy</u> | S |
| | gastro<u>scopy</u> | D |

1. inflammation of the mouth   _____
2. inflammation of the gallbladder   _____
3. a condition of gallstones   _____
4. x-ray image of the gallbladder   _____
5. excision of the gallbladder   _____
6. inflammation of the pancreas   _____
7. instrument used for visual examination of the rectum   _____
8. visual examination of the rectum   _____
9. aspiration of fluid from the abdominal cavity   _____
10. creation of an artificial opening into the colon   _____
11. creation of an artificial opening into the ileum   _____
12. visual examination of the esophagus   _____
13. instrument used for visual examination of the stomach   _____
14. creation of an artificial opening between the esophagus and the intestines   _____
15. inflammation of the stomach   _____
16. suturing of the tongue   _____

17. surgical repair of the lip   _____
18. excision of the colon   _____
19. paralysis of the tongue   _____
20. pertaining to the mouth and stomach   _____
21. pertaining to under the tongue   _____
22. discharge from the rectum   _____
23. enlargement of the liver   _____
24. tumor of the liver   _____
25. pertaining to the pancreas   _____
26. inflammation of the appendix   _____
27. surgical removal of the appendix   _____
28. visual examination of the colon   _____
29. instrument used for visual examination of the colon   _____
30. visual examination of the esophagus, stomach, and duodenum   _____

EXERCISE 6

Define the following medical terms.

1. dysentery

_____

2. upper gastrointestinal (UGI)

_____

3. barium enema

_____

4. cholecystogram

_____

5. jaundice

_____

6. ulcerative colitis

_____

7. gastric ulcer

_____

8. Crohn's disease

_____

EXERCISE 7

Spell each medical term studied in this unit by having someone dictate the terms to you.

1. _____

2. _____

3. _____

4. _____

5. _____

6. _____

7. _____

8. _____

9. _____

10. _____

11. _____

12. _____

13. _____

14. _____

15. _____

16. _____

17. _____

18. _____

19. _____

20. _____

21. _____

22. _____

23. _____

24. _____

25. _____

26. _____

27. _____

28. _____

29. _____

30. _____

31. _____

32. _____

33. _____

34. _____

35. _____

36. _____

37. _____

38. _____

39. _____

40. _____

41. _____

42. _____

43. _____

44. _____

45. _____

46. _____

47. _____

48. _____

49. _____

50. _____

51. _____

52. _____

53. _____

54. _____

55. _____

56. _____

57. _____

58. _____

59. _____

Answer the following questions.

1. A surgical procedure to make an artificial opening from the small intestine to the abdomen is listed on the surgery schedule. Circle the correct surgical term for this procedure and explain your choice:

   a. iliostomy

   b. ileostomy

   c. ileotomy

   _____

   _____

2. A patient enters the hospital with a diagnosis of gall-stones. The admitting diagnosis in medical terms will be _____. The doctor orders a diag-nostic study to visualize the gallbladder to determine the presence of disease or gallstones. He or she orders a _____. The result of the diagnostic study indicates surgery for removal of the gallbladder. The medical term for this operation is _____.

3. The doctor orders a medication to be administered under the patient's tongue. _____ is the word written on the doctors' order sheet to indicate this.

4. List three visual examinations of the digestive tract that the doctor may order and name the instrument used for each examination.

   a. _____

   b. _____

   c. _____

5. A patient enters the hospital with an admitting diagnosis of abdominal pain. The doctor orders two x-rays, of the stomach and small intestine, and one of the colon called a(n) _____ and a(n) _____. Surgery is indicated. The doctor plans to remove the stom-ach, repair the pyloric sphincter, and make an incision into the vagus nerve. The medical terms used to describe the surgery are:

   a. _____

   b. _____

   c. _____

6. The following surgical procedures are listed on the sur-gical schedule, and you are preparing consent forms for them. Circle the terms that are spelled incorrectly, and correctly spell the misspelled terms in the space provided.

   a. laportotomy   _____

   b. appendectomy   _____

   c. herniorraphy   _____

   d. collectomy   _____

   e. gastrostomy   _____

ABBREVIATIONS

Abbreviation	Meaning
BE	barium enema
EGD	esophagogastroduodenoscopy
GE	gastroenterology/gastroenterologist
GERD	gastroesophageal reflux disease
GI	gastrointestinal
PUD	peptic ulcer disease
UGI	upper gastrointestinal

Define the following abbreviations.

1. BE

   _____

2. GI

   _____

3. GE

   _____

4. GERD

   _____

5. EGD

   _____

6. PUD

   _____

7. UGI

   _____

UNIT 8
The Respiratory System

UNIT OBJECTIVES

Upon completion of this unit, you will be able to:

1. Describe the overall function of the respiratory system.
2. Name and locate the organs of the respiratory system and tell the function of each.
3. Compare internal respiration with external respiration.
4. Describe the pathway of air from the outside to the capillary blood in the lungs.
5. Describe pneumothorax, hemothorax, pulmonary embolism, and chronic obstructive pulmonary disease (COPD).
6. Define the unit abbreviations.

THE RESPIRATORY SYSTEM

Organs of the Respiratory System

- Nose
- Pharynx
- Larynx
- Trachea
- Bronchi
- Lungs

Division of the Respiratory System

The upper respiratory system refers to the nose, nasal cavities, sinuses, pharynx, and larynx. The lower respiratory system refers to the trachea, bronchi, alveoli, and lungs (Fig. 23-31).

Function of the Respiratory System

The function of the respiratory system is to exchange gases. Oxygen is taken into the body and carbon dioxide is removed. This process is referred to as *respiration*. The respiratory system also helps to regulate the acid–base balance and enables the production of vocal sounds.

Respiration

External respiration, or breathing, is the exchange of gases between the lungs and the blood. Oxygen is inhaled into the lungs and passes through the capillary wall into the blood to be carried to the blood cells. Carbon dioxide passes out of the capillary blood to the lungs to be exhaled to the outside environment.

An exchange of gases also takes place within the body between the blood in the capillaries and individual body cells. This is called *internal respiration.* Body cells take on oxygen from the blood and at the same time give off carbon dioxide to the blood to be transported back to the lungs, where it is exhaled from the body.

The Nose

Air enters the respiratory system through the nose. The nose is divided into a right and a left nostril by a partition called the *nasal septum.* The nose prepares the air for the body by (1) warming and moistening the air, (2) removing pathogenic microorganisms, and (3) removing foreign particles, such as dust, from the air. Tiny, hair-like growths in the nose called *cilia* trap and move foreign particles toward the outside and away from delicate lung tissue. Particles too large to be handled by the *cilia* produce a sneeze or a cough, which forcibly expels the foreign particles.

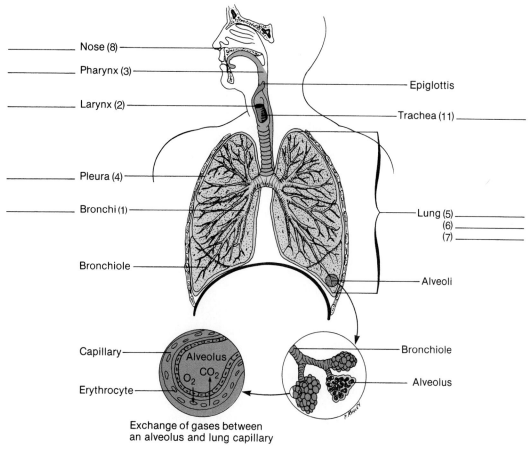

Exchange of gases between
an alveolus and lung capillary

Figure 23-31 The respiratory system.

The Pharynx

Both air and food travel through the *pharynx* (throat). Food passes from the pharynx to the esophagus, while air passes from the pharynx into the larynx, which is located anterior to the esophagus.

The Larynx

The *larynx* (voice box) is a tubular structure located below the pharynx. As was mentioned earlier, the pharynx is a passageway for both food and air. A flap of cartilage, called the *epiglottis*, automatically covers the larynx during the act of swallowing to prevent the passage of food from the pharynx into the larynx. The larynx contains the *vocal cords*. As air is exhaled past the vocal cords, the vibration of the cords produces sound.

The Trachea

The *trachea* (windpipe), a vertical tube 4 to 5 inches (10 to 12.5 cm) long, extends from the larynx to the bronchi. A series of C-shaped cartilage rings prevents the trachea from collapsing. The function of the trachea is the passage of air.

Bronchi

Behind the heart, close to the center of the chest, the trachea branches into two tubes: one leading to the right lung and the other leading to the left lung. These tubes are called *bronchi*

(singular: *bronchus*). The function of the bronchi is the passage of air.

The Lungs

The lungs are cone-shaped organs located in the thoracic cavity. The right lung is the larger of the two and is divided into three lobes. The left lung is divided into two lobes. After the bronchus enters the lung, it divides into smaller tubes and continues to subdivide into even smaller tubes called *bronchioles*. At the end of each bronchiole is a grape-like cluster of air sacs called *alveoli* (singular: *alveolus*). The walls of the alveoli are single celled, which allows for an exchange of gases to take place between the alveoli and the capillaries. The *pleura* is a double sac that surrounds each lung and lines the walls of the thoracic cavity. The *visceral pleura* lines the outer surface of the lungs, whereas the *parietal pleura* covers the chest wall. The small amount of fluid within the sacs allows the lungs to expand and contract without friction.

✎ *TAKE NOTE*

Pathway: air → nose → pharynx → larynx → trachea → bronchi → bronchioles → alveoli, where the exchange of carbon dioxide and oxygen takes place

CONDITIONS OF THE RESPIRATORY SYSTEM

Pneumothorax and Hemothorax

Pneumothorax

Pneumothorax is the collection of air or gas in the pleural cavity, resulting in a collapsed lung, or *atelectasis* (Fig. 23-32). It may be caused by a chest wound, or it may be a spontaneous collapse due to lung disease. The pleural cavity is airtight, with negative pressure. As air enters the pleural cavity, it creates pressure against the lung, causing it to collapse.

Symptoms include sudden sharp chest pain, shortness of breath, cyanosis, and stopping of normal chest movements on the affected side. Treatment ranges from observation and supplemental oxygen for an uncomplicated pneumothorax to a thoracentesis to remove the air or gas from the cavity and a thoracotomy with insertion of chest tubes. The tubes are connected to an underwater drainage system with suction and remain in place until air is no longer expelled from the pleural space.

Hemothorax

A *hemothorax* is the collection of blood in the pleural cavity; it usually is caused by chest trauma. Symptoms include chest pain, shortness of breath, respiratory failure, tachycardia, and anxiety. Treatment includes stabilizing the patient, stopping the bleeding, inserting a chest tube to evacuate blood and air from the pleural space, and reexpanding the lung.

Pulmonary Embolism

Pulmonary embolism (PE) is the most common complication in hospitalized patients. It strikes 6 million adults each year, causing 100,000 deaths. Pulmonary embolism is usually caused by a blood clot that has been dislodged from a leg or pelvic vein—*deep vein thrombosis* (DVT)—and blocks a pulmonary artery. Symptoms include cough, dyspnea (difficulty in breathing), chest pain, cyanosis (blue tinge to the skin), tachycardia, and shock. It is difficult to distinguish between pneumonia and myocardial infarction. Chest x-ray, pulmonary arteriography, arterial blood gases, and lung perfusion scans coupled with a lung ventilation scan are used to diagnose PE. Treatment includes thrombolytic, anticoagulant, and oxygen therapy.

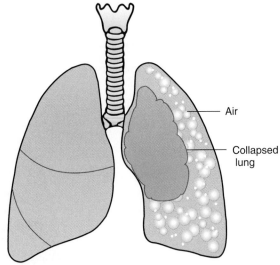

Figure 23-32 Pneumothorax.

Chronic Obstructive Pulmonary Disease

Chronic obstructive pulmonary disease (COPD) is the persistent obstruction of bronchial air flow. This chronic condition of the respiratory system is the second leading cause of hospital admissions in this country. COPD is actually a group of respiratory diseases, of which bronchitis, asthma, and emphysema are the most common.

COPD is attributed to cigarette smoking, environmental pollution, occupational hazards, and chronic infection. Symptoms include shortness of breath, chronic cough, wheezing, increased sputum production, and fatigability upon even mild exertion. Symptoms are progressive and lung damage is irreversible. No cure is known. Treatment focuses on maintaining remaining lung function and relieving symptoms as much as possible.

Acute Respiratory Distress Syndrome

Acute (or adult) respiratory distress syndrome (ARDS) is respiratory failure, usually in the adult patient, that occurs as a result of disease or injury. Symptoms include pulmonary edema (swelling in the lungs), dyspnea (difficulty breathing), tachypnea (rapid respiratory rate), and hypoxemia (decreased oxygen levels in the blood) with cyanosis. The patient with ARDS usually requires intensive medical intervention (in an intensive care unit [ICU]) and the mortality rate is approximately 50% to 60%.

REVIEW QUESTIONS

1. In external respiration, the blood in the capillaries takes on _____ and gives off _____ to the lungs.

2. In internal respiration, the body cells take on _____ from the blood in the capillaries and at the same time give off _____ to the blood in the capillaries to be transported to the lungs.

3. List in sequence the organs through which the air from the outside travels to the blood in the capillaries of the lung.

    a. _____   e. _____
    b. _____   f. _____
    c. _____   g. _____
    d. _____

4. _____ is a passageway for both food and air. _____ is a cartilage flap that prevents food from entering the larynx.

5. List three things that happen to inhaled air in the nose.

a. _____

b. _____

c. _____

6. The vocal cords are located in the _____

7. Describe the lungs.

_____

_____

8.

a. Blood in the pleural cavity is called _____.

b. Air in the pleural cavity is called _____.

c. A collapsed lung is known as _____.

d. A thrombus that blocks a pulmonary artery is called _____.

9. In _____, symptoms are progressive and lung damage is irreversible.

10. List four factors that cause COPD.

a. _____

b. _____

c. _____

d. _____

MEDICAL TERMINOLOGY RELATED TO THE RESPIRATORY SYSTEM

Upon mastery of the medical terminology for this unit, you will be able to:

1. Spell and define the terms related to the respiratory tract.
2. Given the meaning of a medical condition related to the respiratory system, build with word parts the corresponding medical term.
3. Analyze and define medical terms that are built from word parts that relate to the respiratory system.
4. State the meaning of the abbreviations used in this unit.
5. Given a description of a hospital situation in which the HUC may encounter medical terminology, apply the correct medical term to the situation described.

Word Parts

The list below contains word parts for the respiratory system that you need to memorize. The exercises included in this unit will help you with this task. You will continue to use these word parts throughout the course and during your employment. Practice pronouncing each word part aloud.

Combining Forms	Meaning
1. bronch / o (brŏn′-kō)	bronchus (s.); bronchi (pl.)
2. laryng / o (lah-rĭng′-gō)	larynx (voice box)
3. pharyng / o (fah-rĭng′-gō)	pharynx (throat)
4. pleur / o (ploo′-rō)	pleura
5. pneum / o (nū′-mō)	lung (also means air)

Combining Forms	Meaning
6. pneumon / o (nū-mŏn′-ō)	lung
7. pulmon / o (pŭl′-mŏ-nō)	lung
8. rhin / o (rī′-nō)	nose
9. thorac / o (thŏ′-rah-kō)	thorax (chest)
10. tonsill / o (tŏn′-sĭl-ō) (*Note:* The word root for tonsil has a double *l*.)	tonsil
11. trache / o (trā′-kē-ō)	trachea (windpipe)

Prefix

dys- (dĭs)	difficult, labored, painful, abnormal

Suffix

-pnea (nē′-ah)	respiration, breathing

EXERCISE 1

Write the combining forms for the respiratory system in the spaces provided on the diagram in Figure 23-31. The number preceding the combining form in the list above matches the number of the body part on the diagram.

EXERCISE 2

Write the combining forms (and suffix) for each term listed below.

1. lung

_____

2. pharynx

_____

3. larynx

_____

4. trachea

_____

5. tonsil

_____

6. bronchus

_____

7. pleura

_____

8. nose

_____

9. breathing

_____

10. chest

_____

MEDICAL TERMS RELATED TO THE RESPIRATORY SYSTEM

The following list is made up of medical terms for the respiratory system that you will need to know. Exercises following this list will assist you in learning these terms. Practice the pronunciation of these terms aloud.

General Terms	Meaning
adenoids (ăd′-ĕn-oyds)	tissue in the nasopharynx
apnea (ăp′-nē-ah)	without breathing (temporary stoppage of breathing)
bronchotracheal (brŏn-kō-trā′-kē-al)	pertaining to the bronchi and trachea
dyspnea (dĭsp-nē′-ah)	difficulty in breathing
endotracheal (ĕn-dō-trā′-kē-al) (ET)	pertaining to within the trachea
pharyngocele (fah-rĭng′-gō-sēl)	(an abnormal) protrusion in the pharynx
pharyngoplegia (fah-rĭng′-gō-plē′-ja)	paralysis of the pharynx
pulmonary (pŭl′-mŏ-nĕr-ē)	pertaining to the lungs
thoracentesis (thō-rah-sĕn-tē′-sĭs)	surgical puncture and drainage of fluid from the chest cavity (for diagnostic or therapeutic purposes)
thoracic (thō-răs′-ĭk)	pertaining to the chest
thoracocentesis (thō′-rah-kō-sĕn-tē′-sĭs)	surgical puncture and drainage of fluid from the chest cavity (for diagnostic or therapeutic purposes [the same as thoracentesis])
tracheoesophageal (trā′-kē-ō-ĕ-sŏf′-ah-jē′-al)	pertaining to the trachea and esophagus

Surgical Terms	Meaning
adenoidectomy (ăd′-ĕ-noy-dĕk′-to-mē)	surgical removal of the adenoids
laryngectomy (lar-ĭn-jĕk′-to-mē)	excision of the larynx
lobectomy (lō-bĕk′-to-mē)	excision of a lobe (of a lung—also may refer to the brain or liver)
pleuropexy (ploo′-rō-pĕk′-sē)	surgical fixation of the pleura

Surgical Terms	Meaning
pneumonectomy (nū-mŏ-nĕk′-to-mē)	excision of the lung (may be total or partial removal of a lung)
rhinoplasty (rhī-nō-plăs′-tē)	surgical repair of the nose
thoracotomy (thō-rah-kŏt′-o-mē)	incision into the chest cavity
tonsillectomy (tŏn-sĭl-lĕk′-to-mē)	surgical removal of the tonsils
tracheostomy (trā-kē-ŏs′-to-mē)	artificial opening into the trachea (through the neck)

Diagnostic Terms	Meaning
adenoiditis (ăd′-ĕ-noy-dī′-tĭs)	inflammation of the adenoids
asthma (ăz′-mah)	chronic disease characterized by periodic attacks of dyspnea, wheezing, and coughing
bronchitis (brŏn-kī′-tĭs)	inflammation of the bronchi
chronic obstructive pulmonary disease (COPD)	chronic obstruction of the airway that results from emphysema, asthma, or chronic bronchitis
emphysema (ĕm-fĭ-sē′-mah)	degenerative disease characterized by destructive changes in the walls of the alveoli, resulting in loss of elasticity to the lungs
laryngitis (lar-ĭn-jī′-tĭs)	inflammation of the larynx
pharyngitis (fah-rĕn-jī′-tĭs)	inflammation of the pharynx
pleuritis (ploo-rī′-tĭs); pleurisy (ploo′-rĕ-sē)	inflammation of the pleura
pneumonia (nū-mō′-nē-ah)	abnormal condition of the lung
pneumonitis (nū-mō-nī′-tĭs)	inflammation or infection of the lung
pneumothorax (noo-mō-thor′-ăks)	air in the pleural cavity causes the lung to collapse
rhinopharyngitis (rī′-nō-făr-ĭn-jī′-tĭs)	inflammation of the nose and throat
rhinorrhagia (rī-nō-rā′-ja)	bleeding from the nose, also called *epistaxis*
tonsillitis (tŏn-sĭ-lī′-tĭs)	inflammation of the tonsils
upper respiratory infection (rĕs′-pi-rah-tō-rē) (URI)	infection of nose, sinuses, pharynx, larynx, and bronchi

Terms Related to Diagnostic Procedures	Meaning
bronchogram (brŏn′-kō-grăm)	x-ray of the bronchi and lung (with the use of a contrast medium)
bronchoscope (brŏn′-kō-skōp)	instrument used to visually examine the bronchi
bronchoscopy (brŏn-kŏs′-ko-pē)	visual examination of the bronchi
laryngoscope (lăr-răng′-gō-skōp)	instrument used for visual examination of the larynx

EXERCISE 3

Analyze and define each medical term listed below.

1. dyspnea

   _____

2. pharyngocele

   _____

3. apnea

   _____

4. bronchotracheal

   _____

5. tracheoesophageal

   _____

6. endotracheal

   _____

7. pharyngoplegia

   _____

8. rhinopharyngitis

   _____

9. rhinorrhagia

   _____

10. bronchoscope

   _____

11. bronchoscopy

   _____

EXERCISE 4

Using the word parts studied in this unit and in previous units, build a medical term from each definition listed below.

1. inflammation of the bronchi

   _____

2. inflammation of the larynx

   _____

3. artificial opening into the trachea

_____

4. excision of a lung

_____

5. excision of a lobe (of the lung)

_____

6. surgical fixation of the pleura

_____

7. surgical repair of the nose

_____

8. incision into the chest cavity

_____

9. surgical puncture and drainage of the chest cavity

_____

10. inflammation of the tonsils

_____

11. inflammation of the adenoids

_____

EXERCISE 5

Complete the spelling of each medical term listed below.

Medical Term	Meaning
1. pn _ _ _ othor _ _	air in the pleural cavity that causes the lungs to collapse
2. em _ _ _ se _ _	disease of the alveoli of the lung
3. _ _ _ umon _ _	an inflammation or infection of the lung
4. pleuro _ _ _ _	surgical fixation of the pleura
5. phar _ _ _ itis	inflammation of the pharynx

EXERCISE 6

Define each medical term listed below.

1. adenoids

_____

2. lobectomy

_____

3. emphysema

_____

4. pneumonia

_____

5. upper respiratory infection

_____

6. apnea

_____

7. dyspnea

_____

8. pharyngocele

_____

9. laryngectomy

_____

10. pneumothorax

_____

11. rhinorrhagia

_____

12. bronchogram

_____

13. laryngoscope

_____

14. asthma

_____

15. chronic obstructive pulmonary disease

_____

16. tuberculosis

_____

EXERCISE 7

Spell each term studied in this unit by having someone dictate the terms to you.

1. _____

2. _____

3. _____

4. _____

5. _____

6. _____

7. _____

8. _____

9. _____

10. _____

11. _____

12. _____

13. _____

14. _____

15. _____

16. _____

17. _____

18. _____

19. _____

20. _____

21. _____

22. _____

23. _____

24. _____

25. _____

26. _____

27. _____

28. _____

29. _____

30. _____

31. _____

32. _____

33. _____

34. _____

35. _____

36. _____

37. _____

38. _____

39. _____

40. _____

41. _____

42. _____

EXERCISE 8

Answer the following questions.

1. The patient was admitted to the hospital with the diagnosis of hemothorax. The doctor is planning to perform a procedure on the patient to remove fluid from the chest cavity by surgical puncture. This procedure is called a _____.

2. A patient suddenly stops breathing. During this emergency, the doctor may perform the following procedure to ensure the opening of the air passageway. The doctor uses a _____ (an instrument for visual examination of the larynx) to insert a(n) _____ (pertaining to within the trachea) tube. These two items of equipment may be used during an emergency. You may be asked to locate these items for the nursing staff or doctor. Upon assignment to a nursing unit, locate and be able to identify this equipment.

3. The patient is having difficulty breathing (or_____). The doctor performs a procedure called _____ (artificial opening into the trachea) to facilitate breathing. A tube is inserted into the trachea to prevent it from collapsing. It has the same name as the procedure. It is called a(n) _____ tube. A tray that has the same name as the procedure, called a(n) _____, is used by the nursing staff to care for the patient. A patient with a tracheostomy may have difficulty talking; therefore, the HUC should not use the intercom to communicate with this patient.

4. The patient is scheduled for a visual examination of the bronchus, called a _____. _____ is the instrument the doctor uses to perform the examination.

5. The patient is admitted to the hospital with a(n) _____ (a collapsed lung). The patient is having difficulty breathing; the medical term for this is _____. The doctor treats this condition by making a surgical incision into the chest wall, called a(n) _____, for the purpose of inserting tubes. A tray that has the same name as the procedure, a(n) _____ tray, is obtained from the central service department for the doctor's use.

6. T & A is the abbreviation for excision of the tonsils, called _____ and excision of the adenoids, called _____.

ABBREVIATIONS

Abbreviation	Meaning
ARDS	acute respiratory distress syndrome
COPD	chronic obstructive pulmonary disease
ET	endotracheal
NP	nasopharyngeal
PE	pulmonary embolism
RSV	respiratory syncytial virus
SARS	severe acute respiratory syndrome (viral)
TB	tuberculosis (mycobacterial)
URI	upper respiratory infection

EXERCISE 9

Define the following abbreviations.

1. ARDS

_____

2. COPD

_____

3. ET

_____

4. NP

_____

5. PE

_____

6. RSV

_____

7. SARS

_____

8. TB

_____

9. URI

_____

UNIT 9
The Urinary System and the Male Reproductive System

OUTLINE

UNIT OBJECTIVES

Upon completion of this unit, you will be able to:

1. Describe the overall functions of the urinary system and the male reproductive system.
2. Name the organs of the urinary system and tell the function of each organ.
3. Name the components of urine.
4. Name the organs of the male reproductive system and describe the function of each organ.
5. Describe the passageway of sperm from the testes to the outside of the body.
6. State the location and describe the function of the seminal vesicle glands and the prostate gland.
7. Describe pyelonephritis, renal calculi, and tumors of the prostate gland.
8. Define the unit abbreviations.

THE URINARY SYSTEM

Organs of the Urinary System

- Kidneys (2)
- Ureters (2)
- Bladder (1)
- Urethra (1)

Function of the Urinary System

The functions of the urinary system are to monitor and regulate extracellular fluids and to remove waste products from the blood and excrete them from the body. Although toxic substances also are eliminated through the skin, lungs, and intestines, the urinary system is a major contributor to homeostasis in the body because it maintains the proper balance of water, electrolytes, and pH of body fluids. The urinary system also may be referred to as the excretory system.

The Kidneys

The kidneys are two fist-sized, bean-shaped organs located in the lumbar region on either side of the spine, posterior to the abdominal cavity. The primary functions of the kidneys are to remove waste from the blood, to balance the water and electrolytes in the body by removing and retaining water, and to assist in RBC production by releasing erythropoietin (eh-rith′-ro-poy′-eh-tin). Nephrons, the basic functional unit of the kidney, begin to remove waste and water as the blood flows into the kidney through the renal artery. Each kidney contains about one million nephrons. At the entrance of each nephron is a cluster of capillaries called the *glomerulus* (pl. glomeruli), where the process of filtering the blood begins. The antidiuretic hormone (ADH) released by the posterior pituitary gland (neurohypophysis) stimulates the production of urine that contains soluble waste. When danger of dehydration is present, the posterior pituitary gland decreases the amount of ADH that is released. The nephrons continue to remove waste, but the fluid portion of urine decreases. Voided urine is more concentrated and occurs in smaller amounts. This process maintains the fluid

balance in the body. Diuretics commonly prescribed for edema, hypertension, and congestive heart failure are chemicals that serve to increase the rate of urinary output. After urine is produced, it drains into a space in the kidney called the *renal pelvis*. From the renal pelvis, urine is transported to the bladder via the ureters.

The Ureters

The ureters are tubes that provide the drainage system for urine from the renal pelvis of each kidney to the bladder (Fig. 23-33). They are small in diameter and are approximately 10 to 12 inches (25 to 30 cm) long. They extend from the renal pelvis of the kidney and enter the posterior portion of the bladder.

✏ TAKE NOTE

Production and Pathway of Urine
blood flows via the renal artery into the nephrons of the kidneys, where filtering of the blood takes place and urine is produced → renal pelvis → ureter → bladder → urethra → outside

The ureters have muscular walls that contract to keep urine moving toward the bladder. A backup of urine into the kidney is prevented by a flap fold of mucous membrane at the entrance of the ureters into the bladder.

The Urinary Bladder

The urinary bladder is a hollow muscular bag located in the pelvic cavity. The bladder is a temporary reservoir for the urine it receives from the ureters. The need to urinate, or void, is stimulated by distention of the bladder as it fills with urine.

The Urethra

The urethra is the tube through which urine passes from the bladder to the outside of the body. The female urethra is approximately 1 to 2 inches (3.75 cm) long, and the male urethra, which is also a part of the male reproductive system (also carries seminal fluid at the time of ejaculation), is approximately 8 inches (20 cm) long.

Urine

Urine is a straw-colored fluid that is made up of approximately 95% water and 5% waste material (urea, uric acid, creatinine, and ammonia). The amount of urine produced daily by the kidneys is about 1500 mL.

THE MALE REPRODUCTIVE SYSTEM

Organs of the Male Reproductive System

(Fig. 23-34)

- Testes
- Scrotum

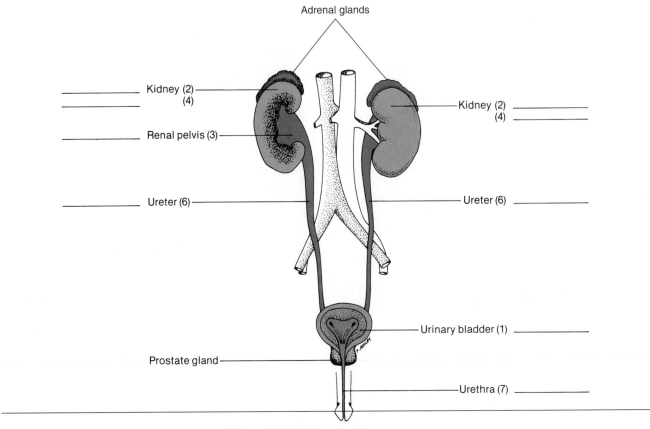

Figure 23-33 The male urinary system.

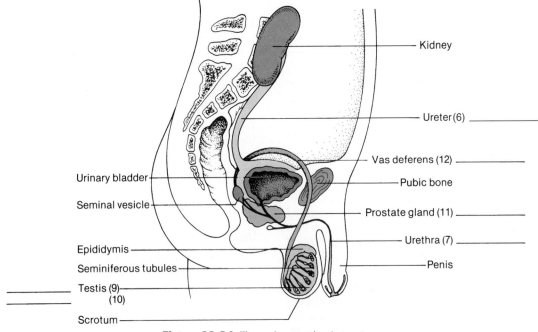

Figure 23-34 The male reproductive system.

- Vas deferens
- Urethra
- Seminal vesicles
- Prostate
- Penis

Functions of the Male Reproductive System

The functions of the male reproductive system are to produce and eject the male reproductive cell (sperm, or spermatozoa) and to secrete the hormone testosterone.

The Testes

The testes (singular: testis), or testicles, are a pair of egg-shaped organs located outside the body, suspended in a sac called the *scrotum*. They are the main sex glands of the male. The function of the testes is to produce sperm (sex cells) and testosterone (hormone). Testosterone is responsible for the development of male secondary sex characteristics, such as beard and deep voice, and for the function of certain reproductive organs.

Production of Sperm

Sperm is produced in coiled tubes, located inside the testes, called *seminiferous tubules*. The sperm passes on to a tiny 20-foot tube called the *epididymis*, which is located in the scrotum. Sperm is stored in the epididymis for a short time, during which it matures and becomes motile (able to move by itself). It then travels through a pair of tubes about 2 feet long called the *vas deferens*. The vas deferens carries sperm to the urethra. The urethra connects with both the bladder and the vas deferens and passes through the penis to the outside. It is a passageway for both semen and urine. The seminal vesicles are glands located near the bladder that open into the vas deferens just prior to its joining with the urethra. The seminal vesicles produce a secretion that nourishes the sperm. This secretion makes up much of the volume of semen (sperm plus secretions). The junction of the vas deferens and the urethra is surrounded by a gland called the *prostate gland*.

The Prostate Gland

The prostate gland secretes a fluid that aids in the motility of sperm. The prostate gland also aids in ejaculation (expulsion of semen from the male urethra). Each ejaculation contains an average of 200 million sperm. Erection (stiffening) of the penis, produced by an increased blood supply to the sponge-like tissue of the penis, allows for the deposit of sperm in the female vagina during ejaculation. A fold of skin called the *prepuce*, or *foreskin*, covers the tip of the penis; this often is removed shortly after birth through the surgical procedure of circumcision.

✎ *TAKE NOTE*

Passageway of Sperm
from the seminiferous tubules (production) → epididymis (sperm matures and becomes motile) → vas deferens (passageway) → seminal vesicles (add nourishing secretions) → prostate (add motility secretions) → urethra (passageway) → to the outside

DISEASES AND CONDITIONS OF THE URINARY SYSTEM AND THE MALE REPRODUCTIVE SYSTEM

Pyelonephritis

Pyelonephritis is an infection of the renal pelvis and the kidney that is caused by bacterial invasion of the urinary tract. Typically, infection spreads from the bladder to the urethra to the kidneys. The three stages of the disease process include pyelitis—inflammation of the renal pelvis; pyelonephritis—inflammation of the renal pelvis and kidney; and pyonephrosis—collection of pus in the renal pelvis. As the disease progresses, the name changes. Symptoms include dysuria (pain or burning during urination), nocturia (excessive urination at night), and hematuria (blood in the urine). Urinalysis and culture and sensitivity of bacterial specimens from the urine are used to diagnose the condition. Treatment includes antibiotic therapy.

Renal Calculi

Renal calculi, or kidney stones, usually form in the renal pelvis, where they may remain, or they may enter the ureter and cause obstruction. Back pain or renal colic, resulting from the obstruction, is usually the key symptom. Kidney, ureter, and bladder x-ray imaging (KUB); intravenous pyelography (IVP); and kidney ultrasonography are used in diagnosing renal calculi. Treatment is to promote normal passage of the stone. Extracorporeal shock wave lithotripsy (ESWL), the crushing of kidney stones by laser beams, is replacing the need for surgery. Endoscopy also is used to remove small calculi from the lower part of the ureters. If indicated, a stone may be removed through a small incision in the skin (percutaneous nephrolithotomy).

Tumors of the Prostate Gland

Tumors of the prostate gland may be malignant (cancer of the prostate) or benign (benign prostatic hyperplasia). Often, the growth is not diagnosed until it is large enough to obstruct urinary outflow. Treatment of choice is surgical removal of the tumor. A radical, or perineal, prostatectomy is the excision of the entire gland and its capsule through an incision in the perineum. Suprapubic prostatectomy is removal of the prostate gland through an incision in the abdomen and the bladder. Retropubic prostatectomy is surgical removal of the prostate gland through an incision in the abdomen, but the bladder is not excised. Transurethral prostatic resection is removal of a portion of the prostate gland through the urethra. No surgical incision is required.

REVIEW QUESTIONS

1. _____ is an organ that is used by both the urinary system and the male reproductive system.

2. Describe the function of the urinary system.

_____

3. The basic functional unit of the kidney is the _____. Its primary functions are

_____.

4. Describe the flow of urine from the renal pelvis of the kidney to the outside of the body.

_____

5. Urine is made up of 95% _____ and 5% _____.

6. The amount of water removed from the blood is determined by the amount of _____ that is released by the _____.

7. Two functions of the testicles are:

a. _____

b. _____

8. Trace the travel of the sperm from the testicles to the outside of the body. Indicate which glands add secretions to the sperm along the passageway.

_____

_____

_____

9. Match the terms in Column 1 with the phrases in Column 2.

Column 1
a. nephrotripsy
b. pyelonephritis
c. renal calculi
d. hydrolithotripsy
e. benign prostatic hyperplasia
f. perineal prostatectomy
g. lithotripsy

Column 2
_____ 1. kidney stone
_____ 2. growth that may obstruct urinary outflow
_____ 3. infection of the renal pelvis and kidney
_____ 4. crushing of a kidney stone

MEDICAL TERMINOLOGY RELATED TO THE URINARY SYSTEM AND THE MALE REPRODUCTIVE SYSTEM

Upon mastery of the medical terminology for this unit, you will be able to:

1. Correctly spell and define the terms related to the urinary system and the male reproductive system.
2. Given the meaning of a medical condition related to the urinary system and the male reproductive system, build with word parts the correct corresponding medical term.
3. Analyze and define medical terms built from word parts that relate to the urinary system and the male reproductive system.
4. Write the meaning of each abbreviation used in this unit.
5. Given a description of a hospital situation in which the HUC may encounter medical terminology, apply the correct medical terms to the situations described.

Word Parts

The list below contains the word parts for the urinary system and the male reproductive system that you need to memorize. The exercises included in this unit will help you with this task. You will continue to use these word parts throughout the course and during employment. Practice pronouncing each word part aloud.

Urinary System

Word Roots/ Combining Forms	Meaning
1. cyst/o (sĭs′-tō)	bladder, sac
2. nephr/o (nĕf′-rō)	kidney
3. pyel / o (pī′-ĕ-lō)	renal pelvis
4. ren / o (rē′-nō)	kidney
5. ur / o (ū′-rō)	urine, urinary tract
6. ureter / o (ū-rē′-ter-ō)	ureter
7. urethr / o (ū-rē′-thrō)	urethra
8. urin / o (ū′-rĭ-nō)	urine (urinary tract, urination)

Male Reproductive System

Word Roots/ Combining Forms	Meaning
9. orchi / o (or′-kē-ō)	testicle, testis
10. orchid / o (or′-kĭ-dō)	testicle, testis
11. prostat / o (prŏs′-tăt-ō)	prostate
12. vas / o (văs′-ō)	vessel, duct

EXERCISE 1

a. Write the combining forms for the urinary system in the spaces provided on the diagram in Figure 23-33 (page 524). The number preceding the combining form in the list above matches the number of the body part on the diagram.

b. Write the combining forms for the male reproductive system in the spaces provided on the diagram in Figure 23-34 (page 524). The number preceding the combining form in the list above matches the number of the body part on the diagram.

EXERCISE 2

Write the combining forms for each term listed below.

1. urine, urinary tract

_____

2. renal pelvis

_____

3. kidney

_____

4. ureter

_____

5. bladder

_____

6. testicle

_____

7. vessel, duct

_____

8. urethra

_____

9. prostate

_____

MEDICAL TERMS RELATED TO THE URINARY SYSTEM AND THE MALE REPRODUCTIVE SYSTEM

The following list is made up of medical terms for the urinary system and the male reproductive system that you will need to know. Exercises following this list will assist you in learning these terms. Practice pronouncing each term aloud.

General Terms	Meaning
hematuria (hēm-ah-tū′-rē-ah)	blood in the urine
scrotum (scrō′-tŭm)	the skin-covered sac that contains the testes and their accessory organs
urethral (ū-rē′-thral)	pertaining to the urethra
urinary (ū′-rĭ-nĕr-ē)	pertaining to urine
urinary catheterization (kăth′-ĕ-ter-ĭ-zā′-shŭn)	insertion of a sterile tube through the urethra into the bladder to remove urine
urination (ū-rĭ-nā′-shŭn)	passage of urine from the body, also called *micturition*
urologist (ū-rŏl′-o-jĭst)	one who specializes in the diagnosis and treatment of (diseases) of the urinary tract (doctor)
urology (ū-rŏl′-o-jē)	study of the urinary tract (the branch of medicine that deals with the diagnosis and treatment of diseases of the male and female urinary tract and of the male reproductive organs)
void (voyd)	to pass urine or feces from the body (generally used with reference to passing urine from the bladder to the outside of the body)

Surgical Terms	Meaning
circumcision (sur′-kŭm-sĭzh′-ŭn)	surgical removal of the foreskin of the penis
nephrectomy (nĕ-frĕk′-to-mē)	excision of the kidney
nephrolithotomy (nĕf′-rō-lĭ-thŏt′-o-mē)	incision into the kidney (to remove a stone)
nephropexy (nĕf′-rō-pĕk-sē)	surgical fixation of a kidney
orchiectomy (ōr-kē-ĕk′-to-mē)	excision of (one or both) testes
prostatectomy (prŏs-tah-tĕk′-to-mē)	surgical removal of the prostate gland
transurethral resection (trăns-ū-rē′-thral) (rē-sĕk′-shŭn) of the prostate gland (TURP)	removal of a portion of the prostate through the urethra by resecting the abnormal tissue in successive pieces
ureterolithotomy (ū-rē′-ter-ō-lĭ-thŏt′-o-mē)	incision into the ureter to (remove) a stone
urethroplasty (ū-rē′-thrō-plăs′-tē)	surgical repair of the urethra
urethrorrhaphy (ū-rē-thrōr′-ah-fē)	suturing of a urethral tear
vasectomy (vah-sĕk′-to-mē)	excision of a duct (vas deferens or a portion of the vas deferens; produces sterility in the male)

Diagnostic Terms	Meaning
cystitis (sĭs-tī′-tĭs)	inflammation of the bladder
cystocele (sĭs′-tō-sēl)	herniation of the urinary bladder
hydrocele (hī′-drō-sēl)	scrotal swelling caused by the collection of fluid in the membrane covering the testes
nephritis (nĕ-frī′-tĭs)	inflammation of the kidney
nephrolithiasis (nĕf′-rō-lĭ-thī′-ah-sĭs)	a kidney stone
pyelonephritis (pī′-ĕ-lō-nĕ-frī′-tĭs)	inflammation of the renal pelvis and kidney
renal calculus (rē′-nal) (kăl′-cū-lŭs)	a kidney stone
uremia (ū-rē′-mē-ah)	urine in the blood (caused by inability of the kidneys to filter out waste products from the blood)
ureteralgia (ū-rē-ter-al′-ja)	pain in the ureter

Terms Related to Diagnostic Procedures	Meaning
blood urea nitrogen (BUN)	laboratory test performed on a blood sample to determine kidney function
creatinine (Cr)	laboratory test usually performed with the BUN to determine kidney function
cystogram (sĭs′-tō-grăm)	x-ray image of the (urinary) bladder; dye is used as a contrast medium
cystoscopy (sĭs-tŏs′-ko-pē)	visual examination of the bladder; usually performed in the operating room so the patient may be anesthetized
intravenous pyelogram (ĭn-trah-vē′-nŭs) (pī′-ĕ-lō-grăm) (IVP)	x-ray image of the kidney, especially the renal pelvis and ureters; contrast medium is used (also called intravenous urogram [IVU])
kidneys, ureters, and bladder (KUB)	x-ray image of the kidneys, ureters, and bladder
urinalysis (ū-rĭ-năl′-ĭ-sĭs) (UA)	a laboratory test to analyze several constituents of urine to assist in the diagnosis of disease

EXERCISE 3

Analyze and define each medical term listed below.

1. uremia

_____

2. urologist

_____

3. nephrolithotomy

_____

4. prostatectomy

_____

5. nephritis

_____

6. urology

_____

7. orchiectomy

_____

8. nephrolithiasis

_____

9. cystocele

_____

10. cystoscopy

_____

11. nephrectomy

_____

12. nephropexy

_____

13. pyelonephritis

_____

14. ureteralgia

_____

15. urethral

_____

16. ureterolithotomy

_____

17. cystitis

_____

18. urethroplasty

_____

19. urethrorrhaphy

_____

Using the word parts studied so far, build a medical term from each definition listed below.

1. visual examination of the urinary bladder

_____

2. inflammation of the kidney

_____

3. excision of the kidney

_____

4. a doctor who specializes in urology

_____

5. blood in the urine

_____

6. urine in the blood

_____

7. suturing of a urethral tear

_____

8. excision of a duct (vas deferens or a portion of it)

_____

9. excision of the prostate gland

_____

10. pain in the ureter

_____

11. herniation of the bladder

_____

12. x-ray image of the bladder

_____

13. inflammation of the kidney and the renal pelvis

_____

14. incision into the kidney to remove a stone

_____

15. surgical repair of the urethra

_____

16. surgical fixation of a kidney

_____

17. branch of medicine that deals with the male and female urinary systems and the male reproductive system

_____

18. excision of the testes

_____

Define each medical term listed below.

1. urinalysis

_____

2. renal calculus

_____

3. hydrocele

_____

4. transurethral resection

_____

5. circumcision

_____

6. urinary

_____

7. urination

_____

EXERCISE 6

Spell each medical term studied in this unit by having someone dictate the terms to you.

1. _____

2. _____

3. _____

4. _____

5. _____

6. _____

7. _____

8. _____

9. _____

10. _____

11. _____

12. _____

13. _____

14. _____

15. _____

16. _____

17. _____

18. _____

19. _____

20. _____

21. _____

22. _____

23. _____

24. _____

25. _____

26. _____

27. _____

28. _____

29. _____

30. _____

31. _____

32. _____

33. _____

34. _____

35. _____

36. _____

EXERCISE 7

Answer the following questions.

1. The patient is unable to void. The doctor writes an order to pass a sterile tube through the urethra into the bladder to remove the urine. This procedure is called a(n) _____. The doctor wants a sample of this urine sent to the lab to be analyzed called a(n) _____.

2. The patient is admitted to the hospital with a diagnosis of inflammation of the bladder, or _____.

3. The doctor orders an image of the kidneys, ureters, and urinary bladder. The abbreviation for this x-ray procedure is _____. The doctor also orders a blood test to determine kidney function called a(n) _____. The abbreviation for this test is _____.

4. The doctor writes an order on the patient's chart for a consultation with a doctor who specializes in the treatment of diseases of the urinary tract and male reproductive system; this specialist is called a(n) _____.

5. The patient is scheduled for the operating room for a procedure to visualize the urinary bladder. The procedure is called _____. The patient may be scheduled for this procedure in the operating room because _____.

ABBREVIATIONS

Abbreviation	Meaning
ADH	antidiuretic hormone
BPH	benign prostatic hyperplasia
BPM	benign prostatomegaly
BUN	blood urea nitrogen
Cr	creatinine
IVP	intravenous pyelogram (x-ray using contrast medium)
IVU	intravenous urogram (x-ray using contrast medium)
KUB	kidneys, ureters, and bladder (x-ray of the abdomen)
TURP	transurethral resection of the prostate
UA	urinalysis
UTI	urinary tract infection

EXERCISE 8

Define the following abbreviations.

1. ADH

   _____

2. BPH

   _____

3. BPM

   _____

4. BUN

   _____

5. Cr

   _____

6. IVP

   _____

7. IVU

   _____

8. KUB

   _____

9. UTI

   _____

10. UA

    _____

11. TURP

    _____

UNIT 10
The Female Reproductive System

OUTLINE

UNIT OBJECTIVES

Upon completion of this unit, you will be able to:

1. Describe the primary functions of the female reproductive system.
2. Name the organs of the female reproductive system and describe the function of each organ.
3. Locate the perineum relative to nearby anatomic structures.
4. Name and describe the functions of two hormones produced by the ovaries.
5. Describe endometriosis, ectopic pregnancy, and pelvic inflammatory disease.
6. Define the unit abbreviations.

THE FEMALE REPRODUCTIVE SYSTEM

Organs of the Female Reproductive System

(Fig. 23-35)

- Uterus (1)
- Ovaries (2)
- Fallopian tubes (2)
- Vagina (1)
- External genitalia
- Mammary and Bartholin's glands

The reproductive organs do not mature and begin to perform reproductive functions until about the age of 11. The maturing of the reproductive organs is called *puberty*.

Functions of the Female Reproductive System

The functions of the female reproductive system are to produce the female reproductive cell (ovum), to produce hormones, and to provide for conception and pregnancy.

The Uterus

The uterus is a thick, muscular, pear-shaped organ that is located in the pelvic cavity between the rectum and the urinary bladder. Three layers make up the uterus: the outer perimetrium, the middle myometrium, and the inner endometrium. In pregnancy, the uterus functions to contain and nourish the unborn child. Rhythmic myometrial contractions during labor assist in the birthing process. The uterus also plays a role in menstruation as the endometrium disintegrates and sloughs off if a fertilized egg is not implanted. The upper rounded region of the uterus is called the *fundus*. The wide, central portion of the uterus is the body, and the lower, narrow end that extends into the vagina is called the *cervix*.

The Ovaries

The ovaries, a pair of small oval organs located within the pelvic cavity, produce the female reproductive cell called the *ovum* (plural: ova). At birth, the female has nearly 1 million ova in the ovaries for which approximately 300,000 remain during the reproductive lifetime. At puberty, the ovaries, in response to the follicle-stimulating hormone (FSH), release a mature ovum about every 28 days. This process is called *ovulation* and it occurs about halfway through the menstrual cycle.

The ovaries, also called *female endocrine glands*, produce two hormones—estrogen and progesterone. Estrogen is responsible for the development of the female reproductive organs and the development of female secondary sex characteristics, such as breasts and pubic hair. The hormone progesterone plays a part in the menstrual cycle by helping to maintain the lining of the uterus for conception and in pregnancy.

The Fallopian Tubes

A pair of tubes, each approximately 5 inches (12.5 cm) long, called the *fallopian tubes*, provide a passageway for the ovum from the ovaries to the uterus. The fallopian tubes are not connected to the ovaries; however, after ovulation, the ovum is swept into one of the fallopian tubes, which are connected to the uterus. Fertilization, the union of the sperm and the ovum, usually takes place within the fallopian tube. It takes approximately 5 days for the ovum to pass through the fallopian tube to the uterus.

The Vagina

The vagina is a muscular tube about 3 inches long that connects the uterus to the outside of the body (Fig. 23-36). The outside opening of the vagina is located between the rectum (posterior) and the urethra (anterior) of the pelvic floor. The vagina receives the penis during sexual intercourse and is the lower part of the birth canal through which the newborn baby passes from the uterus to the outside of the body. Bartholin's glands (or greater vestibular glands), mucus-producing glands at the external opening of the vagina, secrete lubricating substances.

The Perineum

The pelvic floor of both the male and the female is called the *perineum*. However, this term is used most frequently to refer to the area between the vaginal opening and the anus of the female.

Mammary Glands

The mammary glands, specialized organs of milk production, are located within the breasts. Each adult mammary gland contains 15 to 20 glandular lobes. During pregnancy, estrogen and progesterone stimulate development of the mammary glands. The hormone prolactin initiates milk production after birth.

External Reproductive Structures

The vulva (a collective term for the external genitalia) consists of the labia majora and the labia minora, the two folds of adipose tissue surrounding the vagina, as well as the vestibule, the recess formed by the labia minora. The clitoris, a small erectile structure, is located anterior to the urethra.

DISEASES AND CONDITIONS OF THE FEMALE REPRODUCTIVE SYSTEM

Endometriosis

Endometriosis is a condition in which endometrial tissue (lining of the uterus) is found outside of the uterus, especially in the pelvic area, but it can appear anywhere in the body (Fig. 23-37).

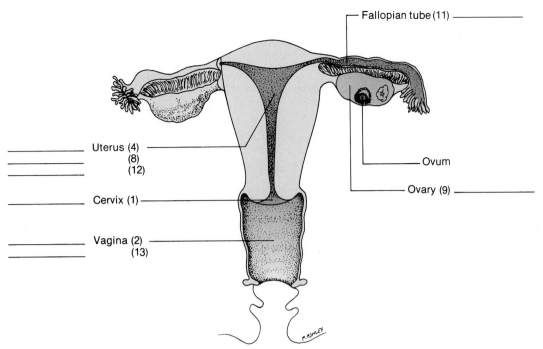

Figure 23-35 The female reproductive system.

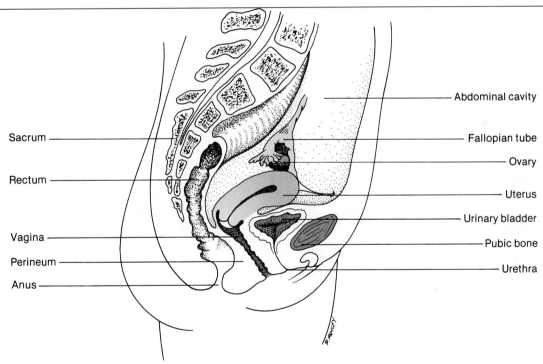

Figure 23-36 Lateral view of the female reproductive system.

The misplaced endometrial tissue undergoes changes, including bleeding, during menstruation. Symptoms include dysmenorrhea (painful menstruation), which causes constant pain in the vagina and the lower abdomen. The cause is unknown.

Treatment varies according to the severity of the disease and according to the age and childbearing desires of the patient. Hormonal treatment may be recommended for milder forms of endometriosis. Endometrial ablation may be performed to suppress ovarian function and to halt the growth of endometrial tissue. Conservative surgery may involve removal of cysts or lysis (freeing) of adhesions. For severe cases and for those women who do not wish to bear children, a total hysterectomy and bilateral salpingo-oophorectomy is recommended (Fig. 23-38).

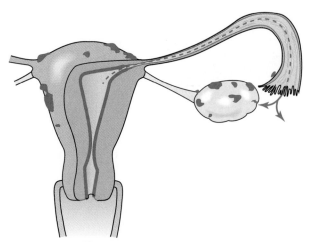

Figure 23-37 Endometriosis.

Pelvic Inflammatory Disease

Pelvic inflammatory disease (PID) is any infection of the female pelvic organs; most often, it is caused by bacterial infection. Early diagnosis and treatment prevent damage to the reproductive organs. If untreated, PID can lead to infertility and to other severe medical complications. Symptoms include vaginal discharge, abdominal pain, and fever. Treatment includes antibiotic therapy.

Ectopic Pregnancy

In an ectopic (tubal) pregnancy, the fertilized ovum is implanted outside of the uterus; more than 90% implant in the fallopian tubes. The fetus may grow large enough to rupture the tube, creating a life-threatening situation. Symptoms of a ruptured fallopian tube include severe abdominal pain on one side and vaginal bleeding. Treatment is surgical repair or removal of the fallopian tube and removal of the products of conception.

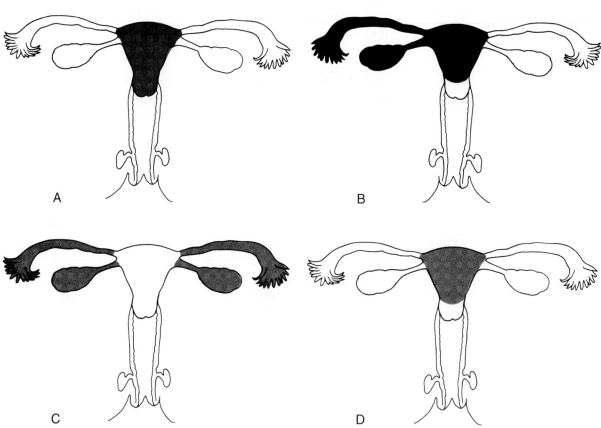

Figure 23-38 A, Total hysterectomy. **B,** Hysterosalpingo-oophorectomy. **C,** Bilateral salpingo-oophorectomy. **D,** Subtotal hysterectomy.

REVIEW QUESTIONS

1. _____ and _____ are the names of two hormones produced by the ovaries. _____ is the hormone responsible for secondary sex characteristics and aids in the development of the female reproductive organs.

2. Fertilization usually takes place in the _____.

3. The _____ is the lower portion of the uterus, which extends into the vagina.

4. Describe the primary functions of the female reproductive system.

   _____

5. List the internal organs of the female reproductive system and write a line or two about the function of each organ.

   a. _____

   b. _____

   c. _____

   d. _____

6. An ovum begins to mature in response to the _____.

7. An infection of the female pelvic organs that if left untreated can lead to infertility is called _____.

8. A pregnancy that occurs outside the uterus is called a(n) _____.

9. A condition in which endometrial tissue is found outside the uterus is called _____.

MEDICAL TERMINOLOGY RELATED TO THE FEMALE REPRODUCTIVE SYSTEM

Upon mastery of the medical terminology for this unit, you will be able to:

1. Spell and define the terms related to the female reproductive system.
2. Given the meaning of a medical condition related to the female reproductive system, build with word parts the correct corresponding medical terms.
3. Analyze and define medical terms that are built from word parts related to the female reproductive system.
4. Define terms related to pregnancy, childbirth, and the newborn.
5. Given a description of a hospital situation in which the HUC may encounter medical terminology, apply the correct medical term to the situation described.

Word Parts

The list below contains the word parts for the female reproductive system that you need to learn. The exercises included in this unit will help you with this task. You will continue to use these word parts throughout the course and during employment. Practice pronouncing each word part aloud.

Word Roots/Combining Forms	Meaning
1. cervic / o (ser′-vĭ-ko)	cervix (the neck-like portion of the uterus)
2. colp / o (kŏl′-pō)	vagina
3. gynec / o (gī′-nĕ-kō, jīn′-ĕ-kō)	woman
4. hyster / o (hĭs′-ter-ō)	uterus (womb)
5. mamm / o (măm′-mō)	breast
6. mast / o (măs′-tō)	breast
7. men / o (mĕn′-ō)	menstruation
8. metr / o (meù′-trō)	uterus (womb)
9. oophor / o (ō-ŏf′-ō-rō)	ovary
10. perine / o (pĕr-ĭ-nē′-ō)	perineum (the pelvic floor); in the female, the area between the vaginal opening and the anus, and in the male, the region between the scrotum and the anus
11. salping / o (săl-pĭng′-gō)	fallopian or uterine tube
12. uter / o (ū′-tĕr-ō)	uterus (womb)
13. vagin / o (văj′-ĭ-nō)	vagina

EXERCISE 1

Write the combining forms for the female reproductive system in the spaces provided on the diagram in Figure 23-35 (page 533). The number preceding the combining forms in the list above matches the number of the body part on the diagram.

EXERCISE 2

Write the combining forms for each of the following.

1. menstruation

   _____

2. woman

   _____

3. vagina

   _____

4. perineum

   _____

5. fallopian or uterine tube

   _____

6. ovary

   _____

7. uterus

   _____

8. cervix

   _____

9. breast

   _____

MEDICAL TERMS RELATED TO THE FEMALE REPRODUCTIVE SYSTEM

The list below contains the medical terms for the female reproductive system that you need to memorize. The exercises included in this unit will help you with this task. You will continue to use these medical terms throughout the course and during your employment. Practice pronouncing each term aloud.

General Terms	Meaning
gynecologist (gī-ně-kŏl′-o-jĭst, jĭn-ě-kŏl′-o-jĭst)	specialist in the diagnosis and treatment of women (doctor)

General Terms	Meaning
gynecology (gī-ně-kŏl′-o-jē, jĭn-ě-kŏl′-o-jē)	study of women (the branch of medicine that deals with diseases and disorders of the female reproductive system)
menopause (měn′-ō-pawz)	the period during which the menstrual cycle slows down and eventually stops
menstrual (měn′-stroo-ăl)	pertaining to menstruation
menstruation (měn-stroo-ā′-shŭn)	discharge of blood and tissue from the uterus, normally occurring every 28 days
ovum (ō′-vŭm) (s.); ova (ō′-vă) (pl.)	female reproductive cell; may be referred to as the female reproductive egg
ureterovaginal (ū-rē′-ter-ō-văj′-ĭ-nal)	pertaining to the ureter and the vagina
uterine (ū′-ter-ĭn)	pertaining to the uterus
vaginal (văj′-ĭ-nal)	pertaining to the vagina
vaginoperineal (văj-ĭ-nō-pěr-ĭ-nē′-al)	pertaining to the vagina and the perineum

Surgical Terms	Meaning
cervicectomy (sěr-vĭ-sěk′-to-mē)	excision of the cervix
colporrhaphy (kŏl-por′-ah-fē)	suturing of the vagina
dilation and curettage (dī-la′-shŭn) (kū-rě-tăhzh′) (D&C)	surgical procedure to dilate the cervix and scrape the inner walls of the uterus (endometrium) for diagnostic and therapeutic purposes
endometrial ablation (en-dō-mē′-trē-al ab-lā′-shun)	use of laser to destroy endometrium in abnormal uterine bleeding
hysterectomy (hĭs-tě-rěk′-to-mē)	surgical removal of the uterus
hysterosalpingo-oophorectomy (hĭs′-ter-ō-săl-pĭng′-gō-ō-ŏf-ō-rěk′-o-mē)	excision of the uterus, fallopian tubes, and ovaries
mammoplasty (măm′-ō-plăs′-tē)	surgical repair of the breast(s) to enlarge (augmentation) or reduce (reduction) in size, or to reconstruct after surgical removal of a tumor
mastectomy (măs-těk′-to-mē)	surgical removal of a breast
oophorectomy (ō-ŏf-ō-rěk′-to-mē)	excision of an ovary; if both ovaries are removed, it is referred to as a bilateral oophorectomy
perineoplasty (pěr-ĭ-nē′-ō-plăs′-tē)	surgical repair of the perineum
perineorrhaphy (pěr′-ĭ-nē-ōr′-ah-fē)	suturing of the perineum
salpingo-oophorectomy (săl-pĭng′-gō-ō-ŏf-o-rěk′-to-mē)	excision of a fallopian tube and an ovary
salpingopexy (săl-pĭng′-gō-pěk-sē)	surgical fixation of a fallopian tube

Diagnostic Terms	Meaning
amenorrhea (ă-měn-ō-rē'-ah)	without menstrual discharge
cervicitis (ser-vĭ-sī'-tĭs)	inflammation of the cervix
dysmenorrhea (dĭs-měn-ō-rē'-ah)	painful menstrual discharge
menometrorrhagia (měn-ō-mět-rō-rā'-ja)	rapid flow of blood from the uterus at menstruation (and between menstrual periods)
metrorrhagia (mě-trō-rā'-ja)	rapid flow of blood from the uterus (bleeding at irregular intervals other than that associated with menstruation)
metrorrhea (mě-trō-rē'-ah)	(abnormal) uterine discharge
oophoritis (ō-ŏf-ō-rī'-tĭs)	inflammation of an ovary
salpingitis (săl-pĭn-jĭ'-tĭs)	inflammation of a fallopian tube
salpingocele (săl-pĭng'-gō-sēl)	herniation of the fallopian tube

Terms Related to Diagnostic Procedures	Meaning
cervical Pap smear	a laboratory test used to detect cancerous cells; commonly performed to detect cancer of the cervix and the uterus
colposcope (kŏl'-pō-skōp)	an instrument used for visual examination of the vagina (and cervix)
colposcopy (kŏl-pōs'-kō-pē)	visual examination of the vagina (and cervix)
hysterosalpingogram (hĭs'-ter-ō-săl-pĭng'-gō-grăm)	x-ray image of the uterus and fallopian tubes
mammogram (măm'-ō-grăm)	x-ray image of the breast
vaginal speculum (spěk'-ū-lŭm)	instrument used for expanding the vagina to allow for visual examination of the vagina and cervix

EXERCISE 3

Analyze and define the following medical terms.

1. gynecology

   _____

2. colporrhaphy

   _____

3. oophorectomy

   _____

4. oophoritis

   _____

5. salpingo-oophorectomy

   _____

6. salpingopexy

   _____

7. hysterectomy

   _____

8. dysmenorrhea

   _____

9. colposcope

   _____

10. mammoplasty

   _____

11. amenorrhea

   _____

12. mammogram

   _____

13. hysterosalpingogram

   _____

14. colposcopy

   _____

EXERCISE 4

Using the word parts you have studied, build a medical term from each definition listed below.

1. excision of the ovary

   _____

2. study of women (branch of medicine that deals with diseases of the reproductive organs of women)

   _____

3. surgical fixation of a fallopian tube

   _____

4. inflammation of an ovary

_____

5. an instrument used for visual examination of the vagina

_____

6. (abnormal) uterine discharge

_____

7. excision of the cervix

_____

8. excision of the uterus, ovaries, and fallopian tubes

_____

9. herniation of a fallopian tube

_____

10. pertaining to the ureter and vagina

_____

11. inflammation of the cervix

_____

12. excision of the uterus

_____

13. suture of the vagina

_____

14. surgical repair of the perineum

_____

15. pertaining to the vagina

_____

16. surgical removal of a breast

_____

17. excision of a fallopian tube and ovary

_____

18. painful menstruation

_____

19. x-ray image of the uterus and fallopian tubes

_____

20. without menstrual discharge

_____

21. x-ray image of the breast

_____

22. surgical repair of the breast

_____

23. visual examination of the vagina (and cervix)

_____

EXERCISE 5

Define the following medical terms.

1. gynecologist

_____

2. uterine

_____

3. vaginal speculum

_____

4. menometrorrhagia

_____

5. dilation and curettage

_____

6. ovum

_____

EXERCISE 6

A surgery schedule lists all the operations to be performed in the hospital on a given day. Information on a surgery schedule includes the patient's name, the operation, and the surgeon. In the sample below, identify the terms spelled incorrectly in the operations listed. Spell the term correctly in the space provided.

Patient Name	Surgery	Doctor
a. Ms. Wallace	dilation and curretage	Dr. Lewis
	_____	
b. Ms. Kelly	histero-solpingo oopherectomy	Dr. Robinowitz
	_____	
c. Ms. Thomas	periniplasty	Dr. Cohen
	_____	
d. Ms. Clark	colporhaphy	Dr. Jacobson
	_____	
e. Ms. Cohen	salpangpexy	Dr. Sheets
	_____	

EXERCISE 7

Spell each medical term studied in this unit by having someone dictate the terms to you.

1. _____
2. _____
3. _____
4. _____
5. _____
6. _____
7. _____
8. _____
9. _____
10. _____
11. _____
12. _____
13. _____
14. _____
15. _____
16. _____
17. _____
18. _____
19. _____
20. _____
21. _____
22. _____
23. _____
24. _____
25. _____
26. _____
27. _____
28. _____
29. _____
30. _____
31. _____
32. _____
33. _____
34. _____
35. _____
36. _____
37. _____
38. _____

TERMS RELATED TO OBSTETRICS

Below is a list of terms commonly used in the field of obstetrics and their definitions.

Obstetric Terms	Meaning
abortion (ah-bor′-shŭn)	termination of pregnancy before the fetus is capable of survival outside the uterus; may be spontaneous or therapeutic abortion
amniotic (ăm-nē-ŏt′-ĭk) fluid	fluid that surrounds the fetus
cesarean (sē-să′-rē-ăn) section (C/S)	incision into the uterus through the abdominal wall to deliver the fetus
congenital (kŏn-jĕn′-ĭ-tal)	term to describe a condition that exists at birth
ectopic (ĕk-tŏp′-ĭk) pregnancy	the fertilized ovum is implanted outside the uterus

Obstetric Terms	Meaning
fetus (fē′-tŭs)	the unborn child in the uterus from the third month of development to birth
natal (nā′-tal)	pertaining to birth
neonatal (nē′-ō-nā′-tal)	pertaining to the first 4 weeks after birth
obstetrician (ŏb-stĕ-trĭsh′-ăn)	a doctor who practices obstetrics
obstetrics (ŏb-stĕt′-rĭks) (OB)	branch of medicine that deals with pregnancy and childbirth
placenta (plah-sĕn′-tah) (afterbirth)	a spongy structure developed during pregnancy through which the unborn child is nourished
postnatal (pōst-nā′-tal)	pertaining to after birth
prenatal (prē-nā′-tal)	pertaining to before birth

EXERCISE 8

Match the word in Column 1 with its meaning in Column 2.

Column 1	Column 2
a. congenital	_____ 1. occurring before birth
b. abortion	_____ 2. present at birth
c. fetus	_____ 3. early termination of pregnancy
d. postnatal	_____ 4. unborn child
e. natal	_____ 5. a branch of medicine
f. prenatal	_____ 6. pregnancy outside the uterus
g. obstetrics	_____ 7. occurring after birth
h. ectopic pregnancy	_____ 8. birth

EXERCISE 9

Define each term listed below.

1. obstetrician

   _____

2. placenta

   _____

3. amniotic fluid

   _____

4. cesarean section

   _____

EXERCISE 10

Answer the following questions.

1. In a large hospital, there is usually a nursing unit for patients who are hospitalized for surgery of the female reproductive tract. This unit is called _____.

A separate nursing unit is used for delivery and care of the newborn and for care of the mothers. This unit is called _____.

2. The doctor plans to perform a pelvic examination of a female patient. The _____ is the instrument she or he uses to expand the vagina. During the pelvic examination, the doctor plans to remove some cells from the cervix to be studied for the presence of cancer. The cells are sent to the laboratory for a _____ test.

ABBREVIATIONS

Abbreviation	Meaning
C/S	cesarean section
D&C	dilation and curettage
EDD	estimated date of delivery
FSH	follicle-stimulating hormone
OB	obstetrics, obstetric
PID	pelvic inflammatory disease
PP	postpartum (after having given birth)
TPAL	term-premature-abortions (terminations)-living

EXERCISE 11

Define the following abbreviations.

1. C/S

   _____

2. D&C

   _____

3. FSH

   _____

4. OB

   _____

5. PID

   _____

6. PP

   _____

7. TPAL

   _____

8. EDD

   _____

UNIT 11
The Endocrine System

OUTLINE

UNIT OBJECTIVES

Upon completion of this unit, you will be able to:

1. Describe the overall function of the endocrine system.
2. Name the glands of the endocrine system and describe the hormones produced by each gland and the function of each of the hormones.
3. Compare endocrine glands with exocrine glands.
4. Describe diabetes mellitus and Graves' disease.
5. Define the unit abbreviations.

THE ENDOCRINE SYSTEM

Primary Organs of the Endocrine System

(Fig. 23-39)

- Hypothalamus
- Pituitary
- Thyroid gland
- Parathyroid gland
- Pancreas (Islets of Langerhans)
- Adrenal glands
- Ovaries (female) and Testes (male)

Functions of the Endocrine System

The functions of the endocrine system are much the same as those of the nervous system—communication, integration, and control; however, endocrine functions are carried out in a much different manner. Both systems use chemicals (hormones and neurotransmitters), but neurotransmitters act immediately and are short-lived, and the effects of endocrine system hormones are farther reaching and longer lasting. The organs of the endocrine system are the endocrine glands, which produce controlling substances called *hormones.* Endocrine, or ductless, glands do not have tubes to carry their secretions to other parts of the body; endocrine secretions go directly into the bloodstream, which carries them to other parts of the body. In contrast to the endocrine glands, the exocrine glands of the body have tubes that carry their secretions from the producing gland to other parts or organs of the body. For example, the saliva produced by the parotid gland (an exocrine gland) flows from the parotid gland through a tube into the mouth. Some nonendocrine organs such as the heart, lungs, kidneys, liver, and placenta also produce and release hormones.

The Pituitary Gland

The pituitary gland, often referred to as the master gland, has a master of its own! Although the pituitary gland produces hormones that stimulate the functions of other endocrine glands, it is the hypothalamus of the brain that directly regulates the secretory activity of the pituitary gland. The pituitary gland, which is attached to the hypothalamus, is a pea-sized gland located in the cranial cavity at the base of the brain. The pituitary gland is divided into two lobes: the anterior and the posterior.

The anterior lobe, or adenohypophysis, produces the following five hormones:

- **Adrenocorticotropic hormone (ACTH):** Stimulates the action of part of the adrenal gland.
- **Thyroid-stimulating hormone (TSH):** Stimulates the action of the thyroid gland.
- **Growth hormone (GH):** Promotes body growth.
- **Prolactin (PRL):** Stimulates and sustains milk production in lactating females. Prolactin has no known effect in males.
- **Gonadotropins:** Stimulate growth and maintenance of the gonads (ovaries [F] and testes [M]). Follicle-stimulating hormone (FSH) stimulates follicles in the ovaries (F) and seminiferous tubes (M), and luteinizing hormone (LH) stimulates ovulation (F) and production of the male sex cell (spermatogenesis).

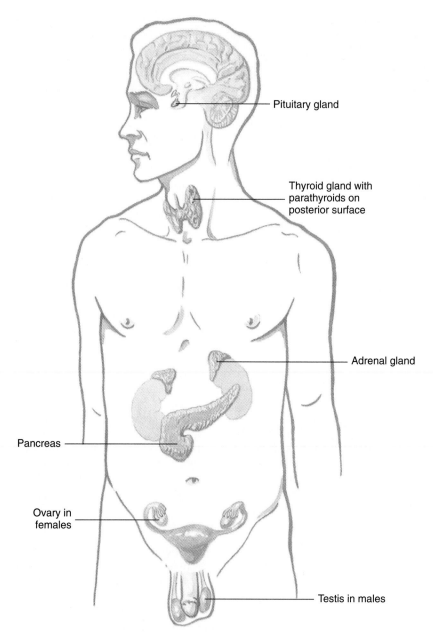

Pituitary gland

Thyroid gland with parathyroids on posterior surface

Adrenal gland

Pancreas

Ovary in females

Testis in males

Figure 23-39 Primary organs of the endocrine system.

The posterior lobe, or neurohypophysis, produces two hormones:

- **Antidiuretic hormone (ADH):** Stimulates reabsorption of water by the kidney
- **Oxytocin:** Stimulates uterine contractions while a woman is in labor

The Thyroid Gland

The thyroid gland, which is shaped like a butterfly, is located in the lower neck on the front and sides of the trachea. It produces the hormone thyroxine, which maintains metabolism of body cells. Iodine is necessary in the body for the production of thyroxine by the thyroid gland, which is critical for normal growth and development.

The Parathyroid Glands

The parathyroid glands are four small bodies that are located posterior to the thyroid gland. They produce parathyroid hormone, which regulates the amount of calcium in the blood.

Pancreas

The pancreas functions as both an exocrine gland and an endocrine gland. The endocrine component, the islets of Langerhans, consists of microscopic bunches of cells scattered throughout the pancreas (refer to Unit 7, p. 503, of this chapter). These cells secrete the hormones insulin and glucagon, which are necessary for the metabolism of carbohydrates in the body. Glucagon works with insulin to regulate blood glucose levels.

The Adrenal Glands

The adrenal glands, situated on top of each kidney, are divided into two parts: the adrenal cortex (outer part) and the adrenal medulla (inner part). The adrenal cortex produces three steroid hormones: mineralocorticoids, glucocorticoids, and androgens. Mineralocorticoids regulate electrolyte balance, which is essential to normal body function and to life itself. Cortisol and cortisone are two glucocorticoids that influence protein, sugar, and fat metabolism. Cortisone, because of its anti-inflammatory effects, is used therapeutically for the treatment of patients with various ailments. During physical or emotional stress, cortisol secretions increase to assist with the body's response. Androgens are hormones that are responsible for the masculinizing effect in males. Testosterone produced by the testes has the same masculinizing effect and is discussed further in Unit 9, p.525, The Urinary System and the Male Reproductive System.

The adrenal medulla produces two hormones—epinephrine (or adrenaline) and norepinephrine—that help the body respond to emergency or stressful situations by increasing the function of vital organs (heartbeat and respiration), raising blood pressure, and providing extra nourishment for the voluntary muscles so they can perform extra work.

Sex Glands

The ovaries of the female and the testes of the male are endocrine glands. Ovaries are described in Unit 10, p.532, and the testes are discussed in Unit 9.

DISEASES OF THE ENDOCRINE SYSTEM

Diabetes Mellitus (Type 1 or Type 2)

Diabetes mellitus, one of the most common endocrine disorders, results in the inability of the body to store and use carbohydrates in the usual manner. Contributing factors are the inability of the islets of Langerhans to produce enough insulin, an increase in the rate at which the body uses insulin, an increase in the rate of insulin storage in the body, and a drop in the efficiency of the use of insulin. In type 1, the beta cells of the pancreatic islets are destroyed and the patient must take regular injections of insulin. In type 2, the body is unable to respond normally to its insulin. Patients tend to be overweight—a factor that is believed to be responsible for the characteristic insulin resistance. Individuals with type 2 diabetes control their blood sugar level with diet, exercise, oral hypoglycemics, and insulin injections.

Symptoms of diabetes mellitus include polyuria, an increase in urine output; polyphagia, an increase in appetite; polydipsia, an increase in thirst; glycosuria, an elevation of sugar in the urine; and hyperglycemia, an elevation of sugar in the blood.

Diagnostic studies include urinalysis, fasting blood sugar, and hemoglobin A1C. Treatment depends on the severity of the disease. Mild diabetes can be controlled by a diet that usually contains limited quantities of sugar, carbohydrates, and fats. Some patients may need to take oral hypoglycemics while adhering to their diet modifications. Moderate to severe diabetes may require insulin therapy. Too much glucose in the blood may cause a condition called *diabetic coma*, whereas too much insulin in the blood may cause a condition called *insulin shock*.

Graves' Disease

Graves' disease, a form of hyperthyroidism, causes overproduction of thyroxine, an increase in the size of the thyroid gland (goiter), and many changes in the other systems. Accompanying symptoms include intolerance to heat, nervousness, loss of weight, and goiter. The cause of Graves' disease is unknown, but it is five times more common in women than in men. It usually occurs between the ages of 20 and 40 years. T_3 and T_4 uptake tests and a thyroid scan may be used to diagnose Graves' disease. Treatment includes antithyroid drugs, radioactive iodine, and subtotal thyroidectomy.

REVIEW QUESTIONS

1. _____ is necessary in the body for the production of thyroxine.

2. Indicate the hormones produced by each endocrine gland by writing the number of the hormone listed in Column 2 by the name of the endocrine gland listed in Column 1. You may wish to write more than one number in each space.

Column 1
a. parathyroid hormone
b. GH
c. TSH
d. FSH
e. oxytocin
f. ACTH
g. cortisone
h. epinephrine
i. insulin
j. PRL
k. thyroxine
l. ADH

Column 2
_____ 1. anterior pituitary gland
_____ 2. adrenal cortex gland
_____ 3. thyroid gland
_____ 4. posterior pituitary gland
_____ 5. parathyroid gland
_____ 6. islets of Langerhans
_____ 7. adrenal medulla gland

3. Explain why the pituitary gland is sometimes referred to as the master gland. Explain the role of the hypothalamus in the secretion of the pituitary.

_____

4. What is the overall function of the endocrine system?

_____

5. Insulin is secreted by the _____ located throughout the _____.

6. What is the function of insulin in the body?

_____

7. List the symptoms of diabetes mellitus.

a. _____

b. _____

c. _____

d. _____

e. _____

8. Graves' disease is a form of _____.

MEDICAL TERMINOLOGY RELATED TO THE ENDOCRINE SYSTEM

Upon mastery of the medical terminology for this unit, you will be able to:

1. Spell and define the terms related to the endocrine system.
2. Given the meaning of a medical condition related to the endocrine system, build with word parts the correct corresponding medical term.
3. Given a description of a hospital situation in which the HUC may encounter medical terminology, apply the correct medical term to the situation described.

Word Parts

The list below contains the word parts for the endocrine system that you need to memorize. The exercises included in this unit will help you with this task. You will continue to use these word parts throughout the course and during employment. Practice pronouncing each word part aloud.

Word Roots/Combining Forms	Meaning
aden / o (ăd′-ĕ-nō)	gland
adren / o (ah-drē′-nō)	adrenal

Word Roots/Combining Forms	Meaning
adrenal / o (ah-drē′-nal-ō)	adrenal
parathyroid / o (păr-ah-thī′-roy-dō)	parathyroid
thyr / o (thī′-rō)	thyroid
thyroid / o (thī′-roy-dō)	thyroid

EXERCISE 1

Write the combining forms for each medical term listed below.

1. gland

_____

2. thyroid

_____

3. adrenal

_____

4. parathyroid

_____

MEDICAL TERMS RELATED TO THE ENDOCRINE SYSTEM

The following list is made up of medical terms for the endocrine system that you will need to know. Exercises following this list will assist you in learning these terms. Practice pronouncing each term aloud.

General Terms	Meaning
adenitis (ăd-ĕ-nī′-tĭs)	inflammation of a gland
adenoid (ăd′-ĕ-noyd)	resembling a gland (adenoids: glandular tissue located in the nasopharynx)
adenoma (ăd-ĕ-nō′-mah)	a tumor of glandular tissue
adenosis (ăd-ĕ-nō′-sĭs)	abnormal condition of a gland
adrenal (ah-drē′-nal)	adrenal gland located near the kidney
adrenalitis (ah-drē-năl-ĭ′-tĭs)	inflammation of the adrenal gland
gland (gland)	a secretory organ that produces hormones or other substances
hormones	chemical messengers produced by the endocrine system
secretion (sē-krē′-shŭn)	a substance produced by a gland

Surgical Terms	Meaning
parathyroidectomy (păr′-ah-th-ī-roy-dĕk′-to-mē)	excision of the parathyroid gland
thyroidectomy (th-ī-roy-dĕk′-to-mē)	surgical removal of the thyroid gland

Diagnostic Terms	Meaning
Addison's (ăd′-i-sŭnz) disease	disease caused by lack of production of hormones by the adrenal gland
Cushing's (koosh′-ĭngz) disease	a disorder caused by overproduction of certain hormones by the adrenal cortex
diabetes insipidus (dī-ah-bē′-tĭs) (ĭn-sĭp′-ĭ-dĭs)	disease caused by inadequate antidiuretic hormone production by the posterior lobe of the pituitary gland
diabetes mellitus (dī-ah-bē′-tĭs) (mĭl-ĭ′-tĭs) (DM)	disease that results in the inability of the body to store and use carbohydrates in the usual manner; may be caused by inadequate production of insulin by the islets of Langerhans

Diagnostic Terms	Meaning
hyperthyroidism (hī-per-thī′-roy-dĭzm)	excessive production of thyroxine and often an enlarged thyroid gland (goiter); also called Graves' disease or exophthalmic goiter
hypothyroidism (hī-pō-thī′-roy-dĭzm)	condition of underproduction of thyroxine by the thyroid gland

Terms Related to Diagnostic Procedures	Meaning
blood glucose monitoring	method of monitoring the patient's glucose level by using a finger stick to obtain blood; performed by nursing staff
fasting blood sugar (FBS)	laboratory test to determine the amount of glucose in the blood after patient has fasted for 8 to 10 hours; may be used to diagnose and/or monitor diabetes mellitus
hemoglobin A1C (HbA$_{1C}$)	laboratory test performed to assess more precisely the control of diabetes; test result shows the percentage of glycated (or glycosylated) hemoglobin in the blood; excess glucose in the bloodstream, which usually occurs when diabetes is poorly controlled, binds (or glycates) with hemoglobin molecules in the RBCs (also called glycohemoglobin [glycoHb])
protein-bound iodine	laboratory test performed on a sample of blood to determine thyroid activity
T$_3$, T$_4$, and T$_7$ uptake	studies performed on a blood sample to determine the function of the thyroid gland
thyroid scan	diagnostic study performed in the nuclear medicine department for thyroid gland function

EXERCISE 2

Using the word parts studied in this unit and in previous units, build a medical term from each definition listed below.

1. inflammation of a gland

_____

2. surgical removal of the thyroid gland

_____

3. surgical removal of the parathyroid gland

_____

4. resembling a gland

_____

5. tumor of glandular tissue

_____

6. abnormal condition of a gland

_____

7. inflammation of the adrenal gland

_____

EXERCISE 3

The following are conditions caused by oversecretion or under-secretion of endocrine glands. In the space provided, write the name of the gland involved with the condition.

1. diabetes mellitus

_____

2. hyperthyroidism

_____

3. Addison's disease

_____

4. hypothyroidism

_____

5. Cushing's disease

_____

6. diabetes insipidus

_____

EXERCISE 4

Complete the following words.

1. dia _ _ t _ _ ins _ p _ d _ _

2. Ad _ _ _ on's dis _ _ se

3. Cu _ _ ing's dis _ _ se

4. h _ poth _ _ oid _ _ m

5. sec _ _ ti _ ns

EXERCISE 5

Spell each term studied in this unit by having someone dictate the terms to you.

1. _____

2. _____

3. _____

4. _____

5. _____

6. _____

7. _____

8. _____

9. _____

10. _____

11. _____

12. _____

13. _____

14. _____

15. _____

16. _____

17. _____

18. _____

19. _____

20. _____

21. _____

22. _____

23. _____

EXERCISE 6

Answer the following questions.

1. The patient is admitted to the hospital with a possible diagnosis of _____, caused by an inadequate amount of insulin in the body. Insulin is produced by the _____. The doctor may order any of these three laboratory tests: _____, _____, or _____, to assist in diagnosing the patient's condition. The doctor also orders _____ to be performed by the nursing staff to determine the patient's glucose level.

2. If the patient is suffering from an insufficiency of a certain hormone in the body, the doctor may order a hormonal medication to be given to the patient to make up for the deficiency. The following is a list of hormonal medications. Indicate which endocrine gland should secrete each hormone.

   a. ACTH_____

   b. cortisone_____

   c. insulin_____

   d. epinephrine _____

   e. Premarin (estrogen) _____

   f. testosterone _____

   g. thyroid preparation_____

3. The patient is admitted to the hospital with a diagnosis of a thyroid condition. List three tests the doctor may order to gather information about the patient's thyroid function.

   a. _____

   b. _____

   c. _____

ABBREVIATIONS

Abbreviation	Meaning
ACTH	adrenocorticotropic hormone
DM	diabetes mellitus
FSH	follicle-stimulating hormone
HbA_{1C}	hemoglobin A1C, or glycosylated hemoglobin
LH	luteinizing hormone
PRL	prolactin
PTH	parathyroid hormone
TSH	thyroid-stimulating hormone

EXERCISE 7

Define the following abbreviations.

1. ACTH

   _____

2. DM

   _____

3. FSH

   _____

4. HbA_{1C}

   _____

5. LH

   _____

6. PRL

   _____

7. PTH

   _____

8. TSH

   _____

Websites of Interest

http://www.merck.com/pubs/mmanual_home/contents.html

http://www.americanheart.org

http://www.niddk.nih.gov

http://www.nlm.nih.gov

http://www.nimh.nih.gov

http://www.epilepsyfoundation.org

http://www.lungusa.org

http://www.cancer.org

http://www.kidney.org

Abbreviations

The following is a list of alphabetized abbreviations that are used frequently in doctors' orders. Most of the abbreviations related to specific departments, such as laboratory and diagnostic imaging, are not included here. For those, please refer to the chapters that discuss those departments.

Abbreviation	Meaning
>	greater than
<	less than
↑	increase or above
/	per or by
Δ	change
@	at
↓	decrease or below
°	degree or hour
A	apical
AA	active assisted
à	before
àà	of each
AAROM	active-assistive range of motion
Ab	antibody
abd	abdominal
ABG	arterial blood gas
ABR	absolute bed rest
ac	before meals
ACL	anterior cruciate ligament repair
ADA	American Diabetic Association
ADE	adverse drug events
ADH	antidiuretic hormone (chemistry)
ADL	activity(ies) of daily living
ad lib	as desired
A-drive	floppy drive
ADS	adult distress syndrome
ADT Log Book	a book used to record all admissions, discharges, and transfers on a nursing unit
ADT Sheet	a form used to record admissions, discharges, and transfers on a nursing unit for each day
AE	antiembolism
AFB	acid-fast bacillus
Ag	antigen
AHA	American Heart Association
AIDS	acquired immunodeficiency syndrome
AKA	above the knee amputation
ALP or alk phos	alkaline phosphatase (chemistry)
A.M.	morning
AMA	against medical advice

Abbreviation	Meaning
amb	ambulate
AMO	against medical orders
amp	ampule
ANA	American Nurses Association; antinuclear antibody (serology)
ANCC	American Nursing Credentialing Center
A&O	alert and oriented
AP	anteroposterior
appt	appointment
APS	Adult Protective Services
ARC	AIDS-related complex
ARDS	acute (adult) respiratory distress syndrome
AROM	active range of motion
ASA	acetylsalicylic acid (aspirin)
ASAP	as soon as possible
as tol	as tolerated
ax	axillary
BAER or AER	brain stem auditory response
BC	blood culture
BCOC	bowel care of choice
BE	barium enema
BIBA	brought in by ambulance
bid	twice a day
bili	bilirubin
BiPap	bilevel positive airway pressure
BiW, biw	twice a week
BKA	below the knee amputation
B/L	bilateral
BLE	both lower extremities
BM	bowel movement
BMI	body mass index
BMP	basic metabolic panel
BNP	brain natriuretic peptide
BP	blood pressure
BR	bed rest
BRP	bathroom privileges
BS	blood sugar
BSC	bedside commode
BUE	both upper extremities
BUN	blood urea nitrogen
Bx	biopsy
c	with
C	Celsius
Ca	cancer
Ca or Ca$^+$	calcium
CABG	coronary artery bypass graft

Abbreviation	Meaning	Abbreviation	Meaning
CAD	coronary artery disease	CVICU	cardiovascular intensive critical care unit
cal	calorie	CVP	central venous pressure
cap	capsule	Cx	culture
CAT	computed axial tomography	CXR	chest x-ray
cath	catheterize	D or E drive	drive/s to read CDs or DVDs
CBC	complete blood cell count	DAT	diet as tolerated; direct antiglobulin test
CBG	capillary blood gas		
CBI	continuous bladder irrigation	D/C or DC	discontinue
CBR	continuous bed rest		discharge
cc or cm^3	cubic centimeter	Diff	differential
CC, creat cl, or cr cl	creatinine clearance (chemistry)	Dig	digoxin
CCM	certified case manager	Disch	discharge
CCU	coronary care unit	D/LR	dextrose in lactated Ringer's solution
CDC	Centers for Disease Control	DME	durable medical equipment
C-drive	hard drive stored inside the computer	DMS	document management system
CDSS	clinical decision support system/s	DNR	do not resuscitate
CE	covered entities	D/NS	dextrose in normal saline
CEA	carcinoembryonic antigen (special chemistry)	DO	doctor of osteopathy
		DOA	dead on arrival
CEO	chief executive officer	DPI	dry powder inhaler
CFO	chief financial officer	dr or ℥	dram
CHF	congestive heart failure	DRG	diagnosis-related group
CHO	carbohydrate	D/RL	dextrose in Ringer's lactate
chol	cholesterol	DSA	digital subtraction angiography
CHUC	certified health unit coordinator	DSS	dioctyl sodium sulfosuccinate (Colace)
CI	clinical indication		
Cl	chloride (chemistry)	DSU	day surgery unit
cl	clear	D/W	dextrose in water
cm	centimeter	DW	distilled water
CMP	comprehensive metabolic panel	D$_5$W	5% dextrose in water
CMS	circulation, motion, sensation	D$_{10}$W	10% dextrose in water
CMT	cardiac monitor technician	Dx	diagnosis
CMV	cytomegalovirus	EBV	Epstein-Barr virus
CNA	certified nursing assistant	EC	enteric coated
c/o	complained of	ECF	extended care facility
CO$_2$	carbon dioxide	ECG or EKG	electrocardiogram
COA or C of A	condition of admission	EchoEG	echoencephalogram
comp or cmpd	compound	ED	emergency department
con't	continue	EEG	electroencephalogram
COO	chief operating officer	EGD	esophagogastroduodenoscopy
COPD	chronic obstructive pulmonary disease	elix	elixir
		EMG	electromyogram
COW	computer on wheels	EMR/EHR	electronic medical (health) record
CP	cold pack	ENG	electronystagmography
CPAP	continuous positive airway pressure	EPC	electronic pain control
CPK or CK	creatine phosphokinase or creatine kinase (chemistry)	EPHI	electronic protected health information
CPM	continuous passive motion	EPS	electrophysiologic study
CPOE	computer physician order entry	ER	emergency room
CPR	cardiopulmonary resuscitation	ERCP	endoscopic retrograde cholangiopancreatography
CPS	Child Protective Services		
CPT	chest physical therapy	ES	electrical stimulation
CPU	central processing unit	ESR	erythrocyte sedimentation rate
CPZ	Compazine	ESRD	end-stage renal disease
CQI	continuous quality improvement	ET	endotracheal tube
C&S	culture and sensitivity	ETS	elevated toilet seat
CSF	cerebrospinal fluid	F	Fahrenheit
CT	computed tomography	FBS	fasting blood sugar
CVA	cerebrovascular accident	Fe	iron
CVC	central venous catheter		

Abbreviation	Meaning	Abbreviation	Meaning
FF	force fluids	ID labels	identification labels
FFP	fresh frozen plasma	IIHI	individually identifiable health information
fib	fibrinogen		
FPG	fasting plasma glucose (chemistry)	IM	intramuscular
FS	full strength	I&O	intake and output
	frozen section	IPG	impedance plethysmography
5-FU	5-fluorouracil	IPPB	intermittent positive-pressure breathing
F/U	follow-up		
FWB	full weight bearing	irrig	irrigate
FWW	front wheel walker	IS	incentive spirometry
Fx, fx	fracture	ISOM	isometric
G, gm, g	gram	IV	intravenous
GB	gallbladder	IVDU	intravenous drug user
GI	gastrointestinal	IVF	intravenous fluids
gluc	glucose	IVP	intravenous pyelogram
gr	grain	IVPB	intravenous piggyback
GTT	glucose tolerance test	IVU	intravenous urogram
gtt(s)	drop(s)	K	potassium
Gyn	gynecology	KCl	potassium chloride
h, hr, hrs	hour/s	kg	kilogram
h or (H)	hypodermic	KO	keep open
HA	heated aerosol	KUB	kidney, ureter, bladder
H/A	headache	L	liter
HBOT	hyperbaric O_2 therapy	lat	lateral
HB$_s$Ag	hepatitis B surface antigen	lb, #	pound(s)
HBV	hepatitis B virus	L&D	labor and delivery
hCG	human chorionic gonadotropin	LDL	low-density lipoprotein
hct	hematocrit	LE	lower extremity
HCTZ	hydrochlorothiazide	liq	liquid
HCV	hepatitis C virus	LLE	left lower extremity
HD	hemodialysis	LLL	left lower lobe
HDL	high-density lipoprotein	LLQ	left lower quadrant
hgb	hemoglobin	L/min	liters per minute
H&H	hemoglobin and hematocrit	LOC	laxative of choice
HIMS	health information management system		leave on chart
			level of consciousness
HIPAA	Health Insurance Portability and Accountability Act		loss of consciousness
		LP	lumbar puncture
HIV	human immunodeficiency virus	LPN	licensed practical nurse
HIVB24Ag	human immunodeficiency virus antigen screen (serology)	LR	lactated Ringer's solution
		L&S	liver and spleen
		LS	lumbosacral
HL or hep-lock	heparin lock	Lt or Ⓛ	left
HMO	health maintenance organization	LTC	long-term care
HNP	herniated nucleus pulposus	LUE	left upper extremity
HO	house officer	LUL	left upper lobe
h/o	history of	LUQ	left upper quadrant
H_2O	water	lytes or e-lytes	electrolytes
H_2O_2	hydrogen peroxide	MAR	medication administration record
HOB	head of bed	MD	doctor of medicine
H&P	history and physical	MDI	metered-dose inhaler
HP	hot packs	Med	medical
hs	bedtime	mEq	milliequivalent
HSV	herpes simplex virus	mets	metastasis
HUC	health unit coordinator	μg, mcg	microgram
	health unit clerk	mg	milligram
HUS	health unit secretary	Mg or Mg$^+$	magnesium
Hx	history	MgSO	magnesium sulfate
ICD	implantable cardioverter-defibrillator	MI	myocardial infarction
	International Classification of Diseases	MICU	medical intensive care unit
ICU	intensive care unit	min	minute

Abbreviation	Meaning	Abbreviation	Meaning
mL	milliliter	PAS	pulsatile antiembolism stockings
MN	midnight	PBZ	pyribenzamine
MOM	Milk of Magnesia	PC	personal computer; packed cell
MR	may repeat	pc	after meals
MRI	magnetic resonance imaging	PCA	patient-controlled analgesia
MRSA	methicillin-resistant *Staphylococcus aureus*	PCN	penicillin
		PCP	primary care physician
MSO_4 or MS	morphine sulfate	PCT	patient care technician
MSSU	medical short-stay unit	PCV	packed-cell volume (hematology; same as hematocrit)
Na or Na^+	sodium		
NAHUC	National Association of Health Unit Coordinators	PCXR	portable chest x-ray
		PD	peritoneal dialysis
NAS	no added salt	PDPV	postural drainage, percussion, ad vibration
NCS	nerve conduction study		
nec	necessary	PDR	*Physicians' Desk Reference*
Neuro	neurology	Peds	pediatrics
NG	nasogastric	PEEP	positive end-expiratory pressure
NICU	neonatal intensive care unit	PEG	percutaneous endoscopic gastrostomy
NINP	no information, no publication		
NKA	no known allergies	PEP	positive expiratory pressure
NKDA	no known drug allergies	PET	positron emission tomography
NKFA	no known food allergies	pH	hydrogen ion concentration (acidity)
NKMA	no known medication allergies		
noc	night	PHI	protected health information reference
non rep	do not repeat		
NP	nasopharynx	PICC	peripherally inserted central catheter
NPO	nothing by mouth		
NS	normal saline	PICU	pediatric intensive care unit
NSA	no salt added	PID	pelvic inflammatory disease
NTG	nitroglycerine	PKU	phenylketonuria (chemistry)
N/V	nausea and vomiting	P.M.	evening, night
NVS or neuro ✓s	neurologic vital signs or checks	PO	by mouth or postoperative
NWB	non–weight-bearing	PO4 or phos	phosphate or phosphorus (chemistry)
O_2	oxygen		
OB	obstetrics	POCT or PCT	point-of-care testing performed on the nursing unit
OBS	observation		
OCG	oral cholecystogram	Postop, postop	after surgery
OD	right eye	PP	postpartum
OOB	out of bed	pp	postprandial (after meals)
O&P	ova and parasites	P&PD	percussion and postural drainage
OPS	outpatient surgery	PPE	personal protective equipment
OR	operating room	PPO	preferred provider organization
ORE	oil-retention enema	pr	per rectum
ORIF	open reduction, internal fixation	Preop, preop	before surgery
Ortho	orthopedics	prn	whenever necessary
OS	left eye	PROM	passive range of motion
OSA	obstructive sleep apnea	PSA	patient support associate
OSHA	Occupational Safety and Health Administration		prostate-specific antigen
		Psych	psychiatry
OSMO	osmolality	PT	physical therapy; prothrombin time
OT	occupational therapy	Pt	patient
OTC	over-the-counter	PTA	physical therapy assistant
OU	both eyes	PTCA	percutaneous transluminal coronary angioplasty
oz	ounce		
p	after	PTHC or PTC	percutaneous transhepatic cholangiography
P	pulse		
PA	posteroanterior	PTT or APTT	partial thromboplastin time or activated partial thromboplastin time
PACS	Picture Archiving and Communication Systems		
		PWB	partial weight bearing
PACU	postanesthesia care unit	q	every
PAP	prostatic acid phosphatase		

Abbreviation	Meaning
qd	every day; daily
qh	every hour (or fill in hour [e.g., q4h])
qid	four times a day
qod	every other day
R	rectal
RA	room air
R *A *C *E	Rescue individuals in danger; Alarm—sound the alarm; Confine the fire by closing all doors and windows; Extinguish the fire with the nearest suitable fire extinguisher
RBC	red blood cell
RBS	random blood sugar
RD	registered dietitian
RDW	red cell distribution width
reg	regular
Retics	reticulocytes (hematology)
RIS	radiology information system
RL	Ringer's lactate
RLE	right lower extremity
RLL	right lower lobe
RLQ	right lower quadrant
R&M	routine and microscopic
RML	right middle lobe
RN	registered nurse
R/O	rule out
ROM	range of motion
Rout	routine
RPR	rapid plasma reagin
RR	recovery room respiratory rate
RSV	respiratory syncytial virus
RT	respiratory therapist
Rt	routine
rt or ®	right
RUE	right upper extremity
RUL	right upper lobe
RUQ	right upper quadrant
Rx	take (e.g., treatment, medication)
s	without
ss̄	semis (one-half)
S&A	sugar and acetone (urinalysis)
SAD	save a day
SaO_2 or O_2 sats	oxygen saturation
SBFT	small bowel follow-through
SBU	small business unit
SC, sq, or sub-q	subcutaneous
SCD	sequential compression device
SDS	same-day surgery
SEP	somatosensory evoked potential
SHUC	student health unit coordinator
SICU	surgical intensive care unit
SIDS	sudden infant death syndrome
SL	sublingual
SNAT	suspected nonaccidental trauma
SNF	skilled nursing facility
SO_4	sulfate
SOB	shortness of breath
sol'n	solution
SOS	if needed (one dose only)

Abbreviation	Meaning
SSE	soap suds enema
SSU	short-stay unit
st	straight
stat	immediately
STM	soft tissue massage
subling, SL	sublingual (under the tongue)
supp	suppository
Surg	surgery
SVN	small volume nebulizer
syr	syrup
T_3, T_4, T_7	thyroid tests
T&A	tonsillectomy and adenoidectomy
tab	tablet
TAH	total abdominal hysterectomy
TB	tuberculosis
TBD	to be done
TBT	template bleeding time
T&C or T & x-match	type and crossmatch
TCDB	turn, cough, deep breathe
TCT or TT	thrombin clotting time or thrombin time
TDWB	touchdown weight bearing
Ted	antiembolism stockings
temp	temperature
TENS	transcutaneous electrical nerve stimulation
THR or THA	total hip replacement/total hip arthroplasty
TIA	transient ischemic attack
TIBC	total iron-binding capacity (chemistry)
TICU	trauma intensive care unit
tid	three times a day
Timed Specimen	to be drawn at specified time
tinct or tr	tincture
TJC	The Joint Commission
TKO	to keep open
TKR or TKA	total knee replacement/total knee arthroplasty
TPN	total parenteral nutrition
TPR	temperature, pulse, respiration
TRA	to run at
Trig or TG	triglycerides (chemistry)
T&S	type and screen
TSH	thyroid-stimulating hormone
T/stat	timed stat
TT	tilt table
TTOT	transtracheal oxygen therapy
TTWB	toe-touch weight bearing
TUR	transurethral resection
TWE	tap water enema
Tx	traction or treatment
U	unit
UA or U/A	urinalysis
UC	urine culture
UCR	usual, customary, and reasonable
UD	unit dose
UGI	upper gastrointestinal
ung	unguent (ointment)
US	ultrasound
USN	ultrasonic nebulizer

Abbreviation	Meaning	Abbreviation	Meaning
VAD	venous access device	WBAT	weight bearing as tolerated
VDRL	Venereal Disease Research Laboratories	WBC	white blood cell
		WHO	World Health Organization
VDT	vi deo display terminal	wk	week
VEP	visual evoked potential	WNL	within normal limits
vib & perc	vibration and percussion	WP	whirlpool
VMA	vanillylmandelic acid	wt	weight
VNS	visiting nurse service	www	World Wide Web
VS	vital sign	x-match	crossmatch
WA or W/A	while awake	Zn	zinc

Word Parts

Each word element present in Chapter 23 is noted in **bold text** along with its meaning and the unit of Chapter 23 in which it is found. Additional word parts that you may encounter in your medical work are provided in normal text, and instead of unit number, a sample medical term incorporating the word part is provided.

Word Element	Meaning	Unit Number (or Sample Medical Term)
a	without	1
abdomin / o	abdomen	7
-ac	pertaining to	*cardiac*
acou / o	hearing	*acoumeter*
acr / o	extremities, height	*acromegaly*
aden / o	gland	11
adren / o	adrenal	11
adrenal / o	adrenal	11
-al	pertaining to	2
-algia	pain	3
amnion / o	amnion, amniotic fluid	*amnionitis*
an-	without	1
angi / o	blood vessel	6
aort / o	aorta	6
-apheresis	removal	*plasmapheresis*
appendic / o	appendix	7
-ar	pertaining to	3
arteri / o	artery	6
arthr / o	joint	3
-ary	pertaining to	*pulmonary*
-asthenia	weakness	*myasthenia*
atel / o	imperfect, incomplete	*atelectasis*
ather / o	yellowish, fatty plaque	*atherosclerosis*
-atresia	absence of normal body opening, occlusion	*hysteratresia*
aut / o	self	*autopsy*
balan / o	glans penis	*balanitis*
bi-	two	*bilateral*
blephar / o	eyelid	5
brady-	slow	6
bronch / o	bronchus	8
cancer / o	cancer	2
carcin / o	cancer	2
cardi / o	heart	2
caud / o	tail or down	*caudal*

Word Element	Meaning	Unit Number (or Sample Medical Term)
-cele	herniation, protrusion	4
-centesis	surgical puncture to aspirate fluid	4
cerebell / o	cerebellum	4
cerebr / o	cerebrum	4
cervic / o	cervix	10
cheil / o	lip	7
cholangi / o	bile duct	*cholangioma*
chol / e, chol / o	bile, gall	7
choledoch / o	common bile duct	*choledocholithiasis*
chondr / o	cartilage	3
clavic / o	clavicle	3
clavicul / o	clavicle	3
-coccus	berry-shaped (form of bacterium)	*Staphylococcus*
col / o	colon	7
colp / o	vagina	10
conjunctiv / o	conjunctiva	5
cost / o	rib	3
crani / o	cranium	3
crypt / o	hidden	*onychocryptosis*
cutane / o	skin	2
cyan / o	blue	6
cyst / o	bladder, sac	7, 9
-cyte	cell	*erythrocyte*
cyt / o	cell	1, 2
derm / o	skin	2
dermat / o	skin	2
diverticul / o	diverticulum	*diverticulosis, diverticulitis*
duoden / o	duodenum	7
dys-	difficult, labored, painful, abnormal	8
ech / o	sound	*echocardiogram*
-ectasis	expansion	*atelectasis*
-ectomy	excision, surgical removal	1, 3
electr / o	electricity, electrical activity	1, 3
-emia	condition of the blood	6
encephal / o	brain	4
endo-	within	6
enter / o	intestine	7

Word Element	Meaning	Unit Number (or Sample Medical Term)	Word Element	Meaning	Unit Number (or Sample Medical Term)
epididym / o	epididymis	*epididymitis*	-lysis	loosening, dissolution, separating	*urinalysis*
episi / o	vulva	*episiotomy*			
epitheli / o	epithelium	2	-malacia	softening	*chondromalacia*
erythr / o	red	6	mamm / o	breast	10
esophag / o	esophagus	7	mast / o	breast	10
eti / o	cause (of disease)	*etiology*	-megaly	enlargement	6
femor / o	femur	3	melan / o	black	*melanoma*
fibr / o	fiber	*fibromyalgia*	men / o	menstruation	10
gastr / o	stomach	7	mening / o	meninges	4
-genic	producing, originating, causing	2	menisc / o	meniscus	3
			meta-	after, beyond, change	*metastasis*
gloss / o	tongue	7	-meter	instrument used to measure	*spirometer*
-gram	record, x-ray image	3			
-graph	instrument used to record	3	metr / o	uterus	10
			-metry	measurement	*pelvimetry*
-graphy	process of recording, x-ray imaging	3	myc / o	fungus	*onychomycosis*
			my / o	muscle	3
			myel / o	spinal cord, bone marrow	4
gravid / o	pregnancy	*gravida*			
gynec / o	woman	10	myring / o	tympanic membrane	5
hem / o	blood	6	nat / o	birth	*prenatal*
hemat / o	blood	6	natr / o	sodium	*hyponatremia*
hepat / o	liver	7	necr / o	death (cells, body)	*necrosis*
herni / o	protrusion of a body part	7	neo-	new	*neonatal*
			nephr / o	kidney	9
hist / o	tissue	2	neur / o	nerve	4
humer / o	humerus	3	noct / i	night	*nocturia*
hyper-	above normal	6	-odynia	pain	*cardiodynia*
hypo-	below normal	6	-oid	resembling	2
hyster / o	uterus	10	olig / o	scanty, few	*oliguria*
-ial	pertaining to	*endometrial*	-oma	tumor	2
-iasis	condition of	7	onc / o	cancer	2
-iatrist	specialist, physician	*physiatrist*	onych / o	nail	*onychomalacia*
iatr / o	physician, treatment	*iatrogenic*	oophor / o	ovary	10
-ic	pertaining to	3	ophthalm / o	eye	5
-ior	pertaining to	*posterior*	-opsy	to view	*biopsy*
ile / o	ileum	7	orchi / o	testicle, testis	9
inter-	between	*intervertebral*	orchid / o	testicle, testis	9
intra-	within	1	organ / o	organ	*organic*
irid / o	iris	5	-osis	abnormal condition	3
isch / o	deficiency, blockage	*ischemia*	oste / o	bone	3
-itis	inflammation	3	ot / o	ear	5
kal / i	potassium	*hyperkalemia*	-oxia	oxygen	*hypoxia*
kerat / o	cornea	5	-ous	pertaining to	2
labyrinth / o	labyrinth	*labyrinthitis*	pancreat / o	pancreas	7
lact / o	milk	*lactorrhea*	parathyroid / o	parathyroid	11
lamin / o	lamina	3	part / o	give birth to, labor, childbirth	*parturition*
lapar / o	abdomen	7			
laryng / o	larynx	8	patell / o	patella	3
lei / o	smooth	*leiomyosarcoma*	path / o	disease	2
leuk / o	white	6	-pathy	disease	*neuropathy*
lingu / o	tongue	7	peri-	surrounding (outer)	6
lip / o	fat	2	perine / o	perineum	10
lith / o	stone, calculus	7	-pexy	surgical fixation	6
-logist	one who specializes in the diagnosis and treatment of	2	-phagia	swallowing	*dysphagia*
			phalang / o	phalange	3
			pharyng / o	pharynx	8
-logy	study of	2	phas / o	speech	4

Word Element	Meaning	Unit Number (or Sample Medical Term)	Word Element	Meaning	Unit Number (or Sample Medical Term)
phleb / o	vein	6	-scopy	visual examination	3
-phobia	fear of	*claustrophobia*	sigmoid / o	sigmoid colon	7
phot / o	light	*photophobia*	-sis	state of	*diagnosis*
-plasty	surgical repair	3	son / o	sound	*sonogram*
-plegia	paralysis, stroke	4	somat / o	body	*psychosomatic*
pleur / o	pleura	8	-spasm	involuntary muscle contraction	*bronchospasm*
-pnea	respiration, breathing	8	spin / o	spine	4
pneum / o	air, lung	8	splen / o	spleen	6
pneumon / o	lung	8	staped / o	stapes	5
-poiesis	formation	*hematopoiesis*	staphyl / o	grape-like clusters	*Staphylococcus*
poli / o	gray matter	4	-stasis	control, stop, standing	*metastasis*
prim / i	first	*primigravida*	-stenosis	narrowing	6
proct / o	rectum	7	stern / o	sternum	3
prostat / o	prostate	9	stomat / o	mouth	7
psych / o	mind	4	-stomy	creation of an artificial opening	7
-ptosis	drooping, sagging, prolapse	*nephroptosis*	streptococcus	twisted chains	*Streptococcus*
puerper / o	childbirth	*peurperal*	sub-	under, below	1
pulmon / o	lung	8	supra-	above	*suprascapular*
pyel / o	renal pelvis	9	tachy-	fast, rapid	6
pylor / o	pylorus, pyloric sphincter	*pyloroplasty*	thorac / o	chest	8
			-thorax	chest	*pneumothorax*
quadr / i	four	*quadriplegia*	thromb / o	clot	6
radic / o, radicul / o, rhiz / o	nerve root	*radiculitis*	thyr / o	thyroid	11
			thyroid / o	thyroid	11
ren / o	kidney	9	tom / o	cut, section	*tomogram*
retin / o	retina	5	-tomy	surgical incision or to cut into	3
rhabd / o	rod-shaped, striated	*rhabdomyolysis*	tonsill / o	tonsil	8
rhin / o	nose	8	trache / o	trachea	8
-rrhagia	rapid flow of blood	4	trans-	through, across, beyond	1
-rrhaphy	surgical repair	4	trich / o	hair	2
-rrhea	excessive discharge, flow	4	-trophy	development, nourishment	3
-rrhexis	rupture	*hysterorrhexis*	ungu / o	nail	2
salping / o	fallopian or uterine tube	10	ur / o	urine, urinary tract	9
sarc / o	connective tissue, flesh	2	ureter / o	ureter	9
			urethr / o	urethra	9
-sarcoma	malignant tumor	*rhabdomyosarcoma*	uria-	urine, urination	*albuminuria*
scapul / o	scapula	3	urin / o	urine	9
scler / o	sclera, hard	5	uter / o	uterus	10
-sclerosis	hardening	6	vagin / o	vagina	10
-scope	instrument used for visual examination	3	vas / o	vessel, duct	9
			ven / o	vein	6
-scopic	pertaining to visual examination	*arthroscopic*	vertebr / o	vertebra	3
			viscer / o	internal organs	2

Answers

CHAPTER 1

Exercise 1

1. CHUC
2. EMR, EHR
3. SHUC
4. pt
5. HUC
6. CDSS
7. CPOE

Exercise 2

1. certified health unit coordinator
2. electronic medical record, electronic health record
3. student health unit coordinator
4. patient
5. health unit coordinator
6. clinical decision support system
7. computer physician order entry

Review Questions

1. a. tasks performed at the bedside or in direct contact with the patient
   b. tasks performed away from the bedside
   c. a pathway of upward mobility
   d. the process of testifying to or endorsing that a person has met certain standards
   e. a process used to communicate the doctors' orders to the nursing staff and other hospital departments; computers or handwritten requisitions are used
2. a. clinical
   b. non-clinical
   c. non-clinical
   d. clinical
   e. non-clinical
   f. clinical
   g. non-clinical
3. a. 1940; implementation of health unit coordinating at Montefiore Hospital in Pittsburgh, Pennsylvania
   b. 1966; one of the first educational programs was implemented in a vocational school in Minneapolis, Minnesota
   c. 1980; the National Association of Health Unit Coordinators was established in Phoenix, Arizona
   d. 1983; first offering of the Health Unit Coordinator Certification Examination by NAHUC
4. a. Any three of the following:
   - Communicate all new doctors' orders to the patient's nurse.
   - Maintain the patient's chart.
   - Perform non-clinical tasks for patient admission, transfer, and discharge.
   - Prepare the patient's chart for surgery.
   - Handle all telephone communication for the nurses' station.
   b. Any three of the following:
   - Transcribe the doctors' orders.
   - Place and receive doctor's telephone calls to and from the doctor's office.
   - Provide information to the physician regarding procedures.
   - Obtain the patient's chart and procedure equipment.
   c. Any three of the following:
   - Schedule diagnostic procedures, treatments, and services.
   - Request services from maintenance and other service departments.
   - Work with the admitting department with patient admission, transfer, and discharge; order the supplies for the nursing unit.
   d. Any three of the following:
   - Advise visitors of patient location.
   - Provide information on location of bathroom, visitors lounge, cafeteria, etc.
   - Inform visitors of visiting rules and special precautions regarding their visit to a patient's room.
   - Receive telephone calls from the patient's relatives and friends regarding patient condition.
   - Handle visitor complaints.
5.
   - an electronic record of patient health information generated by one or more encounters in any care delivery setting
   - a computerized program into which physicians directly enter patient orders, replacing handwritten orders on an order sheet or prescription pad
   - computerized programs that provide suggestions or default values for drug doses, routes, and frequencies. The program also may perform drug allergy checks, drug–laboratory value checks, drug–drug interaction checks, etc.
   a.
   - Monitor and maintain the electronic record.
   - Integrate/scan any paper documents, created by caregivers, into the electronic medical record.
   - Input data for reports and assist in the coordination of mandatory education and assessment.
9. Any three of the following:
   - professional representation format to share ideas and challenges—to be prepared and proactive regarding changes that are taking place in the Health Unit Coordinator profession

- national networking
- national directory
- opportunity to develop leadership skills

10. Any three of the following:
    - increased credibility
    - gaining a broader perspective of health unit coordinating (not just one specialty)—be prepared and proactive regarding changes that are taking place in the health unit
    - coordinator profession
    - increased mobility, geographically and vertically
    - peer and public recognition and respect
    - improved self-image

11. a. telemetry technician
    b. case management technician
    c. patient care assistant (the HUC also may be trained to perform electrograms and/or phlebotomy)

12. a. health unit service manager
    b. health information manager

13. Any four of the following:
    - Complete a Health Unit Coordinator program (if you have not done so).
    - Complete management classes related to health care.
    - Attend in-services that are offered through the hospital or classes that are offered at local colleges that relate to communication or related administrative skills.
    - Complete computer classes to become efficient in or gain a working knowledge of advanced word processing, databases, spreadsheets, and e-mail. (Typing skills are essential.)
    - Become a member of the National Association of Health Unit Coordinators. Receive the newsletter and attend educational conferences.
    - Become certified by taking the National Health Unit Coordinator certification test.

14. August 23rd

CHAPTER 2

Exercise 1

1. ANA
2. ANCC
3. CCM
4. CEO
5. CFO
6. COO
7. DSU
8. DO
9. DRG
10. ECF
11. ED
12. ER
13. HIMS
14. HMO
15. HO
16. ICD
17. JCAHO
18. LTC
19. MD
20. Neuro
21. OB
22. OR
23. Ortho
24. PACU
25. PCP
26. Peds
27. PPO
28. Psych
29. RR
30. SAD
31. SDS
32. SNF
33. Surg
34. UCR
35. WHO
36. www

Exercise 2

1. American Nurses Association
2. American Nursing Credentialing Center
3. certified case manager
4. chief executive officer
5. chief financial officer
6. chief operating officer
7. day surgery unit
8. doctor of osteopathy
9. diagnosis-related groups
10. extended care facility
11. emergency department
12. emergency room
13. health information systems
14. health maintenance organization
15. house officer
16. International Statistical Classification of Diseases and Related Health Problems
17. Joint Commission on Accreditation of Healthcare Organizations
18. long-term care
19. medical doctor
20. neurology
21. obstetrics
22. operating room
23. orthopedics
24. postanesthesia care unit
25. primary care physician
26. pediatrics
27. preferred provider organization
28. psychiatry
29. recovery room
30. save a day
31. same-day surgery
32. skilled nursing facility
33. surgical
34. usual, customary, and reasonable
35. World Health Organization
36. World Wide Web

Review Questions

1. a. improving quality of care
   b. the staggering cost of advanced technology
   c. increasing insurance costs
   d. a growing number of people without health insurance
   e. an increasing demand for care

2. Any eight of the following:
   - more accurate
   - confidential
   - cost effective
   - accessible
   - reduces errors
   - high-quality care
   - reduces length of stay
   - reduces retesting
   - will allow the federal government to track the course and impact of a pandemic in real time
   - will provide local, state, and federal governments with the necessary data to direct therapies, medical personnel, and supplies during an emergency

3. Any four of the following:
   - up-front cost
   - cultural obstacles
   - increased need for advanced privacy and security protection
   - inconsistency among systems
   - lack of standardization
   - increased potential to link health care information to wrong patient
   - widespread interruption if system goes down

4. care and treatment of the sick

5. a. education of physicians and other health care personnel
   b. research
   c. prevention of disease
   d. local health center

6. attending physician

7. resident

8. a. the type of patient service offered
   b. ownership of the hospital
   c. type of accreditation the hospital has been given

9. 1. j
   2. m
   3. l
   4. n
   5. g
   6. a
   7. k
   8. b
   9. e
   10. c
   11. i
   12. f
   13. d
   14. h

10. 1. i
    2. g
    3. j
    4. b
    5. l
    6. a
    7. c
    8. k
    9. f
    10. h
    11. e
    12. d

11. a. business office
    b. admitting department
    c. pathology/clinical laboratory
    d. diagnostic imaging
    e. radiation therapy, or radiation oncology
    f. pharmacy
    g. physical therapy
    h. occupational therapy
    i. respiratory care or cardiopulmonary department
    j. dietary department
    k. endoscopy department
    l. gastroenterology, or GI laboratory
    m. cardiovascular studies department
    n. neurodiagnostics department
    o. health information management, or medical records, department
    p. central service department or supply purchasing department
    q. outpatient department, or clinic
    r. social service department
    s. home care department (also could be handled by Social Services or Case Management)
    t. housekeeping, or Environmental Services
    u. materials management, or purchasing department
    v. pastoral care or chaplain
    w. maintenance department
    x. laundry or linens department
    y. communications department or hospital information systems
    z. security department

12. a. cardiopulmonary resuscitation
    b. infectious disease control
    c. fire and safety
    d. Universal (Standard) Precautions
    e. HIPAA

13. the governing board

14. chief executive officer (CEO) or hospital administrator

15. Any three of the following:
    - Internet
    - newspaper classified advertisements
    - job placement/career counselors
    - employment agencies
    - health care facility bulletin boards
    - networking with professionals in the field
    - instructors
    - health care hotlines
    - library resources

16. the case manager is an expert in <u>managed care</u> and acts as the patient's <u>advocate</u>

17. a. a patient who has been admitted to a health care facility for at least 24 hours for treatment and care
    b. a patient receiving care by a health care facility but not admitted to the facility for 24 hours
    c. an award given by the American Nurses Credentialing Center (ANCC) to hospitals that satisfy a set of criteria designed to measure their strength of quality of nursing
    d. recognition that a health care organization has met an official standard
    e. level of health care, generally provided in hospitals or emergency departments, for sudden, serious illnesses or trauma
    f. care for illnesses of long duration, such as diabetes or emphysema

g. a full-time, acute care specialist whose focus is exclusively on hospitalized patients

h. the combining of individual physician practices and small, stand-alone hospitals into larger networks
  • International Statistical Classification of Diseases and Related Health
  • health maintenance organization
  • a payment method whereby the provider of care receives a set dollar amount per patient, regardless of services rendered

18. hospice
19. home care
20. to provide quality health care for the lowest possible cost
21. Medicare A is hospital insurance.
22. Medicare B is medical insurance (premium and deductible).
23. Medicare D, which started in January of 2006, is a drug plan created for senior citizens who do not have drug coverage.
24. Workers' compensation

CHAPTER 3

Exercise 1

1. CCU
2. CNA
3. CVICU
4. Gyn
5. ICU
6. L&D
7. LPN
8. Med
9. MICU
10. Neuro
11. NICU
12. Ortho
13. PICU
14. PSA
15. Psych
16. RN
17. SICU
18. SSU
19. TICU

Exercise 2

1. coronary care unit
2. certified nursing assistant
3. cardiovascular intensive care unit
4. gynecology
5. intensive care unit
6. labor and delivery
7. licensed practical nurse
8. medical
9. medical intensive care unit
10. neurology
11. neonatal intensive care unit
12. orthopedics
13. pediatric intensive care unit
14. patient support associate
15. psychology
16. registered nurse
17. surgical intensive care unit
18. short stay unit
19. trauma intensive care unit

Review Questions

1. 1. e
   2. c
   3. d
   4. n
   5. g
   6. b
   7. h
   8. m
   9. j
   10. i
   11. a
   12. l
   13. f
   14. k
2. responsible for ensuring the physical and emotional care of the hospitalized patient
3. Any three of the following:
   • nurse or clinical manager: assists the director of nursing in carrying out administrative responsibilities and is usually in charge of one or more nursing units
   • assistant nurse manager: assists the nurse manager in coordinating the activities of the nursing units
   • registered nurse: may give direct patient care or supervise patient care given by others
   • licensed practical nurse: gives direct patient care; functions under the direction of the RN
   • certified nursing assistant: a health care provider who performs basic nursing tasks such as bathing and seeding patients
4. a. preoperative area: area in the hospital where patients are prepared for surgery
   b. intraoperative care: operating room—area in the hospital where surgery is performed
   c. postoperative: postanesthesia care—area in the hospital where patients are cared for immediately after surgery until they have recovered from the effects of the anesthesia
5. A patient who is critically ill in need of constant specialized nursing care would be admitted to ICU and would be transferred to a stepdown unit when his condition improved somewhat, but not enough to be transferred to a regular nursing unit.
6. In the total nursing care delivery model, one RN provides total care to assigned patients, whereas in the team nursing model, a team leader who is an RN and team members provide care for the patients.
7. acuity
8. staff development
9. a. registered nurse
   b. licensed practical nurse
   c. certified nursing assistant
10. used as a method of outlining a patient's path of treatment for a specific diagnosis, procedure, or symptom
11. Holistic nursing care is a system of comprehensive patient care (total patient care) that considers the physical, emotional, social, economic, and spiritual needs of the person, his response to illness, and the effect of the illness on his ability to meet self-care needs.
12. a. facilitates continuous quality improvement
    b. improves patient care
    c. decreases errors

d. provides "total patient care"

e. maximizes resources

f. increases professional satisfaction for health care providers

CHAPTER 4

Exercise 1

1. D or E drive
2. C drive
3. CPU
4. PC
5. VDT
6. COW
7. DMS

Exercise 2

1. drive/s to read CD or DVD
2. hard drive stored inside the computer
3. central processing unit
4. personal computer
5. video display terminal
6. computer on wheels
7. document management system

Review Questions

1. a. Speak slowly and distinctly.
   b. Give first and last names of patient and/or doctor, and spell last names.
   c. State number slowly, and repeat.
   d. Leave your name and number, and repeat both.
2. a. Answer the telephone promptly (before the third ring).
   b. Identify yourself properly by stating location, name, and status.
   c. Speak into the telephone.
   d. Give the caller your undivided attention.
   e. Speak clearly and distinctly.
   f. Be courteous at all times.
   g. When you cannot answer a question, tell the caller that you will get someone who can answer the question; do not say, "I don't know."
   h. If it is necessary to step away or answer another call, place the caller on hold after getting his permission.
3. a. who the message is for
   b. the caller's name
   c. date and time of the call
   d. purpose of the call
   e. phone number to call if a return call is expected
   f. your name
4. a. a list of options projected on the viewing screen
   b. made up of three components: keyboard, viewing screen, and printer
   c. a device that enables a computer to send and receive data over regular phone lines
   d. a computer component that displays information
   e. alphabetical listing of names and telephone numbers, as well as directory of telephone numbers of physicians on staff
   f. a requisition (paper order form) used to process information when the computer is not available for use
   g. a machine that shreds confidential material—usually each nursing station has a barrel or container in which to place documents to be shredded

h. a system by which air pressure transports tubes carrying supplies, requisitions, or messages from one hospital unit or department to another

i. a machine that prints patient labels—located near the health unit coordinator's area

j. a device used to transmit images of paper documents/pictures to be entered into the patient's electronic record

k. a computer on a cart with wheels that can be taken into patients' rooms

l. a computer system (or set of computer programs) used to track and store electronic documents and/or images of paper documents

5. a. to locate information or a person
   b. to answer other telephone lines
   c. to protect patient confidentiality (caller will not hear conversations)
6. Have the chart handy so facts may be located for questions that may be asked. Write down the facts that need to be discussed.
7. posts material in an attractive manner and keeps the posted material current; when material has been read and initialed by nursing personnel, the health unit coordinator removes material and places on the nurse manager's desk
8. (Example) 4 East, Sally, Health Unit Coordinator
9. A. (d)
   B. (c)
   C. (d)
10. a. Access patient information.
    b. Order diagnostic tests and equipment.
    c. Enter discharges and transfers.
11. Doctor—Any three of the following:
    • enter orders directly into the patient's electronic medical record
    • access computerized reports
    • access diagnostic images
    • access diagnostic test results
    • access nurses' notes to review
    Nurse—Any three of the following:
    • enter documentation and notes directly into the patient's medical record.
    • access the doctors' orders.
    • access diagnostic images.
    • access diagnostic test results for evaluation.
    • access computerized reports.
    • send and receive e-mail.
    HUC—Any three of the following:
    • monitors the patient's electronic record for HUC tasks
    • accesses doctors' telephone numbers
    • locates patients for visitors or doctors
    • if requested to do so, enters data into the computer
    • accesses computerized reports
12. for patient confidentiality and your own protection
13. a. Do not use for personal messages or to send inappropriate material such as jokes.
    b. Send or respond to necessary person or department only; refrain from sending to all or using "reply all" unless necessary.
14. a. sending personal messages or jokes
    b. sending or responding to everyone when not necessary or requested

15. Many hospital personnel use the fax machine located in the nurses station; using the re-dial option may send the document or doctors' orders to a different location than intended, possibly violating patient confidentiality.

16. a. handwritten progress notes
    b. electrocardiograms or telemetry strips
    c. outside documents and/or reports

17. a. The HUC may call into a patient's room to communicate with nursing unit personnel.
    b. The nurse may call the nursing unit if help is needed to find SWAT personnel.

18. a. pocket pager
    b. locator device or patient intercom
    c. overhead paging system (hospital operator)

19. An icon such as a telephone would be an indication that there is a health unit coordinator task to be done.

CHAPTER 5

Exercise 1

1. a
2. b
3. b
4. c
5. d
6. d
7. d
8. c
9. a
10. b

Exercise 2

1. AS
2. AG
3. NA
4. NA
5. AS
6. AG
7. AS
8. AG
9. AG
10. AS
11. AG
12. NA
13. AS
14. AG
15. AG
16. NA
17. AS
18. AS

Exercise 3

Answers will vary. Below are examples of responses for each behavior:

1. Assertive: "It upset me when you threw the chart down in front of me and left without giving me a chance to respond."
   * Nonassertive: Be upset and say nothing.
   * Aggressive: "This is a 24-hour facility; what I don't get done, you can do!"

2. Assertive: "I understand that you would prefer someone who is accustomed to working in pediatrics. I may need a little assistance and will do my best to get the job done." (*Fogging*)
   * Nonassertive: "I'm sorry; I know I'm not qualified to work in pediatrics."
   * Aggressive: "You're lucky to have me; if you don't want me to be here, I'll leave."

3. Assertive: "You're right, I did miss that order, I will order it right now." (*Negative assertion*)
   * Nonassertive: "I'm sorry; I'm so stupid! What should I do now?"
   * Aggressive: "Well, maybe if you gave me a little more help, I wouldn't be missing orders!"

4. Assertive: "Only relatives may visit the patient, on the instructions of the physician." Repeat as necessary. (*Broken record*)
   * Nonassertive: "I don't think you're supposed to visit, but maybe just this once we could sneak you in."
   * Aggressive: "You are not allowed to visit; I don't care who you are!"

5. Assertive: "I was not aware that you felt this way. What about my work is sloppy?" (*Negative inquiry*)
   * Nonassertive: "I've always been sloppy. It's just the way I am. I'm sorry."
   * Aggressive: "I'm a lot neater than most of the other people around here!"

6. • Assertive: "I know it must seem that nothing is done right here; however, most things are done very well. I'll scan the report into the patient's record now."
   * Nonassertive: "I'm sorry; I should have scanned it as soon as you asked me too. I am so forgetful sometimes."
   * Aggressive: "You don't understand how hectic it is around here. You doctors always think everyone else is incompetent!"

Review Questions

1. Answers will vary. Below are examples of patient needs.
   a. physiologic—The patient is "NPO" for tests.
   b. safety and security—The patient is concerned about his job and how long he will be unable to work.
   c. belonging and love—The patient's family has not visited or called for 2 days.
   d. esteem—The patient is a quiet, shy gentleman and a nurse calls him "sweetie" and "honey."

2. a. sender
   b. message
   c. receiver
   d. feedback

3. a. translating mental images, feelings, and ideas into symbols to communicate them to the receiver
   b. the process of translating symbols received from the sender to determine the message

4. Answers will vary.

5. a. poor choice of words
   b. contradiction of verbal and nonverbal language used

6. a. poor listening skills
   b. poor feedback skills

7. Any three of the following:
   * clothing
   * hair
   * jewelry

- body art
- cosmetics
- automobile
- house
- perfume or cologne

8. Any three of the following:
   - posture
   - ambulation
   - touching
   - personal distance
   - eye contact
   - breathing
   - hand gestures
   - facial expressions

9. a. 55%
   b. 38%
   c. 7 %

10. a. unsuccessful encoding by sender
    b. unsuccessful decoding by receiver

11. a. unsuccessful decoding: The nurse was not aware of the patient's cultural background (see Table 5-1, p. 71).
    b. unsuccessful encoding: Joe was disrespectful in using the term *honey* and also used medical terms that Mrs. Fredrick did not understand. Mrs. Fredrick by crying was expressing both her esteem and safety and security needs.
    c. unsuccessful decoding: Sue was distracted and failed to listen for the page.
    d. unsuccessful decoding: Cindi was stereotyping Mr. Potter on the basis of his status and personal hygiene.

12. a. Stop talking.
    b. Teach yourself to concentrate.
    c. Take time to listen.
    d. Listen with your eyes.
    e. Listen to what is being said—not only to how it is being said.
    f. Suspend judgment.
    g. Do not interrupt the speaker.
    h. Remove distractions.
    i. Listen for both feeling and content (seek to understand).

13. a. Use paraphrasing (repeat the message to the sender in your own words).
    b. Repeat the last word or words of the message (to allow the speaker to more fully develop the thought).
    c. Use specific rather than general feedback.
    d. Use constructive feedback rather than destructive feedback.
    e. Do not deny senders' feelings.

14. care that involves understanding and being sensitive to a patient's cultural background

15. a. • Understand and evaluate your own values, beliefs, and customs before working with and caring for people of varying cultures.
       • Take the time to learn about the cultural backgrounds of patients, which may involve incorporating their beliefs and practices into their care.
       • Do not judge other people by the standards of your own values and beliefs.
       • Avoid stereotyping or making assumptions about a patient or a coworker that are based on race or ethnicity.

- Treat everyone with respect as unique individuals regardless of their gender, age, economic status, religion, sexual status, education, occupation, physical makeup or limitations, or command of the English language.

16. a. nonassertive
    b. aggresive
    c. assertive

17. a. a skill that allows you to say no over and over again without raising your voice or getting irritated or angry
    b. a skill that allows you to accept manipulative criticism and anxiety-producing statements by offering no resistance and by using a noncommittal reply
    c. a skill that allows you to accept your errors and faults without becoming defensive or resorting to anger
    d. a skill that allows you to actively prompt criticism so you can use the information or, if manipulative, exhaust it

18. a. Always identify yourself by nursing unit, name, and status.
    b. Avoid putting the person on hold.
    c. Listen to what the caller is saying.
    d. Write down what the caller is saying.
    e. Acknowledge the anger.
    f. Do not allow the caller to become abusive.

19. a. the inability to accept other cultures, or an assumption of cultural superiority
    b. discrimination based on social/economic class
    c. subgroups within a culture; people with a distinct identity but who have certain ethnic, occupational, or physical characteristics found in a larger culture
    d. a set of values, beliefs, and traditions that are held by a specific social group
    e. the assumption that all members of a culture or ethnic group act alike (generalizations that may be inaccurate)
    f. an experienced, working health unit coordinator selected to train/teach an HUC student or new employee

20. a. • Provide the student and the student's instructor or the new employee a copy of dates and times that the student or new employee is to be on the nursing unit to complete the clinical experience.
       • Obtain a list of objectives (provided by the hospital or the school).
       • Take the student/new employee on a tour of the nursing unit and hospital, so that he is aware of where rest rooms, cafeteria, and hospital departments are located.
       • Set a positive example.
       • If the student/new employee does not call prior to being late or absent, notify the instructor or nurse manager.
       • Notify the student, nursing unit, new employee, and nurse manager if you are going to be tardy, absent, or transferred to another unit (preferably an hour prior to start of shift).
       • Stay with the student/new employee to monitor his progress and check off objectives as completed, with competence defined as instructed in the clinical/orientation packet.
       • Provide feedback to the student/new employee and provide suggestions for improvement.

- Notify the student's instructor or new employee's nurse manager if the student/new employee is not attired according to hospital/school dress code, is not performing in an appropriate, professional manner, or is having difficulty completing objectives.
- Notify the student's instructor or new employee's nurse manager if there are any questions or concerns.
- Notify the student's instructor or new employee's nurse manager immediately if there are serious concerns.
- Complete an evaluation form regarding the student clinical experience.

21. a. • Be sure you know when and where you are to complete your clinical experience and know the name of your preceptor.
- If you are a student, provide your preceptor with a list of objectives and the instructor's telephone and or pager numbers.
- The student/new employee should notify the nursing unit, the preceptor, and the instructor or nurse manager an hour prior to start of shift (unless emergency) if he is going to be tardy or absent.
- The student must notify the instructor if he will leave the hospital prior to the end of the shift.
- It is the student's responsibility to notify the instructor if the preceptor is going to be late, absent, or transferred to another unit.
- The student or new employee should arrive dressed appropriately and prepared to learn and work each day and should be accountable for his learning.
- The student must be flexible and refrain from saying, "That's not the way we were taught in class," or "That's not the way we did it at Previous Community Hospital."
- The student or new employee should communicate openly with the preceptor, instructor, or nurse manager regarding any problems with his clinical performance.
- The student/new employee should have the list of objectives/evaluation forms completed and signed off by the preceptor 2 days prior to the last day of clinical.
- The student/new employee should complete an evaluation form regarding his clinical experience or orientation.

22. a. obtaining information
   b. providing information
   c. developing trust
   d. showing understanding
   e. relieving stress

23. With the implementation of the electronic medical record, the HUC role is expanding. The HUC assists doctors, nurses, and ancillary personnel in entering and retrieving information regarding the patient's electronic medical record. The HUC has a larger role in listening to visitors, patients, and nursing unit personnel complaints and problem solving.

CHAPTER 6

Exercise 1

1. APS
2. CPS
3. NINP
4. SNAT
5. HIPAA
6. PHI
7. CE
8. CPR
9. EPHI
10. IIHI

Exercise 2

1. Adult Protective Services
2. Child Protective Services
3. no information, no publication
4. suspected non-accidental trauma
5. Health Insurance Portability and Accountability Act
6. protected health information
7. covered entities
8. cardiopulmonary resuscitation
9. electronic protected health information
10. individually identifiable health information

Exercise 3

Personal answers required; answers will vary.

Review Questions

1. Any four of the following:
   - philosophy and standards of the organization
   - leadership style of supervisors
   - how meaningful or important the work is to the person
   - how challenging the work is for the person
   - how the person fits in with coworkers
   - personal characteristics of worker: abilities, interests, aptitudes, values, and expectations

2. Answers will vary. *Example*: A patient is admitted with complications of alcoholism. The health unit coordinator's religion prohibits drinking.

3. Any six of the following:
   - dependability
   - accountability
   - consideration
   - cheerfulness
   - empathy
   - trustworthiness
   - respectfulness
   - courtesy
   - tactfulness
   - conscientiousness
   - honesty
   - cooperation
   - attitude

4. To protect patients' health information. The Privacy Rule mandates that patients must be provided with a copy of privacy practices when treated in a doctor's office or admitted to a health care facility.

5. information about the patient that includes demographic information that may identify the individual and that relates to his past, present, or future physical or mental health condition and related health care services

6. The primary objective of the Security Rule is to protect the confidentiality, integrity, and availability of electronic protected health information (EPHI) when it is stored, maintained, or transmitted.

7. Answers will vary. *Examples*:
   a. It wouldn't be appropriate to discuss this information, especially in the cafeteria.
   b. Walk over to the two members, say "Excuse me," and change the subject. After the wife is out of hearing distance, explain that their discussion could be overheard.
   c. "I appreciate your concern, but I can't discuss her diagnosis or condition with you. I will let the nurse know that you have observed that she hasn't eaten today."
   d. Ask him to hold while you transfer him to the nurse in charge.
   e. Deny knowledge of the patient; if he becomes insistent or rude, ask him to hold while you transfer him to the nurse in charge.
   f. "It would be inappropriate for me to discuss anything that happened at work outside the workplace."
   g. Advise her that you can't discuss any patient with her, and suggest that she could visit or call her friend in the hospital.
8. a. do not discuss patient information
   b. conduct conversations with other health personnel outside of the hearing distance of patients and visitors
   c. do not discuss medical treatment with the patient or relatives
   d. do not discuss general patient information
   e. do not discuss hospital incidents away from the nursing unit
   f. refer all telephone calls from reporters, police personnel, legal agencies, etc., to the nurse manager.
9. a. follow the hospital policy for duplicating portions of the patient's chart
   b. control access to the patient's chart
   c. ask outside agency personnel for picture identification
   d. control transportation of the patient's chart
10. A professional appearance will earn the trust, respect, and confidence of employer, coworkers, patients, and others.
11. a. *quid pro quo*
    b. a hostile working place
12. Advise the person to stop, and explain that you do not like or welcome his behavior.
13. Call security immediately.
14. a. to provide feedback
    b. to make compensation decisions
15. Keep a diary of accomplishments, classes taken, and in-services attended during the evaluation process.
16. a. CPR (cardiopulmonary resuscitation)
    b. fire and safety inservice
    c. infectious disease inservice
    d. HIPAA inservice
17. a. drug testing
    b. finger printing
    c. background checks
    d. immunizations, including TB skin test, hepatitis, and MMR
    Note: Some requirements may vary in facilities
18. 1. b
    2. e
    3. a
    4. f
    5. d
    6. c
19. 1. d
    2. i

3. g
4. c
5. f
6. h
7. a
8. e
20. a. False: Even though a health unit coordinator may be certified but not licensed, he is responsible for his errors.
    b. False: Only authorized personnel should be allowed to read a patient's chart.
    c. False: One should work within his scope of practice.
    d. False: Cell phones are banned for personal use on hospital units.
    e. False: Cell phones are banned for personal use on hospital units.
    f. True: A patient being transported on a stretcher or a member of hospital personnel transporting hospital equipment always has priority for using an elevator.
21. a. confidentiality
    b. nonmaleficence
    c. autonomy
    d. beneficence (one may answer *nonmaleficence*, but the distinction is that *beneficence* is the prevention of harm, whereas *nonmaleficence* indicates that one will not inflict harm)
    e. veracity
22. a. more efficient patient care
    b. greater satisfaction for the patient, the patient's physician, and the health care organization
23. a. Know your job description.
    b. Keep current with the employer's current policies and procedures.
    c. Keep current in your practice.
    d. Do not assume anything.
    e. Do not perform nursing tasks, even as favors.
    f. Be aware of relationships with patients.
24. a. Follow directions carefully.
    b. Be neat, be sure of dates and spelling (if possible, type or use black ink).
    c. Explain gaps in employment reason.
    d. Make reason for leaving last job sound positive.
    e. If you have little work experience, emphasize other strengths. List volunteer jobs.
    f. List the most recent work or educational experience first, not last.
    g. When asked the pay desired, do not identify a specific amount. Often, it is best to write "open" or "negotiable."
    h. If you did not graduate, write "attended" listing institutions.
    i. Be honest.
25. a. Type using a simple font such as Times Roman, size 12.
    b. Use standard 8.5 × 11″ paper in white, ivory, or gray (avoid flashy colors).
       • Keep a 1″ margin on all four sides.
       • Limit resume to one page, if possible.
       • Single-space within sections.
       • Double-space between sections.
       • Bold, underline, or capitalize section headings to make them stand out.
       • Use everyday language; be specific. Give examples.
       • Do a spelling and grammar check.
       • Produce quality photocopies.

26. First impressions are lasting ones, so be sure your appearance and posture demonstrate professionalism. Do not give the interviewer a reason to rule you out because you did not take the time to look your best. A health unit coordinator is responsible for performing at the level of competence of other health unit coordinators who work under similar circumstances This responsibility is one's legal duty as a health care professional and is the *standard of practice.*

27. The standard of care for which the HUC is responsible becomes higher with increased experience and education. The actions of an HUC will be compared with those of a reasonably prudent HUC with the same experience and education under the same circumstances.

28. Answers will vary.

CHAPTER 7

Exercise 1

1. ADT log book
2. ADT sheet
3. CQI

Exercise 2

1. admission, discharge, transfer log book
2. admission, discharge, transfer sheet
3. continuous quality improvement

Exercise 3

Answers will vary.

Review Questions

1. a. management of nursing unit supplies and equipment
   b. management of activities at the nurses' station
   c. management related to the performance of tasks
   d. management of time
   e. management of stress

2. a. Often, it is the health unit coordinator's responsibility to take inventory using the standard supply list and to order supplies. The supply need list also would be used when supplies are ordered.
   b. The health unit coordinator also may have the responsibility to make sure equipment stored on the nursing unit is in working order and is returned to the appropriate storage place.
   c. It is the health unit coordinator's responsibility to keep unit manuals up to date by adding new materials sent to the nursing unit, and to make sure that manuals and textbooks remain on the nursing unit.
   d. It is the responsibility of the health unit coordinator to report and request repair of any maintenance problems regarding the nursing unit (including heating, cooling, plumbing, electrical problems, etc.).
   e. The health unit coordinator enters the order for patients' rental equipment and would report and request repair for any equipment in need of repair.
   f. The health unit coordinator must know where the emergency equipment is kept and must order supplies and replacements as requested.

3. Answers will vary. Examples of acceptable answers follow:
   - A patient has a DNR order.
   - A patient is out on a 2-hour pass.
   - A patient is going to surgery (note time).
   - A patient is in recovery.
   - No visitors for Room 423
   - No phone calls for a patient
   - A patient has an NINP order.

4. The information would be recorded next to the patient's name on the nursing unit census worksheet.

5. Health personnel, doctors, and visitors are constantly asking the health unit coordinator the whereabouts of patients and/or patients' charts. By maintaining the census worksheet, the answer can be found at a glance.

6. a. Listen carefully and attentively to what the person is saying.
   b. Ask pertinent objective questions and gather as many facts as possible.
   c. Respond to the complaint accordingly, saying, "I understand what you are saying," etc.
   d. Refrain from eating or chewing gum.
   e. Avoid answering the telephone if possible; if not, answer the phone and return as soon as possible to the visitor.
   f. Document the complaint and your response after your conversation, and relay the information to the patient's nurse as soon as possible.
   g. If necessary, locate the patient's nurse to speak to the visitor after briefing him of the complaint.

7. a. *Physician's Desk Reference (PDR)*
   b. Hospital Formulary
   c. Policy and Procedure Manual and Disaster Manual
   d. Laboratory Manual and Diagnostic Imaging Manual

8. a. Identify and analyze the problem.
   b. Identify alternative plans for solution.
   c. Choose the best plan.
   d. Put plan for solution in place.
   e. Evaluate plan after in place for a given time.

9. a. Prepare a medical record release form for the patient to sign; after signed, notify the facility or doctor's office of the request, obtain their fax number, provide a fax number for them to use, and fax the release form to them; they then will fax the records or reports to the nursing unit. If paper charts are in use, the signed release form and the faxed documents are placed into the patient's chart.
   b. The procedure is the same when the EMR is in use, except the documents would be scanned into the patient's EMR, and the hard copies of the release and faxed documents would be placed in a basket to be collected by the health records department to be shredded.

10. If tasks are missed or delayed, this could delay the patient's diagnostic tests and/or treatment.

11. a. orders involving a patient in a medical crisis take priority over all other tasks
    b. transcribing stat orders (handwritten orders); placing stat telephone calls
    c. answering the nursing unit telephone (preferably prior to third ring)

12. a. call the code (1)
    b. answer the ringing telephone (2)
    c. check the surgical charts for the necessary reports (3)
    d. process the two discharge orders (4)
    e. order the chest x-ray for today (5)
    f. retrieve objects from the pneumatic tube system (6)

13. a. plan for rush periods
    b. plan a schedule for the routine health unit coordinator tasks
    c. group activities; save time by grouping activities together
    d. complete one task before you begin another
    e. know your job and perform your job
    f. take the breaks assigned to you
    g. avoid unnecessary conversation
    h. delegate tasks to volunteers

14. a. a computerized or written record of the amount of each item that the nursing unit currently needs to last until the next supply order date
    b. a list of patients' names with room and bed numbers located on a nursing unit with blank spaces next to each name (may be printed from a computer menu). This sheet may be used by the health unit coordinator to record patient activities (some hospitals may use a patient information sheet or a patient activity sheet to record patient activity).
    c. the communication process between shifts, in which the nursing personnel going off duty report the nursing unit activities to the personnel coming on duty
    d. a form that is used to credit a patient for items found in the room unused after the patient's discharge, or for items charged to the patient but not used for him
    e. a form that is initiated to charge a discharged patient for any items that were not charged to him or her at the time of use

15. a. Listen to Mrs. Frances with understanding and empathy; tell her that you will ask her husband's nurse to come talk to her. Document what Mrs. Frances said, and advise her husband's nurse of what was said prior to his going in to speak to Mrs. Frances.
    b. Advise the visitor of the rules, and if she persists in taking the child to Mr. Blair's room, ask the patient's nurse to speak to her (there may be extenuating circumstances that you are unaware of).
    c. Go into the room and ask that only two visitors be in the room at one time, or suggest (if possible) that they all go out to the waiting room or to the cafeteria.
    d. Ask the nurse manager if it could be moved to a more convenient place. He may wish to bring it to a health unit coordinator meeting for discussion.
    e. Suggest that you would be glad to help her in any other way, but you are not trained or legally covered by your job description to assist patients in going to the rest room.

16. Any of the following (in detail) would be examples of information that you would communicate during shift report:
    - A patient is out on a pass.
    - There were new admissions and the orders are done.
    - There are pending discharges.
    - A NINP order
    - A patient is scheduled for surgery.
    - A patient is in the recovery room and will be returning to the unit.

17. a. Ask for assistance when necessary.
    b. When returning to the nursing unit from a break, if you see that several charts are lying about, open each chart and check for new orders. Place charts in the chart rack that do not have new orders. Read all of the new orders, notify the patient's nurse of any stats, and provide him with a copy of the orders, fax or send copies to the pharmacy, then proceed to transcribe all other orders, one chart at a time. If the EMR has been implemented, look at the patient census for any HUC tasks that need to be completed.
    c. Always complete a set of orders that you have started transcribing before you take a break.
    d. Follow the ten steps of transcription outlined in Chapter 9 (p. 158) and never sign off on orders until you are sure that you have completed each step.

18. the study of work for the purpose of making the workplace more comfortable and to improve both health and productivity

19. a. acute, which consist of fractures, crushing, or low back strain injuries
    b. cumulative, which occur over time because of repetitive motion activity

20. Any of the following:
    - The computer terminal should be located where it will reduce awkward head and neck postures—Position the terminals so that you must look slightly downward to look at the middle of the screen. The preferred viewing distance is 18 to 24 inches (Fig. 7-6, p. 115).
    - Adjust your chair so that you sit straight yet in a relaxed position, with a backrest supporting the small of your back and your feet flat on the floor.
    - Adjust your chair back to a slightly backward position and extend your legs out slightly so there are no sharp angles that cause pressure to be placed on your hip or knee joints as you work.
    - Your wrists should be straight as you type with forearms level and elbows close to your body. Reduce bending of the wrists by moving the entire arm.
    - Use a computer wrist pad.
    - Eliminate situations that would require constant bending over to complete your tasks.
    - Shift your weight in your chair frequently.
    - Use proper body mechanics when lifting—Do not bend over with legs straight or twist while lifting and avoid trying to lift above shoulder level.
    - Take frequent mini-stretches of your neck (lean your head down in each direction for a 5-second count).
    - Stand, walk, and stretch your back and legs at least every hour. These small breaks in position help avoid neuromuscular strain and alleviate the tension of job stress.
    - Remain drug free, eat a balanced diet, exercise, and get proper rest to be at your best performance level.

21. a. perennial stress: the wear and tear of day-to-day living with the feeling that one is a square peg trying to fit into a round hole. Examples include traffic, difficult relationships, etc.
    b. crisis stress: common, uncontrollable, often unpredictable life experiences that have a profound effect on individuals. Examples include death, divorce, illness, etc.

22. Any five of the following:
    - Effective time management
    - realizing that the nurses, doctors, and other health care workers may be working under a lot of stress, and that their expressions of frustration should not be taken personally—be empathetic and understanding

- saying "no" tactfully when asked to do additional work if you truly don't have the time
- asking for help when you need it
- keeping your sense of humor—humor is a great stress reliever as long as it is timely and appropriate
- taking your scheduled breaks

23. to continuously improve quality at every level of every department of every function of the health care organization

24. Any four of the following:
- The telephone should be within easy reach.
- Frequently used forms should be stored within reaching distance.
- Charts should be located in an area where they can be easily reached.
- The label printer should be in close proximity.
- The document scanner (if EMR used) should be in close proximity.
- The fax machine should be in close proximity.
- The unit reference books and manuals should be kept within reach distance.
- The barrel for documents to be taken to the shredder should be in close proximity.

25. a. assisting doctors, nurses, and ancillary personnel to enter information and orders into the computer system
    b. tracking and maintaining mandatory JCAHO requirement records for nursing unit personnel, including cardiopulmonary resuscitation (CPR), infectious disease control, fire and safety training, Universal (Standard) Precautions, tuberculosis skin test, HIPAA training, etc.
    c. monitoring and maintaining records of certifications and licenses for nursing unit personnel
    d. preparing work schedules for nursing unit personnel
    e. preparing various reports as requested by the nurse manager, and serving on various committees

26. a. electrocardiograms, telemetry strips
    b. handwritten doctors' progress notes
    c. medical records or reports from an outside agency

CHAPTER 8

Exercise 1

1. Hx
2. NKA
3. ID labels
4. H&P
5. MAR
6. NKMA
7. NKDA
8. NKFA

Exercise 2

1. identification labels
2. no known food allergies
3. medication administration record
4. no known allergies
5. no known drug allergies
6. history and physical
7. history
8. no known medication allergies

Review Questions

1. an admission packet
2. a. means of communication
   b. planning patient care
   c. research
   d. educational purposes
   e. legal document
   f. history of patient illnesses, care, treatment, and outcomes
3. a. All paper chart form entries must be made in ink.
   b. The written entries on the paper chart forms must be legible and accurate.
   c. Recorded entries on the paper chart may not be obliterated or erased.
   d. Written entries on the paper chart forms must include the date and time.
   e. Abbreviations may be used according to the health care facility's list of "approved abbreviations."
4. a. All entries into the electronic record/chart must be accurate.
   b. Handwritten progress notes, electrocardiograms, and outside records and reports must be scanned into the electronic record.
   c. Errors made in care or treatment must be documented and cannot be falsified.
   d. All entries into the electronic record must include the date and time (military or traditional) of the entry.
   e. Abbreviations may be used according to the health care facility's list of "approved abbreviations."
5. a. The physicians' order form is the form on which the doctor requests the care and treatment procedures for the patient.
   b. The graphic record is a graphic representation of the patient's vital signs (temperature, pulse, respiration, and blood pressure) for a given number of days.
   c. The physicians' progress record is a form on which the physician records the patient's progress during the period of hospitalization.
   d. The history and physical form is a chart form that usually is dictated by the patient's doctor, hospitalist or resident. The hospital medical transcription department types the dictated report and sends it to the nursing unit to be placed in the patient's chart. It is used to record the medical history and the present symptomatic history of the patient. A review of all body systems or a physical assessment of the patient also is recorded.
   e. Nurses' progress notes is a standard chart form that is used to outline the patient's care and treatment and to record the treatment, progress, and activities of the patient.
   f. The medication administration record (MAR) is a standard chart form that is used to record all medications given by nursing personnel.
6. a. The face sheet or information form contains information about the patient, such as name, address, telephone number, name of employer, admission diagnosis, health care insurance policy information, and next of kin.
   b. The admission/service agreement form is signed by the patient in the admitting department and then is sent to the unit to be placed in the patient's chart. The form provides legal permission to the hospital/doctor to treat the patient and also serves as a financial agreement.

c. The advance directive checklist is a chart form that documents that patients were informed of their choice to declare their health care decisions.

7. a. Supplemental patient chart forms are additional to the standard patient chart forms and are added to patients' charts according to their specific care and treatment.

b. and c. *Examples:* Any of the following:
- clinical pathway form
- anticoagulant record
- diabetic record
- consultation form
- operating room records
- therapy records
- parenteral fluid or infusion record
- frequent vital signs record
- consent forms

8. a. Affix the patient's ID label to the form. Some physicians may have preprinted consent forms for certain procedures or surgeries.

b. Write in black ink the first and last names of the doctor who is to perform the surgery or procedure.

c. All medical terminology should be spelled correctly and all information written legibly.

d. Write in black ink the surgery or procedure to be performed exactly as the physician wrote it on the physician's order sheet, except write out abbreviations.

e. Do not record the date and time. The person who obtains the patient's signature will complete this.

9. a. release of side rails
b. refusal to permit blood transfusion
c. consent form for human immunodeficiency virus
d. consent to receive blood transfusion

10. a. Place all charts in proper sequence (usually according to room number) in the chart rack when they are not in use.

b. Place new chart forms in each patient's chart before the immediate need arises. In many health care facilities, this is referred to as "stuffing the chart." Label each chart form with the patient's ID label before placing it in the chart. New chart forms are placed on top of old chart forms for easy access. The new forms may be folded in half to show the old form has not been completely used.

c. Place diagnostic reports in the correct patient's chart behind the correct divider. Match the patient's name on the report with the patient's name on the front of the chart. (Don't depend on room numbers because patients are often transferred to another room.)

d. Review the patient's charts frequently for new orders (always check each chart for new orders before you returning it to the chart rack).

e. Properly label the patient's chart so that it can be located easily at all times.

f. Check each chart to be sure all forms are labeled with the correct patient's name. Chart forms should be in the proper sequence.

g. Check the chart frequently for patient information forms or face sheets. Usually, five copies are maintained in the chart.

h. Assist physicians or other professionals in locating the patient's chart.

11. a. Monitor the patient's electronic medical record consistently and carry out HUC tasks, as required in a timely manner.

b. Assist nurses, doctors, and ancillary personnel as necessary in entering information and orders into the computer.

c. Report any necessary repairs to nursing unit computers and/or printers to the hospital information systems department.

d. Scan documents such as handwritten progress notes, electrocardiograms, outside medical records, and reports in a timely manner.

e. Place and maintain patient identification labels in a patient label book.

f. Place nursing unit patient face sheets into a notebook to provide to physicians as requested.

12. a. Draw (in black ink) one single line through the error. Record "mistaken entry" with the date, time, your first initial, last name, and status in a blank area near (directly above or next to) the error. Chart forms that are affixed with the wrong or incorrect ID label may be shredded if no notations have been made on them. If the chart form has notations on it, the chart form cannot be shredded. Draw an X with a black ink pen through the incorrect label and write "mistaken entry" with the date, time, your first initial, last name, and status above the incorrect label. Affix the correct patient ID label on the form next to the incorrect label (do not place correct label over incorrect label). It is also permissible to hand print the patient information in black ink next to the incorrect label through which you have drawn an X.

13. 1530

14. 11:45 P.M.

15. a. placing extra chart forms in patients' charts on a nursing unit so they will be available when needed

b. portions of the patient's current chart that are removed when the chart becomes so full that it is unmanageable

c. preprinted labels that contain individual patient information to identify patient records

d. a method of alerting staff when two or more patients with the same or similarly spelled last names are located on a nursing unit

e. labels affixed to the front cover of a patient's chart that indicate a patient's allergies

f. the patient's record from previous admissions stored in the health records department that may be retrieved for review when a patient is admitted to the emergency room, nursing unit, or outpatient department (also may be requested by the patient's doctor)

g. a chart rack located on the wall outside a patient's room, which stores the patient's chart and when unlocked forms a shelf to write upon

CHAPTER 9

Review Questions

1. Symbols are placed on the doctors' order sheet to indicate completion of the task.

2. Answers will vary. *Example*: 0/00/00 0925 Mary Smith/ CHUC

3. a. Read the complete set of doctors' orders.
   b. Send or fax the pharmacy copy of the doctors' order sheet to the pharmacy department.
   c. Complete stat orders.
   d. Place telephone calls as necessary to complete doctors' orders.
   e. Select the patient's name from the census on the computer screen, or collect all necessary forms.
   f. Order diagnostic tests, treatments, and supplies.
   g. Kardex all doctors' orders except medication orders.
   h. Write medication orders on MAR.
   i. Recheck your performance of each step for accuracy and thoroughness.
   j. Sign off the completed set of doctors' orders.

4. It is a legal document. *Note*: The color of ink used would be in accordance with hospital policy.

5. after the step of transcription is completed to document completion of that step

6. a. the absence of symbols
   b. absence of sign-off

7. to communicate new orders to the nursing staff and to update the patient's profile

8. New doctors' orders may involve changing or discontinuing an existing order. Information not subject to change, such as the patient's name, usually is recorded in black ink, and allergies are always recorded in red ink.

9. a. Ordering is the process of inputting the doctors' orders into the computer, or of copying the doctors' order onto a requisition. Whichever method is used, the purpose of ordering is to forward the doctors' orders to the various hospital departments that will execute the order.
   b. Kardexing is the process of recording all new doctors' orders onto the patient's Kardex form.
   c. A requisition is a form used to order diagnostic procedures, treatments, or supplies from hospital departments other than nursing when the computer is down (also called a *downtime requisition*).
   d. Flagging is a method used by the doctor to notify the nursing staff that she or he has written a new set of orders.

10. a. the line directly below the doctors' signature
    b. so there is not a space left and another order cannot be added after sign-off

11. Accuracy in transcribing doctors' orders is essential to avoid errors that may cause harm to a patient.

12. a. ord (or computer order number)
    b. M
    c. K
    d. (*Example*) called Mary 1035
       PCS or PC Faxed 1035 (with time and your initials recorded)
       (*Example*) notified Nancy 1050

13. Ordering is the sixth step of transcription—unless the order is written to be done stat.

14. a. activity
    b. diet
    c. vital sign frequency
    d. treatment
    e. diagnostic studies

15. a. standing: in effect and given routinely until discontinued or changed by the doctor
    b. standing prn: in effect and given as needed by the patient until automatically discontinued or changed by the doctor

c. one-time or short series: in effect for one time or a short period, automatically discontinued when the order has been completed
    d. stat: given immediately, then automatically discontinued

16. a. short-series order
    b. standing prn
    c. one time—stat
    d. standing
    e. standing
    f. short-series order

17. The doctor will write *stat*—"now" usually is considered equivalent to *stat*.

18. Using handwritten requisitions will assist in learning what tests and procedures are performed in each department of the hospital, so when the computer is used it will be easier to know which department to choose from the menu during the ordering process.

19. a. Read and understand each word of doctors' orders. If in doubt, check with a patient's nurse or the doctor. Use symbols and write the appropriate symbol after you have completed each step of transcription. When new orders are recorded at the top of the doctors' order sheet, check the previous order sheet to see if these orders are continued from the previous page. If the set of orders finish near the bottom of the doctors' order sheet, cross through the remaining space with diagonal lines. Record the sign-off information on the line directly below the doctor's signature to avoid leaving space in which future orders could be written and missed. Check for new orders before returning a chart from the counter or elsewhere to the chart rack.
    b. When in doubt about the correct interpretation of doctors' orders, always check with the patient's nurse or the doctor.
    c. Compare the patient's name and the hospital number on the patient's ID label and the number you have placed on the order requisition form and/or selected on the computer screen with the same information on the patient's chart cover. Never select computer labels by the patient's room number only.
    d. Compare the patient's name and the doctor's name on the Kardex form with the same information on the label on the patient's chart cover. Do not use the information on the doctors' order sheet. It may have the wrong information on it. Never select by using room number alone. If the patient has been transferred, the room number printed on the patient ID label on the chart forms may no longer be correct.
    e. When an order cannot be read because of the doctor's handwriting, refer to the progress record form on the patient's chart. Orders often are recorded on this form also, and reading this information may assist you in interpreting the orders on the physicians' order form. If the order remains unclear, ask the doctor who wrote it for clarification. Don't waste time asking others. They may be guessing also. If a doctor has a reputation for poor handwriting, ask him or her to wait while you read the orders so you can clarify orders that you cannot read.

CHAPTER 10

Exercise 1

1. CBR
2. c̄
3. A&O
4. qid
5. °
6. BP
7. q
8. amb
9. ABR
10. ↑
11. BRP
12. RR
13. ad lib
14. q other day
15. bid
16. q day
17. tid
18. q hr
19. temp
20. as tol
21. rt or Ⓡ
22. lt or Ⓛ
23. D/C or DC
24. VS
25. I&O
26. OOB
27. min
28. wt
29. BR
30. R
31. ax
32. TPR
33. P
34. h, hr, hrs
35. prn
36. NVS or neuro ✓s
37. ↓
38. HOB
39. BSC
40. q4h or q4°
41. CMS
42. SOB
43. CVP
44. Rout
45. CMT

Exercise 2

1. left
2. right
3. discontinue or discharge
4. vital signs
5. blood pressure
6. three times a day
7. complete bed rest
8. with
9. temperature, pulse, and respiration
10. bed rest
11. minute
12. bathroom privileges
13. as desired
14. increase, above, or elevate
15. out of bed
16. alert and oriented
17. weight
18. ambulate
19. every other day
20. every day
21. two times a day
22. four times a day
23. every hour
24. absolute bed rest
25. temperature
26. as tolerated
27. intake and output
28. every
29. pulse
30. axillary or axilla
31. rectal
32. as necessary
33. respiratory rate
34. every 4 hours
35. hour, hours
36. neurologic vital signs or neurologic checks
37. decrease, below, or lower
38. routine
39. shortness of breath
40. head of bed
41. bwedside commode
42. circulation, motion, and sensation
43. central venous pressure
44. routine
45. cardiac monitor technician

Review Questions

1. a. activity
   b. positioning
   c. observation
   d. observation
   e. observation
   f. observation
   g. activity
   h. positioning
   i. activity
   j. activity
   k. observation
   l. positioning
   m. activity
   n. observation
2. a. complete bed rest
   b. bed rest with bathroom privileges when alert and oriented
   c. weight every other day
   d. vital signs four times a day
   e. temperature, pulse, and respiration and blood pressure three times a day
   f. elevate head of bed 20 degrees
   g. check dressing for drainage every 2 hours
   h. temperature rectal or axillary only
   i. neurologic vital signs every 4 hours
   j. intake and output every shift
   k. out of bed as desired
   l. up as tolerated

m. temperature, pulse, respiration, and blood pressure every 4 hours

n. ambulate today

o. discontinue vital signs

p. elevate head of bed 30 degrees

q. central venous pressure every hour

r. central venous pressure every 4 hours

s. check circulation, motion, and sensation in toes of left foot

t. Accu-check before meals and at bedtime

u. call me if patient complains of shortness of breath

3. Define the following terms.

a. the patient may sit and dangle his feet over the edge of the bed

b. elevated body temperature (fever)

c. without fever

d. vomit

4. a. temperature   c. respiration

b. pulse   d. blood pressure

5. The nurse would record the patient's blood pressure and pulse rate while the patient is supine (lying) and again while erect (sitting and/or standing).

6. Oxygen saturation (pulse oximetry)

7. a. oral   c. aural (ear)

b. rectal   d. axillary

8. Intake Output

oral liquids   a. urine

intravenous fluids   b. emesis

c. wound drainage (suction)

d. liquid stool

9. telemetry

10. a. diabetics

b. patients receiving nutritional support (total parenteral nutrition)

Note: Total parenteral nutrition (TPN) is discussed in Chapter 13 (pp. 234-235).

CHAPTER 11

Exercise 1

1. SSE
2. KO
3. MR
4. sol'n
5. nec
6. cm
7. TWE
8. NG
9. NS
10. D/LR
11. hs
12. DW
13. @
14. ORE
15. irrig
16. IV
17. cath
18. LR
19. st
20. SCD
21. p
22. abd
23. TCDB
24. min
25. gtts
26. Δ
27. ASAP
28. /
29. H_2O_2
30. ac
31. con't
32. CBI
33. TKO
34. mL
35. IVF
36. ETS
37. PICC
38. VAD
39. CVC
40. D_5W
41. $D_{10}W$
42. B/L
43. HL or hep-lock

Exercise 2

1. 1000 milliliters lactated Ringer's at 125 milliliters per hour, then discontinue
2. Soap suds enema hour of sleep (bedtime), may repeat times one
3. Give oil-retention enema; follow $\bar{c}$ tap water enema if necessary.
4. Irrigate catheter three times a day $\bar{c}$ normal saline solution.
5. 1000 milliliters 5% dextrose in water 0.9 normal saline AT to keep open
6. Insert nasogastric tube.
7. Turn, cough, and deep breathe every 2 hours.
8. Change intravenous tubing as soon as possible.
9. Please obtain elevated toilet seat for patient.
10. Start intravenous fluids of 10% dextrose in water at 120 milliliters per hour.
11. Insert heparin lock.
12. Shave bilateral inguinal groin area.
13. Apply sequential compression device.

Review Questions

1. *Note:* Items may vary depending on type of nursing unit.

Any five of the following:

- Fleets enema
- rectal tube
- irrigation trays
- urinary catheter trays
- IV solutions
- IV catheters and needles
- IV tubing
- suction catheters and tubing
- sterile gloves
- exam gloves
- masks
- syringes and needles
- disposable suture removal kits
- dressings
- abdominal pads
- Telfa pads
- gauze pads in various sizes

- Kling
- Vaseline gauze
- tape (various types)
- alcohol pads
- glycerin swabs
- irrigation solutions, etc.

2. Any five of the following:
   - alternating pressure pad
   - egg-crate mattress
   - Ted hose
   - pneumatic hose
   - colostomy kit
   - stomal bags
   - elastic abdominal binder
   - footboard
   - foot cradle
   - feeding pump and tubing
   - IV infusion pump
   - hypothermia machine
   - K-pad
   - restraints
   - adult disposable diapers
   - sitz bath, disposable
   - sterile trays, including:
     tracheostomy tray
     bone marrow tray
     paracentesis tray
     lumbar puncture (spinal tap) tray
     thoracentesis tray
     central line tray, etc.

Note: Some sterile trays may be found on c-locker or the floor supply closet.

3. Any three of the following:
   - Harris flush
   - oil retention
   - soap suds enema
   - tap water enema
   - Fleets
   - normal saline

4. a. indwelling (retention catheter)—stays in place to drain urine from bladder on a continuous basis
   b. intermittent (straight) catheter—a single-use catheter that is removed after bladder is drained

5. a. amount of solution
   b. name of solution
   c. rate solution is to run

6. a. hemovac
   b. Jackson-Pratt (JP)

7. a. peripherally
   b. central line

8. Any three of the following:
   - D_5LR (dextrose 5% in lactated Ringer's)
   - $D_{10}LR$ (dextrose 10% in lactated Ringer's)
   - 0.45 NS (½ normal saline) (*Note:* Many more answers would be acceptable.)

9. The laboratory would discard the blood, and the patient would need to have his blood redrawn, causing additional discomfort and delaying treatment.

10. Any two of the following:
    - Aquathermia pad
    - hot compresses
    - warm soaks
    - sitz bath

11. Any two of the following:
    - Aquathermia pad
    - alcohol sponge bath
    - ice bag
    - hypothermia mattress/bed

12. a. a vascular access device (also called *intermittent infusion device*) placed on a peripheral intravenous catheter when used intermittently
    b. a disposable suction device (evacuator unit) that is connected to a drain inserted into or close to a surgical wound
    c. a disposable suction device (evacuator unit) that is connected to a drain inserted into or close to a surgical wound
    d. the patient's own blood donated previously for transfusion as needed by the patient; also called *autotransfusion*
    e. blood donated by relatives or friends of the patient to be used for transfusion as needed
    f. insertion of a catheter into a body cavity or organ to inject or remove fluid
    g. a drain that is inserted into or close to a surgical wound and that may lie under a dressing, extend through a dressing, or be connected to a drainage bag or a suction device
    h. A catheter is threaded through to the superior vena cava or the right atrium when used for the administration of intravenous therapy.
    i. a type of commercial blood glucose monitor used to check the glucose level of blood

13. The amount of urine left in the bladder after voiding (emptying their bladder)

14. a. to discontinue a daily charge to the patient
    b. so the item can be cleaned and prepared for another patient's use

15. return the unit of packed cells to the blood bank for proper storage (after confirming this with the nurse)

16. make two trips to pick each unit up separately or ask another person to pick up one unit while you pick up the other

17. The central service department (CSD) distributes the supplies used for nursing procedures.

18. a. true
    b. false
    c. false
    d. true
    e. true

19. a. Have the IV team insert a PICC.
    b. Cont IVF alt 1000 mL of LR c̄ 1000 mL D_5W @ 125 mL/hr via CVC.
    c. Insert NG tube and connect to low gastric suction.

CHAPTER 12

Exercise 1

1. Na or Na1
2. MN
3. NPO
4. reg
5. cl

6. cal
7. ADA
8. liq
9. chol
10. DAT
11. FF
12. CHO
13. NSA
14. FS
15. PEG
16. NAS
17. RD
18. K or K+
19. BMI
20. AHA

Exercise 2

1. sodium
2. nothing by mouth
3. regular
4. midnight
5. liquid
6. calorie
7. no salt added
8. American Diabetic Association
9. diet as tolerated
10. clear
11. cholesterol
12. carbohydrate
13. force fluids
14. full strength
15. percutaneous endoscopic gastrostomy
16. no added salt
17. registered dietitian
18. potassium
19. body mass index
20. American Heart Association

Review Questions

1. a. NPO p MN
   b. cl liq breakfast, then NPO
   c. 1000-cal ADA diet
   d. low-chol diet
   e. DAT
   f. reg diet
   g. low-Na diet
   h. NSA
2. a. a regular diet with modifications or restrictions
   b. a diet that consists of all foods, designed to provide good nutrition
   c. administration of liquids into the stomach, duodenum, or jejunum, through a tube
   d. patient cannot have anything to eat or drink, not even water
3. a. continuous
   b. bolus
   c. cyclic
4. a. standard
   b. therapeutic
   c. therapeutic
   d. standard
   e. therapeutic
   f. standard
   g. therapeutic
   h. therapeutic
5. a. regular
   b. soft
   c. full liquid
   d. clear liquid

(*Note*: Variations such as mechanical soft or pureed also may be ordered for DAT.)

6. The personnel working in the dietary department do not know what the patient could tolerate.
7. a. The patient is scheduled for surgery.
   b. The patient is scheduled for a diagnostic procedure, test, or examination.
8. Any three of the following:
   * Isocal HN
   * Deliver 2.0
   * Ultracal HN Plus
   * Jevity
   * Pulmocare
   * Boost High Nitrogen
   * Boost Plus Respalor
   * Megnacal

(*Note*: Many more are on the market.)

9. a. enteral feeding pump
   b. formula
   c. chest x-ray
10. a. Kosher
    b. vegetarian

(*Note:* Many other diets may be requested by patients.)

11. No: 2.5 g Na would be a modification to the soft diet and is not a diet change.
12. No: Limiting fluids to 1200 mL/day is a modification to the regular diet and is not a diet change.
13. Yes: All dietary orders need to be sent to the dietary department.
14. The patient's food is prepared by the dietary department, and if a patient eats a food that he is truly allergic to, it could cause discomfort or in some cases anaphylactic shock.

CHAPTER 13

Exercise 1

1. L
2. ASA
3. stat
4. cap
5. tab
6. MOM
7. ADE
8. mg
9. KCL
10. G, gm, or g
11. mL or ml
12. mEq
13. pc

14. ung
15. W/A
16. N/V
17. gr
18. IM
19. subling or SL
20. tinct or tr
21. PO
22. oz
23. amp
24. dr or ʒ
25. supp
26. NTG
27. SC, sq, or sub-q
28. μg or mcg
29. noc
30. syr
31. IVPB
32. ac
33. PCN
34. pr
35. TPN
36. PCA
37. CDSS
38. IVP
39. LOC
40. PRN
41. OTC
42. IV
43. BCOC

Exercise 2

1. potassium chloride
2. adverse drug event
3. ampule
4. syrup
5. dram
6. night
7. microgram
8. ounce
9. subcutaneous
10. immediately
11. ante cibum (before meals)
12. milliequivalent
13. post cibum (after meals)
14. unguent (ointment)
15. milliliter
16. per os (by mouth)
17. tincture
18. intramuscular
19. grain
20. milligram
21. suppository
22. gram
23. clinical decision support system
24. nausea and vomiting
25. while awake
26. nitroglycerin
27. acetylsalicylic acid (aspirin)
28. capsule
29. tablet
30. milk of magnesia

31. liter
32. sublingual (under tongue)
33. intravenous piggyback
34. penicillin
35. total parenteral nutrition
36. patient-controlled analgesia
37. per rectum
38. *pro re nata* (as needed)
39. laxative of choice
40. intravenous push
41. over the counter
42. intravenous
43. bowel care of choice

Exercise 3

1. intramuscular, as needed
2. gram, intravenous piggyback
3. milligram, by mouth
4. drops
5. milligram, sublingual, as needed
6. milk of magnesia, milliliters, as needed
7. total parenteral nutrition, milliliters
8. aspirin, milligrams, by mouth, per rectum
9. total parenteral nutrition, milliliters per hour, milliliters per hour
10. before meals. before bedtime

Exercise 4

Answers found by using the *Physicians' Desk Reference.*

Exercise 5

1. gr ii
2. 5 mL
3. 4 dr
4. 0.5 g
5. gr iss
6. 500 mg
7. gr xv
8. 1L
9. 1000 g
10. gr 1/6
11. gr 1/150

Exercise 6

1. a. name of the drug
   b. dosage
   c. routes of administration
   d. frequency of administration
   e. qualifying phrase

2. a.

prochlorperazine supp	5 mg	pr	stat	
1	2	3	4	
b. hydroxyzine	25 mg	IM	q6h prn	anxiety
1	2	3	4	5
c. levofloxacin	500 mg	IV	q day	
1	2	3	4	
d. zolpidem	5 mg	po	hs prn	
1	2	3	4	
e.			after each	
loperamide hydrochloride	2 mg	po	unformed stool	
1	2	3	4	

f. oxycodone	15 mg tab	po	q4h prn	severe pain	
1	2	3	4		5
g. Lente insulin	25 units	sq	qd		
1	2	3	4		
h amoxicillin	500 mg	po	q8h		
1	2	3	4		
i. warfarin sodium	3 mg	po	q day		
1	2	3	4		
j. benazepril	20 mg	po	q day		
1	2	3	4		

Exercise 7

1. Tylenol 500 mg q4h po for pain
2. ciprofloxacin hydrochloride 400 mg IV q12h
3. doxycycline 200 mg po now, then 100 mg @ hs, then 100 mg bid × 3 days
4. Donnatal elixir 5 mL po 3 tid ac
5. Timoptic ophth 0.25% sol gtts 2 in right eye bid
6. Benadryl 50 mg IM stat
7. Coreg 25 mg 1 tab by po q A.M. and hs
8. Coumadin 5 mg po q day

Exercise 8

1. lower blood sugar
2. thin blood—prevent clots from forming in the blood
3. treat a variety of infections; category includes antibiotic, antifungal, and antiviral drugs
4. decrease acid production (digestive system)
5. used to treat cancer
6. to cause relaxation and reduce restlessness without causing sleep
7. used to induce sleep
8. replace or regulate glandular secretions from glands
9. replace potassium
10. to relieve pain
11. assist in drying secretions (respiratory system)
12. to lower cholesterol
13. correct abnormal cardiac beats
14. used to relieve pain caused when the heart muscle does not get enough oxygen and nutrients to meet the demand
15. used to lower blood pressure
16. cause a quick decrease in circulating fluid volume, causing a decrease in pressure demand on the heart
17. used to treat constipation by stimulating a bowel movement; soften the stool for easier passage, or may be a fiber supplement to increase and maintain normal bowel function
18. to treat nausea and vomiting
19. to treat shock and to lower blood pressure

Review Questions

1. a. 1. milligram 2. by mouth 3. every
   b. 1. aspirin
   c. 1. kilogram 2. intravenous 3. hours
   d. 1. each 2. twice a day
   e. 1. milliliter 2. as needed
   f. 1. nitroglycerin 2. sublingual 3. bedside
   g. 1. intramuscular 2. hour
   h. 1. total parenteral nutrition
   i. 1. patient-controlled analgesia
   j. 1. intravenous push
   k. 1. intravenous piggyback
   l. 1. ampule 2. multivitamin
   m. 1. before meals 2. at bedtime
   n. 1. milliequivalent 2. potassium chloride
   o. 1. laxative of choice
   p. 1. nausea and vomiting
   q. 1. three times a day 2. after meals
   r. 1. syrup
2. Any of the following:
   - U (unit)
   - IU (international unit)
   - Q.D., QD, q.d., qd (every day)
   - Q.O.D., QOD. q.o.d., qod (every other day)
   - trailing 0 (X.0 mg)
   - MS (morphine sulfate)
3. Eliminating handwritten will orders reduce errors of misinterpretation of medication.
4. Orders due to poor handwriting. Orders are integrated with patient information, including patient allergies, laboratory results, and prescription data. Clinical decision support systems (CDSS) provide doctors with prompts that warn against the possibility of drug interaction, allergy, or overdose.
   a. name of drug
   b. dose of drug
   c. route
   d. frequency
   e. qualifying phrase
5. a. stat
   b. standing prn
   c. standing
   d. one time
   e. short-series order
6. a. right drug
   b. right dose
   c. right time
   d. right route
   e. right patient
7. 1. m
   2. n
   3. i
   4. l
   5. g
   6. j
   7. c
   8. h
   9. d
   10. e
   11. b
   12. a
   13. k
   14. f
   15. p
   16. o
8. a. narcotic—analgesics with narcotics
   b. hypnotic
   c. antibiotic
   d. anticoagulant
9. a. *Physicians' Desk Reference (PDR)*
   b. The American Hospital Formulary

(*Note:* Nursing drug handbooks also are used.)

10. 1. i
    2. d
    3. f

4. h

5. c

6. a

7. k

8. e

9. l

10. g

11. o

12. j

13. b

14. n

15. p

16. m

11. Any of the following:
- Allergy skin testing—to determine allergies
- PPD (purified protein derivative)—a screening test for tuberculosis
- Cocci skin test—a diagnostic test for coccidioidomycosis (valley fever)
- Histoplasmin skin test—to aid in diagnosing histoplasmosis, a fungal disease

CHAPTER 14

Exercise 1

1. FBS
2. O&P
3. Hgb
4. ESR
5. K
6. AFB
7. RBC
8. PP
9. CSF
10. Fe
11. C&S
12. T&X-match or T&C
13. CBC
14. PAP
15. GTT
16. PC
17. PT
18. Ua or U/A
19. ALP or alk phos
20. HB$_5$Ag
21. FS
22. HIV
23. Mg or Mg+
24. hCG
25. WNL
26. PTT or APIT
27. T$_3$, T$_4$, T$_7$
28. TSH
29. S&A
30. Ag
31. BMP
32. CMV
33. HSV
34. T&S
35. Ab
36. Cx
37. RSV
38. CMP
39. Lytes
40. Bx
41. POCT or PCT
42. PCV
43. RBS or BS
44. RPR
45. Retics
46. PSA
47. Diff
48. WBC
49. PO$_4$ or phos
50. TIBC
51. Hct
52. LP
53. Na
54. NP
55. H&H
56. CO$_2$
57. ANA
58. HDL
59. BUN
60. Ca
61. CC, creat cl, or cr cl
62. Cl
63. CEA
64. BNP
65. LDL
66. ADH
67. CPK or CK
68. EBV
69. Ab
70. RDW
71. Trig or TG
72. Bili

Exercise 2

1. fasting blood sugar
2. ova and parasites
3. hemoglobin
4. erythrocyte sedimentation rate or sedimentation rate
5. potassium
6. acid-fast bacilli
7. red blood cells
8. postprandial
9. cerebrospinal fluid
10. iron
11. culture and sensitivity
12. type and crossmatch
13. complete blood cell count
14. prostatic acid phosphatase
15. glucose tolerance test
16. packed cells
17. prothrombin time
18. urinalysis
19. alkaline phosphatase
20. hepatitis B surface antigen
21. frozen section
22. human immunodeficiency virus
23. magnesium
24. human chorionic gonadotropin
25. within normal limits
26. partial thromboplastin time or activated partial thromboplastin time

27. thyroid tests
28. thyroid-stimulating hormone
29. sugar and acetone
30. antigen
31. basic metabolic chemistry panel
32. cytomegalovirus
33. herpes simplex virus
34. type and screen
35. antibody
36. culture
37. respiratory syncytial virus
38. comprehensive metabolic chemistry panel
39. electrolytes
40. biopsy
41. point-of-care testing
42. packed cell volume
43. random blood sugar or blood sugar
44. rapid plasma reagin
45. reticulocytes
46. prostatic specific antigen
47. differential
48. white blood cell count
49. phosphorus
50. total iron-binding capacity
51. hematocrit
52. lumbar puncture
53. sodium
54. nasopharynx
55. hemoglobin and hematocrit
56. carbon dioxide
57. antinuclear antibody
58. high-density lipoproteins
59. blood urea nitrogen
60. calcium
61. creatinine clearance
62. chloride
63. carcinoembryonic antigen
64. brain natriuretic protein
65. low-density lipoproteins
66. antidiuretic hormone
67. creatine phosphokinase or creatine kinase
68. Epstein-Barr virus
69. Antibody
70. red cell distribution width
71. triglyceride
72. bilirubin

Review Questions

1. a. diagnostic
   b. evaluation of treatment prescribed
2. a. Microbiology studies specimens to determine disease-causing organisms.
   b. Chemistry performs tests related to chemical reactions occurring in living organisms.
   c. Hematology performs tests related to the physical properties of blood.
3. a. voided
   b. clean catch (or midstream)
   c. catheterization
4. a. blood
   b. urine
   c. sputum
   d. stool
   e. spinal fluid

Note: Other specimens include eye/ear drainage, wound drainage, bone marrow, pleural fluid, biopsies, etc.

5. Notify the laboratory by phone or verbally notify the appropriate nursing personnel on the unit. When calling the laboratory, supply the name of the patient, nursing unit, room number, and the test ordered. Enter the order into the computer immediately if the laboratory is going to draw the specimen. The order is entered when the specimen is collected if drawn by nursing personnel on the unit.
6. Ask the nurse to notify you of the time the patient has finished eating and order the blood to be drawn. *Timed:* 2 hours after the patient finished eating.
7. A stat laboratory order must be done immediately. A routine laboratory order can be performed at the next scheduled laboratory draw or when the nursing personnel can draw the blood. The routine laboratory order that requires a blood draw may be collected with a stat but is performed on a routine basis.
8. Any five of the following:
   - lumbar puncture; also called *spinal tap*
   - sternal puncture; also called *bone marrow biopsy*
   - abdominal paracentesis
   - thoracentesis
   - amniocentesis
   - biopsy of a part of the body
9. Type and crossmatch
10. Check to see that the specimen is labeled correctly. Call transport or take the specimen yourself as soon as possible. Do not send specimens that were collected by an invasive procedure (cerebrospinal fluid, cavity fluid, biopsies, etc.) through the tube system.
11. a. sodium (Na)
    b. potassium (K)
    c. chlorides (Cl)
    d. carbon dioxide (CO_2)
12. a. CPK or CK
    b. Troponin
    c. BNP
13. List any six from Appendix F that have "Chemistry" listed in the "Laboratory Division" column.
14. List any six from Appendix F that have "Hematology" listed in the "Laboratory Division" column.
15. List any six from Appendix F that have "Bacteriology, Virology, Mycology, or Parisitology" listed in the "Laboratory Division" column.
16. Fasting means that the patient may have water or other non-nutritional drinks. NPO means no food or liquid by mouth. In both cases, the patient's breakfast tray is held until the test is completed.
17. a. a tissue removed from a living body for examination
    b. a method of obtaining a urine specimen
    c. no solid food or nutritional fluids
    d. a procedure to remove cerebrospinal fluid from the spinal cord
    e. a method of obtaining a urine specimen (same as clean catch)
    f. blood that is undetectable to the eye
    g. after eating

h. a mucous secretion from the lungs

i. a procedure to remove bone marrow from the sternum

j. the physical, chemical, and microscopic examination of urine

k. a specimen obtained by urinating

l. the visual examination of urine using a special commercially treated stick

18. a. chemistry
    b. microbiology
    c. chemistry
    d. hematology
    e. chemistry
    f. hematology
    g. blood bank
    h. hematology
    i. serology
    j. chemistry
    k. serology
    l. microbiology
    m. hematology
    n. chemistry
    o. chemistry
    p. hematology
    q. hematology
    r. chemistry
    s. hematology
    t. chemistry
    u. blood bank
    v. blood bank
    w. chemistry
    x. microbiology
    y. chemistry
    z. chemistry

19. Any three of the following:
    - amikacin
    - cyclosporine
    - digoxin
    - Dilantin
    - gentamicin
    - kanamycin
    - tobramycin
    - vancomycin

20. Read the laboratory values you have recorded back to the person in the laboratory

21. a. CBC and lytes q A.M.
    b. H&H stat
    c. T&X-match 6 U pc—hold for surgery in A.M.
    d. sputum spec for C&S for AFB
    e. LP for CSF tube #1: prot & glu; Tube #2 Cx for CMV& fungus; Tube #3 AFB stain
    f. CMP in A.M.

CHAPTER 15

Exercise 1

1. IVP (also called IVU)
2. RLQ
3. KUB
4. BE
5. PA
6. UGI
7. lat
8. LS
9. LUQ
10. AP
11. GI
12. RUQ
13. CT
14. LLQ
15. GB
16. MRI
17. SBFT
18. CXR
19. DSA
20. PCXR
21. PTC or PTHC
22. Fx
23. H/O
24. F/U
25. CI
26. IVU (also called IVP)
27. US
28. PACS
29. PET
30. L&S
31. RIS
32. abd
33. mets
34. SNAT

Exercise 2

1. barium enema
2. lumbosacral
3. kidneys, ureters, and bladder
4. ultrasound
5. right lower quadrant, left upper quadrant
6. intravenous urogram and upper gastrointestinal
7. computed tomography
8. gastrointestinal
9. posteroanterior, lateral (X-ray)
10. magnetic resonance imaging
11. portable chest X-ray
12. upper gastrointestinal (X-ray), small bowel follow-through
13. liver and spleen
14. positron emission tomography
15. computed tomography, digital subtraction angiogram
16. suspected non-accidental trauma

Review Questions

1. a. radiology
   b. nuclear medicine
   c. radiology
   d. computed tomography
   e. nuclear medicine
   f. ultrasound
   g. radiology
   h. radiology
   i. radiology
   j. radiology
   k. nuclear medicine
   l. radiology
   m. radiology
   n. magnetic resonance imaging

o. special procedures
p. radiology
q. ultrasound
r. special procedures
s. radiology
t. radology
u. radiology
v. radiology
w. special procedures
x. nuclear medicine
y. magnetic resonance imaging
z. special procedures

2. Benefits for the doctor include faster results, ability to compare an image with a previous image (if applicable), ability to share with other physicians, and reduced risk of lost film. Benefits for the patient include reduced delay in treatment, reduced risk of lost film, and protection of confidentiality. There is also a benefit for the environment in that X-ray photographic darkroom chemicals and toxins are eliminated from the process.

3. a. anteroposterior (AP)
   b. posteroanterior (PA)
   c. lateral (lat)
   d. oblique
   e. decubitus

4. These answers may vary between health care facilities—usually these answers apply:
   a. preparation <u>no</u> consent <u>no</u>
   b. preparation <u>yes</u> consent <u>no</u>
   c. preparation <u>no</u> consent <u>yes</u>
   d. preparation <u>no</u> consent <u>no</u>
   e. preparation <u>no</u> consent <u>no</u>
   f. preparation <u>no</u> consent <u>no</u>
   g. preparation <u>no</u> consent <u>no</u>
   h. preparation <u>no</u> consent <u>yes</u>
   i. preparation <u>no</u> consent <u>no</u>
   j. preparation <u>yes</u> consent <u>no</u>
   k. preparation <u>no</u> consent <u>yes</u>
   l. preparation <u>no</u> consent <u>yes</u>

5. routine preparations

6. on-call medications

7. a. pelvic ultrasound
   b. IVU
   c. BE
   d. UGI

8. a. MRI of LS spine CI; fx
   b. PA & Lat CXR CI: pneumonia
   c. UGI, IVU, & BE CI: abd mass
   d. CT of rt shoulder CI: rotator cuff inj
   e. pelvic US CI: age of fetus
   f. CT of head c̄ DSA

9. a. reason for procedure (clinical indication)
   b. transportation required
   c. if patient is receiving intravenous fluids
   d. if patient is receiving oxygen
   e. if patient needs isolation precautions
   f. if patient has a seizure disorder
   g. if patient does not speak English
   h. if patient is diabetic
   i. if patient is sight or hearing impaired
   j. if patient is pregnant or a pregnancy test results are pending

10. Contrast medium is used to differentiate between soft tissue structures.

11. a. water
    b. air
    c. barium
    d. iodinated contrast media
    e. gas

12. magnetic resonance imaging

13. The health unit coordinator when using paper charts would transcribe the handwritten doctors' orders, coordinate the preparation (write on MAR), or put a prep card in Kardex. When the electronic record is implemented, the health unit coordinator would coordinate the scheduling of procedures and the preparations.

14. If the patient is not properly cleaned out or prepared for the procedure, the diagnostic imaging department would have to cancel the procedure. This would cause a delay in the patient's care and treatment.

CHAPTER 16

Exercise 1

1. EEG
2. EKG or ECG
3. EMG
4. RA
5. LOC
6. ABG
7. CBG
8. ERCP
9. EGD
10. EPS
11. NCS
12. OSA
13. BAER
14. ENG
15. SEP
16. VEP
17. DVT
18. TEE
19. PFT
20. IPG
21. ICG

Exercise 2

1. arterial blood gases
2. electrocardiography
3. electroencephalography
4. leave on chart
5. electromyography
6. room air
7. esophagogastroduodenoscopy
8. endoscopic retrograde cholangiopancreatography
9. electrophysiologic study
10. capillary blood gases
11. nerve conduction studies
12. obstructive sleep apnea
13. brainstem auditory evoked response
14. electronystagmography
15. somatosensory evoked potential
16. visual evoked potential
17. deep vein thrombosis

18. transesophageal echocardiography
19. pulmonary function test
20. impedance plethysmography
21. impedance cardiography

Review Questions

1. a. to visualize the heart chambers, arteries, and great vessels to locate the region of coronary occlusion (blockages) and to determine the effects of valvular heart disease. It is used most often to evaluate chest pain or because of abnormalities detected in a cardiac stress test.
    b. to measure the electrical impulses that the heart generates during the cardiac cycle
    c. to monitor patients on ventilators and critically ill non-ventilator patients, and to establish preoperative baseline parameters and regulate electrolyte therapy. Measurement of ABG provides valuable information in assessing and managing a patient's respiratory (ventilation) and metabolic (renal) acid/base and electrolyte homeostasis. It is also used to assess adequacy of oxygenation.
    d. to determine air volumes and air flow rates. Air flow rates provide information about airway obstruction.
    e. to detect lesions in the brainstem that involve the auditory pathway without affecting hearing. This test is commonly used in low-birthweight newborns to screen for hearing disorders; may also be effective in the early detection of posterior fossa brain tumors.
    f. to monitor arterial O_2 saturation levels (SaO_2) in patients at risk for hypoxemia; typically used to monitor oxygenation status during the perioperative period (before, during, and after surgery) and in patients receiving heavy sedation or mechanical ventilation.
2. a. Any two of the following:
    - electrocardiography(EKG or ECG)
    - impedance cardiography (IPG)
    - Holter monitor
    - cardiac stress test (exercise electrocardiogram or treadmill stress test)
    - thallium or sestamibi stress test
    - echocardiography
    - transesophageal echocardiography (TEE)
    - plethysmography
    - Vascular Studies
      Vascular ultrasound studies
      Vascular duplex scans
    b. Any two of the following:
    - electrophysiologic studies (EPS)
    - cardiac catheterization (coronary angiography, angiocardiography, ventriculography)
    - Swan-Ganz catheter insertion
4. cardiovascular
5. Any six of the following:

arthroscopy	joints
bronchoscopy	larynx, trachea, bronchi, alveoli
colonoscopy	rectum, colon
colposcopy	vagina, cervix
cystoscopy	urethra, bladder, ureters, (male) prostate
enteroscopy	upper colon, small intestines
endourology	bladder and urethra
endoscopic retrograde cholangiopancreatography	pancreatic and biliary ducts
esophagogastroduodenoscopy	esophagus, stomach, duodenum
fetoscopy	fetus
gastroscopy	stomach
hysteroscopy	uterus
laparoscopy	abdominal cavity
mediastinoscopy	mediastinal lymph nodes
sigmoidoscopy	sigmoid colon
sinus endoscopy	sinus cavities
thoracoscopy	pleura, lung

6. The presence of stool would obscure visualization of the intestinal walls. Barium studies would have to be performed after GI endoscopies, because barium also would obscure visualization of the intestinal walls. Gastrointestinal endoscopic studies could not be done if the patient was not properly prepared.
7. anticoagulants
8. Any four of the following:
   - oximetry (pulse oximetry, ear oximetry, oxygen saturation)
   - arterial blood gases
   - capillary blood gases
   - pulmonary function tests
   - spirometry
9. Any two of the following:
   - gastric analysis
   - esophageal manometry (esophageal function study, esophageal motility study)
   - secretin test
10. 1. c
    2. d
    3. d
    4. b
    5. c
    6. b
    7. a
    8. a
    9. a
    10. a
    11. e
    12. a
    13. b
    14. a
    15. a
    16. b
    17. c
    18. d
11. Any two of the following:
    - plethysmography vascular studies (venous, arterial impedance [IPG])
    - vascular ultrasound studies (Doppler studies)
    - vascular duplex scans
12. a. to diagnose brain tumors, epilepsy, other brain diseases, or injuries
    b. to confirm brain death or cerebral silence
13. anticonvulsants
14. a. a diagnostic or therapeutic technique that requires entry of a body cavity or interruption of normal body functions

b. a diagnostic or therapeutic technique that does not require the skin to be broken or a cavity or organ of the body to be entered

CHAPTER 17
Exercise 1

1. LUL
2. OT
3. PT
4. L/Min
5. O$_2$
6. IPPB
7. RUL
8. ROM
9. RLL
10. ADL
11. CABG
12. RML
13. USN
14. SVN
15. LLL
16. lbs #
17. NWB
18. WP
19. HP
20. TENS
21. EPC
22. ES
23. CPM
24. IS
25. MDI
26. CPT
27. AA
28. BiW
29. AKA
30. STM
31. LE
32. HD
33. THR, THA
34. ORIF
35. Tx
36. TT
37. ISOM
38. BKA
39. ET
40. HA
41. PEP
42. P & PD
43. SaO or O$_2$ Sats
44. UD
45. >
46. TKR, TKA
47. <
48. CP
49. CPR
50. HBOT
51. TTOT
52. CPAP
53. BUE
54. BLE
55. RUE
56. LUE
57. RLE
58. LLE
59. PTA
60. RT
61. PROM
62. WBAT
63. FWW
64. PD
65. ICD
66. ADS
67. DPI
68. SIDS

Exercise 2

1. oxygen
2. left upper lobe
3. right lower lobe
4. occupational therapy or occupational therapist
5. physical therapy or physical therapist
6. sudden infant death syndrome
7. activities of daily living
8. pounds
9. right upper lobe
10. right middle lobe
11. non–weight bearing
12. range of motion
13. liters per minute
14. small volume nebulizer
15. left lower lobe
16. intermittent positive-pressure breathing
17. ultrasonic nebulizer
18. hot packs
19. whirlpool
20. continuous passive motion
21. electrical stimulation
22. electronic pain control
23. transcutaneous electrical nerve stimulation
24. incentive spirometry
25. chest physiotherapy
26. metered-dose inhaler
27. open reduction, internal fixation
28. tilt table
29. oxygen saturation
30. above the knee amputation
31. unit dose
32. heated aerosol
33. isometric
34. lower extremities
35. soft tissue massage
36. hemodialysis
37. traction
38. percussion and postural drainage
39. greater than
40. total knee replacement/arthroplasty
41. total hip replacement/arthroplasty
42. endotracheal tube
43. peritoneal dialysis
44. less than
45. twice a week
46. positive expiratory pressure
47. cold packs

48. active assisted
49. cardiopulmonary resuscitation
50. hyperbaric oxygen therapy
51. transtracheal oxygen therapy
52. continuous positive airway pressure
53. both upper extremities
54. both lower extremities
55. right upper extremity
56. left upper extremity
57. right lower extremity
58. left lower extremity
59. physical therapist assistant
60. respiratory therapist or respiratory therapist
61. passive range of motion
62. weight bearing as tolerated
63. front wheel walker
64. coronary artery bypass graft
65. dry powder inhaler
66. adult distress syndrome
67. implantable cardioverter-defibrillator
68. peritoneal dialysis

Review Questions

1. angioplasty usually $\bar{c}$ stents
   coronary artery bypass graft
2. a. The cardiopulmonary (respiratory care) department performs treatments that maintain or improve the function of the respiratory system. Diagnostic tests performed by the cardiopulmonary (respiratory care) department are discussed in Chapter 16.
   b. Physical therapy is the division within the hospital that treats patients to improve and restore their functional mobility through methods such as gait training, exercise, water therapy, and heat and ice treatments.
   c. Occupational therapy is the department within the hospital that works toward rehabilitation of patients, in conjunction with other health team members, to return the patient to the greatest possible independence.
3. a. the amount of oxygen
   b. how oxygen is to be administered (delivery device or mode of delivery)
4. a. skin traction
   b. skeletal traction
5. The overhead frame and trapeze is used by the patient to move and support weight during transfer or position change and also may aid in strengthening upper extremities.
6. a. respiratory care
   b. nursing
   c. respiratory care
   d. physical therapy
   e. respiratory care
   f. respiratory care
   g. respiratory care
   h. occupational therapy
   i. nursing
   j. nursing
   k. physical therapy
   l. nursing
   m. physical therapy
   n. physical therapy
   o. respiratory care
   p. physical therapy

7. removal in the blood of wastes usually excreted by the kidneys
8. a. hemodialysis
   b. peritoneal dialysis
9. Hyperbaric oxygen therapy delivers oxygen quickly, systemically, and in high concentrations to injured areas. The increased pressure changes the normal cellular respiration process and causes oxygen to dissolve in the plasma. This stimulates the growth of new blood vessels and a substantial increase in tissue oxygenation that can arrest certain types of infections and enhance wound healing.

CHAPTER 18

Exercise 1

1. wk
2. NINP
3. DME
4. DNR
5. disch
6. Rx
7. appt

Exercise 2

1. appointment
2. durable medical equipment
3. do not resuscitate
4. no information, no publication
5. week
6. take (e.g., treatment, medication) prescription
7. discharge

Review Questions

1. a. a doctors' order requesting that a patient be transferred to another hospital room and/or nursing unit, or to another facility
   b. a doctors' order stating that the patient may leave the hospital
   c. a request by the patient's attending physician for the opinion of a second physician with respect to diagnosis and treatment of the patient
2. a. hospital name
   b. patient's name and age
   c. patient's location (unit and room number)
   d. name of the doctor requesting the consultation
   e. patient's diagnosis
   f. urgency of consultation and any additional information provided in the order
   g. patient's insurance information located on the patient's face sheet
3. The health unit coordinator would place a call to the health information management department of the other hospital to request records and would initiate a consent form for the patient to sign. When signed, this form may be faxed to the health information management department of the other hospital; the requested records then are faxed to the nursing unit. The faxed records are usually placed in the patient's current chart if paper charts are used or are scanned into the patient's electronic medical record, if the electronic medical record is used.
4. The health unit coordinator may be responsible for photocopying the records, or it may be hospital policy that

they must be sent to health information management to be photocopied. If electronic medical records are implemented, the health unit coordinator will print the records from the computer and may fax requested patient records to the facility or doctor's office. The patient would have to sign a consent for the records to be photocopied, printed, or faxed to another facility or to a doctor's office.

5. The health unit coordinator, after scanning patient medical records or documents, would stamp the originals with a "scanned" stamp with the date and time and place them in a bin or box to be picked up by HIMS.

6. a. a different type of room accommodation (e.g., a private room) is desired
   b. more intense nursing care (regular unit to ICU) or less intense nursing care (ICU to regular unit) is called for
   c. the patient's condition requires that he or she be placed in an isolation room

7. a. arrange with the pharmacy for medications the patient is taking
   b. note on the census when the patient leaves and returns
   c. cancel meals for the length of the absence
   d. cancel any hospital treatments for the length of the absence
   e. arrange for any special equipment that the patient may need
   f. provide the nurse with a temporary absence release to have the patient sign

8. Any two of the following:
   • access and prioritize the patient's needs
   • identify and coordinate available resources
   • arrange for home care
   • arrange admission to a long-term care facility
   • arrange for hospice care

9. a. financial assistance for patients
   b. transportation home
   c. arrangement of meals for families staying at hospital or for patients for home after discharge
   d. support for abuse victims (call protective services if necessary)
   e. assistance in planning custodial care
   f. arrangement of home-bound teacher or in-hospital teacher
   g. evaluation of home care providers
   h. arrangement of living assistance for families of patients when necessary

10. No: DNR must be a written doctor's order to be legal.

11. Many pediatric hospitals and/or units have a patient room with a bed for a parent to stay 24 hours a day with his child. The parent after training will assume full care of the child. The child then may be discharged to the parent's care.

12. The doctor may include other orders in a discharge order, such as disch p̄ chest X-ray, disch p̄ CPR training for mother, or disch p̄ Dr. Conrad sees pt, disch c̄ Rx, etc. These orders may be missed if the health unit coordinator does not read the entire discharge order.

CHAPTER 19

Exercise 1

1. MSSU
2. post-op
3. OBS
4. Dx
5. pre-op
6. OPS
7. SSU
8. BIBA
9. DOA
10. IVDU

Exercise 2

1. outpatient surgery
2. before surgery
3. diagnosis
4. observation
5. after surgery
6. medical short stay unit
7. short stay unit
8. brought in by ambulance
9. dead on arrival
10. intravenous drug user

Review Questions

1. 1. c
   2. d
   3. a
   4. b
   5. e

2. a. the number assigned to the patient on or prior to admission; used for records identification and used for all subsequent admissions to that hospital
   b. plastic band with a patient identification label or cardboard insert with patient identification information affixed to it; worn by the patient throughout hospitalization
   c. checklist used to ensure that the paper or the electronic chart and the patient are properly prepared for surgery
   d. list of all the surgeries to be performed on a particular day; the schedule may be printed from the computer or sent to the nursing unit by the admitting department
   e. a number assigned to the patient to access insurance information; usually a unique number is assigned each time the patient is admitted to the hospital
   f. container for storing the patient's jewelry, money, and other valuables, which are placed in the hospital safe for safekeeping
   g. orders written by the doctor before surgery to prepare the patient for the surgical procedure
   h. orders written immediately after surgery; postoperative orders cancel preoperative orders
   i. information obtained from the patient concerning his sensitivity to medications and/or food
   j. a form initiated in the admitting department that is included in the inpatient medical record and contains personal and demographic information; usually computer generated at the time of admission (also may be called the *information sheet*)
   k. a checklist used by the health unit coordinator to ensure that the patient's paper chart is ready for surgery
   l. surgery that is not emergency or mandatory and can be planned at a time of convenience

m. plastic band with a cardboard insert on which allergy information is printed, or a red plastic band that has allergy information written directly on it; worn by the patient throughout the hospitalization

n. the process of obtaining information and partially preparing admitting forms prior to the patient's arrival at the health care facility

o. the process of entering personal information into the hospital information system to enroll a person as a hospital patient and create a patient record; patients may be registered as inpatients, outpatients, or observation patients

3. Any six of the following:
   - admitting diagnosis
   - diet
   - activity
   - diagnostic orders
   - medications—usually, medications are needed for the patient's disease condition, for sleeping, and/or for pain
   - treatment orders
   - request for old records
   - patient care category or code status

(*Note*: The patient care category or code status may be indicated on the patient's admission orders and refers to the patient's wishes regarding resuscitation. Code status may be written as *full code, modified support,* or *do not resuscitate.* The physician must follow any state-specific statute and the hospital's policies and procedures before writing a DNR order.

4. a. admission service agreement
   b. face or front sheet
   c. patient identification bracelet

(Advance directives may or may not be sent to the unit by the registration staff.)

5. See Procedure 19-1, p. 374.
6. See Procedure 19-2, p. 380.
7. Any five of the following:
   - current history and physical record (H&P)
   - surgery consent
   - blood transfusion consent or refusal
   - admission service agreement
   - nursing preoperative checklist
   - MAR
   - diagnostic test results
8. a. name of surgery for surgery consent
   b. enemas
   c. shaves, scrubs, or showers
   d. name of anesthesiologist or anesthesiology group
   e. miscellaneous orders
   f. diet
   g. preoperative medications
9. a. diet
   b. intake and output
   c. intravenous fluids
   d. vital signs
   e. catheters, tubes, and drains
   f. activity
   g. positioning
   h. observation of the operative site
   i. medications

10. See Procedure 19-3, p. 380.
11. documents that intend to indicate a patient's wishes in the event that the patient becomes incapacitated and unable to make his own decisions
12. Any eight of the following:
    - Interview patient or family to obtain personal information.
    - Copy insurance cards.
    - Verify insurance (may be done in advance when admission is scheduled).
    - Ask patient or patient guardian to sign appropriate insurance forms.
    - Prepare admission forms (condition of admission agreement and face sheet) and obtain signatures.
    - Ask patient if he or she has advance directives or would like to create one. (Required in most states)
    - Prepare patient's identification bracelet.
    - Enter information into computer for patient identification labels.
    - Secure patient valuables if necessary. (may be done on nursing unit by admitting nurse)
    - Supply and explain required information, including a copy of the Patients' Bill of Rights and privacy practices of the facility.
    - Include any test results, prewritten orders, or consents that have been sent previously to the admitting department in the packet that accompanies the patient to the nursing unit.
13. A *living will* is a declaration made by the patient to family, medical staff, and all concerned with the patient's care, stating what is to be done in the event of a terminal illness; it directs the withholding or withdrawing of life-sustaining procedures. A *power of attorney* for health care is when the patient appoints a person (called a *proxy* or *agent*) to make health care decisions should the patient be unable to do so.
14. An advance directive becomes effective when the patient becomes incapacitated and unable to make his own decisions.
15. The health unit coordinator does not have the responsibility of transcribing the doctor's orders but will have various tasks that will be indicated by an icon on the computer screen next to the patient's name. Tasks that are missed could cause a delay in the patient's care or preparation for surgery.
16. The health unit coordinator usually prepares the consent form to be signed by the patient and witnessed by the nurse and/or doctor. The consent and other documents as required are scanned into the patient's electronic record.

CHAPTER 20

Exercise 1

1. AMA
2. ECF

Exercise 2

1. against medical advice
2. extended care facility

Review Questions

1. See Procedure 20-1, pp. 388-389.
2. a. The HUC would print the discharge instructions from the computer.

b. The HUC would also print out the medication c̄ medication instruction sheet.

3. Ask the patient to be seated until the nurse is advised.

4. See Procedure 20-1, Task #14, p. xx and Figure 20-4.5. See Procedure 20-2, p. 395.

6. See Procedure 20-3, p. 395.

7. a. an illness ending in death

   b. a death

   c. after death

   d. care and services of a non-medical nature that consist of feeding, bathing, watching, and protecting the patient

   e. an examination of the body after death

   f. donating one's organs and/or tissues after death

   g. a signed consent authorizing a specific funeral home to remove a deceased patient's body from a health care facility

   h. a death that occurs because of sudden, violent, or unexplained circumstances

   i. a medical facility caring for patients who require expert care or custodial care

   j. a meeting that will include the physician or physicians caring for the patient, the primary nurses, the case manager or social worker, and other caregivers involved in the patient's care

   k. centralized, coordinated, multidisciplinary process that ensures that the patient has a plan for continuing care after leaving the hospital.

8. See Procedure 20-4, p. 397.

9. See Procedure 20-6, p. 399.

10. See Procedure 20-5, p. 397.

11. See Procedure 20-7, p. 399.

CHAPTER 21

Exercise 1

1. TPR
2. PP
3. PO day
4. F
5. C
6. BM

Exercise 2

1. postoperative day
2. postpartum
3. Fahrenheit
4. bowel movement
5. Celsius
6. temperature, pulse, respiration

Review Questions

1. Vital signs should be recorded as soon as they are all written on the TPR sheet, so they are available to the doctor when he makes hospital rounds.

2. The doctor may use vital signs data to prescribe treatment for the patient.

3. Write "mistaken entry" on the incorrect, connecting line, mark an x across the dot indicating the incorrect temperature, graph the correct value, and write your first initial and last name next to or above the error.

4. Recopy the entire record showing the correct data. Draw a diagonal line through the old record in ink, and write "mistaken entry" on the line. Write "recopied in ink" with your first and last names, status, and the date on both the old record and the recopied record.

5. The original would be placed behind the recopied record under the graphic divider in the chart; it remains a permanent part of the patient's paper chart.

6. a. 37.0°

   b. 38.5°

   c. 37.6°

   d. 35.9°

7. a. 100.8°

   b. 103.1°

   c. 97.5°

   d. 100.0°

8. a. to have the records available for the attending physician and other health care personnel

   b. to assist the health records department in assembling all patient records for storage

9. a. File at the same time each day.

   b. Separate the records according to the patient's name so that you need to obtain and open the chart binder only once.

   c. Always check the patient's name on the chart back with the name on the record before filing it.

   d. Place the record behind the correct chart divider.

   e. Initial all records you file (check policy of hospital).

10. a. Label each document with the appropriate patient's ID label, and scan the documents as required or requested in a timely manner.

    b. Stamp "scanned" on each document.

    c. Place original documents in a bin or box to be picked up by HIMS.

11. a. purchasing department: non-nursing items, such as pens and pencils

    b. central service department: items used for nursing procedures, such a catheterization tray

    c. pharmacy: all medications

    d. dietary department: food items, such as milk and crackers

    e. laundry department

12. a. the difference between the radial pulse and the apical heartbeat

    b. a scale used to measure temperature in which the freezing point of water is 0° and the boiling point is 100°

    c. body wastes from the digestive tract that are formed in the intestine and expelled through the rectum

    d. a scale used to measure temperature in which 32° is the freezing point of water and 212° is the boiling point

CHAPTER 22

Review Questions

1. a. acquired immunodeficiency syndrome

   b. AIDS-related complex

   c. Centers for Disease Control and Prevention

   d. hepatitis B virus

   e. human immunodeficiency virus

   f. Occupational Safety and Health Administration

   g. personal protective equipment

   h. tuberculosis

   i. *Rescue* individuals in danger; *Alarm*: sound the alarm; *Confine* the fire by closing all doors and windows; *Extinguish* the fire with the nearest suitable fire extinguisher.

2. a. accidents such as a fall of a patient, visitor, or employee
   b. thefts from persons on hospital property
   c. errors of omission of patient treatment or errors of administration of patient treatment
   d. exposure to blood and body fluids such as caused by a needle stick

3. The health unit coordinator may be expected to assist with the evacuation of patients who are endangered by the fire. If the fire is not on the unit, the health unit coordinator may help nursing personnel to close the doors to the patient rooms.

4. a. Avoid the use of extension cords.
   b. Do not overload electrical circuits.
   c. Inspect cords and plugs for breaks and fraying.
   d. Unplug equipment when servicing.
   e. Unplug equipment that has liquid spilled in it.
   f. Unplug and do not use equipment that is malfunctioning.

5. a. *Streptococcus*
   b. *Staphylococcus*
   c. *Pseudomonas*

6. a. division of the U.S. Public Health Service that investigates and controls diseases that have epidemic potential
   b. a precautionary measure taken to prevent a patient with low resistance to disease from becoming infected
   c. when the patient ceases to breathe or when respirations are so depressed that the blood cannot receive sufficient oxygen and therefore the body cells die (may also be referred to as *code arrest*)
   d. another term for isolation
   e. disease-carrying organisms too small to be seen with the naked eye
   f. an emergency that is life threatening
   g. the placement of a patient apart from other patients insofar as movement and social contact are concerned, for the purpose of preventing the spread of infection
   h. an episode that does not normally occur within the regular hospital routine
   i. a disease that may be transmitted from one person to another
   j. a basic hazard communication tool that gives details on chemical dangers and safety procedures
   k. The patient's heart contractions are absent or insufficient to produce a pulse or blood pressure (may also be referred to as *code arrest*).
   l. a planned procedure that is carried out by hospital personnel when a large number of persons have been injured
   m. infections that are acquired from within the health care facility
   n. the creation of a barrier between the health care worker and the patient's blood and body fluids (also may be called *Universal Precautions*)
   o. a department in the hospital that addresses the prevention and containment of liability regarding patient care incidents
   p. required use of mask and ventilated room, in conjunction with Standard Precautions

7. a. Notify the hospital telephone operator to announce the code.
   b. Direct the code arrest team to the patient's room.
   c. Remove the patient information sheet from the patient's chart, and take or send the chart to the patient's room.
   d. Notify all physicians connected with the patient's case when requested to do so by the nurse or doctor.
   e. Notify the patient's family of the situation if requested to do so.
   f. Label any laboratory specimens with the patient's ID label, enter the test ordered in the computer, and send the specimen to the laboratory stat.
   g. Call the appropriate departments for treatments and supplies as needed.
   h. Alert the admissions department and the ICU for possibility of transfer to ICU.
   i. For a successful code, follow the procedure for a transfer to another unit; for an unsuccessful code procedure, follow the procedure for postmortem care.

8. A protective measure is to wear gloves and wash hands after handling specimens (even when bagged).

9. For statistical purposes, records must be kept of infectious diseases; infection control is essential to provide a safe environment for both patients and health care workers. The nurse would have to be tested for HIV if the needle was used for a patient who has not been tested.

10. a. infectious agent or pathogen (bacteria)
    b. a reservoir or source for pathogen to live and grow (human body, contaminated water or food, animals, insects, etc)
    c. means of escape (blood, urine, feces, wound drainage, etc.)
    d. route of transmission (direct contact, airborne)
    e. entry way (mouth, nostrils, and breaks in the skin)
    f. susceptible host (individual who does not have adequate resistance to the invading pathogen)

11. a. air
    b. personal contact
    c. body excretions

12. a. organ transplant recipients
    b. burn victims
    c. patients receiving chemotherapy

13. a. gloves
    b. gowns
    c. goggles
    d. masks

14. an infection in which the infecting organisms take advantage of the patient's weakened immune system

15. a. *Pneumocystis carinii* pneumonia (PCP)
    b. Kaposi's sarcoma (KS)

16. a. Mail is checked and the patient's room and bed numbers are written on each envelope. If patient has been discharged, write "Discharged" in pencil on the envelope and send back to t the mailroom. Deliver when able, or designate to a hospital volunteer.
    b. Sign the receipt slip for flowers only if the patient is still in the hospital and can receive flowers. Send back or give flowers to family if the patient has been discharged or cannot receive them. Pediatric patients cannot receive rubber balloons, and they would have to be sent back or given to family members.

CHAPTER 23

Unit 1

Exercise 1

1. WR   CV   S
   cyt /   o   /   logy
   cell   study of
2. WR   S
   gastr /   ectomy
   stomach   excision, surgical removal of
3. P   WR   S
   sub   /   hepat /   ic
   under   liver   pertaining to
4. WR   CV   WR   CV   S
   electr / o / cardi / o /   gram
   electricity   heart   record of
5. WR   CV   S
   cardi /   o   /   logy
   heart   study of
6. P   WR   S
   trans /   hepat /   ic
   across   liver   pertaining to

Exercise 2

1. cardiology
2. cytology
3. gastrectomy
4. gastroenteritis
5. gastric
6. intragastric
7. nephrectomy

Review Questions

1. a. languages past and present: Greek (Example: nephrology), Latin (Example: maternal), and modern languages, such as lavage from the French
   b. eponyms—generally named after discoverer (Example: Pap smear)
   c. acronyms—words formed from first letter of a descriptive phrase (Example: laser)
2. a. word root: the basic part of a word (Example: gastr/ic)
   b. prefix: the part of the word placed before the word root to alter its meaning (Example: intra/gastric)
   c. suffix: the part of the word added at the end of the word to alter its meaning (Example: gastr/ic)
   d. combining vowel: usually an "o" used between word roots or between a word root and a suffix (Example: gastr/o/enteritis)
3. a. A combining vowel is not used when a prefix and a word root are connected.
   b. When two word roots are connected, the combining vowel usually is used even if the second root begins with a vowel.
   c. When a word root is connected to a suffix, a combining vowel usually is not used if the suffix begins with a vowel.
4. a. dividing medical terms into word parts and identifying each word part
   b. when given a definition of a medical condition, using word parts to build corresponding medical terms

Unit 2

Review Questions

1. a. the basic unit of all living things
   b. a group of similar cells that work together to perform particular functions
   c. made up of two or more tissue types to perform one or more common functions
   d. a group of organs working together in a common purpose to perform complex body functions
2. a. epithelial
   b. connective
   c. muscle
   d. nerve
3. a. cranial—brain
   b. thoracic—heart
   c. abdominal—stomach
   d. pelvic—bladder
   e. spinal—spinal cord

(*Note*: Other organs may be correct answers.)

4. 1. e
   2. d
   3. h
   4. c
   5. a
   6. b
   7. g
   8. f
   9. k
   10. i
   11. l
   12. j
   13. n
   14. m
   15. p
   16. o
5. a. protects the underlying tissues
   b. assists in regulating body temperature
   c. passes messages of pain, cold, and touch to the brain
   d. synthesis of vitamin K
6. epidermis / dermis / subcutaneous (or hypodermis)
7. melanin / albinism
8. oil (sebaceous)
9. sweat glands (sudoriferous)
10. cell membrane—keeps the cell intact and is selectively porous; cytoplasm—main body of the cells, and cell activities take place here; nucleus—control center and plays an important role in reproduction
11. 1. b
    2. a or h
    3. e
    4. f
    5. d
    6. c
    7. h
    8. g

Exercise 1

1. internal organs
2. skin

3. cell
4. tissue
5. skin
6. hair
7. disease
8. cancer
9. connective tissue, flesh
10. epithelium
11. fat
12. cancer
13. skin
14. cancer
15. nail

Exercise 2

1. pertaining to
2. study of
3. one who specializes in the diagnosis and treatment of (specialist, physician)
4. resembling
5. inflammation
6. tumor
7. producing, originating, causing
8. through, across, beyond
9. pertaining to
10. under or below

Exercise 3

1. WR, cyt / o
2. WR, derm / o, dermat / o, cutane / o
3. S, -logist
4. S, -oid
5. WR, viscer / o
6. WR, hist / o
7. S, -al
8. S, -logy
9. P, trans-
10. WR, carcin / o, cancer / o, onc / o
11. P, sub-

Exercise 4

1. WR   CV   S
   cyt   / o   / logy   study of cells
2. WR   S
   trich / oid   resembling hair
3. WR   CV   S
   path   / o   / logy   study of (body changes caused by) disease
4. WR   CV   S
   path   / o   / genic   producing disease
5. WR   S
   dem   / al   pertaining to skin
6. WR   S
   cyt   / oid   resembling a cell
7. WR   S
   viscer / al   pertaining to internal organs
8. WR   CV   S
   hist   / o   / logy   study of tissue
9. WR   CV   S
   dermat / o   / logist one who specializes in the diagnosis and treatment of skin (diseases)

10. WR   S
    dermat / itis   inflammation of the skin
11. WR   CV   S
    carcin / o   / genic   producing cancer
12. WR   S
    epitheli / al   pertaining to epithelium
13. WR   S
    carcin / oma   cancerous tumor
14. WR   S
    epitheli / oma   tumor composed of epithelial (cells)
15. WR   S
    sarc   / oma   tumor composed of connective tissue
16. WR   S
    lip   / oma   tumor (containing) fat
17. WR   CV   S
    path   / o   / logist one who specializes in the diagnosis and treatment of disease
18. WR   S
    dermat / oid   resembling skin
19. WR   CV   S
    dermat / o   / logy   study of skin (branch of medicine that deals with skin diseases)
20. P   WR   S
    trans / derm / al   pertaining to (entering) through the skin
21. WR   CV   S
    onc   / o   / logy   study of cancer
22. P   WR   S
    sub   / ungu / al   pertaining to under the nail
23. P   WR   S
    sub   / cutane / ous   pertaining to under the skin

Exercise 5

1. cytoid
2. trichoid
3. a. dermoid
   b. dermatoid
4. pathologist
5. dermatologist
6. a. dermal
   b. cutaneous
7. visceral
8. histology
9. pathology
10. dermatology
11. pathogenic
12. cytology
13. dermatitis
14. lipoma
15. epithelioma
16. epithelial
17. carcinogenic
18. sarcoma
19. carcinoma
20. a. transdermal
    b. transcutaneous
21. oncology
22. subungual
23. subcutaneous

Exercise 6

Spelling exercise

Exercise 7

- posteroanterior
- right upper quadrant
- anteroposterior
- right lower quadrant
- subcutaneous
- lateral
- cancer
- left lower quadrant
- left upper quadrant

Unit 3

Review Questions

1. a. protects the internal organs
   b. provides the framework for the body
   c. acts with muscles to produce movement
   d. produces blood cells
   e. stores calcium and phosphorus
2. periosteum
3. cranium (8 bones):
   a. frontal, 1
   b. parietal, 2
   c. temporal, 2
   d. ethmoid, 1
   e. sphenoid, 1
   f. occipital, 1
   face (14 bones):
   a. maxilla, 2
   b. mandible, 1
   c. nasal, 2
   d. lacrimal, 2
   e. zygomatic, 2
   f. vomer, 1
   g. inferior nasal concha (2)
   h. palatine (2)
4. hyoid (1 bone)
5. a. malleus(2)
   b. incus (2)
   c. stapes (2)
6. a. cervical (7)
   b. thoracic (12)
   c. lumbar (5)
   d. sacrum (1)
   e. coccyx (1)
7. a. scapula
   b. clavicle
   c. humerus
   d. radius
   e. ulna
   f. carpals
   g. metacarpals
   h. phalanges
8. a. ilium
   b. ischium
   c. pubis
9. a. femur
   b. patella
   c. tibia
   d. fibula
   e. tarsal
   f. metatarsal
   g. phalanges
10. a. skeletal muscles / biceps (voluntary)
    b. cardiac / heart (involuntary)
    c. smooth / stomach (involuntary)
11. a. a place on the skeleton where two or more bones meet
    b. attaches muscles to bones
    c. tough band of tissues that connect bone to bone at a joint
12. a. osteoarthritis
    b. rheumatoid arthritis
13. a. laminectomy
    b. diskectomy
14. a. broken bone, no open wound
    b. broken bone, open wound
    c. bone has been twisted apart
    d. bone is splintered or crushed
    e. bone is partially bent and partially broken
    f. occurs when the vertebrae collapse by trauma or pathology
15. total (name of joint) arthroplasty
16. osteoclasts / osteoblasts
17. a. headaches
    b. ringing in the ears
    c. hearing loss
    d. dizziness
18. osteoporosis
19. Any of the following:
    - calcium supplements and vitamin D
    - weight-bearing exercise
    - hormonal replacement therapy (if appropriate)
    - correct posture
    - drugs to slow down the dissolving process of the osteoclasts

Exercise 1

(*Note:* Not all of the combining forms will be labeled on the diagram.)

3. clavic / o
4. clavicul / o
5. cost / o
6. crani / o
7. femor / o
8. humer/o
12. patell / o
13. phalang / o
14. scapul / o
15. stern / o
16. vertebr / o

Exercise 2

1. joint
2. bone
3. rib
4. skull
5. femur
6. muscle
7. humerus
8. patella

9. sternum
10. clavicle
11. scapula
12. phalange
13. vertebra(e)
14. clavicle
15. electrical activity, electricity
16. lamina
17. cartilage
18. meniscus
19. curved (laterally)

Exercise 3

1. phalang / o
2. arthr / o
3. oste / o
4. femor / o
5. patell / o
6. scapul / o
7. vertebr / o
8. a. clavic / o
   b. clavicul / o
9. crani / o
10. stern / o
11. humer / o
12. cost / o
13. a. my / o
    b. myos / o
14. lamin / o
15. chondr / o
16. menisc / o

Exercise 4

1. -plasty
2. -algia
3. a. -ar
   b. -ic
   c. -al
   d. -ous
4. -tomy
5. -ectomy
6. -graph
7. -graphy
8. -gram
9. -trophy
10. -osis
11. -scope
12. -scopy
13. -centesis
14. -pathy

Exercise 5

1. pain
2. instrument to record
3. record, X-ray image
4. process of recording, X-ray imaging
5. surgical incision or to cut into
6. development, nourishment
7. pertaining to
8. surgical repair
9. surgical removal
10. pertaining to

11. abnormal condition
12. visual examination
13. instrument used for visual examination
14. surgical puncture to aspirate fluid
15. disease of

Exercise 6

1. intra-
2. dys-
3. sub-
4. a. a-
   b. an-
5. inter-
6. supra-

Exercise 7

1. within
2. above
3. below
4. difficult, painful, labored, abnormal
5. without
6. between

Exercise 8

1. WR   CV WR CV   S
   electr / o / my / o / gram   record of electrical activity of muscle

2. WR   S
   my / oma   a tumor (formed of) muscle (tissue)

3. WR   CV   WR   S
   stern / o / clavicul / ar   pertaining to the sternum and clavicle

4. WR   S
   crani / al   pertaining to the cranium

5. WR   CV   WR   S
   vertebr / o / cost / al   pertaining to the vertebrae and ribs

6. WR   S
   arthr / itis   inflammation of a joint

7. P   WR   S
   inter / vertebr / al   pertaining to between the vertebrae

8. WR   S
   humer / al   pertaining to the humerus

9. P   S/WR
   dys / trophy   abnormal development

10. P   WR   S
    sub / scapul / ar   pertaining to below the scapula

11. WR   S
    arthr / osis   abnormal condition of a joint

12. WR   CV WR CV   S
    electr / o / my / o / graphy   process of recording the electrical activity of muscle

13. WR   CV   S
    arthr / o / gram   x-ray image of a joint

14. WR   CV WR CV   S
    electr / o / my / o / graph   instrument to record the electrical activity of muscle

15. WR CV WR S
    stern / o / cost / al   pertaining to the sternum
                                     and ribs

16. WR   S
    arthr / algia   pain in a joint

17. P   WR   S
    sub / cost / al   pertaining to below a rib
                                     (or ribs)

18. WR   S
    femor / al   pertaining to the femur

19. WR CV S
    clavic / o / tomy   surgical incision into the
                                     clavicle

20. WR CV S
    arthr / o / tomy   surgical incision of a joint

21. P   WR   S
    intra / crani / al   pertaining to within the
                                     cranium

22. P   WR
    a / trophy   without development (or
                                     decrease in size of a nor-
                                     mally developed organ)

23. WR CV S
    arthr / o / plasty   surgical repair of a joint

24. WR   S
    oste / oma   tumor (composed of)
                                     bone

25. WR   S
    cost / ectomy   excision of a rib

26. WR CV S
    crani / o / plasty   surgical repair of the
                                     cranium

27. WR   S
    patell / ectomy   excision of the patella

28. WR   S
    vertebr / ectomy   excision of a vertebra

29. WR CV S
    crani / o / tomy   surgical incision into the
                                     cranium

30. P   WR   S
    supra / scapul / ar   pertaining to above the
                                     scapula

31. WR   S
    myos / itis   inflammation of muscle

32. WR CV S
    chondr / o / genic   producing cartilage

33. WR CV S
    arthr / o /scopy   visual examination of the
                                     inside of a joint

34. WR   S
    chondr / itis   inflammation of the
                                     cartilage

35. WR CV S
    arthr / o / scope   instrument used to
                                     visualize a joint

36. WR   S
    chondr / ectomy   excision of cartilage

37. WR   S
    lamin / ectomy   excision of the lamina

38. WR S
    stern / al   pertaining to the
                                     sternum

39. WR   S
    menisc / ectomy   excision of the meniscus

40. WR CV   S
    arthr / o / centesis   surgical puncture to aspirate
                                     fluid from a joint

41. WR   S
    menisc / itis   inflammation of the meniscus

Exercise 9

1. cranial
2. myositis
3. subscapular
4. femoral
5. arthrotomy
6. chondrectomy
7. arthralgia
8. arthritis
9. arthrosis
10. humeral
11. atrophy
12. vertebrocostal
13. craniotomy
14. costectomy
15. subcostal
16. arthrogram
17. vertebrectomy
18. electromyogram
19. clavicotomy
20. electromyography
21. dystrophy
22. myoma
23. electromyograph
24. sternoclavicular
25. intervertebral
26. intracranial
27. sternocostal
28. patellectomy
29. cranioplasty
30. osteoma
31. clavicotomy
32. chondrogenic
33. arthroscopy
34. arthroscope
35. chondritis
36. chondrectomy
37. laminectomy
38. sternal
39. arthrocentesis
40. meniscectomy
41. meniscitis

Exercise 10

1. branch of medicine dealing with the diagnosis and treatment of diseases, fractures, or abnormalities of the musculoskeletal system
2. doctor specializing in orthopedics
3. progressive, crippling disease of the muscles
4. insertion of a hollow needle into the sternum to obtain
   bone marrow sample for laboratory study

Exercise 11

Spelling exercise

Exercise 12

1. orthopedics / orthopedist
2. sternal puncture
3. electromyography
4. a. lower inner leg bone
   b. upper arm bone
   c. neck bone
   d. pelvic bone
   e. collarbone
   f. arm bone, thumb side
5. a. costectomy
   b. (correct)
   c. laminectomy
   d. clavicotomy
   e. (correct)
   f. patellectomy
   g. osteoarthrotomy
   h. (correct)
6. arthrogram / arthrocentesis

Exercise 13

- above the knee amputation
- below the knee amputation
- fracture
- open reduction, internal fixation
- herniated nucleus pulposus
- nonsteroidal anti-inflammatory drugs
- electromyogram, electromyography
- total hip arthroplasty
- total hip replacement

Unit 4

Review Questions

1. a. nerves: transmit impulses from one part of the body to another
   b. brain: the main center for coordinating body activity
   c. spinal cord: the pathway for conducting sensory impulses to the brain and motor impulses down from the brain
2. neuron / sensory / motor
3. a. cerebrum: contains sensory, motor, sight, and hearing centers; memory, judgment, and emotional reactions also take place in the cerebrum
   b. cerebellum: assists in coordination of voluntary muscles and maintains balance
   c. brainstem: contains the control centers for blood pressure, respiration, and heartbeat
4. Extends from the brainstem passing through the spinal cavity to between the first and second lumbar vertebrae. It is the pathway for conducting sensory and motor impulses to and from the brain.
5. dura mater / arachnoid / pia mater
6. 1. a
   2. f
   3. d
   4. c
   5. b
7. a. preictal
   b. interictal
   c. postictal

Exercise 1

(*Note*: Not all of the combining forms will be labeled on the diagram.)

1. cerebell / o
2. cerebr / o
3. encephal / o
4. mening / o
5. myel / o
6. neur / o

Exercise 2

1. cerebrum
2. brain
3. nerve
4. gray matter
5. meninges
6. dura mater
7. spinal cord or bone marrow
8. cerebellum
9. air
10. speech
11. mind

Exercise 3

1. neur / o
2. cerebr / o
3. mening / o
4. myel / o
5. cerebell / o
6. encephal / o
7. dur / o
8. pneum / o
9. poli / o
10. phas / o
11. psych / o

Exercise 4

1. -oma
2. -plasty
3. -ar, -al, -ic, -ous
4. -rrhaphy
5. -rrhea
6. -itis
7. -logist
8. -gram
9. -logy
10. -rrhagia
11. -cele
12. -ectomy
13. -tomy
14. -algia
15. -ia

Exercise 5

1. record, X-ray image
2. inflammation
3. the study of
4. discharge
5. rapid discharge
6. to suture

7. herniation, protrusion
8. pertaining to
9. surgical removal
10. surgical repair
11. surgical incision
12. pain
13. abnormal condition
14. abnormal condition

Exercise 6

1. WR   CV   S
   neur / o / logy   study of nerve (branch of medicine that deals with the nervous system)

2. WR   CV WR   S
   cerebr / o / spin / al   pertaining to the brain and spine

3. WR   S
   neur / algia   pain in a nerve

4. WR   CV WR   S
   poli / o / myel / itis   inflammation of the gray matter and the spinal cord

5. WR   CV   S
   neur / o / plasty   surgical repair of a nerve

6. WR   S
   encephal / itis   inflammation of the brain

7. WR   S
   mening / itis   inflammation of the meninges

8. WR   CV   S
   neur / o / pathy   disease of a nerve

9. WR   CV   S
   neur / o / logist   one who specializes in the diagnosis and treatment of nerves

10. WR   CV   S
    encephal / o / cele   herniation of brain tissue through (a gap in) the skull

11. WR   CV   WR   CV S
    electr / o / encephal / o / gram   recording of electrical activity of the brain

12. WR   CV WR CV S
    mening / o / myel / o / cele   protrusion of the spinal cord and meninges through the vertebral column

13. WR   S
    cerebell / itis   inflammation of the cerebellum

14. WR   S
    cerebr / osis   abnormal condition of the brain

15. WR   S
    neur / oma   tumor of nerve (cells)

16. WR   CV   S
    myel / o / rrhagia   hemorrhage into the spinal cord

17. WR   CV   S
    myel / o / gram   X-ray image of the spinal cord with the use of dye

18. WR   S
    neur / itis   inflammation of a nerve

Exercise 7

1. a disease characterized by hardening patches along the brain and the spine
2. convulsive disorder of the nervous system marked by recurrent or chronic seizures
3. partial paralysis and lack of muscle coordination from a defect, injury, or disease of the brain present at birth or shortly after
4. impaired blood supply to parts of the brain
5. process of recording brain structures with the use of sound recorded on a graph
6. paralysis of the right or left side of the body
7. paralysis of the legs and/or lower part of the body
8. paralysis that affects all four limbs
9. removal of cerebrospinal fluid for diagnostic purposes (in the lumbar area of the spine)
10. accumulation of blood in the subdural space
11. radiologic imaging that produces images of "slices" of the body with the use of X-rays
12. a noninvasive procedure for imaging tissues that uses a magnetic field
13. loss of expression or understanding of speech or writing

Exercise 8

1. neuritis
2. encephalitis
3. meningitis
4. neuroplasty
5. neurologist
6. neuropathy
7. neuroma
8. neuralgia
9. cerebrospinal
10. meningomyelocele
11. cerebellitis
12. encephalocele
13. myelorrhagia
14. electroencephalogram
15. myelogram

Exercise 9

Spelling exercise

Exercise 10

Spelling exercise

Exercise 11

1. neurology / neurologist
2. cerebrovascular / accident / CVA / hemiplegia
3. meningitis / spinal puncture / (lumbar puncture) / spinal puncture (lumbar puncture)
4. a. electroencephalogram
   b. myelogram
   c. pneumoencephalogram
   d. echoencephalogram

Exercise 12

1. central nervous system
2. cerebrospinal fluid
3. computed tomography
4. cerebrovascular accident
5. electroencephalogram

6. evoked potentials
7. lumbar puncture
8. multiple sclerosis
9. peripheral nervous system
10. positron emission tomography
11. magnetic resonance imaging
12. transient ischemic attack

Unit 5

Review Questions

1. a. skull bones
   b. eyelashes
   c. eyelids
   d. lacrimal apparatus
   e. conjunctiva
2. Sound enters the pinna, travels through the auditory canal, and strikes the tympanic membrane, which sends the ossicles into motion. The stapes vibrate the oval window, and the waves continue to travel via the fluid in the cochlea to the auditory nerve and on to the brain.
3. 1. f
   2. h
   3. j
   4. i
   5. b
   6. d
   7. k
   8. a
4. a. conjunctiva
   b. cornea
   c. aqueous humor
   d. pupil
   e. lens
   f. vitreous humor
5. a. cones; adaptation to bright light and color vision
   b. rods; adaptation to dim light
6. a. pinna and auditory canal
   b. tympanic membrane, eustachian tube, malleus, incus, stapes
   c. oval window, cochlea, semicircular canals
7. cloudiness of the lens of the eye
8. abnormal increase in intraocular pressure
9. a. chronic infections
   b. head injuries
   c. prolonged exposure to environmental noise
   d. hypertension
   e. cardiovascular disease
   f. ototoxic drugs
10. a. masking the noise with the use of music
    b. biofeedback
11. separation of the retina from the choroid
12. a. photocoagulation
    b. crysosurgery
    c. scleral buckling

Exercise 1

1. 1. blephar / o
   2. conjunctiv / o
   3. irid / o
   4. kerat / o
   5. ophthalm / o
   6. retin / o
   7. scler / o
2. 1. myring / o
   2. ot / o
   3. staped / o

Exercise 2

1. retina
2. cornea
3. sclera
4. eye
5. conjunctiva
6. ear
7. tympanic membrane
8. eyelid
9. iris
10. stapes

Exercise 3

1. ophthalm / o
2. blephar / o
3. retin / o
4. ot / o
5. myring / o
6. scler / o
7. conjunctiv / o
8. irid / o
9. kerat / o
10. staped / o

Exercise 4

1. WR   CV   S
   ophthalm / o / scope — instrument used for visual examination of the eye
2. WR   CV   S
   ophthalm / o / logist — one who specializes in the diagnosis and treatment of the eye
3. WR   S
   ophthalm / ectomy — excision of the eye
4. WR CV S
   ot / o / rrhea — discharge from the ear
5. WR CV S
   ot / o / scope — instrument used for visual examination of the ear
6. WR CV WR CV S
   irid / o / scler / o / tomy — incision into the iris and sclera
7. WR   S
   irid / ectomy — excision of (part of) the iris
8. WR   CV   S
   blephar / o / plasty — surgical repair of the eyelid
9. WR   CV   S
   blephar / o / rrhaphy — suture of an eyelid
10. WR CV WR   S
    kerat / o / conjunctiv / itis — inflammation of the cornea and conjunctiva
11. WR   CV   S
    kerat / o / cele — herniation of (a layer of the) cornea

12. WR   S
    conjunctiv / itis   inflammation of the
                                 conjunctiva
13. WR   CV   S
    myring / o / tomy   incision of the tympanic
                                 membrane
14. WR   CV   S
    myring / o / plasty   surgical repair of the
                                 tympanic membrane
15. WR   CV   S
    kerat / o / tomy   incision into the cornea

Exercise 5

1. otitis media
2. ophthalmoscope
3. blepharorrhaphy
4. otorrhea
5. iridosclerotomy
6. scleroplasty
7. iridectomy
8. keratocele
9. otoscope
10. ophthalmectomy
11. sclerotomy
12. blepharoplasty
13. myringotomy
14. myringoplasty
15. keratoconjunctivitis
16. conjunctivitis
17. keratotomy

Exercise 6

1. cloudiness of the lens of the eye
2. removal of the clouded lens of the eye
3. separation of the retina from the choroid
4. surgical removal of the eyeball
5. weakness of the eye muscle (crossed eyes)
6. eye disease caused by increased pressure from within the eye
7. a professional person trained to examine the eyes and prescribe glasses
8. transplantation of a donor cornea into the eye of a recipient

Exercise 7

Spelling exercise

Exercise 8

1. ophthalmoscope / otoscope
2. otitis media / myringotomy
3. cataract / cataract extraction
4. enucleation / ophthalmectomy
5. strabismus

Exercise 9

1. pupils equal, round, reactive to light and accommodation
2. otits media
3. photorefractive keratectomy
4. radial keratotomy
5. oculus dexter (right eye)
6. oculus sinister (left eye)
7. oculus uterque (both eyes)

Unit 6

Review Questions

1. and 2. See p. 491 for labeled diagram.
3. a. artery: carries blood away from heart
   b. arterioles: connect arteries to capillaries
   c. capillaries: exchange of substances between the blood
      and the body cells
   d. venules: connect capillaries to veins
   e. veins: carry blood back to the heart
4. plasma:
   a. transports nutrients and waste material
   b. transports hormones
   c. assists in blood clotting
5. a. erythrocytes: carry oxygen
   b. leukocytes: fight against pathogenic microorganisms
   c. platelets: aid in blood clotting
6. a. O
   b. A
   c. B
   d. AB
7. a. destroys old red blood cells, bacteria, and germs
   b. stores blood for an emergency
8. 1. g
   2. b
   3. c
   4. a
   5. d
   6. h
   7. e
   8. i

Exercise 1

	Type	Meaning
1.	P	below normal
2.	P	without
3.	WR	blood
4.	WR	spleen
5.	WR	cell
6.	S/WR	narrowing
7.	P	inside
8.	WR	white
9.	WR	red
10.	WR	blood vessel
11.	WR	heart
12.	WR	artery
13.	P	surrounding (outer)
14.	P	between
15.	P	within
16.	S/WR	hardening
17.	S/WR	condition of the blood
18.	S	enlargement
19.	WR	vein
20.	WR	aorta
21.	WR	clot
22.	P	above normal
23.	P	fast, rapid
24.	P	slow

Exercise 2

	Type	Word Elements
1.	WR	aort/o
2.	S	-megaly
3.	S/WR	-sclerosis
4.	P	inter-
5.	WR	arteri / o
6.	WR	angi / o
7.	WR	leuk / o
8.	S/WR	-stenosis
9.	WR	splen / o
10.	P	a-, an-
11.	S	-pexy
12.	P	endo-
13.	WR	hem / o
14.	WR	cyt / o
15.	P	hypo-
16.	WR	erythr / o
17.	WR	cardi / o
18.	P	peri-
19.	S/WR	-emia
20.	WR	phleb / o
21.	WR	thromb / o
22.	P	tachy
23.	P	brady

Exercise 3

1. WR   S
    aort / ic   pertaining to the aorta
2. WR   CV   S
    splen / o / megaly   enlargement of the spleen
3. WR   CV   S
    hem / o / rrhage   rapid flow of blood
                        (from a blood vessel)
4. WR   S
    thromb / osis   abnormal condition (forma-
                        tion) of a blood clot
5. WR   CV   WR
    leuk / o / cyte   white blood cell
6. WR   CV   WR
    erythr / o / cyte   red blood cell
7. WR   CV   S
    cardi / o / logist   one who specializes in the
                        diagnosis and treatment
                        of the heart
8. WR   CV   S
    cardi / o / megaly   enlargement of the heart
9. WR   CV   S
    phleb / o / tomy   incision into the vein
                        (to withdraw blood)
10. WR   CV   S
    angi / o / rrhaphy   suturing of a blood vessel
11. WR   S
    splen / ectomy   excision of the spleen
12. WR   CV   S
    splen / o / pexy   surgical fixation of the
                        spleen
13. P   WR   S
    endo / card / itis   inflammation of the inner
                        (lining) of the heart

14. WR   CV   S
    arteri / o / sclerosis   hardening of the arteries
15. WR   CV   S
    arteri / o / stenosis   constriction (narrowing)
                            of the arteries
16. WR   CV   WR   S
    thromb / o / phleb / itis   inflammation of a vein due
                                to a clot
17. WR   S
    hemat / oma   tumor-like mass formed
                        from blood in the tissues
18. WR   CV   S
    hemat / o / logy   study of blood
19. WR   S
    leuk / emia   blood condition of white
                        (disease characterized
                        by rapid, abnormal
                        production of white
                        blood cells)
20. P   S (WR)
    an / emia   blood condition of
                        without (deficiency of
                        erythrocytes)
21. WR   CV   WR   CV   S
    electr / o / cardi / o / gram   record of electrical activity
                                    of the heart
22. WR   CV   WR   CV   S
    electr / o / cardi / o / graph   machine used to record elec-
                                    trical activity of the heart
23. WR   CV   WR   CV   S
    electr / o / cardi / o / graphy process of recording electri-
                                    cal activity of the heart
24. WR   CV   S
    angi / o / gram   X-ray image of blood vessels
25. WR   CV   S
    arteri / o / gram   X-ray image of an artery
26. WR   CV   S
    aort / o / gram   X-ray image of the aorta
27. P   WR   S
    peri / card / itis   inflammation of the outer
                        (sac) of the heart
28. P   WR   S
    tachy / card / ia   condition of rapid heart
                        (rate)
29. P   WR   S
    brady / card / ia   condition of slow heart
                        (rate)
30. WR   CV   S
    angi / o / plasty   surgical repair of a blood
                        vessel

Exercise 4

1. aortogram
2. arteriogram
3. angiogram
4. electrocardiogram
5. endocarditis
6. arteriosclerosis
7. thrombophlebitis
8. hematology
9. cardiology
10. cardiologist

11. cardiomegaly
12. phlebotomy
13. splenectomy
14. splenopexy
15. hemorrhage
16. leukocyte
17. erythrocyte
18. pericarditis

Exercise 5

1. laboratory test that measures the volume percentage of red blood cells in whole blood
2. laboratory procedure that measures the oxygen-carrying pigment of the red blood cells
3. sudden stopping of the heartbeat
4. pertaining to the heart and blood vessels
5. excision of hemorrhoids
6. heart attack (damage of the heart muscle from insufficient blood supply to the area)
7. enlarged veins in the rectal area
8. within a vein
9. diagnostic procedure to visualize the heart and to determine the presence of heart disease or heart defects
10. dilation of a weak area of the arterial wall
11. floating mass that blocks a blood vessel
12. high blood pressure
13. low blood pressure
14. inability of the heart to pump enough blood to the body parts
15. blood vessels that supply blood to the heart
16. abnormal accumulation of fluid in the intercellular spaces of the body
17. variation from a normal rhythm
18. condition of rapid heart rate

Exercise 6

Spelling exercise

Exercise 7

1. hematology / hematocrit / hemoglobin
2. a. myocardial infarction
   b. coronary occlusion
   c. coronary thrombosis
3. splen_ectomy,_ hemorrhoid_ectomy_
4. cardiovascular
5. cardiologist
6. cardiac arrest / cardiac arrest (or "code")
7. electrocardiography / electrocardiograph
8. angiogram
9. cardiac catheterization
10. a. WBC
    b. RBC
    c. platelets
11. plasma

Exercise 8

1. blood pressure
2. atherosclerotic heart disease
3. coronary artery bypass graft
4. coronary artery disease
5. congestive heart failure
6. electrocardiogram

7. echocardiogram
8. electrocardiogram
9. human immunodeficiency virus
10. hypertension
11. ventricular fibrillation
12. myocardial infarction
13. percutaneous transluminal coronary angioplasty
14. peripheral vascular disease
15. red blood cell (erythrocyte)
16. white blood cell (leukocyte)
17. deep vein thrombosis

Unit 7

Review Questions

1. a. taking nutrients into the digestive tract through the mouth
   b. the chemical and mechanical breakdown of food for use by the body cells
   c. transfer of digested food from the small intestine to the bloodstream
   d. the removal of solid waste from the body
2. ingestion, digestion, absorption, and elimination
3. mouth; pharynx; esophagus (upper and lower esophageal sphincter); stomach (pyloric sphincter); small intestine—duodenum, jejunum, ileum (ileocecal sphincter between small and large intestine); large intestine—cecum, colon (ascending colon, transverse colon, descending colon, sigmoid colon); rectum (anal sphincter)
4. **Name of**

Digestive Chemical or Enzyme	Organ of Secretion	Organ of Function
a. hydrochloric acid	gastric glands	stomach
b. saliva	salivary glands	mouth
c. bile	liver	small intestine (duodenum)
d. pancreatic enzymes	pancreas	small intestine (duodenum)
e. intestinal enzymes	small intestine	small intestine

5. a. salivary glands
   b. teeth
   c. tongue
   d. liver
   e. gallbladder
   f. pancreas
6. pyloric sphincter
7. a. mastication of food, mixing with salivary juices to start digestion
   b. container for food, and chemically and mechanically aids in the digestive process
   c. digestion is completed
   d. absorption of water and elimination of solid waste from the body
   e. stores bile from the liver and secretes it to the duodenum
8. 1. e
   2. a
   3. b
   4. f
   5. d

Exercise 1

(*Note*: Not all of the combining forms will be labeled in the diagram.)

2. appendic / o
4. chol / o or chol / e
5. col / o
6. duoden / o
8. esophag / o
9. gastr / o
10. gloss / o or lingu / o
11. hepat / o
13. ile / o
15. pancreat / o
18. stomat / o

Exercise 2

1. mouth
2. tongue
3. stomach
4. rectum
5. pancreas
6. intestine
7. liver
8. lip
9. esophagus
10. condition of / S
11. bile, gall
12. bladder
13. duodenum
14. colon
15. ileum
16. abdomen
17. appendix
18. abdomen
19. stone or calculus
20. creation of an artificial opening into / S
21. hernia
22. sigmoid

Exercise 3

1. -tomy—incision into a body part; *laparotomy*: incision into the abdomen
2. -ectomy—surgical removal (of a body part); *appendectomy*: surgical removal of the appendix
3. -stomy—creation of an artificial opening into; *colostomy*: creation of an artificial opening into the colon

Exercise 4

1. WR   CV   S
   gloss / o / plegia   paralysis of the tongue
2. WR   S
   append / ectomy   surgical removal of the appendix
3. R   CV WR S
   chol / e / cyst / ectomy   surgical removal of the gallbladder
4. WR   CV   S
   gastr / o / stomy   creation of an artificial opening into the stomach (for feeding purposes)
5. WR   CV   S
   hepat / o / megaly   enlargement of the liver

6. WR CV S
   ile / o / stomy   creation of an artificial opening into the ileum
7. WR   CV   S
   pylor / o / plasty   surgical repair of the pyloric sphincter
8. WR   CV   S
   proct / o / rrhea   excessive discharge from the rectum
9. WR   CV WR   S
   chol / e / cyst / itis   inflammation of the gallbladder
10. WR   S
    gastr / itis   inflammation of the stomach
11. P   WR   S
    sub / lingu / al   pertaining to under the tongue
12. WR   S
    ile / itis   inflammation of the ileum
13. WR CV WR CV S
    chol / e / cyst / o / gram   x-ray image of the gallbladder
14. WR   CV   S
    sigmoid / o / scopy   visual examination of the sigmoid colon
15. WR   S
    gastr / ectomy   surgical removal of the stomach
16. WR   CV   S
    gastr / o / scopy   visual examination of the stomach
17. WR   CV   S
    gastr / o / scope   instrument used for visual examination of the stomach
18. WR   S
    col / itis   inflammation of the colon
19. WR   S
    hepat / itis   inflammation of the liver
20. WR CV   S
    col / o / stomy   creation of an artificial opening into the colon
21. WR   CV   S
    herni / o / rrhaphy   surgical repair of a hernia (by suturing of the containing structure)
22. WR   CV   S
    colon / o / scope   instrument used for visual examination of the colon
23. WR   CV   S
    colon / o / scopy   visual examination of the colon
24. WR   CV WR CV
    Esophag / o / gastr / o /
    WR   CV   S
    duoden / o / scopy   visual examination of the esophagus, stomach, and duodenum

Exercise 5

1. stomatitis
2. cholecystitis
3. cholelithiasis
4. cholecysto<u>gram</u> / D

5. cholecys<u>tectomy</u> / S
6. pancreatitis
7. proctoscope
8. procto<u>scopy</u> / D
9. abdomino<u>centesis</u> / D
10. colo<u>stomy</u> / S
11. ileo<u>stomy</u> / S
12. esophago<u>scopy</u> / D
13. gastroscope
14. esophagoenterostomy / S
15. gastritis
16. glosso<u>rrhaphy</u> / S
17. cheilo<u>plasty</u> / S
18. col<u>ectomy</u> / S
19. glossoplegia
20. stomatogastric
21. sublingual
22. proctorrhea
23. hepatomegaly
24. hepatoma
25. pancreatic
26. appendicitis
27. append<u>ectomy</u> / S
28. colono<u>scopy</u> / D
29. colonoscope
30. esophagogastroduodeno<u>scopy</u> / D

Exercise 6

1. condition of painful intestines accompanied by diarrhea
2. X-ray image of the esophagus and the stomach
3. X-ray image of the colon
4. X-ray image of the gallbladder
5. yellowness of the skin and eyes
6. inflammation of the colon with the formation of ulcers
7. ulcer in the stomach
8. chronic inflammatory disease that can affect any part of the bowel

Exercise 7

Spelling exercise

Exercise 8

1. b. ileostomy: Ile is the word root for the small intestine; -stomy is the suffix that means artificial opening.
2. cholelithiasis / cholecystogram / cholecystectomy
3. sublingual
4. a. esophagoscopy, esophagoscope
   b. gastroscopy, gastroscope
   c. proctoscopy, proctoscope
5. upper gastrointestinal (UGI) / barium enema (BE)
   a. gastrectomy
   b. pyloroplasty
   c. vagotomy
6. a. laparotomy
   b. (correct)
   c. herniorrhaphy
   d. colectomy
   e. gastrostomy

Exercise 8

1. barium enema
2. gastrointestinal

3. gastroenterology, gastroenterologist
4. gastroesophageal reflux
5. esophagogastroduodenoscopy
6. peptic ulcer disease
7. upper gastrointestinal

Unit 8
Review Questions

1. oxygen / carbon dioxide
2. oxygen / carbon dioxide
3. a. nose
   b. pharynx
   c. larynx
   d. trachea
   e. bronchus
   f. bronchioles
   g. alveoli
4. pharynx / epiglottis
5. a. warmed and moistened
   b. pathogenic microorganisms removed
   c. foreign particles removed
6. larynx
7. Cone-shaped organs located in the thoracic cavity. The right is larger and is divided into three lobes, whereas the left has only two lobes. The bronchus, after entering the lung, continues to subdivide into smaller tubes called bronchioles. At the end of each is a cluster of air sacs or alveoli. The pleura is a double sac that surrounds each lung.
8. a. hemothorax
   b. pneumothorax
   c. atelectasis
   d. pulmonary embolism
9. chronic obstructive pulmonary disease
10. a. cigarette smoking
    b. environmental pollution
    c. occupational hazards
    d. chronic infections

Exercise 1

1. bronch / o
2. laryng / o
3. pharyng / o
4. pleur / o
6. pneum / o
7. pneumon / o
8. pulmon / o
9. rhin / o
12. trache / o

Exercise 2

1. pneum / o, pneumon / o, pulmon / o
2. pharyng / o
3. laryng / o
4. trache / o
5. tonsill / o
6. bronch / o
7. pleur / o
8. rhin / o
9. pnea / o
10. thorac / o

Exercise 3

1. P   WR
    dys / pnea   difficulty breathing
    WR   CV   S
    pharyng / o / cele   abnormal protrusion in
                         the pharynx

3. P   S
    a / pnea   without breathing
                         (temporary stopping
                         of breathing)

4. WR   CV WR   S
    bronch / o / trache / al   pertaining to the bronchi
                               and trachea

5. WR   CV   WR   S
    trache / o / esophag / eal   pertaining to the trachea
                                 and esophagus

6. P   WR   S
    endo / trache / al   pertaining to within the
                         trachea

7. WR   CV   S
    pharyng / o / plegia   paralysis of the pharynx

8. WR   CV WR   S
    rhin / o / pharyng / itis   inflammation of the nose
                                and throat

9. WR   CV   S
    rhin / o / rrhagia   rapid flow of blood
                         from the nose
                         (nosebleed)

10. WR   CV   S
    bronch / o / scope   instrument used for
                         visual examination of
                         the bronchi

11. WR   CV   S
    bronch / o / scopy   visual examination of the
                         bronchi

Exercise 4

1. bronchitis
2. laryngitis
3. tracheostomy
4. pneumonectomy or pneumectomy
5. lobectomy
6. pleuropexy
7. rhinoplasty
8. thoracotomy
9. thoracentesis or thoracocentesis
10. tonsillitis
11. adenoiditis

Exercise 5

1. pneumothorax
2. emphysema
3. pneumonia
4. pleuropexy
5. pharyngitis

Exercise 6

1. tissue in the nasopharynx
2. excision of a lobe of the lung
3. disease of the alveoli of the lung
4. (infection or) inflammation of a lung

5. (infection or) inflammation of the pharynx, larynx, or
    bronchi
6. without breathing (temporary stopping of breathing)
7. difficulty breathing
8. abnormal protrusion in the pharynx
9. excision of the larynx
10. air in pleural cavity (that causes lung to collapse)
11. rapid flow of blood from the nose (nosebleed)
12. X-ray image of the lung and bronchi
13. instrument used for visual examination of the larynx
14. chronic disease characterized by attacks of dyspnea,
    wheezing, and coughing
15. chronic obstruction of the airway
16. chronic infectious disease that commonly affects the lungs

Exercise 7

Spelling exercise

Exercise 8

1. thoracocentesis
2. laryngoscope / endotracheal
3. dyspnea / tracheostomy / tracheostomy / tracheostomy
4. bronchoscopy / bronchoscope
5. pneumothorax / dyspnea / thoracotomy / thoracotomy
6. tonsillectomy, adenoidectomy

Exercise 9

1. acute (adult) respiratory distress syndrome
2. chronic obstructive pulmonary disease
3. endotracheal
4. nasopharyngeal
5. pulmonary embolism
6. respiratory syncytial virus
7. severe acute respiratory syndrome
8. tuberculosis
9. upper respiratory infection

Unit 9
Review Questions

1. urethra
2. to monitor and regulate extracellular fluids and to remove
    some of the waste material from the blood and excrete it
    from the body
3. nephron, to remove waste materials and water from the
    blood; the process of filtration begins at the entrance of the
    nephron in the glomeruli
4. Two ureters drain the urine to the bladder, and then it passes
    from the bladder through the urethra to the outside.
5. water / waste material
6. antidiuretic hormone / anterior pituitary gland
7   a. produce sperm
    b. produce testosterone
8. The sperm passes from the seminiferous tubules to the
    epididymis through the vas deferens, and then through the
    urethra to the outside of the body. The seminal vesicles and
    the prostate gland add solution to the sperm along the pas-
    sageway.
9. 1. c
    2. e
    3. b
    4. g

Exercise 1

1. a. 1. cyst / o
     2. nephr / o or ren / o
     3. pyel / o
     4. nephr / o or ren / o
     6. ureter / o
     7. urethr / o
   b. 6. ureter / o
     7. urethr / o
     9. rchi / o or orchid / o
     10. rchi / o or orchid / o
     11. prostat / o
     12. vas / o

Exercise 2

1. ur / o, urin / o
2. pyel / o
3. ren / o, nephr / o
4. ureter / o
5. cyst / o
6. orchi / o, orchid / o
7. vas / o
8. urethr / o
9. urin / o
10. prostat / o

Exercise 3

1. W   R S
   ur / emia   urine in the blood
2. WR   CV   S
   ur / o / logist   doctor who specializes in the
                                diagnosis and treatment of
                                diseases of the urinary tract
                                and of the male reproduc-
                                tive organs
3. WR   CV WR CV S
   nephr/o/lith/o/tomy   incision into the kidney to
                                remove a stone
4. WR   S
   prostat / ectomy   surgical removal of the pros-
                                tate gland
5. WR   S
   nephr / itis   inflammation of the kidney
6. WR CV   S
   ur / o / logy   study of urine (branch of
                                medicine that deals with
                                the urinary system and the
                                male reproductive system)
7. WR   S
   orchi / ectomy   excision of a testis
8. WR   CV WR   S
   nephr / o / lith / iasis   condition of kidney stone
9. WR   CV   S
   cyst / o / cele   herniation of the urinary
                                bladder
10. WR   CV   S
    cysts / o / scopy   visual examination of the
                                bladder
11. WR   S
    nephr / ectomy   excision of a kidney
12. WR   CV   S
    nephr / o / pexy   surgical fixation of a kidney

13. WR   CV   WR   S
    pyel / o / nephr / itis   inflammation of the kidney
                                and renal pelvis
14. WR   S
    ureter / algia   pain in the ureter
15. WR   S
    urethr / al   pertaining to the urethra
16. WR   CV WR CV S
    ureter / o / lith / o / tomy incision into the ureter to
                                  remove a stone
17. WR   S
    cyst / itis   inflammation of the bladder
18. WR   CV   S
    urethr / o / plasty   surgical repair of the urethra
19. WR   CV   S
    urethr / o / rrhaphy   suture of a urethral tear

Exercise 4

1. cystoscopy
2. nephritis
3. nephrectomy
4. urologist
5. hematuria
6. uremia
7. urethrorrhaphy
8. vasectomy
9. prostatectomy
10. ureteralgia
11. cystocele
12. cystogram
13. pyelonephritis
14. nephrolithotomy
15. urethroplasty
16. nephropexy
17. urology
18. orchiectomy or orchidectomy

Exercise 5

1. a laboratory test to analyze urine to assist in the diagnosis of disease
2. kidney stone
3. swelling of the scrotum caused by the collection of fluid
4. removal of part of the prostate gland through the urethra
5. surgical removal of the foreskin of the penis
6. pertaining to the urine
7. passage of urine from the body

Exercise 6

Spelling exercise

Exercise 7

1. urinary catheterization / urinalysis
2. cystitis
3. KUB / blood urea nitrogen / BUN
4. urologist
5. cystoscopy / he may be anesthetized

Exercise 8

1. antidiuretic hormone
2. benign prostatic hyperplasia
3. benign prostatomegaly
4. blood urea nitrogen

5. creatinine
6. intravenous pyelogram
7. intravenous urogram
8. kidneys, ureters, and bladder
9. urinary tract infection
10. urinalysis
11. transurethral resection of the prostate

Unit 10

Review Questions

1. estrogen / progesterone / estrogen
2. fallopian tubes
3. cervix
4. to produce the female reproductive cell, to provide hormones, to provide for conception, and to provide for pregnancy
5. a. The uterus contains and nourishes the fetus. It also plays a role in menstruation and labor.
   b. The ovaries produce the female reproductive cell, called the *ovum*. They produce the hormones estrogen and progesterone.
   c. The fallopian tubes are a passageway for the ovum from the ovaries to the uterus. Fertilization takes place in the tubes.
   d. The vagina connects the uterus to the outside of the body. It receives the penis during intercourse and is part of the birth canal through which the baby passes from the uterus to the outside of the body.
6. follicle-stimulating hormone
7. pelvic inflammatory disease
8. ectopic pregnancy
9. endometriosis

Exercise 1

1. cervic / o
2. colp / o
4. hyster / o
8. metr / o
9. oophor / o
11. salping / o
12. uter / o
13. vagin / o

Exercise 2

1. men / o
2. gynec / o
3. colp / o or vagin / o
4. perine / o
5. salping / o
6. oophor / o
7. hyster / o, metr / o, or uter / o
8. cervic / o
9. mast / o or mamm / o

Exercise 3

1. WR   CV   S
   gynec / o / logy   study of women (branch of medicine that deals with female reproductive organs)

2. WR   CV   S
   colp / o / rrhaphy   suture of the vagina

3. WR   S
   oophor / ectomy   surgical removal of an ovary

4. WR   S
   oophor / itis   inflammation of an ovary

5. WR   CV WR   S
   salping / o / oophor / ectomy   excision of a fallopian tube and an ovary

6. WR   CV   S
   salping / o / pexy   surgical fixation of a fallopian tube

7. WR   S
   hyster / ectomy   surgical removal of the uterus

8. P   WR CV   S
   dys / men / o / rrhea   painful menstrual discharge

9. WR   CV   S
   colp / o / scope   instrument used for visual examination of the vagina (and cervix)

10. WR   CV   S
    mamm / o / plasty   surgical repair of the breast(s)

11. P   WR CV   S
    a / men / o / rrhea   without menstrual discharge

12. WR   CV   S
    mamm / o / gram   X-ray image of the breast

13. WR   CV WR CV   S
    hyster / o / salping / o / gram   X-ray image of the uterus and fallopian tubes

14. WR   CV   S
    colp / o / scopy   visual examination of the vagina and cervix

Exercise 4

1. oophorectomy
2. gynecology
3. salpingopexy
4. oophoritis
5. colposcope
6. metrorrhea
7. cervicectomy
8. hysterosalpingo-oophorectomy
9. salpingocele
10. ureterovaginal
11. cervicitis
12. hysterectomy
13. colporrhaphy
14. perineoplasty
15. vaginal
16. mastectomy
17. salpingo-oophorectomy
18. dysmenorrhea
19. hysterosalpingogram
20. amenorrhea
21. mammogram
22. mammoplasty
23. colposcopy

Exercise 5

1. physician who specializes in the diagnosis and treatment of women
2. pertaining to the uterus
3. instrument used for expanding the vagina to allow for visual examination of the vagina and cervix
4. excessive uterine bleeding during and between periods.

5. surgical procedure to scrape the uterus and the inner walls
6. female reproductive cell

Exercise 6

a. dilation and curettage
b. hysterosalpingo-oophorectomy
c. perineoplasty
d. colporrhaphy
e. salpingopexy

Exercise 7

Spelling exercise

Exercise 8

1. f
2. a
3. b
4. c
5. g
6. h
7. d
8. e

Exercise 9

1. a doctor who practices obstetrics
2. source of nourishment for the unborn child
3. fluid that surrounds the fetus
4. incision into the uterus through the abdominal wall to deliver the fetus

Exercise 10

1. gynecology / obstetrics
2. vaginal speculum / cervical Pap smear

Exercise 11

1. cesarean section
2. dilation and curettage
3. follicle-stimulating hormone
4. obstetrics, obstetrical
5. pelvic inflammatory disease
6. postpartum
7. term – premature – abortions – living
8. estimated date of delivery

Unit 11

Review Questions

1. iodine
2. a. 2, 3, 4, 6, 10
   b. 7
   c. 11
   d. 5, 12
   e. 1
   f. 9
   g. 8
3. The hormones it produces stimulate the functions of the other endocrine glands. The hypothalamus directly regulates the secretory activity of the pituitary gland.
4. communication, integration, and control
5. islets of Langerhans / pancreas
6. necessary for the metabolism of carbohydrates in the body

7. a. polyuria
   b. polydipsia
   c. glycosuria
   d. hyperglycemia
   e. polyphagia
8. hyperthyroidism

Exercise 1

1. aden / o
2. thyr / o, thyroid / o
3. adren / o, adrenal / o
4. parathyroid / o

Exercise 2

1. adenitis
2. thyroidectomy
3. parathyroidectomy
4. adenoid
5. adenoma
6. adenosis
7. adrenalitis

Exercise 3

1. islets of Langerhans (pancreas)
2. thyroid gland
3. adrenal gland
4. thyroid gland
5. adrenal gland
6. pituitary gland

Exercise 4

1. diabetes insipidus
2. Addison's disease
3. Cushing's disease
4. hypothyroidism
5. secretions

Exercise 5

Spelling exercise

Exercise 6

1. diabetes mellitus / islets of Langerhans / Ua / FBS / GTT / HbA_{1C} / blood glucose monitoring
2. a. pituitary
   b. adrenal cortex
   c. islets of Langerhans
   d. adrenal medulla
   e. ovary
   f. testes
   g. thyroid gland
3. a. protein-bound iodine
   b. T_3, T_4, T_7 uptake
   c. thyroid scan

Exercise 7

1. adrenocorticotropic hormone
2. diabetes mellitus
3. follicle-stimulating hormone
4. glycohemoglobin (glycosylated hemoglobin)
5. luteinizing hormone
6. prolactin

Glossary

Following is a list of terms that are discussed throughout the book. After each definition is the number of the chapter in which the term is introduced. Additional terms may be found in content-specific chapter vocabulary lists. Page numbers for all terms may be located in the Index.

Accepting Assignment Providers of medical services agreeing that the receipt of payment from Medicare for a professional service will constitute full payment for that service (2)

Accountability Taking responsibility for your actions, being answerable to someone for something you have done (6)

Accreditation Recognition that a health care organization has met an official standard (2)

Ace Wraps Elastic gauze used for temporary compression to various parts of the body to decrease swelling and skin breakdown (11)

Active Exercise Exercise performed by the patient without assistance as instructed by the physical therapist (17)

Activities of Daily Living Tasks that enable individuals to meet basic needs (e.g., eating, bathing) (17)

Acuity Level of care a patient would require based on his or her medical condition, used to evaluate staffing needs (3)

Acute Care Short-term care for serious illness or trauma (2)

Admission Day Surgery Surgery for which the patient enters the hospital on the day of surgery; it may be called *same-day surgery* or A.M. *admission* (19)

Admission Service Agreement or Conditions of Admission Agreement Form signed upon the patient's admission that sets forth the general services that the hospital will provide; also may be called *conditions of admission, contract for services,* or *treatment consent* (19)

Admixture The result of adding a medication to a container of intravenous solution (13)

Advance Directives Documents that indicate a patient's wishes in the event that the patient becomes incapacitated (19)

Adverse Drug Event Injury or harmful reaction that results from the use of a drug (13)

Aerobic Living only in the presence of oxygen (17)

Aerosol Liquid suspension of particles in a gas stream for inhalation purposes (17)

Afebrile Without fever (10)

Ageism Discrimination on grounds of age (5)

Aggressive Behavioral style in which a person attempts to be the dominant force in an interaction (5)

Airborne Precautions/Isolation Required use of mask and ventilated room, in conjunction with standard precautions (22)

Allergy Acquired, abnormal immune response to a substance that does not normally cause a reaction; may involve medications, food, tape, and many other substances (8)

Amniocentesis Needle puncture into the uterine cavity performed to remove amniotic fluid, the liquid that surrounds the unborn baby (14)

Ampoule (Ampule) Small glass vial sealed to keep contents sterile; used for subcutaneous, intramuscular, and intravenous medications (13)

Anorexia Nervosa Intense fear of gaining weight or becoming fat, although underweight (12)

Antibody Immunoglobulin (protein) produced by the body that reacts with and neutralizes an antigen (usually a foreign substance) (14)

Antigen Any substance that induces an immune response (14)

Apical Rate Heart rate obtained from the apex of the heart (10)

Apnea Cessation of breathing (16)

Apothecary System Ancient system of weight and volume measurements used to measure drugs and solutions (13)

Aquathermia Pad Waterproof plastic or rubber pad connected to a bedside control used to apply heat or cold (also called a K-Pad or a water flow pad) (11)

Arterial Blood Gases (ABGs) Diagnostic study to measure arterial blood gases (oxygen and carbon dioxide) to gather information needed to assess and manage a patient's respiratory status (16)

Arterial Line (art line) Catheter placed in an artery that continuously measures the patient's blood pressure (11)

Assertive Behavioral style in which a person stands up for his or her own rights and feelings without violating the rights and feelings of others (5)

Attending Physician Term applied to a physician who admits and is responsible for a hospital patient (2)

Auscultation The act of listening for sounds within the body to evaluate the condition of the heart, blood vessels, lungs, pleura, intestines, or other organs, or to detect the fetal heart sound (17)

Autologous Blood The patient's own blood donated previously for transfusion as needed by the patient; also called autotransfusion (11)

Automatic Stop Date Date on which specific categories of medications must be discontinued unless renewed by the physician (13)

Autonomy Independence; personal liberty (6)

Autopsy Examination of a body after death; may be performed to determine the cause of death or for medical research (20)

Axillary Temperature Temperature reading obtained by placing the thermometer in the patient's axilla (armpit) (10)

Bariatric Surgery Surgery performed on part of the gastrointestinal (GI) tract as treatment for obesity (19)

Bariatrics Field of medicine that focuses on the treatment and control of obesity and diseases associated with obesity (19)

Bedside Commode Chair or wheelchair with an open seat, used at the bedside by the patient for the passage of urine and stool (10)

Biopsy Tissue removed from a living body for examination (14)

Blood Gases Diagnostic study to determine the exchange of gases in the blood (16)

Blood Pressure Measure of the pressure of blood against the walls of the blood vessels (10)

Body Mass Index (BMI) Body weight in kilograms divided by height in square meters. This is the usual measurement used to define overweight and obesity (12)

Bolus Concentrated dose of medication or fluid, frequently given intravenously (13)

Brainstorming Structured group activity that allows three to ten people to tap into the creativity of the group to identify new ideas. Typically in quality improvement, the technique is used to identify probable causes and possible solutions for quality problems (7)

Broken Record Assertive skill, wherein a person repeats his or her position over and over again (5)

B-scan Image made up of a series of dots, each indicating a single ultrasonic echo. The position of a dot corresponds to the time elapsed, and the brightness of a dot corresponds to the strength of the echo (16)

Bulimia Nervosa Recurrent episodes of binge eating (rapid consumption of a large amount of food in a discrete period of time) and self-induced vomiting, with use of laxatives or diuretics (12)

Caloric Study Test performed to evaluate the function of cranial nerve VIII. It also can indicate disease in the temporal portion of the cerebrum (16)

Calorie Measurement of energy generated in the body by the heat produced after food is eaten (11)

Capillary Blood Gases (CBG) Diagnostic study performed primarily on infants. Blood is obtained from the infant's capillary arterial vessel, usually from the heel (16)

Capitation Payment method whereby the provider of care receives a set dollar amount per patient regardless of services rendered (2)

Capsule Gelatinous single-dose container in which a drug is enclosed to prevent the patient from tasting the drug (13)

Cardiac Arrest The patient's heart contractions are absent or insufficient to produce a pulse or blood pressure; also may be referred to as *code arrest* (22)

Cardiac Monitor Monitor of heart function that provides a visual and audible record of heartbeat (16)

Cardiac Monitor Technician One who monitors patient heart rhythms and notifies the RN of rhythm changes (additional training required); often done in conjunction with health unit coordinator responsibilities on a telemetry unit (1, 16)

Cardiac Pacemaker Electronic device, temporary or permanent, the regulates the pace of the heart when the heart is incapable of doing so (17)

Cardiac Stress Test Noninvasive study that provides information about the patient's cardiac function (16)

Cardiopulmonary Resuscitation (CPR) Basic life-saving procedure of artificial ventilation and chest compressions done in the event of a cardiac arrest (all health care workers are required to be certified in CPR) (7)

Career Ladder Pathway of upward mobility (1)

C-Arm Mobile fluoroscopy unit used in surgery or at the bedside (15)

Case Manager Health care professional and expert in managed care who assists patients in assessing health and social service systems to ensure that all required services are obtained; also coordinates care with doctor and insurance companies (2)

Catastrophic Coverage Coverage that a Medicare beneficiary has after reaching a certain amount of "out of pocket" monies paid for their medications during the temporary coverage gap. The beneficiary will pay a coinsurance amount (like 5% of the drug cost) or a copayment ($2.15 or $5.35 for each prescription) for the rest of the calendar year (2)

Cathartic Agent that causes evacuation of the bowel (laxative) (15)

Catheterization Insertion of a catheter into a body cavity or organ to inject or remove fluid (11)

Celsius Scale used to measure temperature in which the freezing point of water is 0° and the boiling point is 100° (formerly called *Centigrade*) (21)

Census List of all occupied and unoccupied hospital beds (7, 19)

Centers for Disease Control Division of the U.S. Public Health Service that investigates and controls diseases that have epidemic potential (22)

Central Line Catheter or Central Venous Catheter (CVC) Large catheter that provides access to the veins and/or to the heart to measure pressures; catheter is threaded through to the superior vena cava or right atrium; used for administration of intravenous therapy (13)

Central Service Department Charge Slip Form that is initiated to charge a discharged patient for any items that were not charged to him at the time of use (7)

Central Service Department Credit Slip Form that is used to credit a patient for items found in the room unused after the patient's discharge, or if it is found that a patient was mistakenly charged for an item not used for that patient (7)

Central Service Department Discrepancy Report List of items that are missing from the nursing unit patient supply cupboard or closet that were not charged to a patient; it is sent to the nursing unit from the central service department each day (8)

Certification The process of testifying to or endorsing that a person has met certain standards (1)

Chiropractic Medicine A complementary and alternative health care profession with the purpose of diagnosing and treating mechanical disorders of the spine and musculoskeletal system with the intention of affecting the nervous system and improving health (2)

Chronic Care Care for long-duration illnesses such as diabetes or emphysema (2)

Clean Catch (CC) Method of obtaining a urine specimen through a special cleansing technique; also called a *midstream urine* (14)

Clinical Death Occurs when no brain function is present (20)

Clinical Decision Support System (CDSS) Computerized programs that provide suggestions or default values for drug doses, routes, and frequencies. The program also may perform drug allergy checks, drug–laboratory value checks, drug interaction checks, etc. (1, 2)

Clinical Indications (CI) Notations recorded when diagnostic imaging is ordered, to indicate the reason for doing the procedure (15)

Clinical Pathway Method of outlining a patient's path of treatment for a specific diagnosis, procedure, or symptom (3)

Clinical Tasks Tasks performed at the bedside or in direct contact with the patient (1)

Code Blue Term used in hospitals to announce when a patient stops breathing or when his heart stops beating, or both (7)

Code of Ethics Set of standards for behavior based on values (6)

Code or Crash Cart Cart stocked by the nursing and pharmacy staff with emergency medication, advanced breathing supplies, intravenous solutions and appropriate tubing, needles, a heart monitor and defibrillator, an oxygen tank, and a suction machine (used when a patient stops breathing, when his heart stops beating, or both) (7)

Color Doppler Enhanced form of Doppler echocardiography in which different colors are used to designate the direction of blood flow (16)

Communicable Disease Disease that may be transmitted from one person to another (22)

Community Health Emphasis on prevention and early detection of disease for members of a community (2)

Comorbidity The presence of one or more disorders (or diseases) in addition to a primary disease or disorder, or the effect of such additional disorders or diseases (19)

Compression Garment Tight-fitting, custom-made garment used to put constant pressure on healed wounds to keep down scarring (11)

Compressor Grip (C-GRIP) Tight, stretchy, tubular material used for temporary compression (17)

Computed Tomography (CT) Radiographic process of creating computerized images (scans) of body organs in horizontal slices (15)

Computer on Wheels (COW) Computer on a cart with wheels that can be taken into patients' rooms (4)

Computer Physician Order Entry (CPOE) Computerized program into which physicians directly enter patient orders; replaces handwritten orders on an order sheet or prescription pad (1, 2)

Computerized Medication Cart Storage cart that requires confidential user ID and a password to gain access to medications (13)

Computerized Nurses' Notes Documentation entered directly into the patient's electronic medical record, usually at the patient's bedside on a portable computer (3)

Confidentiality Keeping private any confidential information, spoken or written (6)

Conflict Emotional disturbance—striving for one's own preferred outcome, which, if attained, prevents others from achieving their preferred outcomes (5)

Continuous Quality Improvement (CQI) The practice of continuously improving quality at each level of each department of every function of the health care organization (also called total quality management [TQM]) (7)

Contrast Media Substances (solids, liquids, or gases) used in diagnostic imaging procedures that permit the radiologist to distinguish between different body densities; they may be injected, swallowed, or introduced by rectum or vagina (15)

Coroner's Case A death that occurs because of sudden, violent, or unexplained circumstances, or a patient who expires during the first 24 hours after admission to the hospital (20)

Crackle Common, abnormal respiratory sound that consists of discontinuous bubbling noises heard on auscultation of the chest during inspiration (also called *Rale*) (17)

Crisis Stress Profound effect experienced by individuals as the result of common, uncontrollable, often unpredictable life experiences (e.g., death, divorce, illness) (7)

Cultural Differences Factors such as age, gender, race, socioeconomic status, etc. (5)

Culturally Sensitive Care Care that involves understanding and being sensitive to a patient's cultural background (5)

Culture A set of values, beliefs, and traditions that are held by a specific social group (5)

Culture and Sensitivity The growth of microorganisms in a special medium (culture), followed by a test to determine the antibiotic to which they best respond (sensitivity) (14)

Custodial Care Care and services of a nonmedical nature, which consist of feeding, bathing, watching, and protecting the patient (20)

Cytology The study of cells (14)

Daily Laboratory Tests Tests that are ordered once by the doctor but are carried out every day until the doctor discontinues the order (14)

Damages Monetary compensation awarded by a court for an injury caused by the act of another (6)

Dangle The patient sits and dangles his feet over the edge of the bed (10)

Decoding Process of translating symbols received from the sender to determine the message (5)

Defendant Person against whom a civil or criminal action is brought (6)

Defibrillation Application of an electric shock to the myocardium through the chest wall to restore normal cardiac rhythm (17)

Deposition Pretrial statement of a witness under oath, taken in question-and-answer form as it would be in court, with an opportunity given to the adversary to be present to cross-examine (6)

Diagnosis-Related Group (DRG) Classification system used to determine payments from Medicare based on assignment of a standard flat rate to major diagnostic categories. This flat rate is paid to hospitals regardless of the full cost of the services provided (2)

Dialysis Removal from the blood of wastes usually excreted by the kidneys (17)

Dietary Reference Intake (DRI) Framework of nutrient standards now in place in the United States. These provide reference values for use in planning and evaluating diets for healthy people (12)

Dietary Supplement Product (other than tobacco) taken by mouth that contains a "dietary ingredient" intended to supplement the diet. Dietary supplements come in many forms, including extracts, concentrates, tablets, capsules, gel caps, liquids, and powders (12)

Differential Identification of the types of white cells found in the blood (14)

Dipstick Urine Visual examination of urine with the use of a special chemically treated stick (14)

Direct Admission A patient who was not scheduled to be admitted and is admitted from the doctor's office, clinic, or emergency room (19)

Disaster Procedure Planned procedure that is carried out by hospital personnel when a large number of persons have been injured (22)

Discharge Planning Centralized, coordinated, multidisciplinary process that ensures that the patient has a plan for continuing care after leaving the hospital (20)

Discrimination Seeing a difference; prejudicial treatment of a person (6)

Document Management System (DMS) Computer system (or set of computer programs) used to track and store electronic documents and/or images of paper documents (4)

Document Scanner Device used to transmit images of paper documents/pictures to be entered into the patient's electronic record (4)

Donor-Specific or Donor-Directed Blood Blood donated by relatives or friends of the patient to be used for transfusion as needed (11)

Doppler Ultrasound Procedure used to monitor moving substances or structures, such as flowing blood or a beating heart. Used to locate vessel obstructions, to observe fetal heart sounds, to localize the placenta (afterbirth), and to image heart functions (16)

Downtime Requisition Requisition (paper order form) used to process information when the computer is not available for use (4)

Dumbwaiter Mechanical device used to transport food or supplies from one hospital floor to another (4)

Dysphagia Difficulty eating/swallowing (12)

Dyspnea Difficult or labored breathing (17)

Echocardiogram (2D M-mode Echo) Diagnostic, noninvasive procedure in which ultrasound is used to study the structure and motion of the heart (16)

Egg-Crate Mattress Foam-rubber mattress (11)

Elective Surgery Surgery that is not emergency or mandatory and can be planned at a time of convenience (19)

Electrocardiogram (EKG or ECG) Graphic recording produced by electric impulses of the heart (16)

Electroencephalogram (EEG) Graphic recording of the electric impulses of the brain (16)

Electrolytes Group of tests done in chemistry, which usually includes sodium, potassium, chloride, and carbon dioxide (14)

Electromyogram (EMG) Record of muscle contraction produced by electrical stimulation (16)

Electronic Medical Record (EMR) Electronic record of patient health information generated by one or more encounters in any care delivery setting (1, 2)

Electronystagmography Test used to evaluate nystagmus (involuntary rapid eye movement) and the muscles that control eye movement (16)

Electrophysiologic Study (EPS) Invasive measure of electrical activity (16)

Elevated Toilet Seat Elevated seat that fits over a toilet with handrails for patients who have a problem sitting on a lower seat (11)

Elitism Discrimination based on social/economic class (5)

Emergency Admission Admission necessitated by accident or a medical emergency; such an admission is processed through the emergency department (19)

Emesis Vomit (10)

Empathy Capacity for participating in and understanding the feelings or ideas of another (6)

Encoding Translating mental images, feelings, and ideas into symbols to communicate them to the receiver (5)

Endoscopy Visualization of a body cavity or hollow organ by means of an endoscope. Gastrointestinal (GI) studies also are performed in the endoscopy department (16)

Endotracheal Tube (ET Tube) Tube inserted through the mouth that supplies air to the lungs and assists breathing. The ET tube is connected to a ventilator (17)

Enema The introduction of fluid and/or medication into the rectum and sigmoid colon (11)

Enteral Feeding Set Includes equipment needed to infuse tube feeding; includes plastic bag for feeding solution and may be ordered with or without a pump (12)

Enteral Nutrition The provision of liquid formulas into the gastrointestinal (GI) tract by tube or orally (12)

Epidemiology Study of the occurrence, distribution, and causes of health and disease in humans; the specialist is called an epidemiologist (22)

Ergonomics Branch of ecology concerned with human factors in the design and operation of machines and the physical environment (7)

Erythrocyte Red blood cell (14)

Esteem Needs A person's need for self-respect and for the respect of others (5)

Ethics Behavior that is based on values (beliefs); how we make judgments with regard to right and wrong (6)

Ethnocentrism Inability to accept other cultures, or an assumption of cultural superiority (5)

Evidence All the means by which any alleged matter of fact, the truth of which is submitted to investigation at trial, is established or disproved; evidence includes the testimony of witnesses and the introduction of records, documents, exhibits, objects, or any other substantiating matter offered for the purpose of inducing belief in the party's contention by the judge or jury (6)

Evoked Potential Studies Tests used to evaluate specific areas of the cortex that receive incoming stimuli from the sensory nerves of the eyes, ears, and lower or upper extremities (16)

Expert Witness Witness who has special knowledge of the subject about which he or she is to testify; the knowledge generally must be such that it is not normally possessed by the average person (6)

Expiration A death (20)

Extended Care Facility Medical facility that cares for patients who require expert nursing care or custodial care (20)

Extravasation Leakage of fluid into tissue surrounding a vein (13)

Extubation Removal of a previously inserted tube (such as an endotracheal tube) (17)

Face Sheet Form initiated by the admitting department and included in the inpatient medical record that contains personal and demographic information; usually computer generated at the time of admission (also may be called the *information sheet* or *front sheet*) (19)

Fahrenheit Scale used to measure temperature in which 32° is the freezing point of water and 212° is the boiling point (21)

Fasting No solid foods by mouth and no fluids that contain nourishment (e.g., sugar, milk) (14)

Febrile Elevated body temperature (fever) (10)

Feedback Response to a message (5)

Feeding Tube Small, flexible plastic tube that usually is placed in the patient's nose and that goes down to the stomach or small intestine to provide and/or increase nutritional intake (12)

Fidelity Doing what one promises (6)

Fluoroscopy Observation of deep body structures that are made visible by the use of a viewing screen instead of film; contrast medium is required for this procedure (15)

Fogging Assertive Skill Skill in which a person responds to a criticism by making noncommittal statements that cannot be argued against (5)

Foley Catheter Type of indwelling retention catheter (11)

Food Allergy Negative physical reaction to a particular food involving the immune system (people with food allergies must avoid the offending foods) (12)

Food and Drug Administration (FDA) U.S. Government agency whose purpose is to ensure that foods, drugs, cosmetics, and medical devices are safe and labeled properly (13)

Food Intolerance A more common problem than food allergies involving digestion (people with food intolerances can eat some of the offending food without suffering symptoms) (12)

Fowler's Position Semi-sitting position (10)

Gastric Suction Used to remove gastric contents (11)

Gastritis Inflammation of the stomach (12)

Gastroenteritis Inflammation of the stomach and intestines (12)

Gastrointestinal Study Diagnostic study related to the gastrointestinal system (16)

Gastrostomy Feeding Feeding by means of a tube inserted into the stomach through an artificial opening in the abdominal wall (12)

Gavage Feeding by means of a tube inserted into the stomach, duodenum, or jejunum, through the nose or an opening in the abdominal wall; also called *tube feeding* (12)

GI Study Diagnostic study related to the gastrointestinal system (16)

Guaiac Method of testing stool and urine using guaiac as a reagent for hidden (occult) blood (also may be called a *Hemoccult slide test*) (14)

Harris Flush or Return Flow Enema Mild colonic irrigation that helps expel flatus (11)

Health Maintenance Organization Organization that has management responsibility for providing comprehensive health care services on a prepayment basis to voluntarily enrolled persons within a designated population (2)

Health Records Number Number assigned to the patient on or before admission; it is used for record identification and is used for all subsequent admissions to that hospital (also may be called *medical records number*) (19)

Hemovac Disposable suction device (evacuator unit) that is connected to a drain inserted into or close to a surgical wound (11)

Heparin Lock Intravenous (IV) catheter with a small chamber that is covered with a rubber diaphragm or a specially designed cap and is used to administer medications or to gain venous access in case of an emergency; also called a **Saline Lock** (11, 13)

Hepatitis B Virus (HBV) Infectious blood-borne disease that is a major occupational hazard for health care workers (22)

Holistic Nursing Care Modern nursing practice that expresses the philosophy of total patient care and considers the physical, emotional, social, economic, and spiritual needs of the patient; also called *Comprehensive Care* (3)

Holter Monitor Portable device that records the heart's electrical activity and produces a continuous electrocardiographic (ECG) tracing over a specified period (16)

Home Health Equipment and services made available to patients in the home to provide comfort and care (2)

Homeopathic Medicine Alternative medical system. Belief that "like cures like," meaning that small, highly diluted quantities of medicinal substances are given to cure symptoms, when the same substances given at higher or more concentrated doses would actually cause those symptoms (2)

Hospice Supportive care for terminally ill patients and their families (2)

Hospitalist Full-time, acute care specialist who focuses exclusively on hospitalized patients (2)

Hostile Environment Sexually oriented atmosphere or pattern of behavior that is determined to be sexual harassment (6)

HUC Preceptor Experienced, working health unit coordinator (HUC) selected to train/teach an HUC student or new employee (5)

Human Immunodeficiency Virus (HIV) Virus that causes acquired immunodeficiency syndrome (AIDS) (22)

Hydration Adequate water in the intracellular and extracellular compartments of the body (12)

Hydrotherapy Treatment with water (17)

Hyperbaric Oxygen Therapy (HBOT) Treatment that involves breathing 100% oxygen while in an enclosed system pressurized to greater than one atmosphere (sea level) (17)

Hypertonic Concentrated salt solution (>0.9%) (17)

Hypnotics Drugs that reduce pain or induce sleep; may include sedatives, analgesics, and anesthetics (13)

Hypotonic Dilute salt solution (0.9%) (17)

Impedance Cardiography (ICG) Flexible and fast-acting noninvasive monitoring system that measures total impedance (resistance to the flow of electricity in the heart) (16)

Implied Contract Nonexplicit agreement that affects some aspect of the employment relationship (6)

Incident Episode that normally does not occur within the regular hospital routine (22)

Incontinence Inability of the body to control the elimination of urine and/or feces (11)

Induced Sputum Specimen Sputum specimen obtained by performing respiratory treatment to loosen lung secretions (17)

Indwelling (Retention) Catheter Catheter that remains in the bladder for a longer period until a patient is able to void completely and voluntarily, or as long as hourly accurate measurements are needed (11)

Infiltration The tip of the intravenous (IV) catheter comes out of the vein or pokes through the vein, and the IV solution is released into surrounding tissue. This also could occur if the wall of the vein becomes permeable and leaks fluid (11)

Informed Consent Doctrine that states that before a patient is asked to consent to a risky or invasive diagnostic or treatment procedure, he is entitled to receive certain information: (1) a description of the procedure, (2) any alternatives to it and their risks, (3) the risks of death or serious bodily disability associated with the procedure, (4) probable results of the procedure, including any anticipated problems with recuperation and time needed for recuperation, and (5) anything else that generally is disclosed to patients who are asked to consent to the procedure (6, 19)

Infusion Pump Device used to regulate flow or rate of intravenous fluid; commonly called an *IV pump* (11)

Ingestion Taking in of food by mouth (12)

Injectables Medications that are given by forcing a liquid into the body by means of a needle and syringe (intra-arterial, intradermal, intramuscular, intravenous, and subcutaneous) (13)

Instillation Slow introduction of fluid into a cavity or passage of the body that should remain for a specific length of time before it is drained or withdrawn; purpose is to expose tissues in the area to the solution, to hot or cold, or to a drug or substance in the solution (13)

Insufflate To blow a gas or powder into a tube, cavity, or organ to allow visual examination, to remove an obstruction, or to apply medication (13)

Intake and Output Measurement of the patient's fluid intake and output (10)

Integrated Delivery Networks Health care organizations merged into systems that can provide all needed health care services under a single corporate umbrella (2)

Interdisciplinary Teamwork Well-coordinated collaboration across health care professionals toward a common goal (i.e., improved, efficient patient care) (3)

Intermittent (Straight) Catheter Single-use catheter that is introduced and kept in place long enough to drain the bladder (5 to 10 minutes) and then is removed (11)

International Statistical Classification of Diseases and Related Health Problems Detailed description of known diseases and injuries. Every disease (or group of related diseases) is described along with its diagnosis and is given a unique code, up to six characters long; published by the World Health Organization (2)

Interpreter Person who facilitates oral communication between or among parties who are conversing in different languages (5)

Intervention Synonymous with treatment (17)

Intramuscular (IM) Injection Injection of a medication into a muscle (13)

Intravenous (IV) Administered directly into a vein (13)

Intravenous Hyperalimentation or Total Parenteral Nutrition (TPN) Method used to administer calories, proteins, vitamins, and other nutrients into the bloodstream of a patient who is unable to eat; must be infused into the superior vena cava through a central line catheter—not given through a peripheral IV catheter (13)

Intravenous Infusion Administration of fluid through a vein (11)

Intubation Insertion and placement of a tube (within the trachea, may be endotracheal or tracheostomy) (17)

Invasive Procedure Diagnostic or therapeutic technique that requires entry of a body cavity or interruption of normal body functions (16)

Irrigation Washing out of a body cavity, organ, or wound (11)

Isolation Placement of a patient apart from other patients insofar as movement and social contact are concerned, for the purpose of preventing the spread of infection (22)

Isometric Of equal dimensions; holding ends of contracting muscle fixed so that contraction produces increased tension at a constant overall length (17)

IV (intravenous) Push (IVP) Method of giving concentrated doses of medication directly into the vein (13)

Jackson-Pratt (JP) Disposable suction device (evacuator unit) that is connected to a drain inserted into or close to a surgical wound (11)

Kangaroo Pump Brand name of a feeding pump used to administer tube feeding (12)

K-Pad Electric device used for heat application (also called *K-thermia pad, aquathermia pad,* or *aquamatic pad*) (11)

Kosher Adherence to the dietary laws of Judaism; conventional meaning in Hebrew is "acceptable" or "approved" (12)

Liability Condition of being responsible for damages resulting from an injurious act or for discharging an obligation or debt (6)

Living Will Declaration made by the patient to the family, medical staff, and all concerned with the patient's care, stating what is to be done in the event of a terminal illness; directs the withholding or withdrawing of life-sustaining procedures (19)

Locator Small tracking device worn by nursing personnel and health unit coordinators so that their location may be detected on the interactive console display when necessary (4)

Love and Belonging Needs A person's need to have affectionate relationships with people and to have a place in a group (5)

Lozenge Medicated tablet or disk that dissolves in the mouth (13)

Lumbar Puncture Procedure performed to remove cerebrospinal fluid from the spinal canal (14)

Magnet Status Award given by the American Nurses' Credentialing Center (ANCC) to hospitals that satisfy a set of criteria designed to measure their strength of quality of nursing (2)

Magnetic Resonance Imaging (MRI) Technique used to produce computer images (scans) of the interior of the body with the use of magnetic fields (15)

Managed Care Use of a planned and systematic approach to providing health care, with the goal of offering quality care at the lowest possible cost (2)

Manometric Studies Procedures performed to evaluate certain areas of the body with the use of a manometric device to measure and record pressures; usually performed in the endoscopy department (16)

Material Safety Data Sheet (MSDS) Basic hazard communication tool that provides details on chemical dangers and safety procedures (22)

Medicaid Federal and state program that provides medical assistance for the indigent (2)

Medical Emergency Emergency that is life threatening (22)

Medical Malpractice Professional negligence of a health care professional; failure to meet a professional standard of care, resulting in harm to another, for example, failure to provide "good and accepted medical care" (6)

Medical Savings Accounts (MSAs) Tax-exempt bank accounts that are *owned by an individual* and managed by a financial institution. The individual must have a qualified health plan. An individual cannot use the tax benefits of an MSA until the qualified health plan is in place. The qualified health insurance policy can be completely independent of the MSA (2)

Medicare Government insurance enacted in 1965 for individuals over the age of 65; any person with a disability who has received Social Security for 2 years (some disabilities are covered immediately) (2)

Medicare Supplement Private insurance plan available to Medicare-eligible persons to cover the costs of medical care not covered by Medicare (2)

Medication Administration Record (MAR) List of medications that each individual patient is currently taking; used by the nurse to administer the medications (13)

Medication Nurse Registered nurse or licensed practical nurse who administers medications to patients (13)

Menu List of options that is projected onto the viewing screen of the computer (4)

Merger Combining of individual physician practices and small, stand-alone hospitals into larger networks (2)

Message Images, feelings, and ideas transmitted from one person to another (5)

Metastasis Process by which tumor cells spread to distant parts of the body (15)

Methicillin-resistant Staphylococcus aureus (MRSA) A variation of the common bacteria, *Staphylococcus aureus* (22)

Metric System System of weights and measures based on multiples of 10 (13)

Microfilm Film that contains a greatly reduced photographic image of printed or graphic matter (18)

M-Mode Echo Image obtained with M-mode echocardiography that shows the motion (M) of the heart over time. 2D M-mode would be a two-dimensional study (16)

Modality Method of application or employment of any therapeutic agent; limited usually to physical agents and devices (15)

Modem Device that enables a computer to send and receive data over regular phone lines (4)

Morbid Obesity Excess of body fat that threatens necessary body functions such as respiration (12)

Name Alert Method of alerting staff when two or more patients with the same or similarly spelled last names are located on a nursing unit (8)

Narcolepsy Chronic ailment that consists of recurrent attacks of drowsiness and sleep during the daytime (16)

Narcotic Controlled drug that relieves pain or produces sleep (13)

Nasogastric Tube (NG Tube) Tube that is inserted through the nose into the stomach (11)

Naturopathic Medicine Alternative medical system that proposes the existence of a healing power in the body that establishes, maintains, and restores health. Treatments include nutrition and lifestyle counseling, nutritional supplements, medicinal plants, exercise, homeopathy, and treatments from traditional Chinese medicine (2)

Nebulizer Gas-driven device that produces an aerosol (17)

Needleless IV Hep-lock Safe, sharp device that is placed on a peripheral intravenous catheter when used intermittently (11)

Negative Assertion Assertive skill by which a person verbally accepts the fact that he has made an error, without allowing it to reflect on his worth as a human being (5)

Negative Inquiry Assertive skill by which a person requests further clarification of a criticism to get to the real issue (5)

Negligence Failure to satisfactorily perform one's legal duty, such that another person incurs some injury (6)

Nerve Conduction Studies (NCS) Measures how well individual nerves can transmit electrical signals (often performed with an electromyogram) (16)

Neurologic Vital Signs (Neuro-checks) Measurement of the function of the body's neurologic system; includes checking pupils of the eyes, verbal response, and so forth (10)

Nonassertive Behavioral style by which a person allows others to dictate his self-worth (5)

Non-clinical Tasks Tasks performed away from the bedside (1)

Noninvasive Procedure Procedure that does not require entry into the body, as with puncturing of the skin (16)

Nonverbal Communication Communication that is not written or spoken but that creates a message between two or more people through the use of eye contact, body language, and symbolic and facial expression (5)

Nosocomial Infection Infection that is acquired from within the health care facility (22)

Nuclear Medicine Technique that uses radioactive materials to determine the functional capacity of an organ (15)

Nursing Intervention Any act by a nurse that implements the nursing care plan or clinical pathway, or any specific objective of that plan or pathway (3)

Nutrients Substances derived from food that are used by body cells, for example, carbohydrates, fats, proteins, vitamins, minerals, and water (12)

Obesity Excess amount of body fat usually defined by body mass index (12)

Observation Patient Patient who is assigned to a bed on the nursing unit to receive care for a period of less than 24 hours; also may be referred to as a *medical short stay or ambulatory patient* (19)

Obstructive Sleep Apnea (OSA) Cessation of breathing during sleep (16)

Occlusion Blockage in a canal, vessel, or passage of the body (16)

Occult Blood Blood that is undetectable to the eye (14)

Occupational Safety and Health Administration (OSHA) U.S. government regulatory agency concerned with the health and safety of workers (22)

Old Record Patient's record from previous admissions stored in the health records department that may be retrieved for review when a patient is admitted to the emergency room, nursing unit, or outpatient department (older microfilmed records may be requested by the patient's doctor) (8)

"On Call" Medication Medication prescribed by the doctor to be given prior to the diagnostic imaging procedure; the department notifies the nursing unit of the time the medication is to be administered to the patient (15)

One-Time or Short-Series Order Doctors' order that is executed according to the qualifying phrase, and then is automatically discontinued (9)

Organ Donation Donating or giving one's organs and/or tissues after death; one may designate specific organs (i.e., only cornea) or any needed organs (20)

Organ Procurement Process of removing donated organs; may be referred to as harvesting (20)

Orthostatic Hypotension Temporary lowering of blood pressure (hypotension) usually caused by standing up suddenly; also called *postural hypotension* (10)

Orthostatic Vital Signs Measurement of blood pressure and pulse rate first in supine (lying), then in sitting, and finally in standing position (11)

Over-the-Counter Drugs (OTC) The FDA defines OTC drugs as safe and effective for use by the general public without a doctor's prescription (13)

Oxygen Saturation Noninvasive measurement of gas exchange and red blood cell oxygen-carrying capacity (10, 16)

Parenteral Nutrition Mode of feeding that does not use the gastrointestinal tract; instead, nutrition is provided by intravenous delivery of nutrient solutions (12)

Patent or Patency Term that indicates that no clots are present at the tip of the needle or catheter, and that the needle tip or catheter is not against the vein wall (open) (11)

Pacemaker Electronic device, temporary or permanent, that regulates the pace of the heart when the heart is incapable of doing so (16)

Pap Smear Test performed to detect cancerous cells in the female genital tract; the Pap staining method also can be used to study body secretions and excretions and tissue scrapings (14)

Paracentesis Surgical puncture and drainage of a body cavity (14)

Paraphrase Repeating messages in your own words to clarify their meaning (5)

Parenteral Routes Nonoral methods used for giving fluids or medications (e.g., injection, intravenous approach) (13)

Passive Exercise Exercise in which the patient is submissive and the physical therapist moves the patient's limbs (17)

Patency Term that indicates that no clots are present at the tip of the needle or catheter, and that the needle tip or catheter is not against the vein wall (open) (11)

Pathogenic Microorganisms Disease-carrying organisms that are too small to be seen with the naked eye (22)

Pathology Study of body changes caused by disease (14)

Patient Account Number Number assigned to the patient for access to insurance information; usually, a unique number is assigned each time the patient is admitted to the hospital (19)

Patient Care Conference Meeting that includes the doctor or doctors caring for the patient, the primary nurses, the case manager or social worker, and other caregivers involved in the patient's care (20)

Patient-Controlled Analgesia (PCA) Medications administered intravenously by means of a special infusion pump controlled by the patient within order ranges written by the doctor (13)

Pedal Pulse Pulse rate obtained at the top of the foot (10)

Penrose Drain Drain that that is inserted into or close to a surgical wound and that may lie under a dressing, extend through a dressing, or be connected to a drainage bag or a suction device (11)

Pen Tabs or Tablet PC Computers that may be removed from their base, or portable computers that can be taken into patient rooms; a stylus is used to enter information directly into a patient's electronic record, as in a notebook (4)

Percutaneous Endoscopic Gastrostomy (PEG) Insertion of a tube through the abdominal wall into the stomach under endoscopic guidance (12)

Perennial Stress Wear and tear of day-to-day living with the feeling that one is a square peg trying to fit in a round hole (7, 8)

Perioperative Pertaining to the time of surgery (17)

Peripheral Intravenous Catheter Catheter that begins and ends in the extremities of the body; used for the administration of intravenous therapy (11)

Philosophy Principles; underlying conduct (6)

Physiologic Needs A person's physical needs, such as the need for food and water (5)

Piggyback Method by which drugs usually are administered intravenously in 50 to 100 mL of fluid (13)

Plaintiff Person who brings a lawsuit against another (6)

Plasma Fluid portion of the blood in which the cells are suspended; contains a clotting factor called *fibrinogen* (14)

Plethysmography (Arterial) Usually performed to rule out occlusive disease of the lower extremities; may identify arteriosclerotic disease in the upper extremity (16)

Plethysmography (Venous) Measures changes in the volume of an extremity; usually performed on a leg to exclude DVT (deep vein thrombosis) (16)

Pneumatic Hose Stockings that promote circulation by sequentially compressing the legs from ankle upward, promoting venous return (also called *sequential compression devices*) (11)

Pneumatic Tube System System in which air pressure transports tubes carrying supplies, requisitions, or *some* lab specimens from one hospital unit or department to another (4)

Policy and Procedure Manual Handbook that includes such information as guidelines for practice, hospital regulations, and job descriptions for hospital personnel (1)

Portable X-ray X-ray taken by a mobile x-ray machine that is moved to the patient's bedside (15)

Positive Pressure Pressure greater than atmospheric pressure (17)

Postmortem After death (a postmortem examination is the same as an autopsy) (20)

Postprandial After eating (14)

Power of Attorney for Health Care The patient appoints a person (called a *proxy* or *agent*) to make health care decisions should the patient be unable to do so (19)

Pre-admit Process of obtaining information and partially preparing admitting forms prior to the patient's arrival at the health care facility (19)

Precept To train or teach (a student or new employee) (5)

Primary Care Nursing One nurse provides total care to assigned patients (3)

Primary Care Physician Sometimes referred to as the gatekeepers, these general practitioners are the first physicians to see a patient for an illness (2)

Principles Basic truths; moral code of conduct (6)

Proactive To take action prior to an event to use power, freedom, and ability to choose responses to whatever happens to us, in accordance with personal values (circumstances do not control us, we control them) (7)

Proprietary For profit (2)

Protective Care Another term for *isolation* (22)

Pulse Deficit The difference between the radial pulse and the apical heartbeat (21)

Pulse Oximetry Noninvasive method used to measure the oxygen saturation of arterial blood (10, 16)

Pulse Rate The number of times per minute the heartbeat is felt through the walls of the artery (10)

Quid Pro Quo (Latin) Involves making conditions of employment (hiring, promotion, retention) contingent on the victim who provides sexual favors (6)

Radial Pulse Pulse rate obtained at the wrist (10)

Radiopaque Catheter Catheter coated with a substance that does not allow the passage of x-rays, thus allowing movement of the catheter to be followed on the viewing screen (16)

Random Specimen Body fluid sample that can be collected at any time (14)

Range of Motion Range in which a joint can move (17)

Reactive Taking action or responding after an event happens; circumstances are often in control (7, 8)

Real-Time Imaging Ultrasound procedure that instantaneously displays a rapid sequence of images (like a movie) while an object is being examined (16)

Receiver Person who receives the message (5)

Recertification Process by which certified health unit coordinators exhibit continued personal and professional growth and current competency to practice in the field (1)

Recommended Dietary Allowance (RDA) Average daily intake of a nutrient that will meet the requirements of nearly all (97% to 98%) healthy people of a given age and gender (12)

Rectal Tube Plastic or rubber tube designed for insertion into the rectum; when written as a doctor's order, "rectal tube" means insertion of a rectal tube into the rectum to remove gas and relieve distention (11)

Reduction Correction of a deformity in a bone fracture or dislocation (17)

Reference Range Range of normal values for a laboratory test result (14)

Registration Process of entering personal information into the hospital information system to enroll a person as a hospital patient and create a patient record; patients may be registered as inpatients, outpatients, or observation patients (19)

Rehydration Restoration of normal water balance in a patient by giving fluids orally or intravenously (12)

Release of Remains Signed consent that authorizes a specific funeral home or agency to remove the deceased from a health care facility (20)

Resident Graduate of a medical school who is gaining experience in a hospital (2)

Resistive Exercise Exercise that uses opposition. A T-band or water provides resistance for patient exercises (17)

Respect Holding a person in esteem or honor; having appreciation and regard for another (6)

Respiration Rate Number of times a patient breathes per minute (10)

Respiratory Arrest When the patient ceases to breathe or when respirations are so depressed that the blood cannot receive sufficient oxygen and therefore body cells die (also may be referred to as *code arrest*) (22)

Respondeat Superior (Latin) "Let the master answer." Legal doctrine that imposes liability upon the employer. *Note:* The employee is also liable for his own actions (6)

Restraints Devices used to control patients who exhibit dangerous behavior, or to protect the patient (11)

Retaliation Revenge; payback (6)

Reverse Isolation Precautionary measure taken to prevent a patient with low resistance to disease from becoming infected (22)

Rhythm Strip Cardiac study that demonstrates on the electrocardiogram the waveform produced by electrical impulses (16)

Risk Management Department in the hospital that addresses the prevention and containment of liability regarding patient care incidents (22)

Robotic Surgery Use of robots in performing surgery (2)

Routine Preparation Standard preparation suggested by the radiologist to prepare the patient for a diagnostic imaging study (15)

Scan Image produced with the use of a moving detector or a sweeping beam (scans are produced by computed tomography, magnetic resonance imaging, and ultrasonography) (15)

Scheduled Admission Patient admission that is planned in advance; may be urgent or elective (19)

Scope of Practice Legal description of what a specific health professional may and may not do (6)

Self-Actualization Need Need to maximize one's potential (5)

Self-Esteem Confidence and respect for oneself (5)

Serology Study of blood serum or other body fluids for immune bodies, which are the body's means of defense when disease occurs (14)

Serum Plasma from which fibrinogen, a clotting factor, has been removed (14)

Sexual Harassment Unwanted, unwelcome behavior; sexual in nature (6)

Sheepskin Pad made of lamb's wool or synthetic material; used to prevent pressure sores (used primarily in long-term care) (11)

Sitz Bath Application of warm water to the pelvic area (11)

Skin Tests Tests performed to determine the reaction of the body to a substance by observing the results of injecting the substance intradermally or applying the substance topically to the skin. Skin tests are used to detect allergens, to determine immunity, and to diagnose disease (13)

Spirometry Study undertaken to measure the body's lung capacity and function (16)

Splint Orthopedic device used for immobilization, restraint, or support of any part of the body that may be rigid (metal, plaster, or wood) or flexible (felt or leather) (17)

Splinting Holding the incision area to provide support, promote a feeling of security, and reduce pain during post-surgery coughing. A folded blanket or pillow is helpful to use as a splint (11)

Split or Thinned Chart Portions of the patient's current chart that are removed when the chart becomes so full that it becomes unmanageable (8)

Sputum Mucous secretion from the lungs, bronchi, or trachea (14)

Standard of Care Legal duty one owes to another according to the circumstances of a particular case; the care that a reasonable and prudent person would have exercised in the given situation (6)

Standard Precautions Creation of a barrier between the health care worker and the patient's blood and body fluids (also may be called *universal precautions*) (22)

Standing Order Doctor's order that remains in effect and is executed as ordered until the doctor discontinues or changes it (9)

Standing PRN Order Same as a standing order, except that it is executed according to the patient's needs (9)

Stat Order Doctors' order that is to be executed immediately, then automatically discontinued (9)

Statute Law passed by the legislature and signed by the governor at the state level and the president at the federal level (6)

Statute of Limitations Time within which a plaintiff must bring a civil suit; the limit varies depending on the type of suit, and it is set by the various state legislatures (6)

Stent Tiny metal or plastic tube that is placed into an artery, blood vessel, or other duct to hold the structure open (17)

Stereotyping Assumption that all members of a culture or ethnic group act alike (generalizations that may be inaccurate) (5)

Sternal Puncture Procedure performed to remove bone marrow from the breastbone cavity for diagnostic purposes; also called a *bone marrow biopsy* (14)

Stress Physical, chemical, or emotional factor that causes bodily or mental tension and may be a factor in disease causation (7)

Subculture Subgroups within a culture; people with a distinct identity but who have certain ethnic, occupational, or physical characteristics found in a larger culture (5)

Subcutaneous (SQ) Injection Injection of a small amount of a medication under the skin into fatty or connective tissue (13)

Suppository Medicated substance mixed in a solid base that melts when placed in a body opening; suppositories are used commonly in the rectum, vagina, or urethra (13)

Surgery Schedule List of all the surgeries to be performed on a particular day; the schedule may be printed from the computer or sent to the nursing unit by the admitting department (19)

Suspension Fine-particle drug suspended in liquid (13)

Swan-Ganz Catheter Catheter that is placed in the neck or the chest that measures pressures in the patient's heart and pulmonary artery (11)

SWAT HUC, Nurse, or SWAT Team Health unit coordinator, nurse, or group of health care workers who are on call for all units in the hospital to provide assistance as needed (also may be called *Resource HUC, Nurse,* or *Resource Team*) (3)

Symbols Notations written in black or red ink on the doctors' order sheet to indicate completion of a step of the transcription procedure (9)

Tablet Solid dosage of a drug in disk form (13)

Tact Use of discretion regarding the feelings of others (6)

Tank Room Room in which hydrotherapy is performed (17)

Ted Hose Brand name for antiembolism (A-E) hose (11)

Telemetry Transmission of data electronically to a distant location (16)

Terminal Illness Illness that ends in death (20)

Therapeutic Diet Regular diet with modifications or restrictions (also called a *special diet*) (12)

Thoracentesis Needle puncture into the pleural space in the chest cavity to remove pleural fluid for diagnostic or therapeutic reasons (14)

Timed Specimen Specimen that must be collected at a specific time (14)

Tissue Typing Identification of tissue types to predict acceptance or rejection of tissue and organ transplants (14)

Titer Quantity of substance needed to react with a given amount of another substance; used to detect and quantify antibody levels (14)

Titrate To adjust the amount of treatment to maintain a specific physiologic response (17)

Topical Direct application of medication to the skin, eye, ear, or other parts of the body (13)

Tort Wrong against another person or his property that is not a crime but for which the law provides a remedy (6)

Total Parenteral Nutrition (TPN) Provision of all necessary nutrients via veins (discussed in detail in Chapter 13)

Traction Mechanical pull on part of the body to maintain alignment and facilitate healing; traction may be static (continuous) or intermittent (17)

Transesophageal Echocardiography (TEE) Procedure used to assess the heart's function and structures. A probe with a transducer on the end is inserted down the throat (16)

Trendelenburg Position Position in which the head is low and the body and legs are on an inclined plane (sometimes used in pelvic surgery to displace the abdominal organs upward or out of the pelvis, or to increase blood flow to the brain in hypotension and shock) (10)

Triage Nursing interventions; classification defined as establishing priorities of patient care, usually according to a three-level model: emergent, urgent, and nonurgent (2)

Tube Feeding Administration of liquids into the stomach, duodenum, or jejunum through a tube (12)

Tuberculosis (TB) Disease caused by *Mycobacterium tuberculosis*, an airborne pathogen (22)

Tympanic Membrane Temperature Temperature reading obtained by placing an aural (ear) thermometer into the patient's ear (10)

Type and Crossmatch Patient's blood is typed, then tested for compatibility with blood from a donor of the same blood type and Rh factor (14)

Type and Screen Patient's blood type and Rh factor are determined, and a general antibody screen is performed (14)

Ultrasonography Technique that uses high-frequency sound waves to create an image (scan) of body organs (also may be referred to as *sonography* or *echography*) (15)

Unit Dose Any premixed or prespecified dose; often administered with small volume nebulizer (SVN) or intermittent positive-pressure breathing (IPPB) treatments (17)

Urinalysis Physical, chemical, and microscopic examination of urine (14)

Urinary Catheter Tube used to remove urine or inject fluids into the bladder (11)

Urine Reflex Urine is tested; if certain parameters are met, a culture will be performed (14)

Urine Residual Amount of urine left in the bladder after voiding (11)

Value Clarification Examination of our value system (6)

Values Personal belief about worth of principle, standard, or quality; what one holds as most important (6)

Venipuncture Needle puncture of a vein (11)

Ventilator Machine used to give the patient breaths through the endotracheal or tracheostomy tube (17)

Vital Signs Measurements of body functions, including temperature, pulse, respiration, and blood pressure (10)

Void To empty, especially the urinary bladder (11)

Voluntary Not for profit (2)

WALKaroo Another type of computer on a cart on wheels that may be taken into patients' rooms (4)

WALLaroo Chart rack located on the wall outside of a patient's room that stores the patient's chart and when unlocked forms a shelf to write upon (8)

Work Ethics Moral values regarding work (6)

Workable Compromise Working out a conflict in such a way that the solution is satisfactory to all parties (5)

Index

Page numbers followed by f indicate figures; t, tables; b, boxes.